PSORIASIS

Edited by **Jennifer Soung** and **Bonnie Koo**

Psoriasis
Edited by Jennifer Soung and Bonnie Koo

Published by InTech
Janeza Trdine 9, 51000 Rijeka, Croatia

Publishing Process Manager Marija Radja

Technical Editor Teodora Smiljanic

Cover Designer InTech Design Team

Additional hard copies can be obtained from orders@intechopen.com

Psoriasis, Edited by Jennifer Soung and Bonnie Koo
p. cm.
ISBN 978-953-307-878-6

For EU product safety concerns:
IN TECH d.o.o., Prolaz Marije Krucifikse Kozulić 3, 51000 Rijeka, Croatia, info@intechopen.com or visit our website at intechopen.com.

Meet the editor

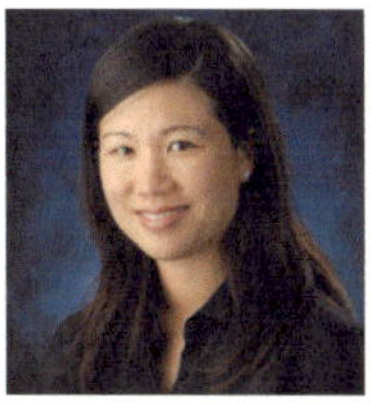

Dr. Jennifer Soung is a board certified dermatologist and Assistant Clinical Professor of Dermatology at the University of California, Irvine. As the director of Dermatology Clinical Research at UC Irvine, Dr. Soung has a broad interest in medical and cosmetic dermatology as well as clinical research. Her clinical and research interest is the treatment of psoriasis. She is currently the Principal Investigator of two large clinical trials focused on examining new medications for the treatment of psoriasis. Besides psoriasis, Dr. Soung plans to explore new treatment options in rosacea and discoid lupus. Dr. Soung treats adult and pediatric skin conditions, including acne, eczema, rosacea, and skin cancer. She is well-versed in techniques for cosmetic rejuvenation of the aging face including Botox, lasers and chemical peels.
Dr. Soung received her Bachelor of Arts at Brown University and earned a medical degree from the Albert Einstein College of Medicine. She completed a medical internship at the West Los Angeles-UCLA Veterans Hospital and a dermatology residency at the University of California, Irvine. Dr. Soung also pursued advanced fellowship training in dermatopharmacology at the Mount Sinai Medical Center, NY and earned top honors for her research on pharmacogenetics.

Contents

Preface

Psoriasis has a worldwide distribution varying according to race and geographic location. This book presents the international experience of psoriasis from pathophysiology to clinical presentation and treatment strategies.

The first section of the volume focuses on research related to the development of therapies for psoriasis. Experimental models and clinical results from immunologically directed therapies have demonstrated the important role and interaction of inflammatory cytokines, chemokines and immune cells in the pathogenesis of psoriasis.

The next segment of the volume presents the varying, and often difficult to treat, clinical manifestations of psoriasis. The role of vitamin D in psoriasis is explored and the role of the metabolic syndrome in psoriasis is reviewed.

The final segment of the volume is a discussion of therapy. The review of topical and biologic treatments discusses the spectrum of therapies available for psoriasis. The efficacy and safety of cyclosporine, a traditional systemic therapy, and the role of diet and nutrition is addressed.

We hope you enjoy and find the information useful in your research or practice. We urge that you continue to keep abreast of the new developments in psoriasis and share your knowledge so that we may advance treatment and cures of psoriasis.

Mona Malakouti (medical student) assisted with editing of the "UVB and Vitamin D in Psoriasis"chapter.

Jennifer Soung, M.D.
Assistant Professor & Director
Dermatology Clinical Research
University of California, Irvine
USA

Bonnie Koo, M.D.
Clinical Research Specialist
University of California, Irvine
USA

Part 1

Pathophysiology

1

Psoriasis and Stem Cells

Kaiming Zhang, Guohua Yin, Xinhua Li,
Xuping Niu, Ruixia Hou, Ruifeng Liu and Junqin Li
*Taiyuan City Central Hospital Affiliated to Shanxi Medical University,
1 Dong San Dao Xiang, Taiyuan, Shanxi Province,
China*

1. Introduction

Psoriasis is a chronic inflammatory skin disorder characterized by hyper-proliferation of basal keratinocytes, thickened and scaly epidermis, and recruitment of inflammatory cells to the skin. It affects approximately 2% of the world's population. The disease follows a pathogenic pathway involving various immunocytes and immune molecules. Activated T cells have been shown to trigger a chain of cellular and molecular reactions leading to the formation of psoriatic lesions. Fusion proteins that can block T cell activation or the function of anergized T cells, and cytokines and biologics that can inhibit T cell migration are effective in the treatment of psoriasis. Intradermal injection of T cells from psoriatic patients into human skin/severe combined immunodeficient (SCID) mice can induce spontaneous psoriatic conversion of skins from healthy human or non-lesional skin from psoriatic patients. Thus, it is widely accepted that psoriasis is a T lymphocyte-mediated autoimmune disease. Although the roles of T cells in psoriasis have been confirmed, the exact mechanisms of psoriasis and the origin of abnormal T cells are still unclear.

Beside T cells, psoriatic patients have a wide variety of other immune abnormalities such as B cells, monocytes, neutrophils and erythrocytes. As the precursor of immune cells, bone marrow hematopoietic stem cells have been suggested to be responsible for immune dysregulation of T cells in psoriasis. Several recent studies have indicated that abnormal T cells may be closely related to anomalous hematopoietic stem cells (HSCs) determined by psoriatic hereditary background. In addition to HSCs, aberrant bone marrow mesenchymal stem cells have also been demonstrated in patients with psoriasis.

2. The clinical cue of relationship between psoriasis and bone marrow cells

Although various exogenous and endogenous factors are believed to activate the immune system leading to imbalance of the system and initiation of psoriasis, increasing evidences suggest that inherent and intrinsic rather than extrinsic factors are more important in psoriasis pathogenesis. These intrinsic factors may be involved in spontaneous T-cell activation or proliferation, regulation of cytokine production, hematopoietic cell development, and T-cell development in the thymus. Allogeneic bone marrow transplantations (BMT) have been reported to either eliminate or aggravate psoriasis.

Leukemia patients with psoriasis reportedly have long-term psoriasis remission or amelioration. On the other hand, non-psoriatic leukemia patients can develop psoriasis after transplanting bone marrow from psoriatic donors. These clinical reports indicate that psoriatic immune abnormalities transferred by BMT may have originated from bone marrow HSC.

3. Bone marrow derived hematopoietic stem / progenitor cells from psoriatic patients are anomalously proliferative

Based on the above evidence, many researchers begin to pay close attention to bone marrow abnormality of psoriatic patients. *In vitro* studies have shown that monocytopoietic activity is enhanced in psoriasis and functional bone marrow scintigraphy using 99Tcm-labelled human serum albumin millimicrospheres has shown hyperplasia of phagocytes in psoriasis.

Bone marrow, with its rapidly renewing cell populations, is one of the most sensitive tissues to various stimulations of exogenous or endogenous factors. Once activated the pathogenic peripheral immunocytes in psoriasis and their released soluble factors, such as gamma-interferon (IFN-γ), interleukin-2 (IL-2), IL-8 and tumor necrosis factor-alpha (TNF-α), may influence hematopoietic microenvironment, and even hematopoiesis. *In vitro* assessment using high proliferative potential colony-forming cell (HPP-CFCs) and colony formation units (CFU) is used as a surrogate marker of hematopoietic activity and can play a key role in linking hematopoiesis to psoriasis. Supernatant of *in vitro* cultured psoriatic peripheral blood mononuclear cells was found to suppress the proliferative activity of normal bone marrow HPP-CFCs, CFU-GM (granulocyte-macrophage colony-forming units) and CFU-E (erythroid colony-forming units). These results support the hypothesis that aberrant psoriatic peripheral immunocytes and cytokines can influence hematopoiesis.

Recently, besides the influence of aberrant peripheral immunocytes and cytokines, researchers began to pay attention to the intrinsic deficiency of psoriatic bone marrow hematopoietic cells. Zhang *et al.* cultured psoriatic bone marrow mononuclear cells in methylcellulose semisolid medium and observed their colony formation ability in the presence of exogenous cytokine combinations. These studies show a decreased colony formation ability of HPP-CFC, CFU-GM but not CFU-E, implying that the proliferative activity of HSCs in patients with psoriasis may be intrinsically decreased. They further investigated the molecular mechanisms of abnormal proliferative activity of HSCs in psoriasis and found that promoter methylation of p15, p16 and p21 genes is significantly decreased and transcription levels of these genes are enhanced in *ex vivo* cultured bone marrow HPP-CFCs from psoriatic patients in comparison to those from healthy volunteers. The P15, P16 and P21 proteins belong to the INK4 kinase family of cyclin-dependent kinase inhibitors and can negatively regulate the cell cycle through competitive inhibition of cyclin-dependent kinases 2, 4 and 6. Higher expression of these genes may contribute to the low proliferative activity of psoriatic hematopoietic cells.

Expression of Notch receptors and their ligands in hematopoietic system has been widely reported, and Notch signaling has been shown to influence hematopoietic cell proliferation and differentiation at several stages. The activation of Notch signaling results in transcriptional activation of *E(spl)/HES* genes, which function as negative regulators of cell proliferation and differentiation. Moreover, Notch1 and Hes-1 expression is significantly enhanced in psoriatic $CD34^+$ bone marrow cells compared to normal controls. Beside *HES* genes, another transcription factor RUNX-1, which is essential for hematopoietic cell development, has long been suspected to be involved in the pathogenesis of psoriasis because loss of RUNX1 binding site located between the SLC9A3R1 and NAT9 genes at 17q25 has been found increased expression in the psoriatic $CD34^+$ cells. These studies suggest that the dysfunction of immune cells in psoriatic patients can be traced back to the early development of hematopoietic cells.

4. T cells differentiated from bone marrow derived hematopoietic cells of psoriatic patients are functionally different from normal T cells

Since T cells are derived from bone marrow hematopoietic cells, it is suggested that hematopoietic cells are partly relevant to the dysfunction of T cells in psoriasis. To demonstrate whether T cells are produced inherently dysfunctional from the immune system, Zhang et al. cultured bone marrow $CD34^+$ cells from psoriatic patients and induced them to differentiate into T cells and $CD4^+CD25^+$ regulatory T cells *in vitro.* A further functional study revealed abnormal characters of these cells compared to normal bone marrow derived ones.

The main hallmark of $CD4^+CD25^+$ T cells is their immune regulatory function by interacting with effector T cells. Several studies have reported that the $CD4^+CD25^+$ T-lymphocyte subpopulation in peripheral blood and lesional skin demonstrates a less inhibitory effect on effector T cells, leading to accelerated proliferation of pathogenic/effector T-cells in autoimmune diseases, especially in psoriasis. Although the proportion of $CD4^+CD25^+$ T cells and FOXP3 gene expression are comparable in both psoriatic and healthy samples, proliferation of psoriatic bone marrow derived $CD4^+CD25^+$ T cells is significantly attenuated and secretion of cytokines IL-2 and IL-10 is decreased compared to normal controls in response to streptococcal superantigen (Strep-A). In particular, $CD4^+CD25^+$ T cells differentiated from psoriatic $CD34^+$ cells are functionally insufficient to restrain proliferation of activated effector T-cells. That is to say, the function of $CD4^+CD25^+$ T cells derived from psoriatic bone marrow $CD34^+$ cells *in vitro* is similar to that of peripheral $CD4^+CD25^+$ T-lymphocytes of psoriatic patient *in vivo.*

In another study, bone marrow $CD34^+$ hematopoietic cells from psoriatic patients with family history were induced into effector T cells and their functions such as in vitro proliferation ability, secretion of cytokines IL-4, IL-8 and IFN-γ, and their ability to induce human keratinocytes producing C-myc, Bcl-xL, and Ki67 proteins were compared with their counterpart from healthy objects. The differentiated T cells from $CD34^+$ cells of psoriatic patients showed higher proliferative activity and stronger capacity to secret Th1 cytokines in response to streptococcal superantigen and could induce expression of C-myc and Ki67, but not Bcl-XL in keratinocytes co-cultured with psoriatic differentiated T cells.

These studies show that regulatory as well as effector T cells differentiated from $CD34^+$ cells of psoriatic patients, but not normal controls, are functionally similar to those psoriatic circulating T cells and suggest that dysfunctional activity of T cells in psoriatic patients can be traced back to the early development of hematopoietic cells.

5. The bionomics of psoriatic bone marrow mesenchymal stem cells

Mesenchymal stem cells, also referred as marrow stromal cells, are another important type of stem cells in bone marrow. Cytokines secreted by bone marrow mesenchymal stem cells (BMSCs) along with extracellular matrix compose the hematopoietic microenvironment and influence hematopoiesis. More than 30 hematopoietic cytokines and growth factors including TNF-a, IL-1, IL-6, IL-7, IL-8, IL-10, IL-12, IFN-γ and IL-18 are reportedly secreted by BMSCs and many of them could influence immune reaction of peripheral blood. Secretion of SCF, granulocyte colony-stimulating factor (G-CSF) and IL-6 is increased in *in vitro* cultured BMSCs from psoriatic patients, while that of IL-1a, IL-1b, IL-3, IL-8, epidermal growth factor (EGF), vascular endothelial growth factor (VEGF), TNF-a, leukaemia inhibitory factor (LIF), hepatocyte growth factor (HGF) and platelet-derived growth factor (PDGF) is decreased and the levels of GM-CSF, IL-11 or IL-7 is not altered. *Pearson* correlation analysis demonstrates that those cytokine levels are not correlated with PASI scores, indicating that abnormal secretion of cytokines is due to anomaly of BMMSCs themselves rather than systemic inflammatory response.

On the other hand, BMSCs are also characterized by their ability to differentiate into multiple mesenchymal lineages, including osteocytes, chondrocytes, adipocytes, endothelial cells and skeletal muscle cells under controlled *in vitro* conditions. Studies have found that BMSCs from psoriatic patients have lower proliferative and passage ability and are more prone to differentiate into vascular endothelial cells (VEC) compared with those from healthy subjects under the same induction conditions. Moreover, this differentiation ability is paralleled with the disease severity. In addition, specimens from a patient whose parents also have psoriasis could spontaneously differentiate into VECs. Further studies on gene expression using RNA sequencing showed a total of 475 genes mostly enriched in prostaglandin (PG) and prostanoid metabolic process (unpublished data) are differentially expressed in this patient.

Studies on differential gene expression of BMSCs from 4 psoriatic patients and 3 healthy subjects found a total of 1617 genes were differently expressed by more than 2-fold between the two groups, among which 324 genes were upregulated and 1293 genes were downregulated in psoriatic patients. GO analysis revealed the first five gene-enriched GO terms were immune response, inflammatory response, antigen processing and presentation of peptide, chemotaxis, and cell adhesion. While the first five highly enriched factor terms were positive regulation of CD4+CD25+ alpha-beta regulatory T cell differentiation, lipoprotein particle clearance, antigen processing and presentation of peptide, negative regulation of peptidase activity, and positive regulation of cholesterol storage (unpublished data). These terms have been confirmed to participate in the onset and development of psoriasis.

Taken together, these studies suggest that BMSCs of psoriatic patients are abnormal in proliferation, differentiation, passage ability, secretion of multiple cytokines and gene expression, and may partly participate in the occurrence and development of psoriasis. In other words, psoriasis is a multi-system disease that involves not only the epidermis, but also the hematopoietic system, immune system, neuroendocrine system, and so on. With continued research, various stem cells may be confirmed to be involved in the generation and development of psoriasis.

6. References

Sabat R, Philipp S, Hoflich C, et al. Immunopathogenesis of psoriasis. Exp Dermatol 2007, 16: 779–798.

Abrams J R, Kelley S L, Hayes E, et al. Blockade of T lymphocyte costimulation with cytotoxic T lymphocyte-associated antigen 4-immunoglobulin (CTLA4Ig) reverses the cellular pathology of psoriatic plaques, including the activation of keratinocytes, dendritic cells, and endothelial cells. J Exp Med 2000, 192: 681–694.

Gordon K B, Papp K A, Hamilton T K, et al. Efalizumab for patients with moderate to severe plaque psoriasis: a randomized controlled trial. JAMA 2003, 290: 3073–3080.

Boyman O, Hefti H P, Conrad C, et al. Spontaneous development of psoriasis in a new animal model shows an essential role for resident T cells and tumor necrosis factor-alpha. J Exp Med 2004, 199: 731–736.

Nickoloff BJ, Schrohder JM, von den Driesch P, et al. Is psoriasis a T- cell disease? [J]. Exp Dermatol, 2000, 9 (5): 359- 375.

Li X, Fan X, Zhang K, Yin G, Liu Y. Influence of psoriatic peripheral blood $CD4^{+}T$ and $CD8^{+}T$ lymphocytes on C-myc, Bcl-xL and Ki67 gene expression in keratinocytes. Eur J Dermatol, 2007, 17: 392-396.

Woods A C, Mant M J. Amelioration of severe psoriasis with psoriatic arthritis for 20 years after allogeneic haematopoietic stem cell transplantation. Ann Rheum Dis 2006, 65: 697.

Snowden J A, Heaton D C. Development of psoriasis after syngeneic bone marrow transplant from psoriatic donor: further evidence for adoptive autoimmunity. Br J Dermatol 1997, 137: 130–132.

Altmeyer P, Munz DL, Chilf G, et al. Morphological and functional findings of fixed phagocytes in psoriatics. Arch Dermatol Res 1983, 275: 95-9.

Zhang K, Zhang R, Li X, et al. The mRNA expression and promoter methylation status of the p16 gene in colony-forming cells with high proliferative potential in patients with psoriasis. Clin Exp Dermatol, 2007, 32: 702.

K. Zhang, R. Hou, X. Niu, *et al.* Decreased colony formation of high proliferative potential colony-forming cells and granulocyte-macrophage colony-forming units and increased Hes-1 expression in bone marrow mononuclear cells from patients with psoriasis. British Journal of Dermatology 2010, 163, 93–101

Yin G, Li J, Wan Y, et al. Abnormality of RUNX1 signal transduction in psoriatic CD34+bone marrow cells. Br J Dermatol. 2011, 164, 1043-1052.

Helms C, Cao L, Krueger J G, et al. A putative RUNX1 binding site variant between SLC9A3R1 and NAT9 is associated with susceptibility to psoriasis. Nat Genet 2003: 35: 349–356.

Zhang K, Zhang R, Li X, et al. Promoter methylation status of p15 and p21 genes in HPP-CFCs of bone marrow of patients with psoriasis. Eur J Dermatol, 2008, 19: 141-146.

Zhang K, Li X, Yin G, et al. Functional characterization of T cells differentiated in vitro from bone marrow-derived $CD34^{+}$ cells of psoriatic patients with family history. Experimental Dermatology, 2010; 19: e128–e135.

Zhang K, Li X, Yin G, et al. Functional characterization of $CD4^{+}CD25^{+}$ regulatory T cells differentiated in vitro from bone marrow-derived haematopoietic cells of psoriasis patients with a family history of the disorder. Br J Dermatol, 2008; 158 (2): 298-305.

Zhang K, Liu R, Yin G, et al. Differential cytokine secretion of cultured bone marrow stromal cells from patients with psoriasis and healthy volunteers. Eur J Dermatol 2010; 20 (1): 1-5.

2

Pathogenesis of Psoriasis: The Role of Pro-Inflammatory Cytokines Produced by Keratinocytes

Anna Balato, Nicola Balato, Matteo Megna,
Maria Schiattarella, Serena Lembo and Fabio Ayala
Department of Dermatology – University of Naples Federico II
Italy

1. Introduction

Psoriasis is a chronic, inflammatory skin disease affecting 2 to 3% of the white population (Gudjonsson & Elder, 2007). It is a multifactorial disease since its development depends on a complex interplay of genetic and environmental factors. As no pathogen has been consistently identified within psoriatic plaques (indeed skin infections are rare in lesions because of antimicrobial peptides) (Nomura et al., 2003), an autoimmune basis for the chronic inflammation is the dogma for this complex disorder. Psoriasis is characterized by macroscopic (clinical) and corresponding microscopic (histological) skin alterations and leads to considerable impairment of the quality of life of the affected patients. Special forms of psoriasis (e.g. arthropathic form) can be accompanied by severe extra-cutaneous changes.

2. Psoriasis pathogenesis

Psoriasis is usually identified by erythematous, raised, scaly skin lesions. These clinical features are explained by impressive growth and dilation of superficial blood vessels (elongated/hyperplastic capillaries in the papillary dermal region) and equally impressive hyperplasia of the epidermis. Epidermal growth occurs in a pattern termed "psoriasiform" hyperplasia, which describes both elongated rete pegs, thickening (acanthosis), and differentiation changes (Krueger & Bowcock, 2005). In psoriatic epidermis, keratinocytes proliferate and mature rapidly so that terminal differentiation, normally occurring in granular keratinocytes and then squamous corneocytes, is incomplete. Hence, squamous keratinocytes aberrantly retain intact nuclei (parakeratosis) and release few extracellular lipids that normally cement adhesions of corneocytes. The failure of psoriatic corneocytes to stack normally and to secrete extracellular lipids cause scaling and a break in the protective barrier whereas marked dilation of blood vessels in the dermis causes the visible redness of psoriatic skin lesions. The extensive infiltration of mononuclear immune cells in the dermis and epidermis (T cells and dendritic cells in the dermis and polymorphonuclear leucocytes such as neutrophils within small foci in the stratum corneum) is another defining feature of psoriasis histopathology and a key point of its pathogenesis. The pathogenesis of psoriasis is considered to be an immunologically mediated process that takes place upon a favourable genetic background. According to this view, the presence of a yet unknown (auto)-antigen causes the generation of effector T-cells that infiltrate the skin and initiate the inflammatory process (Wolk et al., 2009a). Over its course, cutaneous infiltration of various immune cell populations and, subsequently, an activation of numerous immune and tissue cells in the skin take place. Secreted cytokines from activated cells then induce keratinocyte alterations such as excessive growth and aberrant differentiation forming the basis of the epidermal acanthosis, hyperkeratosis and parakeratosis which characterize psoriasis plaques. The trigger of keratinocyte response is thought to be the activation of the cellular immune system, with T cells, dendritic cells and various immune-related cytokines and chemokines implicated in pathogenesis. Rather than viewing psoriasis as a disease caused by a single cell type or a single inflammatory cytokine, it is probably best to conceptualize the disease pathogenesis as linked to many interactive responses among infiltrating leucocytes, resident skin cells, and an array of pro-inflammatory cytokines, chemokines, and chemical mediators produced in the skin (Lowes et al., 2007). Fundamentally two different cell types interact in the formation of a psoriatic lesion: keratinocytes and mononuclear leukocytes. Whereas keratinocytes might be viewed only as bystander cells in terms of immune activation, it is more likely that they are active participants in the recruitment and activation of leukocytes in psoriatic lesions. Thus, there are two sets of interactive cellular responses in the psoriatic lesion that potentially create a ying/yang relationship; the balance between the activation of innate and acquired immune cell types, and the factors produced by epidermal keratinocytes that directly affect T cells and dendritic cells, and vice versa. Psoriasis is considered a T helper 1 (Th1) condition, characterized by the production of interferon-gamma (IFN-γ) and tumor necrosis factor alpha (TNF-α) under the influence of interleukin-12 (IL-12). However, there is increasing evidence of the importance of a novel T cell population, Th17 cells, in this inflammatory disease. Th17 cells are stimulated by IL-23 (which shares the p40 subunit with IL-12) to produce IL-17 and also IL-22, which has recently been shown to be a major driver of acanthosis in psoriasis, and so is a novel target for treatment. Effector cells of innate immunity including neutrophils, plasmacytoid dendritic cells (plasmocytoid DCs) and CD11c+ dendritic cells (myeloid DCs) are involved and present in psoriatic lesions creating a very intricate and complex network of interactions which is the base of the pathogenetic process of psoriasis (Nograles et al., 2010). An interplay between environmental and genetic factors sets the scene for disease-initiating events. Initial triggers such as physical trauma or bacterial products start a cascade of events that include the formation of DNA-LL-37 complexes, activation of plasmocytoid dendritic cells and secretion of interferon-α (IFN-α). IFN-α secreted by plasmocytoid dendritic cells promotes the activation of myeloid dendritic cells (Nestle et al., 2005). Activated myeloid dendritic cells migrate into draining lymph nodes and induce the differentiation of naive T cells into effector cells such as Th17 or type 17 cytotoxic T cells (Tc17) and Th1 or type 1 cytotoxic T cells (Tc1) (Nestle et al., 2010). Effector cells recirculate and slow down in skin capillaries in the presence of selectin-guided and integrin-guided receptor-ligand interactions. Immune cells expressing the chemokine receptors CCR6, CCR4, and CXCR3 emigrate into skin tissue along chemokine gradients. Dendritic cells and T cells form perivascular clusters and lymphoid-like structures around blood vessels in the presence of chemokines such as CCL19 produced by macrophages. A key checkpoint is the migration of T cells from the dermis into the epidermis; this migration is controlled through the interaction of α1β1 integrin (very late antigen 1 [VLA-1]) on T cells and collagen IV at the basement membrane (Conrad et al., 2007). Unconventional T cells, including natural killer T cells (NKT), contribute to the disease process. Key processes during disease maintenance are the presentation of putative (auto)-antigens to T cells, the release of IL-23 by dermal dendritic cells, the production of pro-inflammatory mediators such as IL-17A, IL-17F, IL-22 by Th17 and Tc17 cells and IFN-γ and TNF-α by Th1 and Tc1 cells. These mediators act on keratinocytes leading to the activation, proliferation and production of antimicrobial peptides (AMPs) (e.g., LL-37 cathelicidin and β-defensins) and chemokines (e.g., CXCL1, CXCL9 through CXCL11 and CCL20), and S100 proteins (e.g., S100A7-9) (Nestle et al., 2010). These soluble mediators feed back into the pro-inflammatory disease cycle and shape the inflammatory infiltrate (Fig.1). In fact keratinocyte products influence immune activation, and products of activated lymphocytes alter keratinocyte responses, including the induction of new adhesion molecules for T cells. However although intrinsic alterations in keratinocytes are crucial for the development of psoriatic lesions, a deregulated function of other resident skin cells, such as fibroblasts and endothelial cells, may also contribute to the pathogenesis of psoriasis. Epidermal-dermal cell interaction is a determinant for the maintenance of the psoriatic phenotype because it guarantees the local production of growth factors and cytokines stimulating keratinocyte proliferation. An important paracrine loop

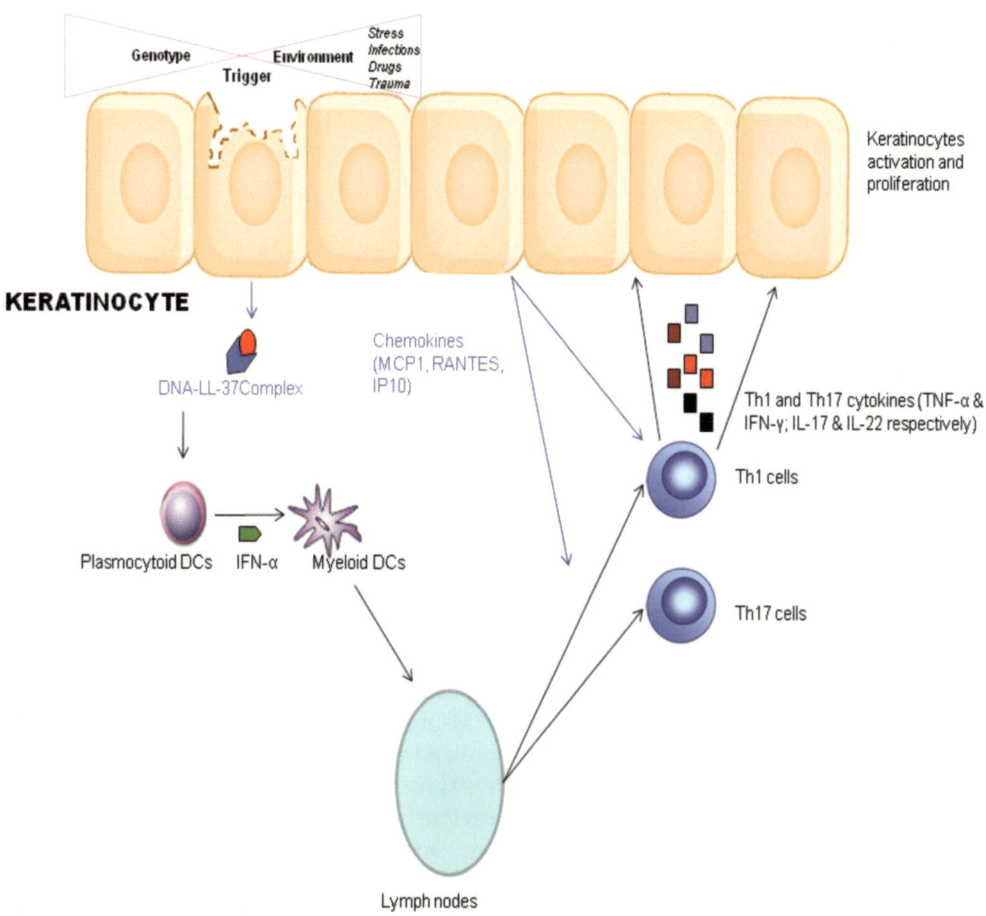

Fig. 1. Main actors of psoriasis pathogenesis.

operating between keratinocytes and fibroblasts that culminates with keratinocyte proliferation is triggered by IL-1: IL-1α and IL-1β neutralization and IL-1 receptor antagonist significantly reduced keratinocyte growth through the abrogation of keratinocyte growth factor (KGF) production by fibroblasts. However, IL-1 is unlikely to be the only regulator of KGF production by fibroblasts, and indeed other keratinocyte-derived factors, such as parathyroid hormone-related protein (PTHrP), induce KGF expression. In addition fibroblast growth factor (FGF) family members and granulocyte-macrophage colony stimulating factor (GM-CSF) also play a particularly important role in the fibroblast-driven regulation of keratinocyte proliferation (Albanesi et al., 2007). Moreover, the activated phenotype of lesional endothelial cells are believed to play a central role in the pathogenesis of psoriasis and are determined by the expression of a variety of membrane and soluble factors mainly responsible for T-cell recruitment in the skin like adhesion molecule 1 (ICAM-1). A key point is the endothelium expression of certain chemokines involved in the arrest of circulating T lymphocytes at inflammatory sites: upon exposure to inflammatory signals, mainly represented by TNF-α and IL-1, endothelial cells express a broad array of chemokines, including CCL20/MIP-3α, CXCL12/SDF-1, CCL21/SLC, CCL17/TARC, CCL2/MCP-1, CXCL10/IL-8, CCL5/RANTES, CXCL1/Gro-α, and CCL4/MIP-1β (Girolomoni et al., 2004).

In summary, feedback loops involving keratinocytes, fibroblast and endothelial cells contribute to tissue reorganization with endothelial cell activation and proliferation and deposition of extracellular matrix. The hypothesis of cytokine/chemokine network in psoriasis proposed a central role of pro-inflammatory cytokines, including TNF-α.

3. A special look at the pathogenetic functions of keratinocytes

Besides erythema, impressive hyperkeratosis manifesting as large, silvery scales, is clinically the most visible pathology and represents a hallmark of psoriasis. This typical and characteristic epidermal involvement has in the past led to discussions on whether hyperproliferation and altered differentiation of epidermal keratinocytes occur indeed only in response to skin inflammation or whether keratinocytes themselves have their share in initiation and/or propagation of psoriasis. Whereas it is widely accepted today that keratinocytes have the potential to actively participate and modulate immune reactions in the skin their role as initiators or amplifiers of the inflammatory reaction in psoriasis is still not so clear (Tschachler, 2007). Some evidence indicates that the exposure of altered auto-antigens by keratinocytes could be directly responsible for the activation and expansion of certain T-cell subpopulations in psoriatic skin (Bos et al., 2005). A keratinocyte-derived candidate auto-antigen is keratin 17. Patients with active psoriasis have an increased frequency of circulating Th1 cells reacting to peptides from keratin 17 that shares ALEEAN aminoacidic sequence with the streptococcus M-protein. Using a new approach termed SErological identification of Recombinant EXpressed antigens (SEREX), new auto-antigens were found in the serum of patients with psoriasis (Jones et al., 2004). Keratin 13, heterogeneous ribonucleprotein-A1, and a previously uncharacterized protein, FLJ00294, were identified by SEREX as representative antigens in psoriatic patients, although auto-reactivity for these proteins was also detected in control subjects without psoriasis. Keratinocytes could be indirectly responsible for the activation of pathogenetic T cells through the exposure to viral or bacterial products. Under the influence of IL-17 and IL-22, keratinocytes, are able to produce AMPs like human beta defensin 2, and S100 proteins

(Nograles et al., 2008). The expression of another antimicrobial peptide, LL-37 cathelicidin, can also be enhanced by IL-17 in the presence of vitamin D3 (Peric et al., 2008). These proteins may function as key inflammation inducers in psoriasis, and at the same time decrease skin infections under conditions of a dysfunctional epidermal barrier. Infections or injury to the skin can promote lesion formation in susceptible individuals and these triggers have been shown to stimulate keratinocyte production of the antimicrobial LL-37 cathelicidin that, when complexed with self-DNA, binds to TLR9 on plasmocytoid DCs. These cells produce massive amounts of IFN-α and are implicated in the initiation of psoriasis lesions (Lande et al., 2007). Accordingly, patients treated with a topical plasmocytoid DCs agonist, imiquimod, up-regulate IFN-α and experience exacerbations in psoriasis. In addition to stimulating plasmocytoid DCs, LL-37 has been shown to complex with self-RNA to trigger the activation of myeloid dendritic cells (myeloid DCs) through TLR8. This leads to production of TNF-α and IL-6, and promotes their differentiation into mature dendritic cells (Ganguly et al., 2009). Because myeloid DCs in psoriasis have been shown to produce IL-23 it is plausible that self-RNA complexes might potentially initiate the inflammatory cascade leading to expansion and activation of Th17 cells (Nograles et al., 2010).

Recent investigations identified high levels of osteopontin (OPN) in psoriatic plaques (Buommino et al., 2009). Osteopontin is produced by both keratinocytes and activated T cells. It is a phosphorylated acidic glycoprotein of pleiotropic properties and has been recently recognized as a potential inflammatory cytokine. A model for the role of OPN in Th1 / Th17 psoriatic disease was so suggested. After activation of myeloid DCs that express OPN, they migrate to skin draining lymph nodes and polarize naive T cells towards a Th1 and Th17 phenotype. In addition OPN secreted by keratinocytes attracts additional inflammatory cells. Moreover OPN inhibits keratinocyte apoptosis thereby supporting enhanced epidermal proliferation, and, through a pro-angiogenic effect on microvascular endothelial cells, OPN also promotes vessel formation subsequently supporting the influx of inflammatory cells (Buback et al., 2009).

3.1 Keratinocytes and cytokines

Cutaneous and systemic over-expression of various pro-inflammatory cytokines has been demonstrated in psoriasis. Psoriatic keratinocytes are able to produce and release IL-1α, IL-1β, IL-6, IL-15, IL-18 and IL-20, all of them involved in the development of different alterations which compose the complex and intricate net of psoriasis pathogenesis (Tab. 1).The cellular composition of the inflammatory infiltrate within the psoriatic plaques as well as hyperproliferation of keratinocytes and so the whole pathogenetic process of psoriasis appears to be mediated by these cytokines (Wojas-Pelc et al., 2006).

3.1.1 Keratinocytes and IL-1α & IL-1β

IL-1 is a pro-inflammatory cytokine stimulating, among others, IL-2 and IFN-γ production through activated T cells. IL-1 activates neutrophils, monocytes, eosinophils and basophils, triggers production of TNF-α, IL-6, IL-8 by macrophages, and in autocrine fashion, IL-1 synthesis. IL-1 promotes proliferation of bone marrow cells, B lymphocytes, neutrophils, macrophages and platelets (Dinariello, 2002). In psoriasis, keratinocytes are the main source of IL-1α and IL-1β in the skin stored in the form of precursor particles (Zepter et al., 1997). Monocytes/macrophages, activated endothelial cells, fibroblasts and

Langerhans cells (LCs) are additional IL-1 sources (Yoshinaga et al., 1995). Normal keratinocytes do not contain a biologically active form of interleukin 1β-converting enzyme (ICE), and almost all IL-1 activity in the healthy epidermis results from the activity of IL-1α. In transgenic mouse models, IL-1α production in the basal layer of the epidermis leads to development of inflammatory lesions characterized by erythema and histology resembling psoriasis (Groves et al., 1995). Although IL-1 expression in the psoriatic epidermis appears altered, data on this finding are often conflicting. Some studies showed that IL-1α levels in psoriatic lesions were decreased or below detection limits in comparison to non-lesional and healthy skin (Okubo & Koga, 1998), whereas others demonstrated increased levels of IL-1β (Debets et al., 1997). Serum levels of IL-1α and IL-1β were low both in patients and in healthy controls. Increased levels of IL-1α and IL-1β were noted in supernatants of monocyte cultures obtained from patients with psoriasis (Okubo & Koga, 1998). Peripheral blood mononuclear cells (PBMCs) of inactive psoriasis patients produced lower levels of IL-1α and IL-1β than the cells obtained from patients with active psoriasis, although still higher than those of healthy controls. The production of IL-1β by PBMCs from psoriatic patients positively correlated with disease severity (Mizutani et al., 1997). Higher levels of IL-1β in blister fluid than in serum support the hypothesis that this cytokine is locally produced in psoriatic lesions. Despite fairly strong arguments for the key role of IL-1 in the activation of psoriasis, there is scarcity of data on the use of IL-1 antagonists in psoriasis treatment.

Cytokines	**Role in psoriasis**
IL-1	Stimulation of IL-2 and IFN-γ production through activated T cells and of TNF-α, IL-6, IL-8 by macrophages, and in autocrine fashion, of IL-1 synthesis.
IL-6	Regulation of growth and differentiation of epidermal cells and stimulation of Th17 cells differentiation.
IL-15	Anti-apoptotic effects on lymphocytes and keratinocytes; stimulation of IL-17 expression, promotion of T cell and monocyte activation, production of cytokines implicated in the pathogenesis of psoriasis, including IFN-γ and TNF-α.
IL-18	Induction of several chemokines in fibroblasts and neutrophils, increased T-cell adhesion to extracellular matrix ligands, induction of angiogenesis, induction of chemotaxis in plasmacytoid dendritic cells.
IL-20	Inhibition of normal terminal differentiation of keratinocytes, induction of anti-bacterial proteins.

Table 1. Roles of cytokines released by psoriatic keratinocytes.

3.1.2 Keratinocytes and IL-6

IL-6 is involved in the growth and differentiation of dermal and epidermal cells (Hirano, 1998), growth and differentiation of cytotoxic cells, activation of natural killer cells (NK) and maturation of hematopoietic stem cells (Pietrzak et al., 1999). Furthermore it acts as a chemotactic factor for T cells, and thus can directly stimulate T-cell migration to the epidermis. Increased levels of mRNA of IL-6 and its receptor were observed in psoriatic lesions, suction blister fluid and in keratinocytes (Krasowska et al., 1998). Previous studies have also shown a high level of IL-6 in plasma/serum of patients with psoriasis (Galadari & Sheriff, 2005; Grossman et al., 1989). Higher IL-6 levels were observed in psoriatic lesions compared to non-lesional and normal healthy skin (Chang et al., 1992; Grossman et al., 1989). Classical anti-psoriatic therapies such as phototherapy (PUVA, UVB), systemic corticosteroids and methothrexate lead to normalization of IL-6 levels (Mizutani et al., 1997). Both non-lesional and lesional psoriatic keratinocytes produce IL-6 (Grossman et al., 1989; Krasowska et al., 1998; Zalewska et al., 2006). IL-1 and TNF-α activate keratinocytes to produce IL-6. Koebner phenomenon is likely to result from the increased activity of IL-6 and its receptor in psoriasis (Grossman et al., 1989). Many studies show that IL-17F is able to induce IL-6 production both in normal human epidermal keratinocytes and in mouse skin (Fujishima et al., 2010). Moreover CD4+ T cells in skin from psoriasis patients express IL-17F and recent studies have demonstrated increased expression of IL-6 in IL-17F-overexpressing mice, thus further supporting a role of IL-17F in the induction of IL-6 (Hurst et al., 2002; Yang et al., 2008). IL-6 could directly contribute to the epidermal hyperplasia seen in psoriatic epithelium as well as affecting the function of dermal inflammatory cells. Moreover, it has been demonstrated that IL-6 induces Th17 cell differentiation in humans (Ishigame et al., 2009). Taken together, all these data suggest that IL-17F-induced IL-6 produced by keratinocytes promotes the development of Th17 cells as an autocrine regulator. Thus, the IL-17F/IL-6 axis may enhance inflammation of the lesional skin in psoriasis (Fujishima et al., 2010).

3.1.3 Keratinocytes and IL-15

IL-15 is a pro-inflammatory cytokine involved in chronic inflammatory processes. It is a key factor controlling the activation, proliferation and survival of NK cells (Fehniger & Caligiuri, 2001; Liu et al., 2000). IL-15 is also a strong chemotactic factor for leukocytes. This cytokine triggers angiogenesis and exerts strong anti-apoptotic effects, especially on lymphocytes, hepatocytes and keratinocytes (Berard et al., 2003; Rückert et al., 2000). Furthermore, it stimulates the expression of IL-17 by T cells (Elder, 2007). Elevated levels of IL-15 were noted in the lesional psoriatic skin (Elder, 2007; Rückert et al., 2000; Yano et al., 2003). Monocytes and macrophages represent the main source of IL-15 (Fehniger & Caligiuri, 2001; Musso et al., 1999) in lesional psoriatic skin, as well as keratinocytes (McInnes & Gracie, 2004; Yano et al., 2003). Lesional keratinocytes are strong producers of IL-15, which not only appears critical in the promotion of T cell and monocyte activation and, hence, in the maintenance of the local pro-inflammatory milieu, but also in the keratinocyte self-protection from apoptosis (Rückert et al., 2000); the pathogenic effect of this cytokine in psoriasis probably results from the stimulation of proliferation and activation of T cells and pro-inflammatory cytokines release (including TNF-α). Recent genetic studies (Elder, 2007) further supported the role of IL-15 as an important factor in psoriasis pathogenesis: IL-15 acts as a growth factor for CD8+ T cells, which infiltrate the epidermis during the development of psoriatic lesions, triggers inflammatory cell recruitment, angiogenesis, and production of other cytokines implicated in the pathogenesis of psoriasis, including IFN-γ and TNF-α.

3.1.4 Keratinocytes and IL-18

IL-18 exerts its activity on the human defense system in inflammatory, infectious and autoimmune diseases (Dinarello, 2006). IL-18 over-production stimulates the recruitment of dendritic cells to the site of inflammation (Gutzmer et al., 2003). IL-18, especially together with IL-12, triggers the production of IFN-γ in many immunocompetent cells, including NK cells, T helper and cytotoxic cells. Subsequently, IFN-γ decreases Th2 response and enhances Th1 response by stimulating cytotoxic T cells (Ericson et al., 2004). Thus, IL-18 possesses the capacity to stimulate innate immunity as well as Th1-mediated responses (Nakanishi et al., 2001). IL-18 overproduction is characteristic for many diseases including psoriasis (Nakanishi et al., 2001). The role of IL-18 in psoriasis has not been fully elucidated. It is speculated that IL-18 produced by human keratinocytes enhances IFN-γ production in inflammation and thus IL-18 seems to be a promising target in Th1-type inflammatory diseases, like psoriasis (McKenzie et al., 2002; Ohta et al., 2001). Its expression in psoriasis is significantly enhanced in supra-basal keratinocytes (Flisiak et al., 2006; McKenzie et al., 2002; Ohta et al., 2001). Reverse transcription polymerase chain reaction (RT-PCR) revealed IL-18 mRNA levels to be two to eight times higher in psoriatic skin biopsies than in the non-lesional psoriatic skin and healthy controls. Overexpression of IL-18 was observed in keratinocytes of the whole epidermis in psoriatic lesions and in the basal layer of non-lesional epidermis compared to only slight IL-18 expression in the epidermis of healthy controls (McKenzie et al., 2002). McKenzie et al. reported six to eight-fold higher levels of the IL-18 receptor mRNA in the epidermis of psoriatic lesions compared to non-lesional and healthy control skin. Moreover total IL-18 protein levels were found to be 3.5 times higher in the active and progressive psoriatic epidermis compared to the normal and stable, plaque-type psoriatic epidermis. To date, there are only a few studies on IL-18 in the blood of psoriatic patients (Flisiak et al., 2006, Gangemi et al., 2003), which revealed increased plasma IL-18 levels in psoriatic patients in comparison to controls. IL-18 might act in the early phases of psoriasis via IFN-γ independent routes, such as: a) induction of several chemokines in fibroblasts and neutrophils (Leung et al., 2001; Morel et al., 2001); b) increased T-cell adhesion to extracellular matrix ligands (Ariel et al., 2002); c) induction of angiogenesis (Park et al., 2001); d) induction of chemotaxis in plasmacytoid dendritic cells (Kaser et al., 2004). Thus, IL-18 could be involved in the regulation of early inflammatory events by promoting the recruitment and adhesion of the immune system cells to the inflamed sites. However, whether IFN-γ-dependent or independent mechanisms are responsible for the IL-18 activity in early stages of psoriatic plaque development remains to be elucidated.

3.1.5 Keratinocytes and IL-20

IL-20 was demonstrated to promote hyperproliferation of keratinocytes by activating IL-20 receptor to modulate skin inflammation. It was also reported that IL-20 induced IL-6 and TNF-α in monocytes, stimulated the expression of keratinocytes growth factor (KGF), IL-6, TNF-α and reactive oxygen species (ROS) in CD8+ T cells (Wei et al., 2006). In psoriasis, the two most important effects of IL-20 are the inhibition of normal terminal differentiation of keratinocytes and the induction of anti-bacterial proteins (Wolk et al., 2009a). Keratinocyte terminal differentiation is the apoptosis-like process that generates corneocytes for the desquaming stratum corneum from living keratinocytes of the upper (granular) epidermis layer (Candi et al., 2005). In psoriatic lesions, which contain high levels of IL-20, this process is altered. Furthermore, IL-20 simultaneously enhance the K16 expression, a keratin known to be up-regulated in psoriatic lesions and associated with keratinocyte regeneration (Wolk et al., 2006, 2009b). Apart from the inhibition of normal terminal differentiation of keratinocytes, IL-20 in addition to other mediators (Kanda & Watanabe, 2008), induce a state of enhanced antimicrobial defence of the epidermis by inducing a range of antimicrobial proteins (Sa et al., 2007; Wolk et al., 2004, 2006). In psoriatic lesions IL-20 expression was found preferentially in basal and supra-basal keratinocytes above the dermal papillae (Romer et al., 2003; Wolk et al., 2009a). Most interestingly, IL-17 and TNF-α amplified the IL-22 induced production of IL-20 in keratinocytes. In summary, the T/NK cell cytokine IL-22 induces the keratinocyte secretion of IL-20 as a second mediator that has very similar effects to its own. IL-20, therefore, may, to some extent, further amplify and/or prolong the IL-22 action on the keratinocyte differentiation that leads to the characteristic epidermal changes observed in psoriasis.

3.1.6 Keratinocytes and other cytokines

TNF-α is a key pro-inflammatory cytokine with an important pathogenetic role in psoriasis and psoriatic arthritis. The evidence includes further observations that a variety of anti-TNF-α approaches such as monoclonal antibodies and fusion proteins of soluble TNF-α receptors are effective therapies both in psoriasis and psoriatic arthritis. As for TNF-α itself, production of this cytokine is mainly attributed to immune cells (Lowes et al., 2007); however, it is noteworthy that keratinocytes are also able to elaborate TNF-α (Gottlieb at al., 2005). In psoriasis, the inflammatory response to TNF-α could be self-sustaining: activated dendritic cells are the major source of TNF-α in psoriasis lesions (Boyman et al., 2004) and at the same time TNF-α mRNA is induced in keratinocytes after TNF-α exposure (Gottlieb et al., 2005). Low level of TNF-α is present in the upper layer of the healthy epidermis, but its synthesis and release from keratinocytes are greatly augmented by injury, infection and UV irradiation. Of the two distinct cell-surface receptors for TNF-α, TNFR1 and TNFR2, keratinocytes mainly express TNFR1 (Kondo & Sauder, 1997). The binding of TNF-α to TNFR1 triggers a series of intracellular events resulting in the activation of transcription factors, including NF-KB, AP-1, CCAAT enhancer-binding protein-β, and others, which are responsible for the induction of genes important for diverse biological processes, including cell growth and death and immune, inflammatory, and stress responses (Banno et al., 2004). TNF-α activates the immune responses through inducing the production of additional signals, such as IL-1 and IL-8, transforming growth factor type-β (TGF-β) and ICAM-1. Psoriatic keratinocytes are also an important source of IL-7. Increased IL-7 levels were observed in both the psoriatic skin and serum of psoriatic patients (Bonifati et al., 1997; Pietrzak et al., 2008). However, no correlation between IL-7 levels and psoriasis area severity index (PASI) score was observed. In addition, IL-7 levels did not decrease after effective anti-psoriatic treatment, which suggests that this cytokine could not be regarded as a marker of the disease activity. IL-7 is a pleiotropic cytokine playing an essential role in the development and differentiation of T cells. IL-7 regulates survival, proliferation and cytotoxicity of maturation of T cells at the periphery. Furthermore, IL-7 together with IL-2 and IL-12, can induce the synthesis of IFN-γ, while, in turn, IFN-γ induces IL-7 secretion by keratinocytes (Ariizumi et al., 1995). In psoriasis IL-7 seems to play a key role in driving reciprocal interactions between epithelial cells (keratinocytes) and T-lymphocytes. The concomitant T-lymphocyte activation may be dependent on IL-7, and therefore the subsequent events driving toward the clinical expression and persistence of psoriasis may be IL-7 mediated (Bonifati et al., 1997). All these findings suggest an involvement of IL-7 in psoriasis, although further studies are warranted to elucidate the exact role of this molecule in the cytokine network of psoriasis pathogenesis.

3.2 Keratinocytes and chemokines

Keratinocytes produce many different types of chemokines involved in the recruitment of immune cells in the skin. For this reason epidermal cells can play a fundamental role in collecting all the immune cells which are implicated in the beginning of the cutaneous inflammation process that characterize psoriatic disease. Specifically, keratinocytes release IL-8 (CXCL8) and related chemokines which are responsible for the intra-epidermal collection of neutrophils and so to the formation of subcorneal microabscesses, a characteristic feature of psoriasis (Nickoloff & Turka, 1994); CCL2 (MCP-1), CCL5 (RANTES), CXCL10 (IP-10), and other CXCR3 ligands are responsible to attract predominantly monocytes and Th1 cells, (Gillitzer et al., 1993; Gottlieb et al., 1998), whereas CCL20 (MIP-3α) recruits immature Langerhans cells, dendritic cells, and CLA+ T cells (Dieu-Nosjan et al., 2000; Homey et al., 2000) (Tab. 2).

Chemokines	Roles
IL-8 (CXCL8)	Intra-epidermal recruitment of neutrophils
CCL-2 (MCP-1) CCL5 (RANTES) CXCL10 (IP-10)	Recruitment of monocytes and Th1 cells
CCL20 (MIP-3α)	Recruitment of dendritic cells, CLA+ T cells and immature Langherans cells

Table 2. Roles of chemokines produced by psoriatic keratinocytes.

3.3 Keratinocytes and other products

Psoriatic keratinocytes are a reservoir of inflammatory mediators. Under the influence of pro-inflammatory cytokines such as IFN-γ, TNF-α, IL-23, and IL-17, keratinocytes express a plethora of mediators, not only cytokines, thereby contributing to amplifying the inflammatory response implicated in the pathogenesis of psoriasis (Albanesi et al., 2005). Apart from pro-inflammatory cytokines as IL-1α, IL-1β, IL-6, IL-15, IL-18 and IL-20 psoriatic keratinocytes are able to produce other important factors involved in the development of the psoriatic process like vascular endothelial growth factor (VEGF) and CD1d (Tab. 3).

Factors	Functions
VEGF	Stimulation of angiogenesis, enhancement of vascular permeability, induction of keratinocytes hyperproliferation in an autocrine manner.
CD1d	Activation of CD161+ NK T cells and their stimulation to secrete IFN-γ.

Table 3. Roles of VEGF and CD1d in psoriasis.

3.3.1 Keratinocytes and VEGF

The typical erythema of psoriatic lesions is due to the increased, dilated, and tortuous capillaries that extend between the epidermal columns protruding into the dermis. The formation of new blood vessels starts with early psoriatic changes and disappears with disease clearance. Several angiogenic mediators like VEGF, hypoxia inducible factors, angiopoietins and pro-angiogenic cytokines, such as TNF-α, IL-8 and IL- 17, are involved in psoriasis development (Heidenreich et al., 2009). Interestingly, already in uninvolved, non-lesional skin significant over-expression of several VEGF isoforms was observed in patients as compared to healthy skin of normal volunteers (Henno et al., 2009). These findings suggest that angiogenesis is also one of the key features in the pathogenesis of psoriasis and various recent studies focused on the identification and role of pro-angiogenic mediators in psoriatic skin. In general, angiogenesis is tightly regulated by a balance between pro- and anti-angiogenic mediators (Heidenreich et al., 2009). VEGF, hypoxia-inducible factor-1α (HIF-1α), TNF-α, IL-8 and angiopoietins are considered to be the main players responsible for the increased vessel formation in psoriasis (Creamer et al., 2002; Heidenreich et al., 2008). Interestingly, several small molecules as well as modern biologics used for systemic therapy of psoriasis have been shown to provide not only immune regulatory effects but also influence endothelial cell biology (Heidenreich et al., 2008). Thus, direct targeting of angiogenesis could help both to dissect psoriasis pathogenesis and to develop new therapeutic strategies for psoriasis treatment by blocking angiogenic pathways driving cutaneous inflammation. Strongly increased production of VEGF by keratinocytes has been found in psoriasis (Detmar et al., 1994). Furthermore, over-expression of VEGF in the epidermis of mice triggered sub-epidermal angiogenesis and increased leukocyte adhesion to these vessels (Detmar et al., 1998), and later in life, these animals develop hyperkeratotic skin lesions with a resemblance to psoriasis (Xia et al., 2003). VEGF signaling often represents a critical rate-limiting step in physiological angiogenesis (Ferrara et al., 2003). Under physiological conditions, VEGF promotes growth of endothelial cells (ECs) derived from arteries, veins and lymphatic vessels. VEGF delivery also induces lympho-angiogenesis in mice and it is known to be a survival factor for endothelial cells both in vitro and in vivo. However, VEGF is also known as a vascular permeability factor, based on its ability to induce vascular leakage. In the meantime it is well established that such permeability enhancing activity underlies significant roles of this molecule in inflammation and other pathological circumstances (Ferrara et al., 2003). Besides its potential role in causing aberrant angiogenesis and vascular leakage in the upper dermis, VEGF may also contribute to keratinocyte proliferation and epidermal barrier homeostasis (Elias et al., 2008; Heidenreich et al., 2009). In psoriatic skin, the VEGF receptors VEGFR-1 and -2 are detectable and functional in keratinocytes (Man et al., 2006). As VEGF is secreted by keratinocytes and induces VEGFR expression in the same cells, VEGF may also contribute to keratinocyte hyperproliferation in psoriasis in an autocrine manner. This could be relevant when psoriasis is triggered by external injury (Koebner phenomenon) and interestingly disruption of the epidermal barrier homeostasis induces VEGF expression (Elias et al., 2008). Further evidence for a role of VEGF in keratinocyte proliferation comes from transgenic mice deficient in epidermal VEGF: these animals have delayed permeability barrier recovery after acute perturbation, decreased density of dermal blood vessels and lack epidermal hyperplasia as well as angiogenesis in response to sustained barrier disruption (Elias et al., 2008). Thus, physiological production of VEGF contributes to normal proliferation, differentiation and function of the epidermis (Heidenreich et al., 2009). Consequently, VEGF over-expression in psoriasis might contribute to the epidermal changes observed in this disease. Although immune cells are also able to secrete VEGF, the findings of VEGF over-expression in psoriatic epidermis together with the data reported from the transgenic animals strongly suggest that VEGF derived from epidermal keratinocytes acts as a key cytokine driving angiogenesis in psoriasis and as a central paracrine growth factor contributing to the pathology seen in psoriasis.

3.3.2 Keratinocytes and C1d

The expression of CD1d by normal human skin and its pronounced over-expression in psoriatic skin lesions is well documented (Bonish et al., 2000) as well as the presence of NK-T cells in the epidermis of acute and chronic psoriatic plaques (Nickoloff & Wrone-Smith, 1999; Nickoloff et al., 2000). A hallmark of NK-T cells is their expression of certain C-type lectin NK cell receptors (NKRs)4 such as CD94 and CD161. Classical NK-T cells may plan an immunoregulatory role for recognition of both self and foreign antigens and are implicated in the pathogenesis of autoimmune and inflammatory diseases like psoriasis. An important clue to the function of NK-T cells is provided by their interaction with professional antigen presenting cells (APCs) via CD1d (Huang et al., 1999). CD1d has some similarities in structure to the major histocompatibility complex class II (MHC II) molecules. While initially CD1d was believed to bind and present peptide antigens to T cells (Castano et al., 1995), more recent studies highlight its ability to present glycolipids and GPI-linked proteins (Huang et al., 1999). NK-T cells can become activated in a CD1d-restricted fashion with subsequent proliferation and cytokine production, including IFN-γ and IL-4. Keratinocytes in vitro and in vivo synthesize and express CD1d, which is capable of triggering CD161+ NK-T cells to produce high levels of IFN-γ, but not IL-4. The stimulation by CD1d of T cells bearing NK receptors preferentially induces a cytokine switch to IFN-γ (Arase et al., 1996, 1997). Moreover, the differential induction of IFN-γ production, but not IL-4, after the NK-T cell clones recognized CD1d on keratinocytes has potentially important implications for psoriasis. Not only is there over-expression of CD1d by psoriatic epidermal keratinocytes and the presence of NK-T cells bearing CD94 and CD161, but the cytokine IFN-γ has been shown to trigger psoriatic lesions (Fierlbeck et al., 1990). Therefore a positive feedback loop could be established in skin due to the presence of NK-T cells being activated to produce IFN-γ upon contact with CD1d-positive keratinocytes, leading to further CD1d expression and subsequent NK-T cell release of more IFN-γ. The lack of a proliferative response by NK-T cells to CD1d keratinocytes is also consistent with the general number and distribution of CD94- and CD161-positive NK-T cells in psoriasis. Thus, the NK-T cells are never observed in tight clusters or in very large numbers as might be expected if they were undergoing a local proliferative response; rather, they are found as more evenly distributed single cells throughout a psoriatic plaque. In normal human skin CD1d is generally restricted to the outermost keratinocyte layers in the stratum granulosum just beneath the lipid-rich stratum corneum. In addition to epidermal keratinocytes, CD1d is detected on upper dermal dendritic cells, endothelium, eccrine ducts, acrosyringium, and the pilo-sebaceous unit, except for the dermal papillae and hair matrix cells. In psoriatic plaques CD1d expression was increased compared with that in normal and symptomless skin, beginning in the supra-basilar layer and extending to the outermost keratinocytes immediately beneath the parakeratotic layer juxtaposed to the stratum corneum. CD161-positive T cells were frequently observed in direct contact with keratinocytes expressing CD1d in psoriatic plaques. Given this anatomical juxtaposition, it is possible for various types of glycolipids in the psoriatic scale to be directly exposed to the abundant keratinocyte cell surface CD1d. Moreover, given the large hydrophobic binding pockets in CD1d, the presence of CD1d on the outer layers of epidermis in psoriatic plaques opens up the possibility that various glycolipids present in the stratum corneum could play a role in triggering a response by NK-T cells or other T cell subsets capable of recognizing such glycolipids in the context of CD1d. During epidermal differentiation keratinocytes produce different amounts and types of various glycolipids, including glucosylceramides (Holleran et al., 1993). Alterations in these glycolipids in the stratum corneum can have a significant impact on the barrier function of skin. However, it is also clear that barrier perturbation can initiate cytokine cascades and thus influence inflammatory and mononuclear cell activation (Nickoloff & Naidu, 1994). A cycle can be envisioned in which pathogenic NK-T cells initiate barrier abnormality, which, in turn, would generate glycolipids that could be presented by keratinocyte CD1d and further activate CD161+ T cells in psoriasis (Kalish et al., 1994). Taken together, these findings support the idea that NK-T cells may play an important patho-physiological role in psoriasis. Besides the ability of keratinocytes to initiate (Barker et al., 1991), perpetuate (Nickoloff & Turka, 1994), and terminate (Guttierrez-Steil et al., 1998) immune reactions involving conventional T cell responses to nominal antigens and super-antigens, CD1d expression may also imbue the keratinocyte with the capacity to interact with NKR-bearing T cells. As a member of a non-classical, MHC independent, antigen-presenting system, CD1d expression as seen in psoriasis provides a novel opportunity for therapeutic targeting and for understanding the immunologic and genetic basis of psoriasis as well as the potential role for innate immunity in psoriasis (Nickoloff, 1999a, 1999b).

4. Conclusion

The pathogenesis of psoriasis is considered to be an immunologically mediated process that takes place upon a favourable genetic background. According to this view, the presence of a yet unknown (auto)-antigen causes the generation of effector T-cells that infiltrate the skin and initiate the inflammatory process. Over its course, cutaneous infiltration of various immune cell populations and, subsequently, an activation of numerous immune and tissue cells in the skin takes place. Two fundamentally different cell types interact in the formation of a psoriatic lesion: epidermal keratinocytes and mononuclear leukocytes. Whereas keratinocytes might be viewed only as bystander cells in terms of immune activation, it is more likely that they are active participants in the recruitment and activation of leukocytes in psoriatic lesions: the interplay between keratinocytes and immune cells can be considered the main feature of the psoriasis pathogenesis. In facts whatever the sequence of events that leads to the induction of the mentioned cytokines and mediators in epidermal keratinocytes, it is highly likely that they significantly contribute to the typical changes observed in psoriatic lesions; cytokine or growth factor secretion by epidermal keratinocytes can be sufficient to recruit immune cells into the skin and induce a hyperplastic epidermis with hyperkeratosis and reproduce features of psoriatic disease. Regulation of the inflammatory events initiated or perpetuated by keratinocytes could so represent an important strategy for the treatment of psoriasis and other chronic inflammatory skin diseases.

5. References

Albanesi, C., Scarponi, C., Giustizieri, M.L., et al. (2005). Keratinocytes in inflammatory skin diseases. *Curr Drug Targets Inflamm Allergy,* 4, 3, (Jun 2005), 329-334.

Albanesi, C., De Pità, O. & Girolomoni, G. (2007). Resident skin cells in psoriasis: a special look at the pathogenetic functions of keratinocytes. *Clin Dermatol,* 25, 6, (Nov-Dec 2007), 581-588.

Arase, H., Arase, N. & Saito, T. (1996). Interferon γ production by natural killer cells and NK1.1+ T cells upon CD161 cross-linking. *J Exp Med,* 183, 5, (May 1996), 2391-2396.

Arase, N., Arase, H., Park, S., et al. (1997). Association with FeRg is essential for activation signal through NKR-P1 (CD161) in natural killer cells and NK1.1+ T cells. *J Exp Med,* 186, 15, (Dec 1997), 1957-1963.

Ariel, A., Novick, D., Rubinstein, M., et al. (2002). IL-12 and IL-18 induce MAP kinase-dependent adhesion of T cells to extracellular matrix components. *J Leukoc Biol,* 72, 1, (Jul 2002), 192–198.

Ariizumi, K., Meng, Y., Bergstresser, P.R., et al. (1995). IFN-gamma-dependent IL-7 gene regulation in keratinocytes. *J Immunol,* 154, 11, (Jun 1995), 6031–6039.

Banno, T., Gazel, A. & Blumenberg, N. (2004). Effects of Tumor Necrosis Factor-α (TNF-α) in epidermal keratinocytes revealed using global transcriptional profiling. *J Biol Chem,* 279, 31, (Jul 2004), 32633-32642.

Barker, J.N.W., Mitra, R.S., Griffith, C.E.M., et al. (1991). Keratinocytes as initiators of inflammation. *Lancet,* 337, 8735, (Jan 1991), 211-214.

Berard, M., Brandt, K., Bulfone-Paus, S., et al. (2003). IL-15 promotes the survival of naïve and memory phenotype CD8+ T cells. *J Immunol,* 170, 10, (May 2003), 5018–5026.

Bonifati, C., Trento, E., Cordiali-Fei, P., et al. (1997). Increased interleukin-7 concentrations in lesional skin and in the sera of patients with plaque-type psoriasis. *Clin Immunol Immunopathol,* 83, 1, (Apr 1997), 41-44.

Bonish, B., Jullien, D., Dutronc, Y., et al. (2000). Overexpression of CD1d by keratinocytes in psoriasis and CD1d-dependent IFN-gamma production by NK-T cells. *J Immunol,* 165, 7, (Oct 2000), 4076-4085.

Bos, J.D., de Rie, M.A., Teunissen, M.B.M., et al. (2005). Psoriasis: dysregulation of innate immunity. *Br J Dermatol,* 152, 6, (Jun 2005), 1098-1107.

Boyman, O., Hefti, H.P., Conrad, C., et al. (2004). Spontaneous development of psoriasis in a new animal model shows an essential role for resident T cells and tumor necrosis factor α. *J Exp Med,* 199, 5, (Mar 2004), 731–736.

Buback, F., Renkl, A.C., Schulz, C., et al. (2009). Osteopontin and the skin: multiple emerging roles in cutaneous biology an pathology. *Exp Dermatol,* 18, 9, (Sep 2009), 750-759.

Buommino, E., Tufano, M.A., Balato, N., et al. (2009). Osteopontin: a new emerging role in psoriasis. *Arch Dermatol Res,* 301, 6, (Jul 2009), 397-404.

Candi, E., Schmidt, R. & Melino, G. (2005). The cornified envelope: a model of cell death in the skin. *Nat Rev Mol Cell Biol,* 6, 4, (Apr 2006), 328–340.

Castano, A.R., Tangari, S., Miller, J.E.W. et al. (1995). Peptide binding and presentation by mouse CD1. *Science,* 269, 5221, (Jul 1995), 223-226.

Chang, E.Y., Hammerberg, C., Fisher, G., et al. (1992). T-cell activation is potentiated by cytokines released by lesional psoriatic, but not normal, epidermis. *Arch Dermatol,* 128, 11, (Nov 1992), 1479–1485.

Conrad, C., Boyman, O., Tonel, G., et al. (2007). Alpha1beta1 integrin is crucial for accumulation of epidermal T cells ant the development of psoriasis. *Nat Med,* 13, 7, (Jul 2007), 836-842.

Creamer, D., Sullivan, D., Bicknell, R., et al. (2002). Angiogenesis in psoriasis. *Angiogenesis,* 5, 4, 231-236.

Debets, R., Hegmans, J.P., Croughs, P., et al. (1997). The IL-1 system in psoriatic skin. IL-1 antagonist sphere of influence in lesional psoriatic epidermis. *J Immunology,* 158, 6, (Mar 1997), 2955-2963.

Detmar, M., Brown, L.F., Claffey, K.P., et al. (1994). Overexpression of vascular permeability factor/vascular endothelial growth factor and its receptors in psoriasis. *J Exp Med,* 180, 3, (Sep 1994), 1141-1146.

Detmar, M., Brown, L.F., Schön, M.P., et al. (1998). Increased microvascular density and enhanced leukocyte rolling and adhesion in the skin of VEGF transgenic mice. *J Invest Dermatol,* 111, 1, (Jul 1998), 1-6.

Dieu-Nosjan, M.C., Massacrier, C., Homey, B., et al. (2000). Macrophage inflammatory protein 3alpha is expressed at inflamed epithelial surfaces and is the most potent chemokine known in attracting Langerhans cell precursors. *J Exp Med,* 192, 5, (Sep 2000), 705-718.

Dinarello, C.A. (2002). The IL-1 family and inflammatory diseases. *Clin Exp Rheumatol,* 20, 5, (Sep-Oct 2002), S1-S13.

Dinarello, C.A. (2006). Interleukin 1 and interleukin 18 as mediators of inflammation and the aging process. *Am J Clin Nutr,* 83, 2, (Feb 2006), 447S-455S.

Elder, J.T. (2007). IL-15 and psoriasis: another genetic link to Th17? *J Invest Dermatol,* 127, 11, (Nov 2007), 2495-2497.

Elias, P.M., Arbiser, J., Brown, B.E., et al. (2008). Epidermal vascular endothelial growth factor production is required for permeability barrier homeostasis, dermal angiogenesis and the development of epidermal hyperplasia: implications for the pathogenesis of psoriasis. *Am J Pathol,* 173, 3, (Sep 2008), 689-699.

Ericson, P., Linden, A. & Riise, G.C. (2004). BAL levels of interleukin-18 do not change before or during acute rejection in lung transplant recipients. *Respir Med,* 98, 2, (Feb 2004), 159-163.

Fehniger, T.A. & Caligiuri, M.A. (2001). Interleukin 15: biology and relevance to human disease. *Blood,* 97, 1, (Jan 2001), 14-32.

Ferrara, N., Gerber, H.P. & LeCouter, J. (2003). The biology of VEGF and its receptors. *Nat Med,* 9, 6, (Jun 2003), 669-676.

Fierlbeck, G., Russner, G. & Muller, C. (1990). Psoriasis induced at the injection site of recombinant interferon g results of immunohistologic investigation. *Arch Dermatol,* 126, 3, (Mar 1990), 351-355.

Flisiak, I., Klepacki, A. & Chodynicka, B. (2006). Plasma and scales levels of interleukin 18 in comparison with other possible clinical and laboratory biomarkers of psoriasis activity. *Biomarkers,* 11, 2, (Apr 2006), 194-200.

Fujishima, S., Watanabe, H., Kawaguchi, M., et al. (2010). Involvement of IL-17F via the induction of IL-6 in psoriasis. *Arch Dermatol Res,* 302, 7, (Sep 2010), 499-505.

Galadari, I. & Sheriff, M.O. (2005). Estimation of interleukin-6 level in psoriasis patients. *Eur Ann Allergy Clin Immunol,* 37, 2, (Feb 2005), 63-65.

Gangemi, S., Merendino, R.A., Guarneri, F., et al. (2003). Serum levels of interleukin-18 and s-ICAM-1 in patients affected by psoriasis: preliminary considerations. *J Eur Acad Dermatol Venereol*, 17, 1, (Jan 2003), 42–46.

Ganguly, D., Chamilos, G., Lande, R., et al. (2009). Self-RNA-antimicrobial peptide complexes activate human dendritic cells through TLR7 and TLR8. *J Exp Med*, 206, 9, (Aug 2009), 1983-1994.

Gillitzer, R., Wolff, K., Tong, D., et al. (1993). MCP-1 mRNA expression in basal keratinocytes of psoriatic lesions. *J Invest Dermatol*, 101, 2, (Aug 1993), 127-131.

Girolomoni, G., Pastore, S., Cavani, A., et al. (2004). The role of chemokines in inflammatory skin diseases. *Ernst Schering Res Found Workshop*, 44, 191-225.

Gottlieb, A.B., Luster, A.D., Posnett, D.N., et al. (1998). Detection of a gamma interferon-induced protein IP-10 in psoriatic plaques. *J Exp Med*, 168, 1, (Sep 1998), 941-948.

Gottlieb, A.B., Chamian, F., Masud, S., et al. (2005). TNF inhibition rapidly downregulates multiple proinflammatory pathways in psoriasis plaques. *J Immunol*, 175, 4, (Aug 2005), 2721-2729.

Grossman, R.M., Krueger, J., Yourish, D. et al. (1989). Interleukin 6 is expressed in high levels in psoriatic skin and stimulates proliferation of cultured human keratinocytes. *Proc Natl Acad Sci USA*, 86, 16, (Aug 1989), 6367–6371.

Groves, R.W., Mizutani, H., Kieffer, JD., et al. (1995). Inflammatory skin disease in transgenic mice that express high levels of interleukin 1α in basal epidermis. *Proc Natl Acad Sci USA*, 92, 25, (Dec 1995), 11874–11878.

Gudjonsson, J.E. & Elder, J.T. (2007). Psoriasis: epidemiology. *Clin Dermatol*, 25, 6, (Nov-Dec 2007), 535-546.

Guttierrez-Steil, C., Wrone-Smith, T., Sun, X. et al. (1998). Sunlight-induced basal cell carcinoma tumor cells and ultraviolet-B irradiated psoriatic plaques express Fas ligand (CD95L). *J Clin Invest*, 101, 1, (Jan 1998), 33-39.

Gutzmer, R., Langer, K., Mommert, S., et al. (2003). Human dendritic cells express the IL-18R and are chemoattracted to IL-18. *J Immunol*, 171, 12, (Dec 2003), 6363–6371.

Heidenreich, R., Rocken, M. & Ghoreschi K. (2008). Angiogenesis: the new potential target for the therapy of psoriasis. *Drug New Perspect*, 21, 2, (Mar 2008), 97–105.

Heidenreich, R., Rocken, M. & Ghoreschi, K. (2009). Angiogenesis drives psoriasis pathogenesis. *Int J Exp Pathol*, 90, 3, (Jun 2009), 232–248.

Henno, A., Blacher, S., Lambert, C., et al. (2009). Altered expression of angiogenesis and lymphoangiogenesis markers in the uninvolved skin of plaque-type psoriasis. *Br J Dermatol*, 160, 3, (Mar 2009), 581–590.

Hirano, T. (1998). Interleukin 6 and its receptor: ten years later. *Int Rev Immunol*,16, 3-4, 249–284.

Holleran, W.M., Takagi, Y., Menon, G.K., et al. (1993). Processing of epidermal glucosylceramides is required for optimal mammalian cutaneous permeability barrier function. *J Clin Invest*, 91, 4, (Apr 1993), 1656-1664.

Homey, B., Wang, W., Soto, H., et al. (2000). Cutting edge: the orphan chemokine receptor G protein-coupled receptor-2 (GPR-2, CCR10) binds the skin associated chemokine CCL27 (CTACK/ALP/ILC). *J Immunol*, 164, 7, (Apr 2000), 3465-3470.

Huang, S., Scherer, D.C., Singh, N., et al. (1999). Lipid antigen presentation in the immune system: lessons learned from CD1d knockout mice. *Immunol Rev*, 169, (Jun 1999), 31-44.

Hurst, S.D., Muchamuel, T., Gorman, D.M. et al. (2002). New IL-17 family members promote Th1 or Th2 responses in the lung: in vivo function of the novel cytokine IL-25. *J Immunol*, 169, 1, (Jul 2002), 443–453.

Ishigame, H., Kakuta, S., Nagai, T. et al. (2009). Differential roles of interleukin-17A and -17F in host defense against mucoepithelial bacterial infection and allergic responses. *Immunity*, 30, 1, (Jan 2009), 108–119.

Jones, D.A., Yawalkar, N., Suh, Ki-Y., et al. (2004). Identification of autoantigens in psoriatic plaques using expression cloning. (2004). *J Invest Dermatol*, 123, 1, (Jun 2004), 93-100.

Kalish, R.S., Wood, J.A. & LaPorte, A. (1994). Processing of urushiol (poisonivy) antigen by both endogenous and exogenous pathways for presentation to T cells in vitro. *J Clin Invest*, 93, 5, (May 1994), 2039-2047.

Kanda, N. & Watanabe, S. (2008). IL-12, IL-23, and IL-27 enhance human betadefensin-2 production in human keratinocytes. *Eur J Immunol*, 38, 5, (May 2008), 1287–1296.

Kaser, A., Kaser, S., Kaneider, N.C., et al. (2004). Interleukin-18 attracts plasmacytoid dendritic cells (DC2s) and promotes Th1 induction by DC2s through IL-18 receptor expression. *Blood*, 103, 2, (Jan 2002), 648–655.

Krasowska, D., Pietrzak, A., Kądzielewski, J., et al. (1998). Plasma concentration of IL-6 and soluble interleukin-6 receptor versus selected acute phase proteins in patients with stationary psoriasis. *Med Sci Monit*, 4, 628–632.

Kondo, S. & Sauder, D.N. (1997). Tumor necrosis factor (TNF) receptor type 1 (p55) is a main mediator for TNF-alpha-induced skin inflammation. *Eur J Immunol*, 27, 7, (Jul 1997), 1713-1718.

Krueger, J.G. & Bowcock, A. (2005). Psoriasis pathophysiology: current concepts of pathogenesis. *Ann Rheum Dis*, 64, 2, (Mar 2005), 30-36.

Lande, R., Gregorio, J., Facchinetti, V., et al. (2007). Plasmacytoid dendritic cells sense self-DNA coupled with antimicrobial peptide. *Nature*, 449, 7162, (Sep 2007), 564-569.

Leung, B.P., Culshaw, S., Gracie, J.A., et al. (2001). A role for IL-18 in neutrophil activation. *J Immunol*, 167, 5, (Sep 2001), 2879–2886.

Liu, C.C., Perussia, B. & Young, J.D. (2000). The emerging role of IL-15 in NK-cell development. *Immunol Today*, 21, 3, (Mar 2000), 113–116.

Lowes, M.A., Bowcock, A.M. & Krueger J.G. (2007). Pathogenesis and therapy of psoriasis. *Nature*, 445, 7130, (Feb 2007), 866-873.

Man, X.Y., Yang, X.H., Cai, S.Q., et al. (2006). Immunolocalization and expression of vascular endothelial growth factor receptors (VEGFRs) and neuropilins (NRPs) on keratinocytes in human epidermis. *Mol Med*, 12, 7-8, (Jul-Aug 2006), 127–136.

Mclnnes, I.B. & Gracie, J.A. (2004). Interleukin-15: a new cytokine target for the treatment of inflammatory diseases. *Curr Opin Pharmacol*, 4, 4, (Aug 2004), 392–397.

McKenzie, R.C., Boyce, F., Szepietowski, J., et al. (2002). Psoriatic epidermis expresses high levels of interleukin 18 (IL-18), IL-18 receptor mRNA and IL-18. *Derm Klin*, 1, 4, 17–23.

Mizutani, H., Ohmoto, Y., Mizutani, T., et al. (1997). Role of increate production of monocytes TNF-α, IL-1 β and IL-6 in psoriasis: relation to focal infection, disease activity and responses to treatments. *J Dermatol Sci*, 14, 2, (Feb 1997), 145–153.

Morel, J.C., Park, C.C., Woods, J.M., et al. (2001). A novel role for interleukin-18 in adhesion molecule induction through NF kappa B and phosphatidylinositol (PI) 3-

kinasedependent signal transduction pathways. *J Biol Chem,* 276, 40, (Oct 2001), 37069–37075.

Musso, T., Calosso, L., Zucca, M., et al. (1999). Human monocytes constitutively express membrane-bound, biologically active, and interferon-γ-upregulated interleukin-15. *Blood,* 93, 10, (May 1999), 3531–3539.

Nakanishi, K., Yoshimoto, T., Tsutsui, H., et al. (2001). Interleukin-18 is a unique cytokine that stimulates both Th1 and Th2 responses depending on its cytokine milieu. *Cytokine Growth Factor Rev,* 12, 1, (Mar 2001), 53–72.

Nestle, F.O., Conrad, C., Tun-Kyi, A., et al. (2005). Plasmocytoid predendritic cells initiate psoriasis through interferon-alpha production. *J Exp Med,* 202, 1, (Jul 2005), 135-143.

Nestle, F.O., Kaplan, D.H. & Barker J. (2009). Psoriasis. *N Engl J Med,* 361, 5, (Jul 2009), 496-509.

Nickoloff, B.J. & Turka, L.A. (1994). Immunological functions of non-professional antigen-presenting cells: new insights from studies of T-cell interactions with keratinocytes. *Immuno Today,* 15, 10, (Oct 1994), 464-469.

Nickoloff, B.J., &. Naidu, Y. (1994). Perturbation of epidermal barrier function correlates with initiation of cytokine cascade in human skin. *J Am Acad Dermatol,* 30, 4, (Apr 1994), 535-546.

Nickoloff, B.J., & Wrone-Smith, T. (1999). Injection of pre-psoriatic skin with CD41 T cells induces psoriasis. *Am J Pathol,* 155, 1, (Jul 1999), 145-158.

Nickoloff, B.J. (1999). The immunological and genetic basis of psoriasis. *Arch Dermatol,* 135, 9, (Sep 1999), 1104-1110.

Nickoloff, B.J. (1999). Skin innate immune system in psoriasis: friend or foe? *J Clin Invest,* 104, 9, (Nov 1999), 1161-1164.

Nickoloff, B.J., Bonish, B., Huang, B., et al. (2000). Characterization of a T cell line bearing natural killer receptors and capable of creating psoriasis in a SCID mouse model system. *J Dermatol Sci,* 24, 3, (Dec 2000), 212-225.

Nograles, K.E., Zaba, L.C., Guttman-Yassky, E., et al. (2008). Th17 cytokines interleukin(IL)-17 and IL-22 modulate distinct inflammatory and keratinocyte-response pathways. *Br J Dermatol,* 159, 5, (Nov 2008), 1092-1102.

Nograles, K.E., Davidovici, B. & Krueger, J.G. (2010). New insights in immunologic basis of psoriasis. *Semin Cutan Med Surg,* 29, 1, (Mar 2010), 3-9.

Nomura, I., Goleva, E., Howell, M.D., et al. (2003). Cytokine milieu of atopic dermatitis, as compared to psoriasis, skin prevents induction of innate immune response genes. *J Immunol,* 171, 6, (Sep 2003), 3262-3269.

Ohta, Y., Hamada, Y. & Katsuoka, K. (2001). Expression of IL-18 in psoriasis. *Arch Dermatol Res,* 293, 7, (Jul 2001), 334–342.

Okubo, Y. & Koga, M. (1998). Peripheral blood monocytes in psoriatic patients overproduce cytokines. *J Dermatol Sci,* 17, 3, (Jul 1998), 223–232.

Park, C.C., Morel, J.C., Amin, M.A., et al. (2001). Evidence of IL-18 as a novel angiogenic mediator. *J Immunol,* 167, 3, (aug 2001), 1644–1653.

Peric, M., Koglin, S., Kim, S.M., et al. (2008). IL-17A enhances vitamin D3-induced expression of cathelicidin antimicrobial peptide in human keratinocytes. *J Invest Immunol,* 181, 12, (Dec 2008), 8504-8512.

Pietrzak, A., Krasowska, D., Kozioł-Montewka, M., et al. (1999). IL-8, IL-6 levels and IL-6R in the blood of psoriasis vulgaris patients. *Przegl Dermatol,* 86, 115–121.

Romer, J., Hasselager, E., Norby, P.L., et al. (2003). Epidermal overexpression of interleukin-19 and -20 mRNA in psoriatic skin disappears after short-term treatment with cyclosporine a or calcipotriol. *J Invest Dermatol,* 121, 6, (Dec 2003), 1306–1311.

Rückert, R., Asadullah, K., Seifert, M., et al. (2000). Inhibition of keratinocyte apoptosis by IL-15: a new parameter in the pathogenesis of psoriasis? *J Immunol,* 165, 4, (Aug 2000), 2240-2250.

Sa, S.M., Valdez, P.A., Wu, J., et al. (2007). The effects of IL-20 subfamily cytokines on reconstituted human epidermis suggest potential roles in cutaneous innate defense and pathogenic adaptive immunity in psoriasis. *J Immunol,* 178, 4, (Feb 2007), 2229–2240.

Tschachler, E. (2007). Psoriasis: the epidermal component. *Clin Dermatol,* 25, 6, (Nov-Dec 2007), 589-595.

Wei, C.C., Hsu, Y.H., Li, H.H., et al. (2006). IL-20: biological functions and clinical implications. *J Biomed Sci,* 13, 5, (Sep 2006), 601-612.

Wollenberg, A., Wagner, M., Günther, S., et al. (2002). Plasmacytoid dendritic cells: a new cutaneous dendritic cell subset with distinct role in inflammatory skin diseases. *J Invest Dermatol,* 119, 5, (Nov 2002), 1096–1102.

Wojas-Pelc, A., Ciszek, M., Kurnyta, M., et al. (2006). Cytokine network in psoriasis. Cross-talk between keratinocytes and cells of the skin immune system. *Centr Eur J Immunol,* 31, 111–116.

Wolk, K., Kunz, S., Witte, E., et al. (2004). IL-22 increases the innate immunity of tissues. *Immunity,* 21, 2, (Aug 2004), 241–254.

Wolk, K., Witte, E., Wallace, E., et al. (2006). IL-22 regulates the expression of genes responsible for antimicrobial defense, cellular differentiation, and mobility in keratinocytes: a potential role in psoriasis. *Eur J Immunol,* 36, 5, (May 2006), 1309–1323.

Wolk, K., Witte, E., Warszawska, K., et al. (2009). The Th17 cytokine IL-22 induces IL-20 production in keratinocytes: a novel immunological cascade with potential relevance in psoriasis. *Eur J Immunol,* 39, 12, (Dec 2009), 3570-3581.

Wolk, K., Haugen, H.S., Xu, W., et al. (2009). IL-22 and IL-20 are key mediators of the epidermal alterations in psoriasis while IL-17 and IFN-gamma are not. *J Mol Med,* 87, 5, (May 2009), 523–536.

Xia, Y.P., Li, B., Hylton, D., et al. (2003). Transgenic delivery of VEGF to mouse skin leads to an inflammatory condition resembling human psoriasis. *Blood,* 102, 1, (Jul 2003), 161-168.

Yang, X.O., Chang, S.H., Park, H. et al. (2008). Regulation of inflammatory responses by IL-17F. *J Exp Med,* 205, 5, (May 2008), 1063–1075.

Yano, S., Komine, M., Fujimoto, M., et al. (2003). Interleukin 15 induces the signals of epiderma proliferation through ERK and PI 3-kinase In a human epiderma keratinocyte cell line, HaCaT. *Biochem Biophys Res Commun,* 301, 4, (Feb 2003), 841–847.

Yoshinaga, Y., Higaki, M., Terajima, et al. (1995). Detection of inflammatory cytokines in psoriatic skin. *Arch Dermatol Res,* 287, 2, 158–164.

Zalewska, A., Głowacka, E., Wyczółkowska, J., et al. (2006). Interleukin 6 and 8 levels in plasma and fibroblast cultures in psoriasis. *Mediators Inflamm,* 1, 1, 81767-81773.

Zepter, K., Haffner, A., Soohoo, L.F., et al. (1997). Induction of biologically active IL-1β - converting enzyme and mature IL-1β in human keratinocytes by inflammatory and immunologic stimuli. *J Immunol,* 159, 12, (Dec 1997), 6203–6208.

3

Wound Repair Studies Reveal New Insights to Psoriasis

Chee Ren Ivan Lam[1], Ming Jie Tan[1], Yan Yih Goh[1],
Mark Boon Yang Tang[2] and Nguan Soon Tan[1]
[1]*School of Biological Sciences, Nanyang Technological University, Nanyang Drive*
[2]*National Skin Centre*
Singapore

1. Introduction

Psoriasis, a chronic relapsing inflammatory skin disease with a disturbing global incidence of approximately 2%, is an afflicting and disfiguring skin disease with high morbidity (Lomholt, 1964). The disease is characterized by the well-demarcated erythematous plaques with silvery white scales and a predilection for body areas such as the elbows, knees, umbilicus and lumbar area (Schön & Boehncke, 2005). In contrast to normal skin, the dermal vasculature in psoriasis dermis is dramatically increased with large, tortuous blood vessels, accounting for the erythematous appearance or redness of the affected skin regions/psoriatic plaques (Nestle et al, 2009). In addition, the psoriatic epidermis is significantly thickened and acanthotic, due to hyperproliferative keratinocytes with an approximate seven-fold increase in the number of dividing cells in the basal and suprabasal epidermal layers (Castelijns et al, 2000). Keratinocytes of the psoriatic skin are prematurely differentiated, as evident in the incomplete cornification of the stratum corneum, characterized by the retention of nuclei (i.e., parakeratosis) and the loss of the granular layer. The stratum corneum of psoriasiform skin is also thickened (i.e., hyperkeratosis). This heavy disruption of epidermal differentiation and skin barrier homeostasis coupled with altered levels of intercellular adhesion molecules result in the widespread scaling of psoriatic lesions (Christensen et al, 2006). While psoriasis primarily affects the epidermis, the disease has a strong immunopathological basis, with the psoriatic skin being significantly infiltrated with immune cells. Notably, this immune infiltrate has a characteristic distribution and is composed mainly of dendritic cells and macrophages in the dermis, neutrophils in the epidermis and T cells in both layers. Another immunologic feature of the disease is its extracutaneous manifestation of an arthritic condition, which affects approximately 5% of the population and approximately 20% of psoriasis patients (Zachariae et al, 2002; Hueber & McInnes, 2007). However, the direct involvement of the skin and immune system in psoriasiform features complicates and confounds studies of psoriasis. Therefore, despite the detailed documented pathological observations of psoriasis and the vast research efforts aimed at understanding the disease, a key question remains unanswered: is psoriasis provoked by an epidermal or an immunological trigger?

2. Background

It is well accepted that the pathology of psoriasis involves the participation of both the immune system and skin tissue; therefore a rational research approach would include studying the disease from an *in vivo* rather than an *in vitro* perspective. Hence, most psoriasis studies have been in the context of animal models which continue to serve as an invaluable platform for drug testing and development. While there is an absolute need for an *in vivo* platform, an ideal animal model is still lacking as no naturally and frequently occurring animal disease is known to exhibit every complex disease feature of psoriasis (Schön, 1999). Hence the study of psoriasis is narrowly limited to the artificial induction of the disease in laboratory animals. Nevertheless, several animal models have been developed in recent decades to meet the demands of psoriasis research. Study approaches include spontaneous mutants, T cell transfer models and xenografts.

2.1 Spontaneous mutants

The earliest psoriasis models were laboratory-bred mutant mice that were found to manifest skin lesions resembling psoriasis. These animals were spontaneous mutants of known allelic mutations. One such mutant strain was mice carrying the homozygous asebia mutation ($Scd1^{ab}$/ $Scd1^{ab}$). The skin of the asebia mouse is typified by hair loss (i.e., alopecia) and the complete absence of sebaceous glands. Like psoriatic human skin, asebia mouse skin displayed hyperkeratosis, epidermal acanthosis, increased dermal vascularity and an immune cell infiltrate (Gates & Karasek, 1965). However, unlike human psoriatic skin, the leukocytic infiltrate of asebia mouse skin was devoid of neutrophils and T cells. Because the immune system is strongly believed to account for a substantial portion of the pathogenesis of psoriasis, this difference in the inflammatory response in asebia mouse skin reduces the reliability of this disease model. Moreover, lipid metabolism in asebia mouse skin was significantly altered, implying a distinctly different disease mechanism from psoriasis, which further undermined its value as a psoriasis model (Wilkinson & Karasek, 1966). Two other homozygous mouse mutants, chronic proliferative dermatitis (*cpd*) and the flaky skin (*fsn*), also display a hyperproliferative epidermis, increased dermal vascularity and a mixed immune cell infiltrate including neutrophils in micro-abscesses of lesions. These similarities with human psoriatic skin make these animal models slightly superior to the asebia mouse model as disease models for psoriasis (Morita et al, 1995). However, the psoriasiform-like phenotype of both *fsn* and *cpd* critically lack a T cell-based immunopathogenesis. This was demonstrated by the ability of glucocorticosteroid treatment to improve the *fsn* lesions, which targets the innate immune response, but not with cyclosporine A, a licensed psoriasis drug which inhibits T cell-mediated immune responses (Sundberg et al, 1994). Cyclosporin A treatment also did not improve *cpd* skin lesions (HogenEsch et al, 1994). *Fsn* mice that were double homozygous for the severe combined immunodeficiency mutation (*scid/scid*) and lacked mature T and B lymphocytes also developed skin lesions nonetheless (Sundberg et al, 1994). Furthermore, the transfer of hemopoietic T cell precursors from *cpd* to syngeneic recipients did not pass on the psoriasiform condition (HogenEsch et al, 1994). *Cpd* and *fsn* are also far more complex than psoriasis; both involve pathologies that extend to other organ systems. This complexity confounds the study of psoriasis when these models are used. Critically, the psoriasiform-like phenotype of *cpd* and *fsn* could both develop without the participation of T cells, which are known key effectors in psoriasis (HogenEsch et al,

1994; Sundberg et al, 1994). Given these limitations, spontaneous mutants still fall short of being an ideal psoriasis model. The greatest concern about using this type of animal model for psoriasis research is that researchers are essentially deriving conclusions about the causes of psoriasis from diseases with another unknown basis.

2.2 T cell transfer models

The disqualification of the early animal models (i.e., *fsn* and *cpd*) as psoriatic models highlights the strong growing recognition of psoriasis as a T cell-mediated disease. Several clinical observations support this theory, including how psoriasis can be significantly improved with drugs targeting T cell-mediated immunity (Weinshenker et al, 1989). Streptococcal infection of the upper respiratory tract, which is remote from the skin, is known to trigger psoriasis via T cell-mediated responses to bacterial superantigens that mimic keratins. This process initiates a pseudo-autoimmune reaction responsible for the psoriasiform outcome (Prinz et al, 1991; Leung et al, 1995; Valdimarsson et al, 2009). Interestingly, psoriasis was shown to be transferrable when the bone marrow of an affected individual was transplanted into a previously unaffected recipient (Snowden & Heaton, 1997). Conversely, psoriasis in a previously affected individual was completely cured after bone marrow ablation prior to transplant (Eedy et al, 1990). While phagocytic immune cells (i.e., neutrophils, macrophage and dendritic cells) are responsible for indiscriminate immune functions such as the engulfment of pathogens or cellular debris and antigen presentation (Delves & Roitt, 2000), T cells have a more specific molecular recognition role in the immune system. In summary, every cytotoxic CD8 T cell clone possesses antigen specificity, allowing it to recognize a unique antigen presented on the major histocompatibility complex (MHC) of non-immune cells. For example, this antigen could be a viral peptide in the context of an infected cell, a foreign peptide in the context of an allograft, or a self peptide in the event of an autoimmune response. In any of these cases, CD8 T cells would mount a cytotoxic response against the target cell. The CD8 T cells can mediate a necrotic cell killing through the targeted secretion of lytic proteins, perforin and granzyme, onto the target cells. These proteins drastically destabilize the target cell membrane, eventually leading to osmotic stress and colloid osmotic lysis (Delves & Roitt, 2000).

The classic study of tissue graft rejection showed that the adoptive transfer of normal T cells into nude mice *scid* would lead to an immune rejection of the host animal's skin (Roopenian & Anderson, 1988). An experimental proof of T cell pathogenesis for psoriasis would require a T cell-mediated response directed against skin cells. Using principles of tissue graft rejection, MHC compatible naïve CD4+/CD45RB^{Hi} T lymphocytes that were minor histocompatibility complex mismatched were transplanted into *scid/scid* mice. The minor histocompatibility mismatch was aimed at minimizing the severity of the immune response and hence prolonging the rejection process. Without fail, this procedure led to the development of clinically consistent psoriasiform skin within 4-8 weeks. The resulting mouse skin lesions were markedly similar to those of human psoriatic skin; they shared the key histopathological features of acanthosis, parakeratosis, leukocytic infiltrate and dermal angiogenesis. Remarkably, pro-inflammatory cytokine expression in the lesional skin was also similar to that of human psoriatic skin, with elevated expressions of tumor necrosis factor-α (TNF-α), interleukin-6 (IL-6), interferon-γ and granulocyte macrophage colony stimulating factor (GM-CSF). These lesions also responded well to immunosuppressive treatments such as cyclosporine A and ultraviolet B (310 nm) phototherapy (Schön et al, 1997). Taken together, these features suggest that an epidermal abnormality is unnecessary for the formation of psoriatic lesions and that a T cell-invoked immune response results in psoriasiform skin. However, this model cannot rule out the involvement of an epidermal trigger, as T cells were deliberately mismatched to the host skin cells. Hence, this T cell transfer model can only be used to study cutaneous psoriatic events post-T cell activation and not those processes preceding T cell activation.

2.3 Xenografts

Although animal and T cell transfer models offer a convenient bench approach to studying psoriasis, they still do not reflect the genuine pathogenesis of the disease. Animal models may have typical psoriasiform-like skin lesions but closer analysis has revealed critical cellular differences from the human disease. In addition, T cell transfer models exhibit only the immune aspects of psoriasis after T cell activation, and they lack all aspects of the preliminary events leading to T cell activation. Furthermore, the vast differences between mouse and human skin further complicate the ability to extrapolate animal models to the actual human disease (Gudjonsson et al, 2007). Hence, another approach is to study every *in situ* event of human psoriatic skin *in vivo*. This has been made possible by xenotransplantation, whereby human diseased skin is grafted across species to an immunocompromised murine host. With xenotransplantation, psoriatic features of diseased human skin can be maintained for more than 2 months, providing sufficient study time (Krueger et al, 1975). Apart from T cells originating in the systemic circulation, resident T cells and other immune cells in psoriatic skin may also contribute to pathogenesis, which is not possible using T cell models. Xenotransplantation models circumvent this shortcoming, as all forms of resident immune cells in the transplanted diseased skin may be continually studied post-transplantation (Boehncke & Schön, 2007). Altogether, xenotransplantation models allow the study of *in situ* events in the context of actual human psoriatic skin. This approach has helped elucidate the role of resident T cells in disease pathogenesis and helped identify the molecules involved in the epidermal recruitment of T cells, such as integrin $\alpha_1\beta_1$ (Conrad et al, 2007). Importantly, the xenotransplantation method allows for comparisons between involved and uninvolved skin (Boehncke et al, 1994; Nickoloff et al, 1995). Xenotransplantation models may also be used to study other components of the immune system, such as the role of natural killer cells in psoriasis. The immune background of the host could be modified by cross-breeding mouse strains that carry mutations to different immunity-related genes. For example, non-obese diabetic (NOD) mice with impaired natural killer and antigen presenting cells could be combined with *scid* through cross-breeding to generate a host animal with a modified immune background to enhance the study of natural killer cells in psoriasis (Roder & Duwe, 1979; Shultz et al, 1995). With this concept, many other combinations of immune backgrounds have since been innovated to support novel studies. Regarding drug discovery studies, xenotransplantation models facilitate the testing of human directed antibodies or biologics because of the limited cross-species reactivity (Boehncke, 2005). However, xenotransplantation models do have their own shortcomings and limitations, including the challenge of assessing T cell homing processes since human T cells in the transplanted xenograft may not transit normally to mouse lymph nodes in the hybrid natured "two-species-systems" (Garcia et al, 1997). Also, xenotransplantation is limited by a lack of diseased skin donors. In response to this issue, a bioengineered skin-humanized mouse model was recently developed. Healthy human skin biopsies were engrafted onto mice and allowed to regenerate. T cells isolated from blood samples of the same donors were cultured *in vitro* and transfected with recombinant IL-17 and IL-22 expression vectors. The regenerated skin graft was then reconstituted with this T cell population through intradermal injections. The stratum corneum surface of the graft was also removed by mild abrasion, which then triggered psoriasiform features. The bioengineered skin was claimed to accurately represent human psoriatic skin (Guerrero-Aspizua et al, 2010).

2.4 Transgenic animal models

With the advent of genetic engineering, another approach using transgenic expression of individual molecules in the mouse epidermis has allowed scientists to identify possible psoriatic triggers. To assess the relevance of a protein factor, researchers induce an overexpression of the factor in the epidermis. By varying the promoter used, scientists can localize and target the epidermal overexpression to either the basal or the suprabasal layer, taking advantage of distinct promoters found in the different skin layers. For example, there is exclusive expression of keratin 14 in the basal layer and involucrin in the suprabasal keratinocytes. Epidermal overexpression helps enhance the presence of the protein of interest in the skin which enables investigations of the effects of the proteins on the immune system (Schön, 2008). To date, most of the proteins shortlisted for studies are related to the immune system or angiogenesis (e.g., TNF-α, IL-1α, IL-6, IL-8, IFN-γ, ICAM-1, VEGF, etc.). Comparatively few proteins studied are of epidermal origin (i.e., TGF-α, KGF, etc.) because previous studies using animal or T cell transfer models have identified a more immunological etiology of psoriasis (Schön, 1999). While the compilation of these studies suggests a strong immunopathogenic basis for psoriasis, an epidermal trigger of psoriasis cannot be completely discounted, as these *in vivo* disease models also involve the immune and cutaneous systems of animal models.

3. New players in psoriasis identified from wound repair studies

While the current evidence suggests that dysregulation of the immune system, particularly abnormal Th1 and Th17 immune responses, is the primary and predominant pathogenic basis for psoriasis, it is still debatable how epidermal barrier dysfunction contributes as a primary and secondary etiological factor in psoriasis. It is noteworthy that psoriasis susceptibility has been linked to a large number of genes, including those involving epidermal and immunological functions. While psoriasis has been associated with key adaptive immune genes like the *PSORS1* MHC locus antigen cluster (Allen et al, 2005), it has also been linked to epidermal proteins like the S100 proteins (Wolf et al, 2010). These genetic associations reinforce the mechanistic complexity of psoriasis, which cannot be reduced simply to either an epidermal or immunological mode of causation. This uneven balance of research attention could also stem from the natural difficulty of studying cutaneous factors in animal models. While immune cells can be studied by their transfer into an *in vivo* system, the same cannot be said for keratinocytes. Moreover, immune responses are always obligate and inseparable from the *in vivo* context of an animal model. Skin grafting, for example, inevitably leads to wounding and subsequent inflammation in the grafted skin region. In every study performed on an animal host, immune responses are inevitable after manipulation or perturbation of the epidermal barrier. The heavy influx of immune responses and their corresponding mediators would obscure any genuine causal triggers, especially if the cause may be of a subtle epidermal origin. A similar obfuscation of epidermal causes could happen in the actual human disease, confounding the continual search for an initiating factor. Moreover, the concept of skin as a immunological tissue has gradually gained importance over the last two decades, supported by the notion of skin-associated lymphoid tissue (SALT) that was conceptualized in the early eighties. This SALT concept supports a specialized exclusive circulation of immune cells between the skin, the draining lymph nodes and the systemic circulation, which facilitates the priming of the T cell-mediated response in the skin (Streilein, 1983; Streilein, 1989). This helps highlight the importance of the adaptive immune response in psoriasis. Furthermore, to effectively safeguard the extensive cutaneous barrier against the external environment, immunosurveillance of the skin cannot rely solely on skin-residing immune scavenger cells (i.e., Langerhans cell). Rather, the average keratinocyte can capably assume the versatile role of an immune sentinel in the epidermis (Nestle et al, 2009). Armed with Toll-like receptors (TLRs) on their surfaces, keratinocytes recognize pathogen-associated molecular patterns on invading microorganisms and activate both cell-mediated immune responses and the production of type I interferons (IFNs) (Baker et al, 2003; Mempel et al, 2003; Pivarcsi et al, 2004). Keratinocytes are also constitutive producers of pro-inflammatory cytokines (i.e., IL-1, TNF-α, IL-6, IL-10, etc.) (Pivarcsi et al, 2004; Nestle et al, 2009) and can express MHC class II molecules (Nickoloff & Turka, 1994). It is thus feasible for keratinocytes to serve as adjunct antigen-presenting cells (Nickoloff & Turka, 1994). As such, the keratinocyte, despite being a non immune cell, can trigger both the innate and adaptive immune responses, suggesting that it can act as a peripheral extension of the immune system. Importantly, the role of epidermal barrier dysfunction in psoriasis should not be overlooked given the inextricable relationship between the skin and the immune system.

3.1 A neglected aspect of psoriasis research: The relevance of wound healing

3.1.1 Koebner phenomenon

Although psoriasis is strongly believed to have an underlying genetic predisposition, psoriatic plaque formation is demarcated and usually does not cover or affect the patient's entire skin area (Schön & Boehncke, 2005). The unexpected outbreak of psoriatic lesions in most patients gives the impression of an unpredictable skin condition and has greatly complicated the study of psoriasis. With an unknown trigger for psoriasis, it is difficult to rationally attribute a direct or indirect causation to either the epidermal or the immune systems. Thus, to understand the epidermal role in psoriasis, it is advantageous to trigger psoriatic plaque formation on uninvolved skin with a specific epidermal perturbation and subsequently study the molecular changes in keratinocytes corresponding to the known perturbation. This is, however, impossible in animal models in which psoriasis does not naturally occur (Schön, 1999).

The Koebner phenomenon is a well recognized clinical finding in psoriasis, whereby new psoriastic lesions can be induced in previously uninvolved skin after skin wounding or trauma. Such psoriatic lesions usually form within 10-20 days of the wounding event, coinciding with the duration of the wound healing phase. This strongly suggests that skin in predisposed individuals may still develop normally until substantial triggering by key epidermal perturbations (Weiss et al, 2002). Wounding stands out as the only known epidermal perturbation with the predictable ability to trigger psoriasis, thus offering a unique opportunity to study pathogenetic mechanisms in psoriasis. While the molecular basis for koebnerized psoriasis remains largely unexamined (Weiss et al, 2002), wound healing studies have been comparatively well established. Considering the obligate coincidence and connection between wounding and psoriasis, an adequate understanding of koebnerized psoriasis requires a solid understanding of wound healing. The Koebner phenomenon was initially described after animal bite wounds and incision wounds. However, with accumulated observation and documentation, the Koebner phenomenon was later broadened to more accurately and extensively include psoriasis arising from all other forms of skin injury such as insect bites, friction, pressure wounds, excoriations, burns, contact dermatitis, chemical irritation, infections, tattoo and sunburns (Sagi & Trau, 2011). Some interesting exceptions were also made and accordingly, not every form of trauma resulted in koebnerization. Some interesting exceptions have been observed that did not result in koebnerization, such as experimentally inflicted knife blade injury to the dermis that did not produce psoriatic lesions on the overlying epidermis above the wounded dermal portion, but only at the incisional point where the epidermis was damaged (Farber et al, 1965). Likewise, the dermal injection of potent inflammatory stimulators like hyaluronidase and chymotrypsin did not initiate a Koebner response (Farber et al, 1965). The key conclusion from both experiments was that koebnerization must involve epidermal traumatic damage (Farber et al, 1965). This finding was further confirmed by suction blistering experiments, resulting in epidermal and dermal separation without epidermal rupture, which did not induce koebnerization (Miller, 1982; Pedace et al, 1969). The criterion of an epidermal rupture needed for koebnerization is crucial and on a microscopic level, necrotic damage of keratinocytes will activate the innate inflammatory cascade leading to psoriasis (Chen et al, 2007). Thus, it is conceivable that some forms of wounds, perturbations and traumas to the skin are not as visibly obvious as others. These subtle forms of epidermal injuries could lead to koebnerized psoriasis but still display the misleading outward appearance and impression of a spontaneous psoriatic outbreak. This revelation will shed light on many of our clinical and scientific observations concerning psoriasis. As mentioned earlier, adoptive T cell transfer experiments in *scid* mice have demonstrated the independent ability of T cells to promote the complex pathogenesis of psoriasis (Schön et al, 1997). It is likely that transplanted minor histocompatibility complex mismatched T cells would direct a T cell-mediated cytotoxic response against host keratinocyte cells leading to widespread necrotic epidermal damage, hence fueling the onset of koebnerized psoriasis. Furthermore, the injured epidermis may expose putative self antigens to the adaptive immune system, triggering an autoimmune inflammatory reaction. The importance of undetected, insidious micro-trauma to the skin as a possible initiating and aggravating factor in psoriasis cannot be over-emphasized and may explain the predilection for psoriasis over sites of frequent trauma such as the knees and elbows (Schön & Boehncke, 2005). Recent advances in wound healing research has enhanced our understanding and allowed better insight into the role of wound healing in the pathogenesis of psoriasis.

3.2 Events in wounding

Wounding or skin injury results in keratinocyte disruption leading to an epidermal gap that may expose the dermis if sufficiently large or deep. With the epidermal barrier being the key protective barrier against various insults of the external environment, re-epithelialization of the breached epidermis is an urgent priority to close the wound gap and restore epidermal integrity. Keratinocytes at the edge of the wound are required to proliferate and migrate to fill up the epidermal gap to effectively seal it (Stadelmann et al, 1998).

The wound and psoriatic lesional microenvironment in the initial stages appear to be largely similar in terms of the abundant production of pro-inflammatory cytokines, such as TNF-α, IFN-γ and IL-1 (Nickoloff et al, 2006). Keratinocytes in wound sites and psoriatic lesions are also similarly differentiated; both express keratin 6 (K6), keratin 16 (K16) and keratin 17 (K17) instead of the standard keratin 1 (K1) and keratin 10 (K10) expressed by normal differentiating suprabasal keratinocytes (de Jong et al, 1991; Mommers et al, 2000; Wang & Chang, 2003). This suggests that transcriptional regulation responsible for both wound healing and psoriasis are similar. It is thus relevant to identify the key transcriptional regulators responsible for wound healing to evaluate its impact on psoriatic skin.

3.3 Nuclear hormone receptors as prospective transcriptional regulators in wounded skin

Among transcriptional regulators, nuclear hormone receptors are of particular interest. Nuclear hormone receptors (NRs), such as the retinoid acid receptors, are one of the largest known classes of transcription factors, several have significant transcriptional activities in the skin and are responsible for skin homeostasis (Redfern & Todd, 1992). In humans, this superfamily comprises 48 ligand-dependent or "orphan" transcription factors (Robinson-Rechavi et al, 2003). Unlike conventional transmembrane receptors, NRs are intracellular and locked in an inactive conformation by means of a bound chaperone (i.e., heat shock proteins, immunophilins) (Young & Hartl, 2002). Upon ligand binding in the cytosol, the chaperone is displaced, and the nuclear receptor is freed to undergo an active conformation, enabling its translocation into the nucleus where it subsequently binds specific DNA recognition elements present in the promoter sequence of target genes, inducing their transcription (Gronemeyer et al, 2004). As such, NRs are dual functional, serving as both a receptor and a transcription factor. The active conformation of NRs possesses a hydrophobic pocket as the ligand-binding site (Gronemeyer et al, 2004). Hence, ligands of NRs are necessarily small hydrophobic molecules (e.g., fatty acids, steroid hormones, thyroid hormones, vitamin D, retinoids, etc.), which eases their diffusion-based passage through the hydrophobic cell membrane and their subsequent binding to intracellular receptors (Friedmann et al, 2005). Furthermore, the skin is increasingly recognized as an endocrine tissue because it synthesizes and modifies steroidal hormones, which subsequently has autocrine, paracrine or endocrine signaling functions (Zouboulis, 2009). As such, significant research attention has been paid to NRs and their transcriptional regulatory role in the skin. Agonist and antagonist drugs that target the NR family constitute one of the largest and most potent groups of pharmaceuticals currently in use, and thus hold great potential for use in improved wound treatment strategies (Sladek, 2003).

3.3.1 PPARβ/δ as wound healing transcription regulator and psoriasis trigger

Recent research by various groups including our laboratory has highlighted the crucial role of a distinct member group of the NR superfamily, the peroxisome proliferator-activated receptors (PPARs), in wound healing (Tan et al, 2004). PPARs consist of three isotypes, namely α, β/δ and γ (Tan et al, 2004). Specifically, studies of adult murine skin wounds have shown that wounding rapidly elevates the expression of PPAR β/δ from an initially undetectable range to very high levels in wound-edge keratinocytes located at the interfollicular regions of the epidermis (Tan et al, 2004). Apart from the epidermis, dermal PPAR β/δ levels were also up-regulated (Tan et al, 2004). In addition to wounding, the up-regulation of PPAR β/δ in interfollicular keratinocytes was also observed upon hair plucking and treatment with chemical irritants like phorbol esters, which can induce skin inflammation, epidermal hyperplasia and act as tumor promoting agents (TPAs) (Fürstenberger et al, 1981; Tan et al, 2003). The common underlying theme of these three skin perturbation events is that they all involve a preliminary phase of inflammation followed by epidermal proliferation. Wounding and hair plucking which are examples of koebnerization, both involve damage to the epidermis that initiate inflammation, followed by keratinocyte proliferation in order to re-epithelialize the breached epidermis. Inflammation and a hyperproliferative epidermis are also hallmark features of psoriasis, thus suggesting the possible involvement of PPAR β/δ in the transcription regulatory process of psoriasis. We conducted *in vitro* studies on mouse primary keratinocytes to evaluate the means of PPAR β/δ up-regulation during wounding. A mixed leukocyte reactions (MLR) procedure was used to mimic the inflammatory environment in the wound. MLR involves exposing immature bone marrow-derived dendritic cells (DCs) and T cells to a necrotic cellular mixture of minced skin. DCs activated by the necrotic cellular mixture will induce T cells to synergistically produce pro-inflammatory cytokines equivalent to those produced in a wound environment (i.e., TNF-α, IFN-γ, IL-1, etc.). Incubation of keratinocytes with the conditioned MLR media led to the up-regulation of PPAR β/δ. In fact, TNF-α and IFN-γ were confirmed to be the signaling inducers responsible for this PPAR β/δ up-regulation. TNF-α and IFN-γ were also found to up-regulate the endogenous ligand of PPAR β/δ, hence enhancing the transcriptional activity of PPAR β/δ in the wounded skin. Without this production of the ligand, transcription through PPAR β/δ would have been futile despite a deliberate overexpression of PPAR β/δ (Tan et al, 2001).

In summary, wounding and skin injury lead to epidermal damage, which trigger innate skin inflammation. Excessive pro-inflammatory cytokines in the inflamed skin induce the up-regulation of PPAR β/δ and its endogenous ligand, which subsequently counter the apoptotic consequences of inflammation, favoring epidermal hyperproliferation (Tan et al, 2001). This relationship was first established in wounding studies and bears clear resemblances to the pathological manifestation of psoriasis. This insight into PPAR β/δ's involvement in wound healing prompted further investigation into its probable role in psoriasis. Immunohistochemistry and expression profiling studies have revealed that PPAR β/δ is overexpressed in the psoriatic lesions of most patients (Romanowska et al, 2010). The overexpression of PPAR β/δ in mouse skin also resulted in an inflammatory skin disease that was phenotypically similar to psoriasis (Romanowska et al, 2010).

Other epidermal factors have also been linked to psoriasis. One emerging area of interest is the S100 proteins, a multigene family of low molecular weight calcium binding proteins encoded within a well known psoriasis susceptibility locus (PSOR4) on chromosome 1q21 (Semprini et al, 2002). S100A7 (psoriasin) and S100A15 (koebnerisin), prominent members of this protein family, are up-regulated in skin inflammation and psoriasis (Semprini et al, 2002). Uninvolved psoriatic skin was found to have more constitutively enhanced S100A7/A15 expression than healthy skin (Wolf et al, 2010). In lesional psoriatic skin, the level of S100A7/A15 was further elevated, suggesting its significant role in the disease. This up-regulated S100A7/A15 expression was also retained when psoriatic keratinocytes were isolated and cultured *in vitro* (Wolf et al, 2010). S100A7/A15 was found to prime psoriatic keratinocytes, thereby increasing their susceptibility to inflammation (Wolf et al, 2010). This has been largely attributed to its autocrine effect on keratinocytes with recent studies confirming the intracellular presence of S100A7 (Broome et al, 2003). Moreover, S100A7 expression was also correlated with epidermal fatty acid binding protein (E-FABP), a keratinocyte protein that is distinctly up-regulated in psoriasis (Ruse et al, 2003). As it is difficult for lipophilic ligands to traverse through the hydrophilic cytosolic environment enroute the nucleus, E-FABP eases this transition by binding the endogenous ligands and transferring them to the PPAR β/δ receptor (Kannan-Thulasiraman et al, 2010). Notably, S100A7 has been found to bind and co-localize with E-FABP in keratinocytes (Broome et al, 2003). This interaction effectually stabilizes intracellular E-FABP levels (Broome et al, 2003). Hence, E-FABP is necessary for PPAR β/δ to stabilize and function effectively as a nuclear receptor (Kannan-Thulasiraman et al, 2010). This relationship explains how increased levels of S100A7 predisposes keratinocytes to inflammation and psoriasis, possibly via the stabilization of PPAR β/δ receptors for their relevant transcriptional activity. As S100 proteins interact with their target proteins in a calcium-dependent manner, it is also possible that calcium released from the endoplasmic reticulum during inflammation activates S100A7 which acts together with PPAR β/δ to induce transcription of anti-apoptotic features in psoriatic keratinocytes. Herein, the role of PPAR β/δ in psoriasis is reinforced.

3.4 ROS-induced oxidative damage of keratinocytes as initiating event of psoriasis

Psoriatic lesions are associated with up-regulated levels of reactive oxygen species (ROS) (Zhou et al, 2009). Using dichlorodihydrofluorescein diacetate (DCF) staining, we assessed levels of intracellular ROS in mouse wounds and found ROS levels in wound epithelial tissue peaking at 3-7 days post-injury (Lam et al, 2011). This ROS up-regulation is likely secondary to the strong pro-inflammatory wound microenvironment, supported by TNF-α, which can up-regulate cellular ROS (Kim et al, 2010). ROS-induced oxidative damage can trigger both apoptotic and necrotic cell death through multiple mechanisms including DNA fragmentation (Higuchi, 2003) and mitochondria cytochrome c release (Kirkland & Franklin, 2001). While all previously mentioned forms of skin trauma involve external perturbation to the epidermis, this endogenous ROS-triggered necrotic cell death secondary to epidermal trauma may theoretically be the initializing cause of koebnerized psoriasis. Such an ROS-triggered skin trauma could arise in apparently unwounded psoriatic skin based on intracellular signaling dysregulation and could help explain the spontaneous occurrence of psoriatic lesions. However, key questions remain as to how this death-promoting ROS signal is regulated.

Interestingly, we have found that the wound expression of transforming growth factor-β (TGF-β) activated kinase 1 (TAK1), a downstream signaling player of TNF-α, coincides with the pattern of ROS production, with peak expression also at 3-7 days post-injury (Lam et al, 2011). Like PPARβ/δ, TAK1 activity is most likely affected by TNF-α induction in wounding. A known signal transducer in the innate immune response, TAK1 in keratinocytes may serve as both an epidermal and an immune factor responsible for the pathogenesis of psoriasis. Another separate study reported that mice with an epidermal specific deletion of TAK1 suffered massive keratinocyte death attributed to elevated ROS levels which subsequently resulted in severe psoriasiform-like skin inflammation (Omori et al, 2008). These findings strongly suggest that the dysregulation of epidermal homeostasis could trigger inflammation and initiate/sustain psoriasis of the skin and death by the 7th post-natal day (Omori et al, 2008). This precise role of TAK1 in psoriasis needs further elucidation.

To circumvent the limitations of *in vivo* models, we generated lentiviral-mediated TAK1 knockdown (TAK1 kd) human keratinocytes and cultured them in organotypic co-cultures (OTC). OTC consists of seeded keratinocytes cultured on a dermal-like fibroblast embedded collagen layer. The bottom fibroblast/collagen dermal layer contacts the OTC medium, while the top keratinocyte layer is exposed to the air. This mimics the *in vivo* positions of keratinocytes and fibroblasts in the intact skin, whereby nutrients are solely supplied to the dermis through the dermal blood circulation with nutrients reaching the epidermal layer only through diffusion (Stark et al, 2004). The advantage of using OTC models in the study of psoriasis is that it allows us to study the behavior and development of keratinocytes at the tissue level without the confounding influences of the immune system. This is especially useful in psoriasis research so that epidermal factors can be isolated and studied alone, without any immune related effects. Using this setup, we found that TAK1 kd OTC epidermis displayed significantly higher ROS levels with an increased incidence of keratinocyte cell death (Lam et al, 2011). This suggests that TAK1 kd keratinocytes succumbed to ROS-induced keratinocyte death even in normal tissue development. A unique feature of keratinocytes is that they are naturally subjected to anoikis-induced death after detachment from the basement membrane during skin homeostasis. Through flow cytometric analyses of DCF and annexin V staining, we found that either TNF-α induction or anoikis could enhance ROS production and subsequently induce cell death in TAK1 kd keratinocytes (Lam et al, 2011).

Importantly, we found that TAK1 protects healthy keratinocytes from ROS-mediated death by inducing epidermal expression of stem cell factor (SCF) through transcription factor c-Jun. SCF is secreted in an autocrine manner to bind and activate its c-Kit receptor on neighboring keratinocytes (Lam et al, 2011). The activation of c-Kit further leads to the activation of phosphoinositide-3 kinase (PI3K)/protein kinase B (PKB)α to initiate cell survival and anti-apoptotic effects (Lam et al, 2011). Incidentally, epidermal deletion of c-Jun in mice has been shown to produce a realistic psoriatic model (Zenz et al, 2005), further substantiating the role of TAK1 in psoriasis pathogenesis. As the skin is frequently exposed to oxidative stress from the external environment (Zhou et al, 2009), additional protection of keratinocytes is necessary to ensure that epidermal cells do not succumb to a fatal, massive cell death fate, similar to mice with epidermal specific TAK 1 deletion (Omori et al, 2008). Likewise, the constant microbial insults the skin confronts may lead to inflammatory responses like TNF-α induction, which will enhance ROS production in keratinocytes (Omori et al, 2008). Without the protective effects of TAK1, the epidermis may undergo necrotic degeneration especially during episodes of skin infection. We postulate that the pathogenesis of psoriasis may involve the suppression of TAK1 mediated protective mechanisms against ROS in psoriatic keratinocytes, leading to keratinocyte death and inflammation. The degree of this suppression may vary with the severity of psoriasis, with mild cases having lower levels of suppression compared to severe cases. Keratinocytes with strong suppression would undergo anoikis-triggered ROS elevation and necrotic cell death, triggering psoriasis even without any external wounding. Several clinically approved psoriasis drugs have been found to have a therapeutic effect on ROS-induced oxidative stress, further favoring the ROS aspect of psoriasis pathogenesis (Zhou et al, 2009). A primary example is dimethylfumarate (DMF), which is known to up-regulate glutathione (Ghashghaeinia et al, 2010) and the induction of NADPH:quinine oxidoreductase 1 (NQO1) (Begleiter et al, 2004), two antioxidative pathways in the cell. Vitamin D analogues also increase the production and activity of glucose-6-phosphate dehydrogenase (G6PD), which reduces ROS-induced oxidative stress (Bao et al, 2008).

4. Conclusion

Chronic psoriasis has a complex pathogenesis, involving both epidermal barrier and immune mediated dysfunction. While much of the recent advances have been in the area of the immunopathogenesis of psoriasis, the role of epidermal disruption as an initiating event and perpetuating cause of psoriasis certainly warrants further investigation and understanding. In this chapter, we have highlighted wound healing studies that support the key role of epidermal dysfunction in psoriasis and the koebner phenomenon. In particular, the role of nuclear receptor S100 proteins and the protective role of TAK1 against ROS induced stress were highlighted and discussed. It is noteworthy that the wound healing studies using novel organotypic skin cocultures have been crucial in further enhancing our understanding of the epidermal dysfunction in psoriasis and complementing existing *in vivo* models.

5. Acknowledgment

The work done in authors' laboratories is supported by National Medical Research Council (IRG10MAY017).

6. References

Allen, M.H., Ameen, H., Veal, C., Evans, J., Ramrakha-Jones, V.S., Marsland, A.M., Burden, A.D., Griffiths, C.E., Trembath, R.C. & Barker, J.N. (2005). The major psoriasis susceptibility locus PSORS1 is not a risk factor for late-onset psoriasis. *Journal of Investigative Dermatology,* Vol. 124, No. 1, pp. 103-106.

Baker, B.S., Ovigne, J.M., Powles, A.V., Corcoran, S. & Fry, L. (2003). Normal keratinocytes express Toll-like receptors (TLRs) 1, 2 and 5: modulation of TLR expression in chronic plaque psoriasis. *British Journal of Dermatology,* Vol. 148, No. 4, pp. 670-679.

Bao, B.Y., Ting, H.J., Hsu, J.W. & Lee, Y.F. (2008). Protective role of 1 alpha, 25-dihydroxyvitamin D3 against oxidative stress in nonmalignant human prostate epithelial cells. *International Journal of Cancer,* Vol. 122, No. 12, pp. 2699-2706.

Begleiter, A., Leith, M.K., Thliveris, J.A. & Digby, T. (2004). Dietary induction of NQO1 increases the antitumour activity of mitomycin C in human colon tumours in vivo. *British Journal of Cancer,* Vol. 91, No. 8, pp. 1624-1631.

Boehncke, W.H. (2005). The psoriasis SCID mouse model: a tool for drug discovery? *Ernst Schering Res Found Workshop,* pp. 213-234.

Boehncke, W.H. & Schön, M.P. (2007). Animal models of psoriasis. *Clinics in Dermatology,* Vol. 25, No. 6, pp. 596-605.

Boehncke, W.H., Sterry, W., Hainzl, A., Scheffold, W. & Kaufmann, R. (1994). Psoriasiform architecture of murine epidermis overlying human psoriatic dermis transplanted onto SCID mice. *Archives in Dermatological Research,* Vol. 286, No. 6, pp. 325-330.

Broome, A.M., Ryan, D. & Eckert, R.L. (2003). S100 protein subcellular localization during epidermal differentiation and psoriasis. *Journal of Histochemistry and Cytochemistry.,* Vol. 51, No. 5, pp. 675-685.

Castelijns, F.A., Gerritsen, M.J., van Erp, P.E. & van de Kerkhof, P.C. (2000). Cell-kinetic evidence for increased recruitment of cycling epidermal cells in psoriasis: the ratio of histone and Ki-67 antigen expression is constant. *Dermatology.,* Vol. 201, No. 2, pp. 105-110.

Chen, C.J., Kono, H., Golenbock, D., Reed, G., Akira, S. & Rock, K.L. (2007). Identification of a key pathway required for the sterile inflammatory response triggered by dying cells. *Nature Medicine,* Vol. 13, No. 7, pp. 851-856.

Christensen, T.E., Callis, K.P., Papenfuss, J., Hoffman, M.S., Hansen, C.B., Wong, B., Panko, J.M. & Krueger, G.G. (2006). Observations of psoriasis in the absence of therapeutic intervention identifies two unappreciated morphologic variants, thin-plaque and thick-plaque psoriasis, and their associated phenotypes. *Journal of Investigative Dermatology,* Vol. 126, No. 11, pp. 2397-2403.

Conrad, C., Boyman, O., Tonel, G., Tun-Kyi, A., Laggner, U., de Fougerolles, A., Kotelianski, V., Gardner, H. & Nestle, F.O. (2007). Alpha1beta1 integrin is crucial for accumulation of epidermal T cells and the development of psoriasis. *Nature Medicine,* Vol. 13, No. 7, pp. 836-842.

de Jong, E.M., van Vlijmen, I.M., van Erp, P.E., Ramaekers, F.C., Troyanovski, S.M. & van de Kerhof, P.C. (1991). Keratin 17: a useful marker in anti-psoriatic therapies. *Archives in Dermatological Research,* Vol. 283, No. 7, pp. 480-482.

Delves, P.J. & Roitt, I.M. (2000). The immune system. First of two parts. *New England Journal of Medicine,* Vol. 343, No. 1, pp. 37-49.

Delves, P.J. & Roitt, I.M. (2000). The immune system. Second of two parts. *New England Journal of Medicine,* Vol. 343, No. 2, pp. 108-117.

Eedy, D.J., Burrows, D., Bridges, J.M. & Jones, F.G. (1990). Clearance of severe psoriasis after allogenic bone marrow transplantation. *British Medical Journal,* Vol. 300, No. 6729, pp. 908.

Farber, E.M., Roth, R.J., Aschheim, E., Eddy, D.D. & Epinette, W.W. (1965). Role of Trauma in Isomorphic Response in Psoriasis. *Archives in Dermatology,* Vol. 91, pp. 246-251.

Friedmann, P.S., Cooper, H.L. & Healy, E. (2005). Peroxisome proliferator-activated receptors and their relevance to dermatology. *Acta Dermato-Venereologica,* Vol. 85, No. 3, pp. 194-202.

Fürstenberger, G., Berry, D.L., Sorg, B. & Marks, F. (1981). Skin tumor promotion by phorbol esters is a two-stage process. *Proceedings of the National Academy of Sciences of the United States of America,* Vol. 78, No. 12, pp. 7722-7726.

Garcia, S., Dadaglio, G. & Gougeon, M.L. (1997). Limits of the human-PBL-SCID mice model: severe restriction of the V beta T-cell repertoire of engrafted human T cells. *Blood,* Vol. 89, No. 1, pp. 329-336.

Gates, A.H. & Karasek, M. (1965). Hereditary Absence of Sebaceous Glands in the Mouse. *Science,* Vol. 148, No. 3676, pp. 1471-1473.

Ghashghaeinia, M., Bobbala, D., Wieder, T., Koka, S., Brück, J., Fehrenbacher, B., Rocken, M., Schaller, M., Lang, F. & Ghoreschi, K. (2010). Targeting glutathione by dimethylfumarate protects against experimental malaria by enhancing erythrocyte cell membrane scrambling. *American Journal of Physiology. Cell Physiology,* Vol. 299, No. 4, pp. C791-C804.

Gronemeyer, H., Gustafsson, J.Å. & Laudet, V. (2004). Principles for modulation of the nuclear receptor superfamily. *Nature Reviews Drug Discovery,* Vol. 3, No. 11, pp. 1474-1776

Gudjonsson, J.E., Johnston, A., Dyson, M., Valdimarsson, H. & Elder, J.T. (2007). Mouse models of psoriasis. *Journal of Investigative Dermatology,* Vol. 127, No. 6, pp. 1292-1308.

Guerrero-Aspizua, S., García, M., Murillas, R., Retamosa, L., Illera, N., Duarte, B., Holquín, A., Puig, S., Hernández, M.I., Meana, A., Jorcano, J.L., Larcher, F., Carretero, M. & Del Río, M. (2010). Development of a bioengineered skin-humanized mouse model for psoriasis: dissecting epidermal-lymphocyte interacting pathways. *American Journal of Pathology,* Vol. 177, No. 6, pp. 3112-3124.

Higuchi, Y. (2003). Chromosomal DNA fragmentation in apoptosis and necrosis induced by oxidative stress. *Biochemical Pharmacology,* Vol. 66, No. 8, pp. 1527-1535.

HogenEsch, H., Gijbels, M.J.J. & Zurcher C. (1994). The chronic proliferative dermatitis (cpd) mutation chromosome?, *In: Handbook of Mouse Mutations with Skin, Hair Abnormalities. Animal Models, Biomedical Tools.,* Sundberg, J.P. , pp. 217-220. CRC Press, Boca Raton.

Hueber, A.J. & McInnes, I.B. (2007). Immune regulation in psoriasis and psoriatic arthritis--recent developments. *Immunology Letters.,* Vol. 114, No. 2, pp. 59-65.

Kannan-Thulasiraman, P., Seachrist, D.D., Mahabeleshwar, G.H., Jain, M.K. & Noy, N. (2010). Fatty acid-binding protein 5 and PPARbeta/delta are critical mediators of epidermal growth factor receptor-induced carcinoma cell growth. *Journal of Biological Chemistry,* Vol. 285, No. 25, pp. 19106-19115.

Kim, J.J., Lee, S.B., Park, J.K. & Yoo, Y.D. (2010). TNF-alpha-induced ROS production triggering apoptosis is directly linked to Romo1 and Bcl-X(L). *Cell Death and Differentiation,* Vol. 17, No. 9, pp. 1420-1434.

Kirkland, R.A. & Franklin, J.L. (2001). Evidence for redox regulation of cytochrome C release during programmed neuronal death: antioxidant effects of protein synthesis and caspase inhibition. *Journal of Neuroscience.,* Vol. 21, No. 6, pp. 1949-1963.

Krueger, G.G., Manning, D.D., Malouf, J. & Ogden, B. (1975). Long-term maintenance of psoriatic human skin on congenitally athymic (nude) mice. *Journal of Investigative Dermatology,* Vol. 64, No. 5, pp. 307-312.

Lam, C.R., Tan, M.J., Tan, S.H, Tang, M.B, Cheung, P.C. & Tan, N.S. (2011). TAK1 regulates SCF expression to modulate PKBα activity that protects keratinocytes from ROS-induced apoptosis. *Cell Death and Differentiation,* Vol. 18, No. 7, pp. 1120-1129.

Leung, D.Y., Travers, J.B., Giorno, R., Norris, D.A., Skinner, R., Aelion, J., Kazemi, L.V., Kim, M.H., Trumble, A.E. & Kotb, M. (1995). Evidence for a streptococcal superantigen-driven process in acute guttate psoriasis. *Journal of Clinical Investigation,* Vol. 96, No. 5, pp. 2106-2112.

Lomholt, G. (1964). Prevalence of Skin Diseases in a Population; A Census Study from the Faroe Islands. *Danish Medical Bulletin,* Vol. 11, pp. 1-7.

Mempel, M., Voelcker, V., Köllisch, G., Plank, C., Rad, R., Gerhard, M., Schnopp, C., Fraunberger, P., Walli, A.K., Ring, J., Abeck, D. & Ollert, M. (2003). Toll-like receptor expression in human keratinocytes: nuclear factor kappaB controlled gene activation by Staphylococcus aureus is toll-like receptor 2 but not toll-like receptor 4 or platelet activating factor receptor dependent. *Journal of Investigative Dermatology,* Vol. 121, No. 6, pp. 1389-1396.

Miller, R.A. (1982). The Koebner phenomenon. *International Journal of Dermatology,* Vol. 21, No. 4, pp. 192-197.

Mommers, J.M., van Rosum, M.M., van Erp, P.E. & van De Kerkhof, P.C. (2000). Changes in keratin 6 and keratin 10 (co--)expression in lesional and symptomless skin of spreading psoriasis. *Dermatology,* Vol. 201, No. 1, pp. 15-20.

Morita, K., Hogan, M.E., Nanney, L.B., King, L.E.Jr, Manabe, M., Sun, T.T & Sundberg, J.P. (1995). Cutaneous ultrastructural features of the flaky skin (fsn) mouse mutation. *J Dermatol.,* Vol. 22, No. 6, pp. 385-395.

Nestle, F.O., Di Meglio, P., Qin, J.Z. & Nickoloff, B.J. (2009). Skin immune sentinels in health and disease. *Nature Reviews. Immunology,* Vol. 9, No. 10, pp. 679-691.

Nickoloff, B.J., Kunkel, S.L., Burdick, M. & Strieter, R.M. (1995). Severe combined immunodeficiency mouse and human psoriatic skin chimeras. Validation of a new animal model. *American Journal of Pathology,* Vol. 146, No. 3, pp. 580-588.

Nickoloff, B.J. & Turka, L.A. (1994). Immunological functions of non-professional antigen-presenting cells: new insights from studies of T-cell interactions with keratinocytes. *Immunology Today,* Vol. 15, No. 10, pp. 464-469.

Nickoloff, B.J., Bonish, B.K., Marble, D.J., Schriedel, K.A., DiPietro, L.A., Gordon, K.B. & Lingen, M.W. (2006). Lessons Learned from Psoriatic Plaques Concerning Mechanisms of Tissue Repair, Remodeling, and Inflammation. *Journal of Investigative Dermatology Symposium Proceedings,* Vol. 11, No. 1, pp. 16-29.

Omori, E., Morioka, S., Matsumoto, K. & Ninomiya-Tsuji, J. (2008). TAK1 regulates reactive oxygen species and cell death in keratinocytes, which is essential for skin integrity. *Journal of Biological Chemistry,* Vol. 283, No. 38, pp. 26161-26168.

Pedace, F.J., Muller, S.A. & Winkelmann, R.K. (1969). The biology of psoriasis. An experimental study of the Koebner phenomenon. *Acta Dermato-Venereologica,* Vol. 49, No. 4, pp. 390-400.

Pivarcsi, A., Kemény, L. & Dobozy, A. (2004). Innate immune functions of the keratinocytes. A review. *Acta Microbiologica et Immunologica Hungarica.,* Vol. 51, No. 3, pp. 303-310.

Prinz, J., Braun-Falco, O., Meurer, M., Daddona, P., Reiter, C., Rieber, P. & Riethmüller, G. (1991). Chimaeric CD4 monoclonal antibody in treatment of generalised pustular psoriasis. *Lancet,* Vol. 338, No. 8762, pp. 320-321.

Redfern, C.P. & Todd, C. (1992). Retinoic acid receptor expression in human skin keratinocytes and dermal fibroblasts in vitro. *Journal of Cell Science,* Vol. 102, No. Pt1, pp. 113-121.

Robinson-Rechavi, M., Escriva Garcia, H. & Laudet, V. (2003). The nuclear receptor superfamily. *Journal of Cell Science,* Vol. 116, No. Pt 4, pp. 585-586.

Roder, J. & Duwe, A. (1979). The beige mutation in the mouse selectively impairs natural killer cell function. *Nature,* Vol. 278, No. 5703, pp. 451-453.

Romanowska, M., Reilly, L., Palmer, C.N., Gustafsson, M.C. & Foerster, J. (2010). Activation of PPARbeta/delta causes a psoriasis-like skin disease in vivo. *PLoS One.*, Vol. 5, No. 3, pp. e9701.

Roopenian, D.C. & Anderson, P.S. (1988). Adoptive immunity in immune-deficient scid/scid mice. I. Differential requirements of naive and primed lymphocytes for CD4+ T cells during rejection of minor histocompatibility antigen-disparate skin grafts. *Transplantation,* Vol. 46, No. 6, pp. 899-904.

Ruse, M., Broome, A.M. & Eckert, R.L. (2003). S100A7 (psoriasin) interacts with epidermal fatty acid binding protein and localizes in focal adhesion-like structures in cultured keratinocytes. *Journal of Investigative Dermatology,* Vol. 121, No. 1, pp. 132-141.

Sagi, L. & Trau, H. (2011). The Koebner phenomenon. *Clinics in Dermatology,* Vol. 29, No. 2, pp. 231-236.

Schön, M.P. (1999). Animal models of psoriasis - what can we learn from them? *Journal of Investigative Dermatology,* Vol. 112, No. 4, pp. 405-410.

Schön, M.P. (2008). Animal models of psoriasis: a critical appraisal. *Experimental Dermatology,* Vol. 17, No. 8, pp. 703-712.

Schön, M.P. & Boehncke, W.H. (2005). Psoriasis. *New England Journal of Medicine,* Vol. 352, No. 18, pp. 1899-1912.

Schön, M.P., Detmar, M. & Parker, C.M. (1997). Murine psoriasis-like disorder induced by naive CD4+ T cells. *Nature Medicine,* Vol. 3, No. 2, pp. 183-188.

Semprini, S., Capon, F., Tacconelli, A., Giardina, E., Orecchia, A., Mingarelli, R. Gobello, T., Zambruno, G., Botta, A., Fabrizi, G. & Novelli, G. (2002). Evidence for differential S100 gene over-expression in psoriatic patients from genetically heterogeneous pedigrees. *Human Genetics,* Vol. 111, No. 4-5, pp. 310-313.

Shultz, L.D., Schweitzer, P.A., Christianson, S.W., Gott, B., Schweitzer, I.B., Tennent, B., McKenna, S., Mobraaten, L., Rajan, T.V. & Greiner, D.L. (1995). Multiple defects in innate and adaptive immunologic function in NOD/LtSz0scid mice. *Journal of Immunology,* Vol. 154, No. 1, pp. 180-191.

Sladek, F.M. (2003). Nuclear receptors as drug targets: new developments in coregulators, orphan receptors and major therapeutic areas. *Expert Opinion on Therapeutic Targets,* Vol. 7, No. 5, pp. 679-684.

Snowden, J.A. & Heaton, D.C. (1997). Development of psoriasis after syngeneic bone marrow transplant from psoriatic donor: further evidence for adoptive autoimmunity. *British Journal of Dermatology,* Vol. 137, No. 1, pp. 130-132.

Stadelmann, W.K., Digenis, A.G. & Tobin, G.R. (1998). Physiology and healing dynamics of chronic cutaneous wounds. *American Journal of Surgery,* Vol. 176, No. 2A Suppl, pp. 26S-38S.

Stark, H.J., Szabowski, A., Fusenig, N.E. & Maas-Szabowski, N. (2004). Organotypic cocultures as skin equivalents: A complex and sophisticated in vitro system. *Biological Procedures Online,* Vol. 6, pp. 55-60.

Streilein, J.W. (1983). Skin-associated lymphoid tissues (SALT): origins and functions. *Journal of Investigative Dermatology,*Vol. 80, pp. 12-16.

Streilein, J.W. (1989). Skin-associated lymphoid tissue. *Immunology Series,* Vol. 46, pp. 73-96.

Sundberg, J.P, Boggess, D., Shultz, L.D. & Dunstan, R.W. (1994). The Flaky Skin (fsn) mutation chromosome?, *In: Handbook of Mouse Mutatins with Skin, Hair*

Abnormalities. Animal Models, Biomedical Tools, Sundberg, J.D., pp. 253-268. CRC Press, Boca Raton.

Tan, N.S., Michalik, L., Desvergne, B. & Wahli, W. (2003). Peroxisome proliferator-activated receptor (PPAR)-beta as a target for wound healing drugs: what is possible? *American Journal of Clinical Dermatology,* Vol. 4, No. 8, pp. 523-530.

Tan, N.S., Michalik, L., Desvergne, B. & Wahli, W. (2004). Peroxisome proliferator-activated receptor-beta as a target for wound healing drugs. *Expert Opinion on Therapeutic Targets.,* Vol. 8, No. 1, pp. 39-48.

Tan, N.S., Michalik, L., Di-Poï, N., Desvergne, B. & Wahli, W. (2004). Critical roles of the nuclear receptor PPARbeta (peroxisome-proliferator-activated receptor beta) in skin wound healing. *Biochemical Society Transaction,* Vol. 32, No. Pt 1, pp. 97-102.

Tan, N.S., Michalik, L., Noy, N., Yasmin, R., Pacot, C., Heim, M. Fluhmann, B., Desvergne, B. & Wahli, W. (2001). Critical roles of PPAR beta/delta in keratinocyte response to inflammation. *Genes & Development,* Vol. 15, No. 24, pp. 3263-3277.

Valdimarsson, H., Thorleifsdottir, R.H., Sigurdardottir, S.L., Gudjonsson, J.E. & Johnston, A. (2009). Psoriasis--as an autoimmune disease caused by molecular mimicry. *Trends in Immunology,* Vol. 30, No. 10, pp. 494-501.

Wang, Y.N. & Chang, W.C. (2003). Induction of disease-associated keratin 16 gene expression by epidermal growth factor is regulated through cooperation of transcription factors Sp1 and c-Jun. *Journal of Biological Chemistry,* Vol. 278, No. 46, pp. 45848-45857.

Weinshenker, B.G., Bass, B.H., Ebers, G.C. & Rice, G.P. (1989). Remission of psoriatic lesions with muromonab-CD3 (orthoclone OKT3) treatment. *Journal of American Academy of Dermatology,* Vol. 20, No. 6, pp. 1132-1133.

Weiss, G., Shemer, A. & Trau, H. (2002). The Koebner phenomenon: review of the literature. *Journal of the European Academy of Dermatology and Venereology.,* Vol. 16, No. 3, pp. 241-248.

Wilkinson, D.I. & Karasek, M.A. (1966). Skin lipids of a normal and mutant (asebic) mouse strain. *Journal of Investigative Dermatology,* Vol. 47, No. 5, pp. 449-455.

Wolf, R., Mascia, F., Dharamsi, A., Howard, O.M., Cataisson, C., Bliskovski, V., Winston, J., Feigenbaum, L., Lichti, U., Ruzicka, T., Chavakis, T. & Yuspa, S.H. (2010). Gene from a psoriasis susceptibility locus primes the skin for inflammation. *Science Translational Medicine,* Vol. 2, No. 61, pp. 61-90.

Young, J.C. & Hartl, F.U. (2002). Chaperones and transcriptional regulation by nuclear receptors. *Nature Structural Biology,* Vol. 9, No. 9, pp. 640-642.

Zachariae, H., Zachariae, R., Blomqvist, K., Davidsson, S., Molin, L., Mørk, C. & Sigurgeirsson, B. (2002). Quality of life and prevalence of arthritis reported by 5,795 members of the Nordic Psoriasis Associations. Data from the Nordic Quality of Life Study. *Acta Dermato-Venereologica,* Vol. 82, No. 2, pp. 108-113.

Zenz, R., Eferl, R., Kenner, L., Florin, L., Hummerich, L., Mehic, D., Scheuch, H., Angel, P., Tschachler, E. & Wagner, E.F. (2005). Psoriasis-like skin disease and arthritis caused by inducible epidermal deletion of Jun proteins. *Nature,* Vol. 437, No. 7057, pp. 369-375.

Zhou, Q., Mrowietz, U. & Rostami-Yazdi, M. (2009). Oxidative stress in the pathogenesis of psoriasis. *Free Radical Biology & Medicine.,* Vol. 47, No. 7, pp. 891-905.

Zouboulis, C.C. (2009). The skin as an endocrine organ. *Dermato-endocrinology*, Vol. 1, No. 5, pp. 250-252.

4

Psoriatic Skin Models: A Need for the Pharmaceutical Industry

Jessica Jean, Martha Estrella Garcia-Pérez and Roxane Pouliot
Centre LOEX de l'Université Laval, Génie Tissulaire et Régénération : LOEX - Centre de Recherche FRSQ du Centre Hospitalier Affilié Universitaire de Québec
Faculté de Pharmacie, Université Laval
Canada

1. Introduction

1.1 Skin

Skin is composed of three layers: epidermis, dermis and hypodermis (Sugihara *et al.*, 1991). Epidermis is divided into five layers namely, *stratum basale, spinosum, granulosum, lucidum,* and *corneum* (Bragulla & Homberger, 2009, Nagarajan *et al.*, 2009). The differentiation process implies that keratinocytes are transformed through the different cell layers to reach their complete maturation in the *stratum corneum* (Harding, 2004). In this process, various proliferation and differentiation markers are expressed in a well-orchestrated sequence of events (Fig. 1). When the differentiation process is negatively affected, skin pathologies such as psoriasis can appear (Rashmi *et al.*, 2009, Karlsson *et al.*, 2004).

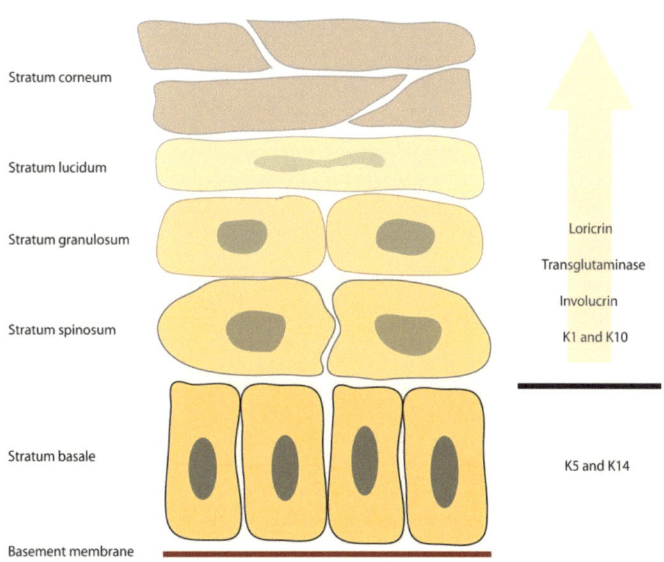

Fig. 1. Differentiation process

1.2 Psoriasis

1.2.1 Prevalence

Psoriasis is a severe skin disease affecting men and women worldwide. It affects about 2 % of the world population (Baker *et al.*, 2008, Wippel-Slupetzky & Stingl, 2009). Previous studies have demonstrated that psoriasis prevalence varies as a result of two factors: (1) geographical localization and (2) ethnic group. Firstly, psoriasis shows a significant geographical variability with the lowest incidence seen at the equator and increasing frequency towards the poles (Kormeili *et al.*, 2004, Krueger & Bowcock, 2005, Lowes *et al.*, 2007) (Fig. 2). Secondly, even if psoriasis is universal, it does not affect all ethnic groups in a similar way. In fact, various studies have demonstrated that psoriasis prevalence can be modified in function of ethnic factors. They established that, in the United States, the prevalence was of 0.5 to 0.7 % in African population compared with 1.4 to 4.6 % for Caucasian population (Schon & Boehncke, 2005). Furthermore, some populations, such as Samoan population (Polynesia), are exempt from psoriasis, whereas other ethnic groups show a high percentage of affected peoples such as observed in Kazach'ye population (12.0 %).

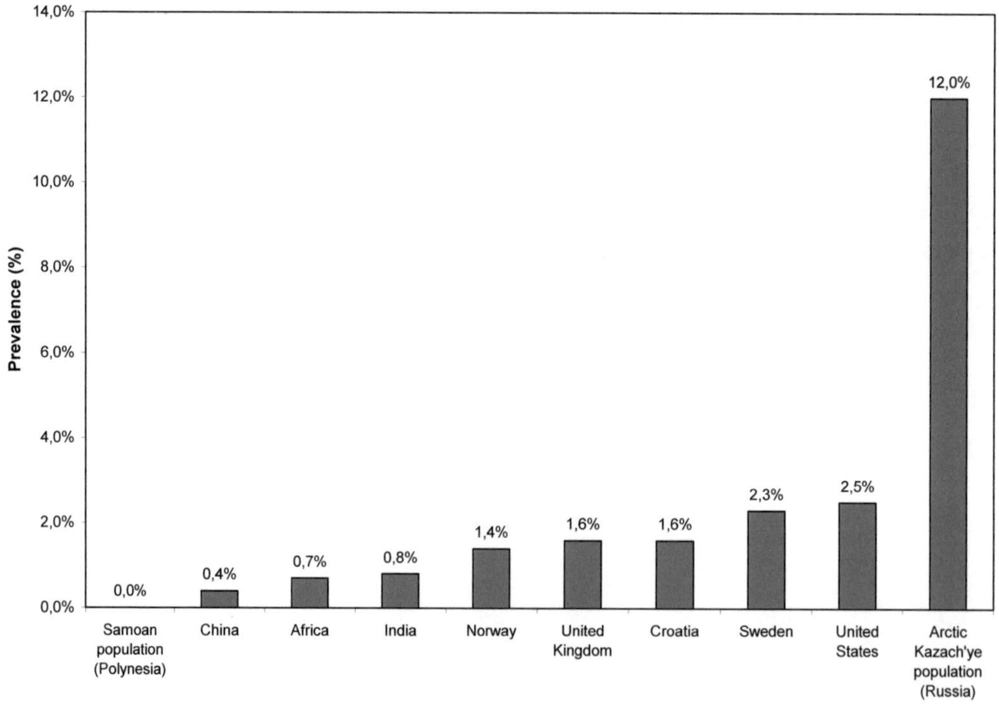

Fig. 2. Worldwide psoriasis prevalence

Psoriasis prevalence shows a significant geographical variability. A lower incidence can be observed at the equator while the frequency increases towards the poles. Studies suggest that the incidence may be related with the time and/or the intensity exposure to the ultraviolet wavelengths of sunlight (Menter & Stoff, 2010).

1.2.2 Physiopathology

Psoriatic skin is characterized by remarkable hyperplasia of the epidermis (acanthosis), loss of the granular layer, increased vascularization in the dermis, and thickening of the cornified layer (hyperkeratosis). Additionally, the incomplete keratinocyte differentiation (parakeratosis) and the leukocyte infiltration in skin are hallmarks of this disease (Tonel & Conrad, 2009).

So far, the pathogenesis of psoriasis constitutes a matter of scientific debate. Controversy exists about whether this disease starts as a primary abnormality of altered keratinocytes or as a result of an altered immune response against an undetermined antigen. According to the first hypothesis, epidermal alterations could be sufficient for the initiation of psoriasis in genetically predisposed individuals. Moreover, it has been demonstrated that the abrogation of JunB/activator protein (AP-1) in epidermal mouse keratinocytes leads to a phenotype that notably mimics psoriasis with inflammation, disturbances in epidermal differentiation and dermal changes, including the expression of chemokines/cytokines, which are able to recruit neutrophils and macrophages in the epidermis (Zenz *et al.*, 2005).

According to the second hypothesis, psoriasis could be a result of an altered immune response to an undetermined antigen. However, it is still not clear where the psoriatic immune response begins. This theory arises from evidences obtained using xenograft psoriatic models, where uninvolved psoriatic skin is transformed into a psoriatic lesion under the action of skin resident cells present in the graft (Boyman *et al.*, 2004, Conrad *et al.*, 2007). The failure to generate a psoriatic lesion after the administration of an anti-CD3 mAb, demonstrated that T cells and not keratinocytes alone were necessary to generate the psoriatic phenotype (Boyman *et al.*, 2004, Conrad *et al.*, 2007). Thus, psoriatic lesions could be initiated by an initial trigger which activates dendritic cells (DCs) and induces their migration to skin-draining lymph nodes. DCs thus prime antigen-specific T cells to differentiate into effector T cells bearing the skin addressing CLA (Cutaneous Lymphocyte Antigen). Activated T cells then traffic to the skin, where they induce together with DCs and other cells, the release pro-inflammatory cytokines, which in turn stimulate keratinocytes to synthesize other cytokines, chemokines and pro-inflammatory molecules, thereby causing the typical epidermal changes observed in psoriasis (Bowcock & Krueger, 2005). Furthermore, migration of T cells in the epidermis seems to be connected with the disturbances of desmosome connection between keratinocytes, thereby contributing to the disruption of epidermal integrity (Krueger, 2002). That could be interpreted by keratinocytes as an injury with a further wound repair response, and the release of cytokines leading to a regenerative epidermal growth.

Psoriasis is considered to be an immune-mediated disease characterized by a predominantly Th1-type cytokine profile in lesional skin with elevated levels of interferon-γ (INF-γ), tumour necrosis factor-alpha (TNF-α), IL-12, and IL-18, among others. Thus, the secretion of the INF-α from DCs and the production of TNF-α by cells of the innate and adaptive immune system are considered to be one of the earliest events leading to psoriasis (Nestle *et al.*, 2005). Cytokines released by T cells, DCs, macrophages and neutrophils such as IL-1, IL-6 and INF-γ have been shown to directly induce epidermal hyperplasia (Krueger, 2002). Additionally, other inflammatory cytokines such as IL-23, have gained attention for their role in psoriasis pathogenesis. IL-23 leads to the production of IL-17 and IL-22, contributing to the enhancement and maintenance of inflammation as well as epidermal proliferation

(Chan *et al.*, 2006, Wolk *et al.*, 2004). Intradermal injection of this IL-23 contributes to the development of epidermal acanthosis in mice (Chan *et al.*, 2006, Zheng *et al.*, 2007). Other evidence supporting its role in psoriasis includes the clinical efficacy of anti-p40 monoclonal antibody (Krueger *et al.*, 2007).

Overall, psoriasis involves a complex interplay between various cells of the immune system and skin, including dendritic cells, T cells, neutrophils, and keratinocytes, which leads to the release of numerous cytokines and chemokines that signal keratinocytes to hyperproliferate and undergo abnormal differentiation (Gottlieb *et al.*, 2003).

1.2.3 Treatment satisfaction: Results of worldwide surveys

Previous worldwide surveys of psoriasis affected individuals have revealed widespread dissatisfaction with available treatments, as well as frustration with current management strategies, thereby demonstrating the need for more appropriate forms of therapy (Nijsten *et al.*, 2005, Stern *et al.*, 2004) and the importance for an improved access for patients to health care services (Klotz *et al.*, 2005, Simpson *et al.*, 2006).

In 1998, a self-administered questionnaire was mailed to the entire membership of the National Psoriasis Foundation in the United States (n=40,350) and followed by a telephone survey of patients with severe psoriasis. Of the 40,350 questionnaires mailed out, a response rate of 43 % was realized. Although 48 % of responders were very or fairly satisfied with psoriasis treatments, a nearly similar number of patients (49 %) reported that they were only somewhat or not at all satisfied (Krueger *et al.*, 2001). Additionally, 46 % of patients responded that their treatment functioned "just somewhat well" or "not well at all" and a high degree of dissatisfaction with the capacity of treatments to control the symptoms was reported. In the case of patients with severe disease, 78 % reported that their treatment did not function well enough, thereby leading them to a frustration with their medications (Krueger *et al.*, 2001). In fact, 32 % of these patients replied that the treatment they received was not aggressive enough. As a consequence, many of the responders (43 %) had tried over-the-counter medications or alternative therapies such as herbs, relaxation or acupuncture in order to control their psoriasis (Krueger *et al.*, 2001). Another survey, conducted with 77 psoriatic patients in Israel also demonstrated that 62 % of patients used complementary and alternative medicines including herbal medicines and nutritional treatments followed by homeopathy and traditional Chinese medicine. The main reasons for complementary and alternative medicines were: the less toxic indications, disappointment with conventional treatments and stress reduction (Ben-Arye *et al.*, 2003).

In order to assess the satisfaction of psoriatic patients with four systemic medications (methotrexate, PUVA-therapy, cyclosporin and acitretin), 1,197 patients were interviewed in the United States between 2001 and 2002 (Nijsten *et al.*, 2005). Of these patients, only 26 % (n=311) indicated the use of these systemic treatments for their psoriasis. Less than 40 % of these patients were very satisfied with their treatment, while a comparable proportion indicated being dissatisfied. Low levels of satisfaction were related with treatment resistance, toxicity, convenience, costs and unrealistic patients' expectations (Nijsten *et al.*, 2005). Patients were more satisfied with methotrexate and PUVA-therapy than with acitretin and cyclosporine. Furthermore, PUVA-therapy had the highest satisfaction rate and cyclosporine the lowest compared with other therapies.

In 2002, the European Federation of Psoriasis Patient Associations (EUROPSO) carried out a Europe-wide survey investigating quality of life of psoriatic patients, as well as their satisfaction with available treatments (Dubertret *et al.*, 2006). Self-administered questionnaires were thus mailed to members of psoriasis associations in Germany, Belgium, Finland, France, Czech Republic, Italy and Netherlands. From 18,386 responders, 17,990 had psoriasis. At the time of the survey, 32 % of all participants used a topical treatment, 17 % a systemic treatment and 13 % phototherapy treatment. Although many patients were satisfied with the information and care offered by their physicians (40 % highly satisfied), available treatment modalities were less satisfactory, with over 70 % reporting low or moderate satisfaction. Higher satisfaction (score of 8–10) was observed for treatments with methotrexate (30 %), cyclosporin (28 %) and fumarates (26 %) followed by PUVA-therapy (38 %). Lower satisfaction (score of 1–4) was observed for tazarotene (42 %) and etretinate (38 %). Responders (50 %) reported that the time consumed during therapies was the most troublesome aspect, followed by ineffectiveness of treatments (32 %). Patients with severe psoriasis reported side effects as a problem (31 %), whereas only 23 % of patients with mild psoriasis considered this aspect (Dubertret *et al.*, 2006). Furthermore, another survey conducted in 2003 with 301 psoriatic patients in Europe, also demonstrated that 42 % of patients were dissatisfied with their treatment (Christophers *et al.*, 2006). Lack of satisfaction was lower among the patients receiving treatment with more than one agent, and in those who had more frequent psoriasis relapses, demonstrating the high need for safe and effective therapies for management of this disease (Christophers *et al.*, 2006).

Patients diagnosed with psoriasis in the United States between 2006 and 2007 were contacted to complete an online survey ("Psoriasis Patient Study Wave 1") related to their psoriasis diagnosis, treatment and treatment satisfaction (total of patients=1,006). Of those who had ever taken a prescription (topical, phototherapy, systemic oral or biologics, n=557), 31.8 % (n=177) reported that their current treatment was not able to satisfactorily clear their psoriasis. When patients were separated by treatment, 20.8 % (n=33) of those using biologics, 31.1 % (n=33) of those using systemic oral, 46.4 % (n=13) of those using phototherapy, and 34.2 % (n=163) of those using topical treatments reported that their current treatment was not able to satisfactorily clear their psoriasis. Patients with severe disease were less satisfied than those with mild and moderate disease (47.9 % *vs.* 32.9 % *vs.* 27.6 % respectively) (DiBonaventura *et al.*, 2010).

An online Canadian survey conducted in December 2007 with 514 patients diagnosed with moderate, severe and very severe plaque psoriasis demonstrated that awareness of available treatment options ranged from 98 % for topical treatments to 75 % for phototherapies, 49 % for oral treatments and 35 % for injectable medications. Satisfaction with treatments were generally low, and only 24 % of patients reported to be "very satisfied" with their current therapy. Satisfaction decreased with the increase of psoriasis severity, 39 % of patients with mild/very mild psoriasis reported to be "very satisfied", compared with 16 % of those diagnosed with moderate/severe/very severe psoriasis (Wasel *et al.*, 2009). In this survey, dissatisfaction with the efficacy of antipsoriatic treatment was highlighted by the majority of patients (68 %) reporting that "No medication works really well for my psoriasis". Additionally, patients with severe psoriasis more frequently complained that "medication was very ineffective for my psoriasis" compared to those less affected (49 %, 69 % and 77 % for respondents with 0–2 %, > 3%, and > 10% of body surface area (BSA) involvement, respectively) (Wasel *et al.*, 2009). Additionally, most affected patients were concerned about side effects from medication to treat psoriasis (54 %, 64 % and 69 % of psoriatic patients with 0-2 %, > 3% and > 10% BSA involvement, respectively). Patients also manifested that the reasons for treatment discontinuation were as following: lack of efficacy (60 %), inconvenience (23 %) and improvement of symptoms (22 %), side effects (20 %), cost (14 %) and doctor's advice (14 %) (Poulin *et al.*, 2010).

Overall, results of worldwide surveys demonstrate that a substantial proportion of psoriatic patients are highly dissatisfied with current therapies, particularly those with greater psoriasis severity. A perceived lack of efficacy of available treatments suggests the importance of the development of more relevant treatments, in order to allow the establishment of more individualized therapies.

2. Challenges for antipsoriatic drug development

The most significant challenge for antipsoriatic drug development is to provide safe and effective long-term management of this disease. In general, a conventional vision of this process starts with the study of disease in relevant model systems, in order to determine cellular and molecular mechanisms involved in pathogenesis. Afterwards, new therapeutic approaches are developed in these models before clinical trials in humans (Guttman-Yassky & Krueger, 2007). The comprehension that psoriasis is an immune-mediated disease, which involves a complex interplay of T cells, natural killer cells, dendritic cells, macrophages and other leukocytes, has led to the development of new biological treatments. The positive results obtained with these agents have expanded our understanding on psoriasis pathogenesis. However, many questions remain regarding psoriasis pathogenesis, and other medications should be developed to offer individualized treatments able to improve patient's quality of life. Some of the challenges for this field include the improvement of efficacy and safety of new drugs, the solution of problems related to formulation/administration/costs of new agents, and the development of more relevant psoriatic skin models.

2.1 Efficacy

Many psoriatic patients are unresponsive to current therapies or have aggressive disease that is not addressed by current approaches. The determination of relevant biomarkers directly related to psoriasis pathogenesis to be targeted with effective treatments could allow quantitative assessment of treatment response (Rashmi *et al.*, 2009).

2.2 Safety

The challenge of improving the safety of new antipsoriatic drugs is a very important aspect for long-term therapies, and can be overcome through the understanding of the toxicity mechanisms of new agents at early stages of drug development. Unfortunately, this is not always feasible during the drug development process, and the "safety question" should respond to what constitutes an acceptable risk. Thus, it is important to carefully analyse the risk/benefit rate of new antipsoriatic agents, mainly in the case of severe disease.

2.3 Practical issues

In the case of drugs approved for clinical use, their specific immunogenicity, costs, patient access and inconveniences for administration should be considerate. Other challenges include the optimization of the new drug delivery to give maximum effects to its intended biological targets.

2.4 Development of more relevant psoriatic skin models

Maybe the most important challenge for antipsoriatic drug development is the inexistence of validated *in vivo* and *in vitro* skin models. Psoriasis is a complex disease in which interactions with 30 or more upregulated cytokines and chemokines implies the formation of interactive circuits that are not completely reproduced by *in vivo* and *in vitro* models. In the case of animal models, which are very important in pre-clinic stages of drug development, no one can fully mimic the genomic signature of this disease in which expression than more of 1,300 genes is altered (Guttman-Yassky & Krueger, 2007). Other problems are related to the fact that murine skin is different from human skin, and often the immune infiltrates are less intense and contain different mixtures of leucocytes compared with psoriatic plaques (Gudjonsson *et al.*, 2007). Furthermore, animal models of epidermal hyperplasia are not selective enough, being also used for the study of other diseases, such as atopic dermatitis, even when different inflammatory genes are implied in these two diseases. Thus, it is not a surprise that targeted therapies such as the antibody efalizumab, are effective in both diseases (Farshidi & Sadeghi, 2006). The lack of representative *in vivo* and *in vitro* skin models could also be related to failures of clinical trials at late stages. Hence, some psoriatic models are of questionable value for the development of selective antipsoriatic treatments. A detailed explanation of these models will be provided in subsequent sections.

3. *In vivo* and *in vitro* psoriatic skin models

3.1 *In vivo* models

3.1.1 Spontaneous mutations

Psoriasis is a typical human skin disease. Even if spontaneous mutation models do not exhibit every features found in psoriasis, various pathology-like characteristics can be observed, including hyperkeratosis and scaly formation (Mizutani *et al.*, 2003). Hundred of these spontaneous mutation models have been described in the literature (Sundberg *et al.*, 1990), but no one shows all the characteristics of psoriasis. However, these models can be really practical for studying individual characteristics such as hyperkeratosis (Schon, 2008). A comparison between the characteristics observed in the three major models of spontaneous mutations is presented in table 1.

3.1.2 Xenotransplantation

Animal models based on transgenic technology have been used extensively to study the pathogenesis of various skin diseases, including psoriasis (Raychaudhuri *et al.*, 2001, Jean & Pouliot, 2010). Xenotransplantation approach consists of grafting a piece of *in vivo* psoriatic skin (or an *in vitro* psoriatic substitute) on a genetically modified mouse. Currently, three major models are used: athymic nude mice (Fraki *et al.*, 1983), severe combined immunodeficient mice (SCID) (Raychaudhuri *et al.*, 2001), and spontaneous AGR129 model (Boyman *et al.*, 2004). The main difference between each model is the immunological potential of the immune system. Athymic nude mice have no thymus and therefore no T cells, whereas severe combined immunodeficient mice have no T and no B cells

Model	Characteristics		References
	Psoriasis-like	Psoriasis-unlike	
Homozygous *asebia* ($Scd1^{ab}/Scd1^{ab}$)	Epidermal acanthosis Increased dermal vascularization Dermal infiltrate (mast cells and macrophages)	Alterations of the cutaneous lipid metabolism different from psoriasis Lack of T cells and neutrophils	(Schon, 2008, Zheng *et al.*, 1999)
Flaky skin mice (Ttc^{fsn}/Ttc^{fsn})	Best spontaneous model of psoriasis described Proliferation and hyperkeratosis of stratified squamous epithelia Positive Koebner reaction after tape-stripping	Comprises aspects not find in psoriasis Lack of the immunological side	(Sundberg *et al.*, 1990, Danilenko, 2008, Stratis *et al.*, 2006, Sundberg *et al.*, 1994, Schon, 1999)
Spontaneous chronic proliferative dermatitis mutation ($Sharpin^{cpdm}/Sharpin^{cpdm}$)	Hyperproliferative skin Infiltration of inflammatory cells in the skin Dilation of blood vessels in the dermis	Lack of T cells	(Schon, 1999)

Table 1. Examples of spontaneous mutation models and their characteristics

(Raychaudhuri *et al.*, 2001). As for AGR129 model, it is characterized by the absence of T and B cells and by the presence of immature natural killer (NK) cells, less cytotoxic than mature NK cells (Boyman *et al.*, 2004). A weaker system is potent to dwell skin transplants for a longer time on a compromised mouse upon rejection. Thus, the amount of transplant rejection is reduced in the AGR129 model compared to the others. Boyman *et al.* demonstrated that human uninvolved psoriatic skin grafted onto AGR129 mice spontaneously developed psoriatic plaques without the injection of any activated immune cells or any other exogenous factor, suggesting that uninvolved psoriatic skin is not exactly comparable to the normal human skin of healthy patients (Boyman *et al.*, 2004, Gudjonsson *et al.*, 2007, Jean & Pouliot, 2010). However, the absence of an inflammatory system could be a significant weakness of these models, since the importance of the immunology has been described by many research groups.

3.1.3 Genetically modified models

Development of rat and mouse transgenic models was an important step in the field of *in vivo* models. These genetically modified animals allow the observation of psoriasis-like characteristics in rodents following the overexpression or underexpression of cytokines (or enzymes) (Bullard *et al.*, 1996, Danilenko, 2008, Keith *et al.*, 2005). It is important to note that psoriasis is a multisystemic skin disease, and that transgenic models consider only a single gene at the time. Thus, even if these models are interesting to observe isolated psoriasis-like features, they do not allow the study of all the characteristics of the pathology. There exist a broad variety of genetically modified *in vivo* models. An exhaustive list can be seen in table 2 (Jean & Pouliot, 2010).

Model	Epidermal thickness	Abnormal differentiation	Increased vascularization	Epidermal T cell infiltration	References
Targeting the immune system					
HLA-B27/β2 microglobulin rat	+	+	+	+	(Keith *et al.*, 2005, Breban *et al.*, 1996)
Hypomorphic CD18	+	+	+	+	(Bullard *et al.*, 1996, Kess *et al.*, 2003)
αE (CD103)	+	+	?	+	(Schon *et al.*, 2000)
K14/p40	+	?	?	+	(Kopp *et al.*, 2001)
Targeting vascular endothelium					
pTek-*tTA*/Tie2	+	+	+	+	(Voskas *et al.*, 2005)
K14/VEGF	+	+	+	+	(Xia *et al.*, 2003)
Targeting epidermal proteins					
K5/Stat3C	+	+	+	+	(Sano *et al.*, 2005)
IKK2	+	+	?	-	(Pasparakis *et al.*, 2002)
c-Jun/JunB	+	+	+	+	(Zenz *et al.*, 2005)
K14/KGF	+	+	+	-	(Guo *et al.*, 1993)
K14/TGF-α	+	+	?	Some animals	(Vassar & Fuchs, 1991)
K14/IL-20	+	+	-	-	(Blumberg *et al.*, 2001)
K14/amphiregulin	+	+	+	+	(Cook *et al.*, 1997)
K14/IL-1α	+	+	-	?	(Groves *et al.*, 1995)
K14/IL-6	+	-	-	-	(Turksen *et al.*, 1992)
K10/BMP-6	+	+	+	+	(Blessing *et al.*, 1996)
Involucrin/integrins	+	+	+	+	(Carroll *et al.*, 1995)
Involucrin/MEK1	+	+	?	+	(Hobbs *et al.*, 2004)
Involucrin/amphiregulin	+	+	+	+	(Cook *et al.*, 2004)
Involucrin/IFN-γ	+	+	+	-	(Carroll *et al.*, 1997)
Chymotryptic enzyme	+	+	?	+	(Hansson *et al.*, 2002)

Table 2. *In vivo* genetically modified models of psoriasis

Reproduced and modified from Jean *et al.*, 2010 according to the copyright policy of the publisher.

3.2 *In vitro* models

3.2.1 Monolayer

By using only a small skin biopsy, monolayer techniques allow the attainment of a large number of cells (normal or pathological) supporting the production of many experiments. In monolayer models, only one cell type is studied. Thus, keratinocytes (or fibroblasts) can be used to test different conditions or to observe psoriatic skin features such as hyperproliferation or abnormal differentiation of keratinocytes. These models allow the isolation of one cell type for step by step dissection of the implied mechanisms. Even if it was not possible to observe direct interaction between cell types, these models allowed the discovery of many interesting facts about psoriasis, and favoured a better understanding of the pathology (Jean & Pouliot, 2010).

3.2.2 Collagen gels

Despite the absence of a complete *in vitro* model allowing the observation of interactions between different cell types, such as keratinocytes and fibroblasts, some teams have developed specialized techniques which imply an exogenous matrix: the collagen gel.

3.2.2.1 Organ culture

Some teams decided to put down complete skin biopsies on collagen gel, containing fibroblasts, to observe cell proliferation. Total surface recovered by keratinocytes was used to calculate cell proliferation percentage (Saiag *et al.*, 1985). Higher keratinocyte proliferation values were obtained in the presence of psoriatic fibroblasts (Saiag *et al.*, 1985). Furthermore, this model led to the conclusion that normal fibroblasts are unable to suppress the hyperproliferative growth of psoriatic keratinocytes, and that hyperproliferation of normal epidermis can be induced both by uninvolved and involved psoriatic fibroblasts (Saiag *et al.*, 1985, Jean & Pouliot, 2010).

3.2.2.2 Models using many cellular types

Other teams developed skin substitutes composed of two cell types, in order to observe the effects of psoriatic keratinocytes on fibroblasts and *vice versa*. In a global way, these models consist of isolating normal and pathological cells from a small biopsy. Fibroblasts are extracted from dermis, expanded and seeded in collagen gel. Keratinocytes are extracted in a similar way and are placed on the pre-prepared collagen gel (Konstantinova *et al.*, 1996). Barker *et al.* developed and characterized an *in vitro* psoriatic skin model using collagen gel. This model was very representative of the pathology (Barker *et al.*, 2004). In fact, they have demonstrated that the model kept many characteristics of psoriasis such as hyperproliferation and abnormal differentiation of keratinocytes, augmentation of the interleukin 6 and 8 concentrations, as well as the overexpression or underexpression of some proliferation, differentiation and inflammatory markers observed in psoriatic skin. Researchers concluded that involved and uninvolved skins seem to have the same pathological characteristics as psoriatic human skin (Barker *et al.*, 2004, Jean & Pouliot, 2010). Barker, Konstantinova and Saiag models are interesting *in vitro* models for studying psoriasis, but they are produced with a contractile exogenous material (collagen gel).

3.2.3 Self-assembly approach

Facing the absence of exogenous material-free models, our group developed a new pathological skin model to study psoriasis *in vitro* by using the self-assembly approach (Michel *et al.*, 1999) (Fig. 3). Briefly, normal and pathological fibroblasts are thawed and cultured with ascorbic acid for a period of time of four weeks. Then, dermal sheets are produced and removed from flasks. Two fibroblast sheets are superimposed to form a new dermal equivalent. Seven days later, normal or pathological keratinocytes are seeded on the dermal equivalent to obtain a new epidermal equivalent. After another 7 days of culture, the substitutes are raised to the air-liquid interface to favour cell differentiation and stratification. Finally, biopsies are taken after 21 days of culture at the air-liquid interface, and samples are analyzed using histological, immunohistochemical, physico-chemical or permeability techniques (Jean *et al.*, 2009).

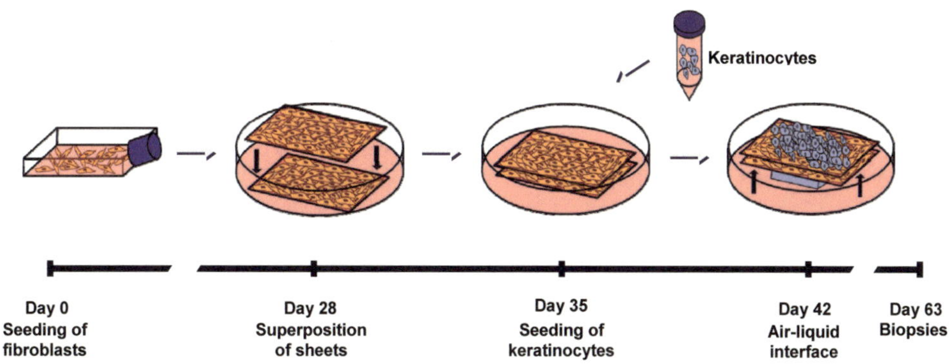

Fig. 3. The self-assembly approach for the production of skin substitutes

Schematic representation of the various steps of skin substitutes production in function of time. Reproduced and modified from Jean *et al.*, 2010 according to the copyright policy of the publisher. © 2010 InTech.

In 2009, Jean *et al.* showed that self-assembled skin substitutes partially maintained psoriasis-like features such as a thick epidermis, hyperproliferation as well as abnormal cell differentiation of epidermal cells (Jean *et al.*, 2009). In 2011, they demonstrated for the first time that pathological substitutes produced by the self-assembly approach can be treated with an anti-psoriatic molecule and react positively to the treatment such as observed in psoriatic skin *in vivo*. This functional study suggests that the self-assembled skin substitutes could be useful to better understand the mechanisms through which retinoic acid regulates cellular physiology in psoriatic skin, and could become an effective and innovative dermopharmaceutical tool for the screening of new treatments (Jean *et al.*, 2011).

4. Conclusion

Psoriasis is characterized by the presence of physical and psychological pains, which can severely affect the quality of life of psoriatic patients. Currently, a broad spectrum of anti-psoriatic treatments, both topical and systemic, is available for the management of psoriasis. These treatments only allow to control psoriasis without curing it. Challenges for antipsoriatic-drugs development are numerous, and the pharmaceutical industry strongly needs highly predictive *in vivo* and *in vitro* models to improve the success rate of the development of new drugs. Effectively, the lack of representative *in vivo* and *in vitro* models could be related with failures of clinical trials. Thus, the elaboration of these models represents a key component in the fight against psoriasis.

5. References

Baker, B.S., Owles, A.V. & Fry, L. (2008). A possible role for vaccination in the treatment of psoriasis? *G Ital Dermatol Venereol,* Vol. 143, No. 2, (Apr), pp. 105-117.

Barker, C.L., McHale, M.T., Gillies, A.K., Waller, J., Pearce, D.M., Osborne, J., Hutchinson, P.E., Smith, G.M. & Pringle, J.H. (2004). The development and characterization of an in vitro model of psoriasis. *J Invest Dermatol,* Vol. 123, No. 5, (Nov), pp. 892-901.

Ben-Arye, E., Ziv, M., Frenkel, M., Lavi, I. & Rosenman, D. (2003). Complementary medicine and psoriasis: linking the patient's outlook with evidence-based medicine. *Dermatology,* Vol. 207, No. 3, pp. 302-307.

Blessing, M., Schirmacher, P. & Kaiser, S. (1996). Overexpression of bone morphogenetic protein-6 (BMP-6) in the epidermis of transgenic mice: inhibition or stimulation of proliferation depending on the pattern of transgene expression and formation of psoriatic lesions. *J Cell Biol,* Vol. 135, No. 1, (Oct), pp. 227-239.

Blumberg, H., Conklin, D., Xu, W.F., Grossmann, A., Brender, T., Carollo, S., Eagan, M., Foster, D., Haldeman, B.A., Hammond, A., Haugen, H., Jelinek, L., Kelly, J.D., Madden, K., Maurer, M.F., Parrish-Novak, J., Prunkard, D., Sexson, S., Sprecher, C., Waggie, K., West, J., Whitmore, T.E., Yao, L., Kuechle, M.K., Dale, B.A. & Chandrasekher, Y.A. (2001). Interleukin 20: discovery, receptor identification, and role in epidermal function. *Cell,* Vol. 104, No. 1, (Jan 12), pp. 9-19.

Bowcock, A.M. & Krueger, J.G. (2005). Getting under the skin: the immunogenetics of psoriasis. *Nat Rev Immunol,* Vol. 5, No. 9, (Sep), pp. 699-711.

Boyman, O., Hefti, H.P., Conrad, C., Nickoloff, B.J., Suter, M. & Nestle, F.O. (2004). Spontaneous development of psoriasis in a new animal model shows an essential role for resident T cells and tumor necrosis factor-alpha. *J Exp Med,* Vol. 199, No. 5, (Mar 1), pp. 731-736.

Bragulla, H.H. & Homberger, D.G. (2009). Structure and functions of keratin proteins in simple, stratified, keratinized and cornified epithelia. *J Anat,* Vol. 214, No. 4, (Apr), pp. 516-559.

Breban, M., Fernandez-Sueiro, J.L., Richardson, J.A., Hadavand, R.R., Maika, S.D., Hammer, R.E. & Taurog, J.D. (1996). T cells, but not thymic exposure to HLA-B27, are required for the inflammatory disease of HLA-B27 transgenic rats. *J Immunol,* Vol. 156, No. 2, (Jan 15), pp. 794-803.

Bullard, D.C., Scharffetter-Kochanek, K., McArthur, M.J., Chosay, J.G., McBride, M.E., Montgomery, C.A. & Beaudet, A.L. (1996). A polygenic mouse model of psoriasiform skin disease in CD18-deficient mice. *Proc Natl Acad Sci U S A,* Vol. 93, No. 5, (Mar 5), pp. 2116-2121.

Carroll, J.M., Crompton, T., Seery, J.P. & Watt, F.M. (1997). Transgenic mice expressing IFN-gamma in the epidermis have eczema, hair hypopigmentation, and hair loss. *J Invest Dermatol,* Vol. 108, No. 4, (Apr), pp. 412-422.

Carroll, J.M., Romero, M.R. & Watt, F.M. (1995). Suprabasal integrin expression in the epidermis of transgenic mice results in developmental defects and a phenotype resembling psoriasis. *Cell,* Vol. 83, No. 6, (Dec 15), pp. 957-968.

Chan, J.R., Blumenschein, W., Murphy, E., Diveu, C., Wiekowski, M., Abbondanzo, S., Lucian, L., Geissler, R., Brodie, S., Kimball, A.B., Gorman, D.M., Smith, K., de Waal Malefyt, R., Kastelein, R.A., McClanahan, T.K. & Bowman, E.P. (2006). IL-23 stimulates epidermal hyperplasia via TNF and IL-20R2-dependent mechanisms with implications for psoriasis pathogenesis. *J Exp Med,* Vol. 203, No. 12, (Nov 27), pp. 2577-2587.

Christophers, E., Griffiths, C.E., Gaitanis, G. & van de Kerkhof, P. (2006). The unmet treatment need for moderate to severe psoriasis: results of a survey and chart review. *J Eur Acad Dermatol Venereol,* Vol. 20, No. 8, (Sep), pp. 921-925.

Conrad, C., Boyman, O., Tonel, G., Tun-Kyi, A., Laggner, U., de Fougerolles, A., Kotelianski, V., Gardner, H. & Nestle, F.O. (2007). Alpha1beta1 integrin is crucial for accumulation of epidermal T cells and the development of psoriasis. *Nat Med,* Vol. 13, No. 7, (Jul), pp. 836-842.

Cook, P.W., Brown, J.R., Cornell, K.A. & Pittelkow, M.R. (2004). Suprabasal expression of human amphiregulin in the epidermis of transgenic mice induces a severe, early-onset, psoriasis-like skin pathology: expression of amphiregulin in the basal epidermis is also associated with synovitis. *Exp Dermatol,* Vol. 13, No. 6, (Jun), pp. 347-356.

Cook, P.W., Piepkorn, M., Clegg, C.H., Plowman, G.D., DeMay, J.M., Brown, J.R. & Pittelkow, M.R. (1997). Transgenic expression of the human amphiregulin gene induces a psoriasis-like phenotype. *J Clin Invest,* Vol. 100, No. 9, (Nov 1), pp. 2286-2294.

Danilenko, D.M. (2008). Review paper: preclinical models of psoriasis. *Vet Pathol,* Vol. 45, No. 4, (Jul), pp. 563-575.

DiBonaventura, M., Wagner, S., Waters, H. & Carter, C. (2010). Treatment patterns and perceptions of treatment attributes, satisfaction and effectiveness among patients with psoriasis. *J Drugs Dermatol,* Vol. 9, No. 8, (Aug), pp. 938-944.

Dubertret, L., Mrowietz, U., Ranki, A., van de Kerkhof, P.C., Chimenti, S., Lotti, T. & Schafer, G. (2006). European patient perspectives on the impact of psoriasis: the EUROPSO patient membership survey. *Br J Dermatol,* Vol. 155, No. 4, (Oct), pp. 729-736.

Farshidi, A. & Sadeghi, P. (2006). Successful treatment of severe refractory atopic dermatitis with efalizumab. *J Drugs Dermatol,* Vol. 5, No. 10, (Nov-Dec), pp. 994-998.

Fraki, J.E., Briggaman, R.A. & Lazarus, G.S. (1983). Transplantation of psoriatic skin onto nude mice. *J Invest Dermatol,* Vol. 80 Suppl, No. (Jun), pp. 31s-35s.

Gottlieb, A.B., Casale, T.B., Frankel, E., Goffe, B., Lowe, N., Ochs, H.D., Roberts, J.L., Washenik, K., Vaishnaw, A.K. & Gordon, K.B. (2003). CD4+ T-cell-directed antibody responses are maintained in patients with psoriasis receiving alefacept: results of a randomized study. *J Am Acad Dermatol,* Vol. 49, No. 5, (Nov), pp. 816-825.

Groves, R.W., Mizutani, H., Kieffer, J.D. & Kupper, T.S. (1995). Inflammatory skin disease in transgenic mice that express high levels of interleukin 1 alpha in basal epidermis. *Proc Natl Acad Sci U S A,* Vol. 92, No. 25, (Dec 5), pp. 11874-11878.

Gudjonsson, J.E., Johnston, A., Dyson, M., Valdimarsson, H. & Elder, J.T. (2007). Mouse models of psoriasis. *J Invest Dermatol,* Vol. 127, No. 6, (Jun), pp. 1292-1308.

Guo, L., Yu, Q.C. & Fuchs, E. (1993). Targeting expression of keratinocyte growth factor to keratinocytes elicits striking changes in epithelial differentiation in transgenic mice. *Embo J,* Vol. 12, No. 3, (Mar), pp. 973-986.

Guttman-Yassky, E. & Krueger, J.G. (2007). Psoriasis: evolution of pathogenic concepts and new therapies through phases of translational research. *Br J Dermatol,* Vol. 157, No. 6, (Dec), pp. 1103-1115.

Hansson, L., Backman, A., Ny, A., Edlund, M., Ekholm, E., Ekstrand Hammarstrom, B., Tornell, J., Wallbrandt, P., Wennbo, H. & Egelrud, T. (2002). Epidermal overexpression of stratum corneum chymotryptic enzyme in mice: a model for chronic itchy dermatitis. *J Invest Dermatol,* Vol. 118, No. 3, (Mar), pp. 444-449.

Harding, C.R. (2004). The stratum corneum: structure and function in health and disease. *Dermatol Ther,* Vol. 17 Suppl 1, No. pp. 6-15.

Hobbs, R.M., Silva-Vargas, V., Groves, R. & Watt, F.M. (2004). Expression of activated MEK1 in differentiating epidermal cells is sufficient to generate hyperproliferative and inflammatory skin lesions. *J Invest Dermatol,* Vol. 123, No. 3, (Sep), pp. 503-515.

Jean, J., Lapointe, M., Soucy, J. & Pouliot, R. (2009). Development of an in vitro psoriatic skin model by tissue engineering. *J Dermatol Sci,* Vol. 53, No. 1, (Jan), pp. 19-25.

Jean, J. & Pouliot, R. (2010), In vivo and in vitro models of psoriasis, In: *Tissue engineering,*pp. 359-382,

Jean, J., Soucy, J. & Pouliot, R. (2011). Effects of Retinoic Acid in Keratinocyte Proliferation and Differentiation in a Psoriatic Skin Model. *Tissue Eng Part A,* Vol. No. (Mar 18),

Karlsson, T., Rollman, O., Vahlquist, A. & Torma, H. (2004). Immunofluorescence localization of nuclear retinoid receptors in psoriasis versus normal human skin. *Acta Derm Venereol,* Vol. 84, No. 5, pp. 363-369.

Keith, J.C., Jr., Sainz, I.M., Isordia-Salas, I., Pixley, R.A., Leathurby, Y., Albert, L.M. & Colman, R.W. (2005). A monoclonal antibody against kininogen reduces inflammation in the HLA-B27 transgenic rat. *Arthritis Res Ther,* Vol. 7, No. 4, pp. R769-776.

Kess, D., Peters, T., Zamek, J., Wickenhauser, C., Tawadros, S., Loser, K., Varga, G., Grabbe, S., Nischt, R., Sunderkotter, C., Muller, W., Krieg, T. & Scharffetter-Kochanek, K. (2003). CD4+ T cell-associated pathophysiology critically depends on CD18 gene dose effects in a murine model of psoriasis. *J Immunol,* Vol. 171, No. 11, (Dec 1), pp. 5697-5706.

Klotz, J., Muir, L., Cameron, C. & Delaney, L. (2005). Monitoring a remote phototherapy unit via telemedicine. *J Cutan Med Surg,* Vol. 9, No. 2, (Apr), pp. 47-53.

Konstantinova, N.V., Duong, D.M., Remenyik, E., Hazarika, P., Chuang, A. & Duvic, M. (1996). Interleukin-8 is induced in skin equivalents and is highest in those derived from psoriatic fibroblasts. *J Invest Dermatol,* Vol. 107, No. 4, (Oct), pp. 615-621.

Kopp, T., Kieffer, J.D., Rot, A., Strommer, S., Stingl, G. & Kupper, T.S. (2001). Inflammatory skin disease in K14/p40 transgenic mice: evidence for interleukin-12-like activities of p40. *J Invest Dermatol,* Vol. 117, No. 3, (Sep), pp. 618-626.

Kormeili, T., Lowe, N.J. & Yamauchi, P.S. (2004). Psoriasis: immunopathogenesis and evolving immunomodulators and systemic therapies; U.S. experiences. *Br J Dermatol,* Vol. 151, No. 1, (Jul), pp. 3-15.

Krueger, G., Koo, J., Lebwohl, M., Menter, A., Stern, R.S. & Rolstad, T. (2001). The impact of psoriasis on quality of life: results of a 1998 National Psoriasis Foundation patient-membership survey. *Arch Dermatol,* Vol. 137, No. 3, (Mar), pp. 280-284.

Krueger, G.G., Langley, R.G., Leonardi, C., Yeilding, N., Guzzo, C., Wang, Y., Dooley, L.T. & Lebwohl, M. (2007). A human interleukin-12/23 monoclonal antibody for the treatment of psoriasis. *N Engl J Med,* Vol. 356, No. 6, (Feb 8), pp. 580-592.

Krueger, J.G. (2002). The immunologic basis for the treatment of psoriasis with new biologic agents. *J Am Acad Dermatol,* Vol. 46, No. 1, (Jan), pp. 1-23; quiz 23-26.

Krueger, J.G. & Bowcock, A. (2005). Psoriasis pathophysiology: current concepts of pathogenesis. *Ann Rheum Dis,* Vol. 64 Suppl 2, No. (Mar), pp. ii30-ii36.

Lowes, M.A., Bowcock, A.M. & Krueger, J.G. (2007). Pathogenesis and therapy of psoriasis. *Nature,* Vol. 445, No. 7130, (Feb 22), pp. 866-873.

Menter, A. & Stoff, B. (2010). *Psoriasis* London

Michel, M., L'Heureux, N., Pouliot, R., Xu, W., Auger, F.A. & Germain, L. (1999). Characterization of a new tissue-engineered human skin equivalent with hair. *In Vitro Cell Dev Biol Anim,* Vol. 35, No. 6, (Jun), pp. 318-326.

Mizutani, H., Yamanaka, K., Konishi, H. & Murakami, T. (2003). Animal models of psoriasis and pustular psoriasis. *Arch Dermatol Res,* Vol. 295 Suppl 1, No. (Apr), pp. S67-68.

Nagarajan, P., Parikh, N., Garrett-Sinha, L.A. & Sinha, S. (2009). Ets1 induces dysplastic changes when expressed in terminally-differentiating squamous epidermal cells. *PLoS One,* Vol. 4, No. 1, pp. e4179.

Nestle, F.O., Conrad, C., Tun-Kyi, A., Homey, B., Gombert, M., Boyman, O., Burg, G., Liu, Y.J. & Gilliet, M. (2005). Plasmacytoid predendritic cells initiate psoriasis through interferon-alpha production. *J Exp Med,* Vol. 202, No. 1, (Jul 4), pp. 135-143.

Nijsten, T., Margolis, D.J., Feldman, S.R., Rolstad, T. & Stern, R.S. (2005). Traditional systemic treatments have not fully met the needs of psoriasis patients: results from a national survey. *J Am Acad Dermatol,* Vol. 52, No. 3 Pt 1, (Mar), pp. 434-444.

Pasparakis, M., Courtois, G., Hafner, M., Schmidt-Supprian, M., Nenci, A., Toksoy, A., Krampert, M., Goebeler, M., Gillitzer, R., Israel, A., Krieg, T., Rajewsky, K. & Haase, I. (2002). TNF-mediated inflammatory skin disease in mice with epidermis-specific deletion of IKK2. *Nature,* Vol. 417, No. 6891, (Jun 20), pp. 861-866.

Poulin, Y., Papp, K.A., Wasel, N.R., Andrew, R., Fraquelli, E., Bernstein, G. & Chan, D. (2010). A Canadian online survey to evaluate awareness and treatment satisfaction in individuals with moderate to severe plaque psoriasis. *Int J Dermatol,* Vol. 49, No. 12, (Dec), pp. 1368-1375.

Rashmi, R., Rao, K.S. & Basavaraj, K.H. (2009). A comprehensive review of biomarkers in psoriasis. *Clin Exp Dermatol,* Vol. 34, No. 6, (Aug), pp. 658-663.

Raychaudhuri, S.P., Dutt, S., Raychaudhuri, S.K., Sanyal, M. & Farber, E.M. (2001). Severe combined immunodeficiency mouse-human skin chimeras: a unique animal model for the study of psoriasis and cutaneous inflammation. *Br J Dermatol,* Vol. 144, No. 5, (May), pp. 931-939.

Saiag, P., Coulomb, B., Lebreton, C., Bell, E. & Dubertret, L. (1985). Psoriatic fibroblasts induce hyperproliferation of normal keratinocytes in a skin equivalent model in vitro. *Science,* Vol. 230, No. 4726, (Nov 8), pp. 669-672.

Sano, S., Chan, K.S., Carbajal, S., Clifford, J., Peavey, M., Kiguchi, K., Itami, S., Nickoloff, B.J. & DiGiovanni, J. (2005). Stat3 links activated keratinocytes and immunocytes required for development of psoriasis in a novel transgenic mouse model. *Nat Med,* Vol. 11, No. 1, (Jan), pp. 43-49.

Schon, M.P. (1999). Animal models of psoriasis - what can we learn from them? *J Invest Dermatol,* Vol. 112, No. 4, (Apr), pp. 405-410.

Schon, M.P. (2008). Animal models of psoriasis: a critical appraisal. *Exp Dermatol,* Vol. 17, No. 8, (Aug), pp. 703-712.

Schon, M.P. & Boehncke, W.H. (2005). Psoriasis. *N Engl J Med,* Vol. 352, No. 18, (May 5), pp. 1899-1912.

Schon, M.P., Schon, M., Warren, H.B., Donohue, J.P. & Parker, C.M. (2000). Cutaneous inflammatory disorder in integrin alphaE (CD103)-deficient mice. *J Immunol,* Vol. 165, No. 11, (Dec 1), pp. 6583-6589.

Simpson, G.L., Yelverton, C.B., Rittenberg, S. & Feldman, S.R. (2006). Do utilization management controls for phototherapy increase the prescription of biologics? *J Dermatolog Treat,* Vol. 17, No. 6, pp. 359-361.

Stern, R.S., Nijsten, T., Feldman, S.R., Margolis, D.J. & Rolstad, T. (2004). Psoriasis is common, carries a substantial burden even when not extensive, and is associated with widespread treatment dissatisfaction. *J Investig Dermatol Symp Proc,* Vol. 9, No. 2, (Mar), pp. 136-139.

Stratis, A., Pasparakis, M., Rupec, R.A., Markur, D., Hartmann, K., Scharffetter-Kochanek, K., Peters, T., van Rooijen, N., Krieg, T. & Haase, I. (2006). Pathogenic role for skin macrophages in a mouse model of keratinocyte-induced psoriasis-like skin inflammation. *J Clin Invest,* Vol. 116, No. 8, (Aug), pp. 2094-2104.

Sugihara, H., Toda, S., Miyabara, S., Kusaba, Y. & Minami, Y. (1991). Reconstruction of the skin in three-dimensional collagen gel matrix culture. *In Vitro Cell Dev Biol,* Vol. 27A, No. 2, (Feb), pp. 142-146.

Sundberg, J.P., Beamer, W.G., Shultz, L.D. & Dunstan, R.W. (1990). Inherited mouse mutations as models of human adnexal, cornification, and papulosquamous dermatoses. *J Invest Dermatol,* Vol. 95, No. 5, (Nov), pp. 62S-63S.

Sundberg, J.P., Dunstan, R.W., Roop, D.R. & Beamer, W.G. (1994). Full-thickness skin grafts from flaky skin mice to nude mice: maintenance of the psoriasiform phenotype. *J Invest Dermatol,* Vol. 102, No. 5, (May), pp. 781-788.

Tonel, G. & Conrad, C. (2009). Interplay between keratinocytes and immune cells--recent insights into psoriasis pathogenesis. *Int J Biochem Cell Biol,* Vol. 41, No. 5, (May), pp. 963-968.

Turksen, K., Kupper, T., Degenstein, L., Williams, I. & Fuchs, E. (1992). Interleukin 6: insights to its function in skin by overexpression in transgenic mice. *Proc Natl Acad Sci U S A,* Vol. 89, No. 11, (Jun 1), pp. 5068-5072.

Vassar, R. & Fuchs, E. (1991). Transgenic mice provide new insights into the role of TGF-alpha during epidermal development and differentiation. *Genes Dev,* Vol. 5, No. 5, (May), pp. 714-727.

Voskas, D., Jones, N., Van Slyke, P., Sturk, C., Chang, W., Haninec, A., Babichev, Y.O., Tran, J., Master, Z., Chen, S., Ward, N., Cruz, M., Jones, J., Kerbel, R.S., Jothy, S., Dagnino, L., Arbiser, J., Klement, G. & Dumont, D.J. (2005). A cyclosporine-sensitive psoriasis-like disease produced in Tie2 transgenic mice. *Am J Pathol,* Vol. 166, No. 3, (Mar), pp. 843-855.

Wasel, N., Poulin, Y., Andrew, R., Chan, D., Fraquelli, E. & Papp, K. (2009). A Canadian self-administered online survey to evaluate the impact of moderate-to-severe psoriasis among patients. *J Cutan Med Surg,* Vol. 13, No. 6, (Nov-Dec), pp. 294-302.

Wippel-Slupetzky, K. & Stingl, G. (2009). Future perspectives in the treatment of psoriasis. *Curr Probl Dermatol,* Vol. 38, No. pp. 172-189.

Wolk, K., Kunz, S., Witte, E., Friedrich, M., Asadullah, K. & Sabat, R. (2004). IL-22 increases the innate immunity of tissues. *Immunity,* Vol. 21, No. 2, (Aug), pp. 241-254.

Xia, Y.P., Li, B., Hylton, D., Detmar, M., Yancopoulos, G.D. & Rudge, J.S. (2003). Transgenic delivery of VEGF to mouse skin leads to an inflammatory condition resembling human psoriasis. *Blood,* Vol. 102, No. 1, (Jul 1), pp. 161-168.

Zenz, R., Eferl, R., Kenner, L., Florin, L., Hummerich, L., Mehic, D., Scheuch, H., Angel, P., Tschachler, E. & Wagner, E.F. (2005). Psoriasis-like skin disease and arthritis caused by inducible epidermal deletion of Jun proteins. *Nature,* Vol. 437, No. 7057, (Sep 15), pp. 369-375.

Zheng, Y., Danilenko, D.M., Valdez, P., Kasman, I., Eastham-Anderson, J., Wu, J. & Ouyang, W. (2007). Interleukin-22, a T(H)17 cytokine, mediates IL-23-induced dermal inflammation and acanthosis. *Nature,* Vol. 445, No. 7128, (Feb 8), pp. 648-651.

Zheng, Y., Eilertsen, K.J., Ge, L., Zhang, L., Sundberg, J.P., Prouty, S.M., Stenn, K.S. & Parimoo, S. (1999). Scd1 is expressed in sebaceous glands and is disrupted in the asebia mouse. *Nat Genet,* Vol. 23, No. 3, (Nov), pp. 268-270.

Part 2

Clinical Presentation

5

Detecting Psoriasis Arthritis Early in the Disease Course – Why This is Important and How Dermatologists and Rheumatologists Can Successfully Cooperate?

Peter Härle
Katholisches Klinikum Mainz, Klinik für Rheumatologie und Physikalische Therapie
An der Goldgrube 11, Mainz
Germany

1. Introduction

Psoriatic arthritis (PsA) was first recognized as a specific rheumatic entity in 1964 by the American Rheumatism Association (later American College of Rheumatology) (Blumberg, 1964). In the forthcoming years it has become clear that PsA belongs to the spondyloarthritis (SpA) family that comprises several heterogeneous clinical conditions. These are Ankylosing Spondylitis, Reactive Arthritis (which occurs after bacterial infections), Spondyloarthritis associated to Chronic Inflammatory Bowel Diseases (Crohn´s disease and Ulcerative Colitis), Undifferentiated Spondyloarthritis, and juvenile forms (figure 1). The term spondyloarthritis relates to inflammatory manifestations of peripheral and spinal joint structures. The Spondyloarthitides are defined by classification criteria (Sieper, 2009; Zeidler 2011, Rudwaleit 2011). The main clinical manifestation will trigger the main group for each disease entity may have varying degrees of articular, spinal, and extraaticular manifestations. Furthermore, extraarticular inflammatory manifestations may also occur at different intensity levels. However, it needs to emphasized that classification criteria are not diagnostic criteria. Classification criteria were developed for clinical studies in order to include rather homogenous disease manifestations. In daily clinical practice it may occur that although the classification criteria are not fully met, the patient still may be allocated to a certain disease entity.

Peripheral joint manifestations	Spinal manifestations	Extra-articular Manifestations
Arthritis	Spondylitis	Uveitis, Scleritis, Conjunctivitis
Enthesitis	Enthesitis	Psoriasis
Bursitis	Sacroiliac joint arthritis	Urethritis
Tendosynovitis	Facet joint arthritis	Inflammatory bowel disease
Erosive-proliferative joint destruction	Bony ankylosis	Periodontitis with dental loss

Table 1. Clinical manifestation of the Spondyloarthritides, which may be present in all the different disease entities (Fig. 1).

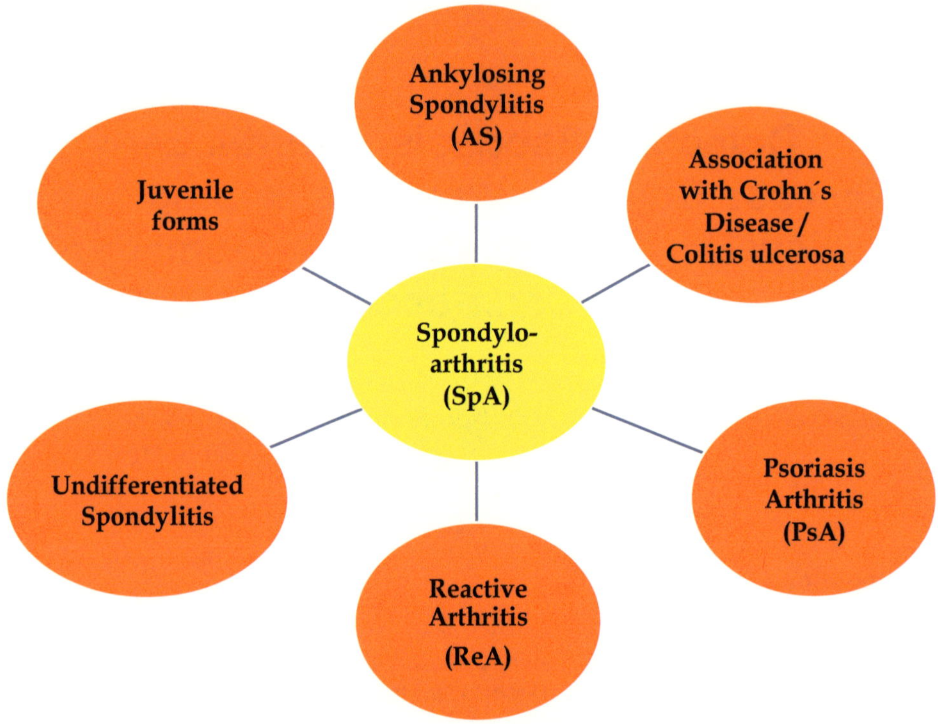

Fig. 1. Clinical entities of Spondyloarthritis. The overall disease group is the Spondyloarthritis, which comprises 6 distinct diseases. Psoriasis Arthritis is one disease entity of the group. Common abbreviations are given in parenthesis.

In clinical practice, articular and extraarticular manifestations overlap quite frequently among the SpA diseases. Initially, the clinical manifestations of PsA were collected and a set of manifestations was proposed as classification criteria by Moll and Wright in 1973 (Moll, 1973). These described clinical features were considered to be "Psoriatic Arthritis". However, over the following years, 6 modified classification criteria for PsA (Bennet, 1979; Dougados, 1991; Fournie, 1999; Gladman, 1987; McGonagle, 1999; Vasey, 1984) have been proposed by different research groups in order to differentiate between the different disease entities (Taylor, 2002). As in the Moll and Wright criteria proposal, these criteria mainly have been established in groups of patients with classical and fully developed disease manifestations. The validity of these criteria have never been formally proven in studies. Formal prove of PsA criteria was done in 2006 with the publication of the CASPAR (Classification of Psoriasis Arthritis Study Group)-Criteria (Taylor, 2006) as a joint project of the EUAR and ACR. As with the other above mentioned 7 criteria sets, the CASPAR criteria also were established in a group of patients with long standing psoriasis arthritis (mean disease duration of greater than 10 years (Taylor, 2006). As we know that chronic inflammatory arthritis like Rheumatoid Arthritis (RA) and PsA can destroy joints and cause significant disability (see Tab. 1) we need to diagnose arthritis before destruction of tissue has taken place. For this reason, in RA, arthritis classification criteria have just been revised to also classify early RA (Aletaha, 2010). Next to the new RA early classification criteria, the newly proposed classification criteria for spinal spondyloarthritis now include MRI diagnostics of the sacroiliac joints (Rudwaleit, 2009). Bone marrow edema around the sacroiliac joints seen in MRI in water sensitive squences, i.e. STIR (short tau inversion recovery, T1 plus contrast media) detects inflammatory processes significantly earlier than actual joint destruction can be seen on conventional X-ray films.

However, we still do not have validated early PsA criteria and early PsA most times does not present with the classical, fully developed clinical picture as is described in our textbooks.

This book chapter is dedicated to discuss why we need to detect PsA early and will answer the question of how patients with psoriasis can be screened for possible early peripheral and spinal arthritis manifestations. Suggestions on how cooperation between dermatologists and rheumatologists can be effectively set up will be given at the end.

2. Why is early detection of inflammatory processes important?

2.1 The earlier the better or time is joint function

Early detection and treatment of chronic inflammatory joint disease has been shown in numerous reports to correlate with better long-term outcome in rheumatoid arthritis (van der Bijl, 2007; Verstappen, 2007). Severity of joint destruction and loss of quality of life in PsA has been shown to be similar to RA (Husted, 2001; Rahman, 2001). Therefore, many aspects in PsA may be compared with aspects in RA. As depicted in figure 2, the chronic inflammatory process begins with an undulating situation of clinical and subclinical manifestations of joint pain with or without swelling. A trigger event then sets off the clinical manifest chronic inflammatory course. Joint destruction begins very early after this event. If the inflammatory process is not stopped, the natural disease course will occur with more or less destruction of joint structures.

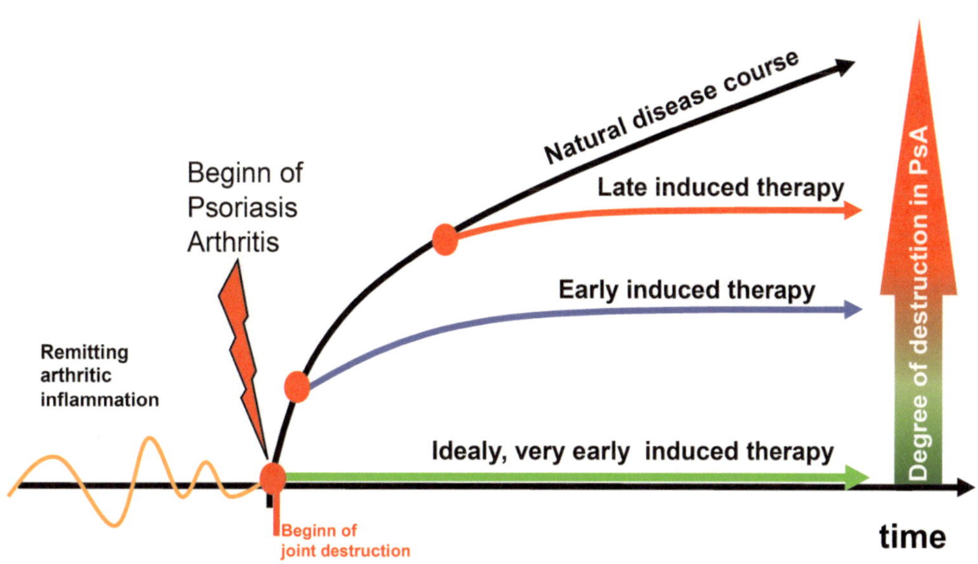

Fig. 2. Time course of the development of PsA. The earlier detection and treatment of arthritis takes place, the better the outcome in the following years will be, adapted according to (Machold, 1998).

However, if we treat to the target of remission and control the inflammatory process, it is possible to prevent or slow down the destructive process. We have plenty of evidence for this targeted approach for RA as reviewed elsewhere (Schoels, 2010). Furthermore, recommendations for physicians (Smolen, 2010) and patients (de Wit, 2011) on how to treat to the target of remission have recently been published. Very likely, the targeted approach is also true for PsA, because PsA also shows destructive disease courses and we use the same outcome measures than for RA. However, this has not yet been formally proven as has been for RA.

Inflammation of articular structures always is coupled with loss of function. Early in the disease course inflammation and loss of function correlate very well. This means, if inflammation is suppressed, function is completely regained. However, the longer the inflammatory process goes on, the more fibrotic and destructive changes occur which are not reversible (Aletaha, 2006). This implies that effective suppression of inflammation will not result in full regain of function anymore (figure 3). Furthermore, fibrotic tissue may cause destruction by itself thus uncoupling the destructive process from classic immune mediated mechanisms (Neumann, 2006).

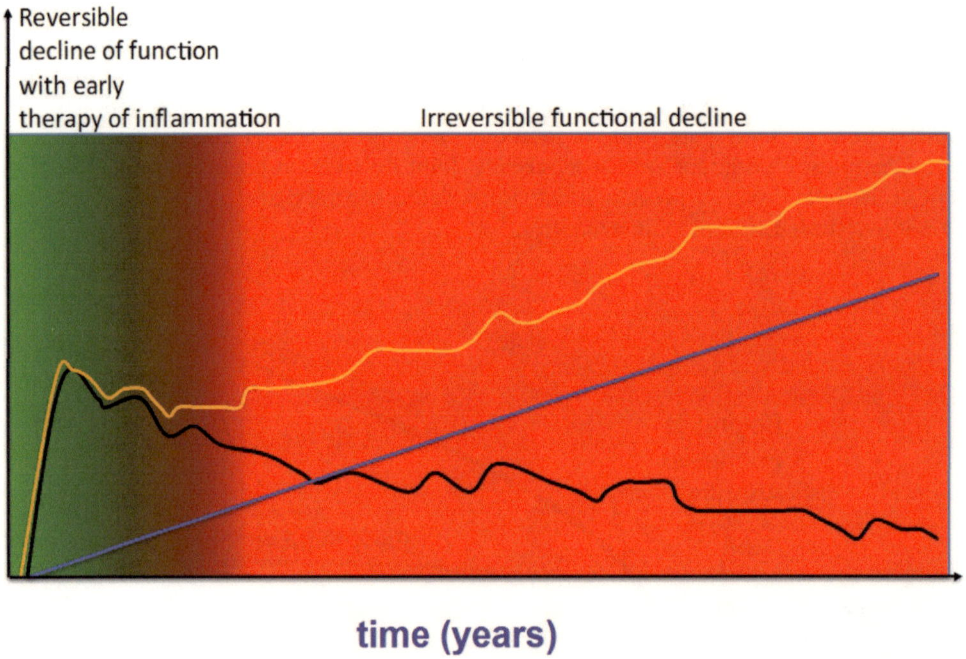

Fig. 3. Correlation of inflammation (black), loss of function (yellow) and joint destruction (blue) with time. Very early in the inflammatory process loss of joint function is tightly correlated with the degree of inflammation. In this phase, complete reduction of joint inflammation will restore joint function. However, the longer the inflammatory process goes on, the more destruction of joint structures will occur along with continuously more irreversible loss of function and destruction. Finally, there may occur an uncoupling of inflammation and irreversible joint destruction with loss of function, adapted according to (Kirwan, 2001).

2.2 Chronic inflammation confers a cardiovascular risk factor by itself

An upcoming discussion is that chronic inflammatory processes enhance the cardiovascular risk to a similar extend like the classical known risk factors diabetes, hypertension, hyperlipidemia, obesity, smoking and genetics (van Halm, 2009). This implies that treatment of inflammation may be similar important to the treatment of the classical cardiocascular risk factors in order to reduce the overall cardiovascular risk. Prospective studies on reduction of cardiovascular risk by anti-inflammatory treatment are still pending but it was shown retrospectively that effective reduction of inflammation with combination therapy of methotrexate and anti-TNF (Tumor Necrosis Factor) medication may reduce the risk for the first cardiovascular event (Cugno, 2010).

As in RA the cytokine TNF plays an important role in the pathophysiological mechanism of Ps and PsA. The prothrombotic effects of TNF in cardiovascular disease are discussed in a recent review and may play an important role in the about 4 fold enhanced cardiovascular risk compared with the normal population (Jacobsson, 2005). However, Ps and PsA patients seem to additionally have an increased prevalence of cardiovascular risk factors such as smoking, hypertension, raised levels of homocysteine, excessive alcohol consumption and metabolic syndrome compared to the normal population (Tobin, 2010). Therefore, it cannot be finally answered to what extend chronic inflammation of the skin, joints, and spine in Ps/PsA add to an enhanced cardiovascular risk.

2.3 Health care costs of PsA are high

Another reason for early detection of PsA is health care costs. PsA shows increasing costs with the duration of the disease. This seems to mainly be due to the rising risk of work disability. However, the association of work disability and disease duration has not very well been studied up to day. Only 3 studies were published on this topic (Mau, 2005; Verstappen, 2010) and one review gets to the conclusion that the data is too heterogeneous to draw hard conclusions (Tillett, 2011). Nevertheless the study of Mau et al. describes a reduction of the standard employment rate in PsA patients from 0,94 to 0,7 within 5 years. Functional status seems to be the most important factor to predict total costs. Zink et al. summarize that patients with a poor functional status of 50% (HAQ of more than 1,7) cost more than double compared to patients with a good functional status (functional status of 70% or HAQ less than 1,2) (Zink, 2006).

2.4 Psychosomatic comorbidity is important to consider

Finally, the psychological and psychiatric comorbidities resulting from the cutaneous stigmatization and the painful, debilitating arthritic manifestations of joint and spine add to the disease burden of PsA (Devrimci-Ozguven, 2000; Esposito, 2006). There seems to be no difference in depression rate among sex and age of patients with PsA. Effective therapy of cutaneous manifestations and arthritis may reduce depressive disorders, which will significantly reduce health costs and therefore needs to be balanced against the high costs of modern treatment with biologics.

3. How can patients with PsA be identified in daily clinical routine?

In clinical practice, psoriatic patients with a dominant skin manifestation primarily consult dermatologists and patients with a dominant peripheral or spinal manifestation primarily consult rheumatologists or orthopedics. However, the vast majority of Ps patients gather within the dermatology setting. Therefore, it seems rational to screen patients for arthritic manifestations in the dermatology setting.

From July 2005 until October 2008, we validated and established the self-administered patient-screening questionnaire GEPARD (GErman Psoriasis ARthritis Diagnostic questionnaire) to detect PsA in psoriatic patients seeking primarily dermatologic care (Härle, 2010) (Tab. 2 and www.kkm-mainz.de/rheumatologie). In order to keep the questionnaire simple, only dichotomous answers (yes/no) were used. The twelve questions were derived from discussions about appropriate questions among the authors and additional advice provided by other experienced rheumatologists. Questions number 1 to 4 relate to clinical signs of arthritis but do not necessarily impose a momentary active state of arthritis by asking if the patient ever had these signs. It was considered that these questions take into account the remitting and relapsing nature of PsA. We considered the detection of these patients being especially important in the context of a longitudinal follow-up of fluctuating arthritis, which might eventually lead to establishing prognostic parameters for PsA. Questions number 5 to 8 pertain to arthritis in a more indirect way by relating to the discomfort caused by joint pain or dysfunction. Questions number 9 to 13 relate to the clinical signs of inflammatory back pain which can be associated with PsA. An additional

#	Question	Yes	No
1	*Have you ever had joint pain accompanied by swelling?*		
2	*Have you ever had a completely swollen digit or toe?*		
3	*Have you ever had joint pain accompanied by redness of that joint?*		
4	*Do your joints feel stiff after waking up in the morning?*		
5	*Have you ever thought of having a joint disease?*		
6	*Have you ever consulted a doctor because of your joint problems?*		
7	*Have you ever received the diagnosis of "arthritis"?*		
8	*Do you take pain medication for your joint pain?*		
9	*Do you suffer from back- or buttock pain? If yes, does/is this pain.... (please, answer questions 8a to 8d)*		
10	*... most intense in the early morning hours?*		
11	*... improve through exercising or moving around?*		
12	*... persist while resting?*		
13	*... accompanied by back stiffness in the morning hours?*		
14	*If you answered one of the above questions with "**YES**": Since when do you have these complaints?*		

More than 1 week	More than 1 month	More than 3 months	More than 6 months	More than 1 year	More than 3 years	More than 5 years

Table 2. The GEPARD questionnaire targets arthritic complaints of peripheral joints and spinal manifestations in addition of duration of arthritic symptoms thus enableing early detection of PsA. The patient alone answers the questionnaire. The physician or assistant counts the positive answers. The cut-off value of equal or more than 4 positive answers showed a sensitivity of 89% and a specificity of 73% to detect PsA in Ps patients

question related to the time period since the first occurrence of complaints lasting from one week up to more than 5 years in order to detect early PsA manifestations. In the statistical evaluation of the study, we calculated a cut-off value of greater than or equal to 4 positive answered questions. This cut-off showed a sensitivity of 89% and a specificity of 73% to detect PsA in Ps patients (Härle, 2010).

In the final evaluation, we clinically evaluated 54 patients. These patients were selected by the GEPARD questionnaire from dermatology outpatient clinics. We found 43 patients who had some arthritic manifestations according to clinical examination, ultrasound, x-ray, MRI, and Technecium-Szintigraphy. This accounts for 79,6% patients being positive for PsA manifestation. This percentage of PsA among patients with Ps is in line with earlier publications (Sadek, 2007). Furthermore, 23 patients were first diagnosed as having PsA.

According to the time duration of arthritic complaints we found 57% suffering over 4 years but 43% of patients below 4 years (figure 4) which may still be considered as being early arthritis. From these patients with complaints of less than 4 years 80% could be classified for PsA just by clinical examination according the CASPAR criteria without the use of sonography, x-ray, MRI, or szintigraphy (figure 5). Considering that the initial screening process was exclusively based on patients' answers, without evaluation by a physician, the GEPARD patient - questionnaire is well suited for routine clinical usage. In addition, the screening tool does not consume additional time from the dermatologist but still enables him to identify patients who need to be referred to a rheumatologist for further evaluation of arthritic manifestation.

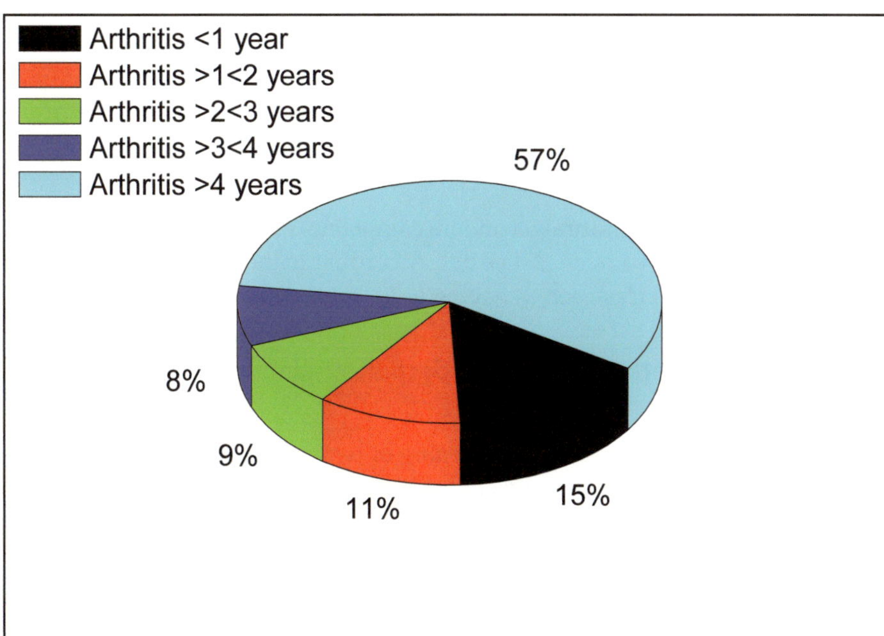

Fig. 4. Pie chart of arthritis duration according to the GEPARD patient-questionnaire. Forty-three percent suffered of symptoms of less than 4 years. Less than 4 years is considered to be early arthritis.

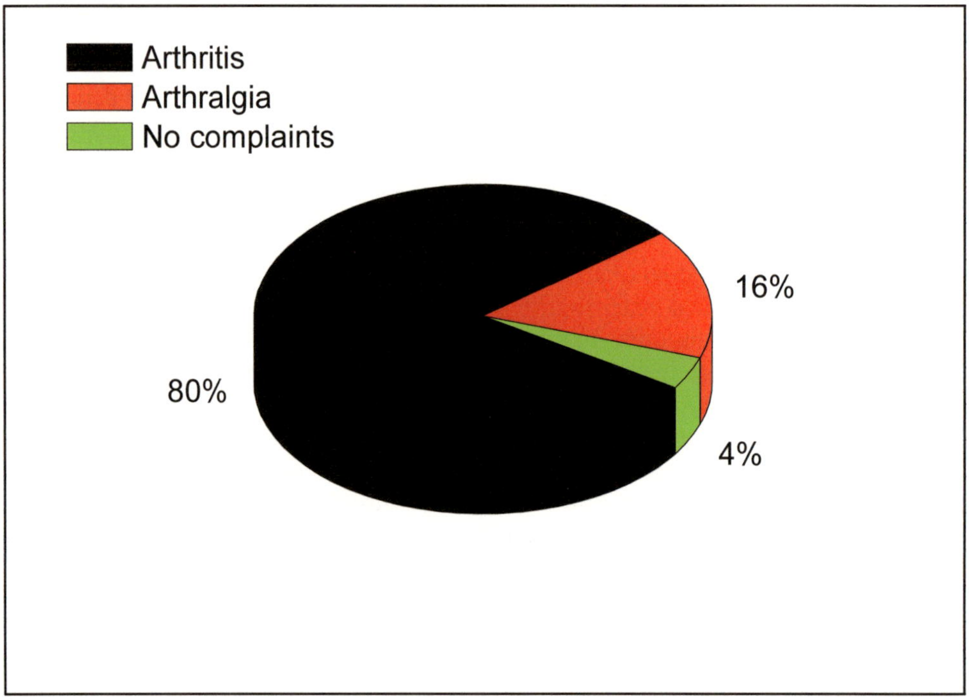

Fig. 5. Distribution of arthritis, arthralgia and no complaints in percent of GEPARD patient-questionnaire early arthritis patients (≤ 4 years). According to the CASPAR classification criteria, eighty percent were classified as having PsA.

4. How could the cooperation between dermatologist and rheumatologist be set up?

As described in the previous paragraphs screening of patients with Ps can easily be done by using the GEPARD patient self-administered questionnaire. In the case of equal or more than 4 positive answers in the questionnaire, the dermatologist may refer the patient to a cooperating rheumatologist. Since the end of the 90s most rheumatologists have set up an early arthritis schedule. With the GEPARD questionnaire the patient is already screened for arthritis and is more likely to have an arthritic manifestation. After the rheumatologic assessment the decision has to be made which discipline is advantageous to take the lead in guidance and treatment of the patient. Usually a cooperative way is chosen, taken into consideration that the general practitioner is the stearing physician for the other comorbid and social problems of the individual patient (figure 6).

In the case of leading arthritis, the consultation of the dermatologist is necessary to confirm the diagnosis of Ps by clinical means or by biopsy in unclear situations (figure 7). Furthermore, topical treatment may be instituted if systemic therapy of PsA does not lead to full treatment success of the skin. The same treatment cycle as described before is necessary in order to treat all facets of PsA.

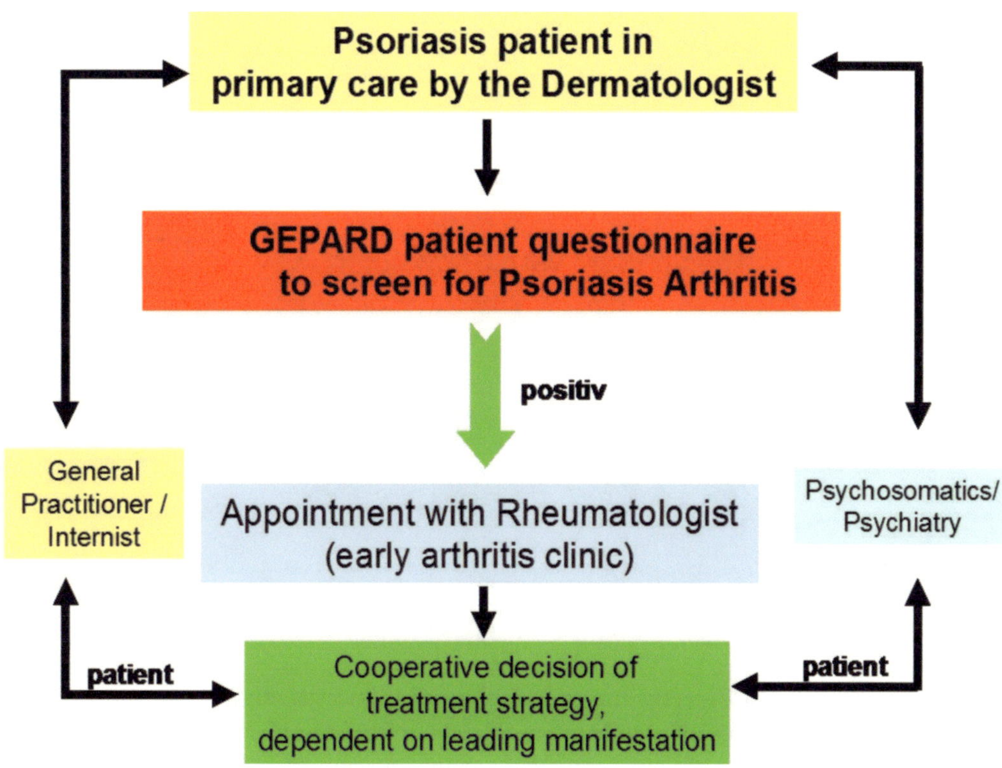

Fig. 6. Flow chart of possible cooperation among the medical disciplines. Screening starts in the dermatology practice by using the GEPARD patient self-administered questionnaire.

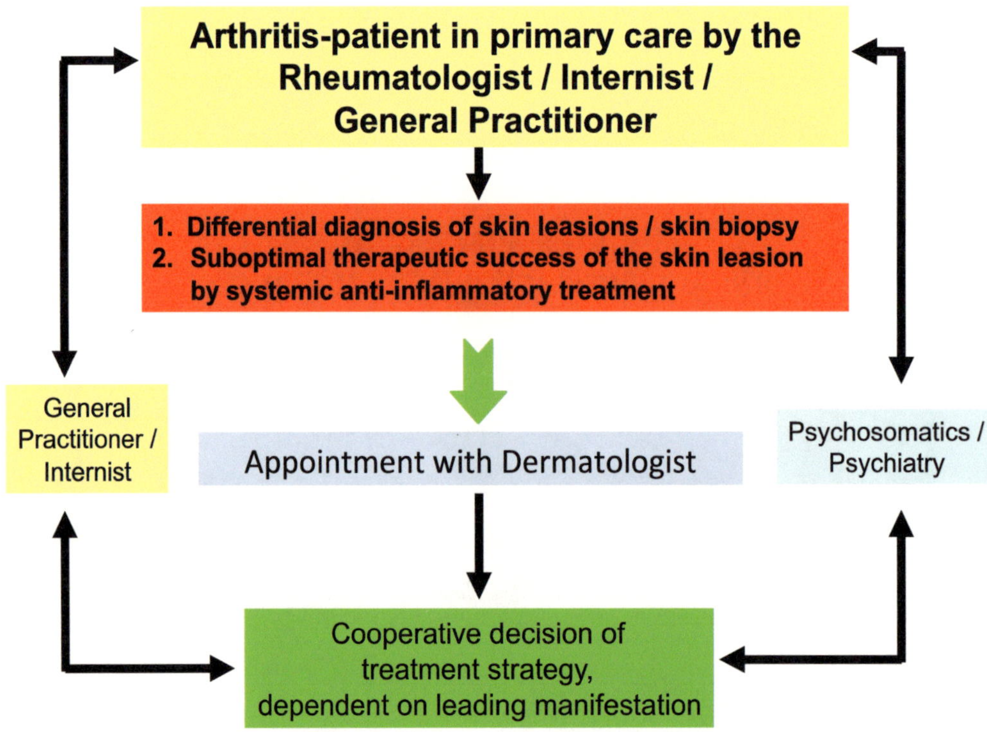

Fig. 7. Flow chart of possible cooperation among the medical disciplines. In the case of suspected psoriatic manifestation or in the case of suboptimal treatment response of Ps by systemic therapy the rheumatologist confers the patient to the dermatologist for further evaluation.

5. Summary

Considering all the many facets of PsA and the different diagnostic and therapeutic strategies is the art of modern medicine and good clinical practice. We need to understand the context of inflammatory skin, joint, and spine manifestations with mental health, extra articular problems and economical considerations. This can only be accomplished by good cooperation between dermatologist and rheumatologist in addition to the comprehensive care by the general practitioner, internist, and psychological disciplines (figure 8).

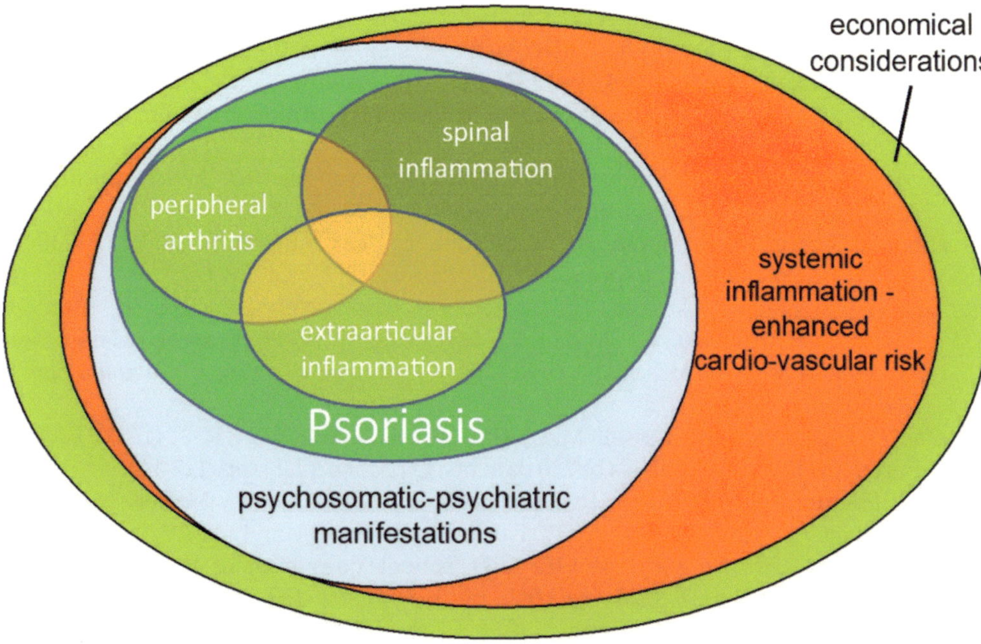

Fig. 8. Interdisciplinary, holistic view of Ps and PsA.

6. References

Aletaha, D., Neogi, T., Silman, A. J., Funovits, J., Felson, D. T., Bingham, C. O., 3rd, Birnbaum, N. S., Burmester, G. R., Bykerk, V. P., Cohen, M. D., Combe, B., Costenbader, K. H., Dougados, M., Emery, P., Ferraccioli, G., Hazes, J. M., Hobbs, K., Huizinga, T. W., Kavanaugh, A., Kay, J., Kvien, T. K., Laing, T., Mease, P., Menard, H. A., Moreland, L. W., Naden, R. L., Pincus, T., Smolen, J. S., Stanislawska-Biernat, E., Symmons, D., Tak, P. P., Upchurch, K. S., Vencovsky, J., Wolfe, F., & Hawker, G. (2010). 2010 rheumatoid arthritis classification criteria: an American College of Rheumatology/European League Against Rheumatism collaborative initiative. *Ann Rheum Dis* 69(9), pp. 1580-1588.

Aletaha, D., Smolen, J., & Ward, M. M. (2006). Measuring function in rheumatoid arthritis: Identifying reversible and irreversible components. *Arthritis Rheum* 54(9), pp. 2784-2792.

Bennet, R. M. (1979). Psoriasis Arthritis. Philadelphia, Lea & Febiger.

Blumberg, B., Bunim, J., & Calkins, E. (1964). Nomenclature and classification of arthritis and rheumatism accepted by the American Rheumatism Association. *Bull Rheum Dis* 14, pp. 339-340.

Cugno, M., Ingegnoli, F., Gualtierotti, R., & Fantini, F. (2010). Potential effect of anti-tumour necrosis factor-alpha treatment on reducing the cardiovascular risk related to rheumatoid arthritis. *Curr Vasc Pharmacol* 8(2), pp. 285-292.

de Wit, M. P., Smolen, J. S., Gossec, L., & van der Heijde, D. M. (2011). Treating rheumatoid arthritis to target: the patient version of the international recommendations. *Ann Rheum Dis* 70(6), pp. 891-895.

Devrimci-Ozguven, H., Kundakci, T. N., Kumbasar, H., & Boyvat, A. (2000). The depression, anxiety, life satisfaction and affective expression levels in psoriasis patients. *J Eur Acad Dermatol Venereol* 14(4), pp. 267-271.

Dougados, M., van der Linden, S., Juhlin, R., Huitfeldt, B., Amor, B., Calin, A., Cats, A., Dijkmans, B., Olivieri, I., Pasero, G., & et al. (1991). The European Spondylarthropathy Study Group preliminary criteria for the classification of spondylarthropathy. *Arthritis Rheum* 34(10), pp. 1218-1227.

Esposito, M., Saraceno, R., Giunta, A., Maccarone, M., & Chimenti, S. (2006). An Italian study on psoriasis and depression. *Dermatology* 212(2), pp. 123-127.

Fournie, B., Crognier, L., Arnaud, C., Zabraniecki, L., Lascaux-Lefebvre, V., Marc, V., Ginesty, E., Andrieu, V., Dromer, C., & Fournie, A. (1999). Proposed classification criteria of psoriatic arthritis. A preliminary study in 260 patients. *Rev Rhum Engl Ed* 66(10), pp. 446-456.

Gladman, D. D., Shuckett, R., Russell, M. L., Thorne, J. C., & Schachter, R. K. (1987). Psoriatic arthritis (PSA)--an analysis of 220 patients. *Q J Med* 62(238), pp. 127-141.

Härle, P., Hartung, W., Lehmann, P., Ehrenstein, B., Schneider, N., Müller, H., Müller-Ladner, U., Tarner, I., Vogt, T., Fleck, M., & Bongartz, T. (2010). [Detection of psoriasis arthritis with the GEPARD patient questionnaire in a dermatologic outpatient setting]. *Z Rheumatol* 69(2), pp. 157-160, 162-153.

Husted, J. A., Gladman, D. D., Farewell, V. T., & Cook, R. J. (2001). Health-related quality of life of patients with psoriatic arthritis: a comparison with patients with rheumatoid arthritis. *Arthritis Rheum* 45(2), pp. 151-158.

Jacobsson, L. T., Turesson, C., Gulfe, A., Kapetanovic, M. C., Petersson, I. F., Saxne, T., & Geborek, P. (2005). Treatment with tumor necrosis factor blockers is associated with a lower incidence of first cardiovascular events in patients with rheumatoid arthritis. *J Rheumatol* 32(7), pp. 1213-1218.

Kirwan, J. R. (2001). Links between radiological change, disability, and pathology in rheumatoid arthritis. *J Rheumatol* 28(4), pp. 881-886.

Machold, K. P., Eberl, G., Leeb, B. F., Nell, V., Windisch, B., & Smolen, J. S. (1998). Early arthritis therapy: rationale and current approach. *J Rheumatol Suppl* 53, pp. 13-19.

Mau, W., Listing, J., Huscher, D., Zeidler, H., & Zink, A. (2005). Employment across chronic inflammatory rheumatic diseases and comparison with the general population. *J Rheumatol* 32(4), pp. 721-728.

McGonagle, D., Conaghan, P. G., & Emery, P. (1999). Psoriatic arthritis: a unified concept twenty years on. *Arthritis Rheum* 42(6), pp. 1080-1086.

Moll, J. M., & Wright, V. (1973). Psoriatic arthritis. *Semin Arthritis Rheum* 3(1), pp. 55-78.

Neumann, E., Lefevre, S., Zimmermann, B., Gay, S., & Müller-Ladner, U. (2006). Rheumatoid arthritis progression mediated by activated synovial fibroblasts. *Trends Mol Med* 16(10), pp. 458-468.

Rahman, P., Nguyen, E., Cheung, C., Schentag, C. T., & Gladman, D. D. (2001). Comparison of radiological severity in psoriatic arthritis and rheumatoid arthritis. *J Rheumatol* 28(5), pp. 1041-1044.

Rudwaleit, M., van der Heijde, D., Landewe, R., Listing, J., Akkoc, N., Brandt, J., Braun, J., Chou, C. T., Collantes-Estevez, E., Dougados, M., Huang, F., Gu, J., Khan, M. A., Kirazli, Y., Maksymowych, W. P., Mielants, H., Sorensen, I. J., Ozgocmen, S., Roussou, E., Valle-Onate, R., Weber, U., Wei, J., & Sieper, J. (2009). The development of Assessment of SpondyloArthritis international Society classification criteria for axial spondyloarthritis (part II): validation and final selection. *Ann Rheum Dis* 68(6), pp. 777-783.

Rudwaleit, M., Van der Heijde, D., Landewé, N., Akkoc, N., Brandt, J.,Chou, C.T., Dougados, M., Huang, F., Gu, J., Kirazli, Y., Van den Bosch, F., Olivieri, I., Roussou, E., Scarpato, S., Sorensen, I.J., Valle-Onate, R., Weber, U., Wei, J., Sieper, J. (2011). The Assessment of SpondyloArthritis international Society classification criteria for peripheral spondyloarthritis and for spondyloarthritis in general. Ann Rheum Dis 70(1), pp.25-31.

Sadek, H. A., Abdel-Nasser, A. M., El-Amawy, T. A., & Hassan, S. Z. (2007). Rheumatic manifestations of psoriasis. *Clin Rheumatol* 26(4), pp. 488-498.

Schoels, M., Knevel, R., Aletaha, D., Bijlsma, J. W., Breedveld, F. C., Boumpas, D. T., Burmester, G., Combe, B., Cutolo, M., Dougados, M., Emery, P., van der Heijde, D., Huizinga, T. W., Kalden, J., Keystone, E. C., Kvien, T. K., Martin-Mola, E., Montecucco, C., de Wit, M., & Smolen, J. S. (2010). Evidence for treating rheumatoid arthritis to target: results of a systematic literature search. *Ann Rheum Dis* 69(4), pp. 638-643.

Sieper, J., Rudwaleit, M., Baraliakos, X., Brandt, J., Braun, J., Burgos-Vargas, R., Dougados, M., Hermann, K. G., Landewe, R., Maksymowych, W., & van der Heijde, D. (2009). The Assessment of SpondyloArthritis international Society (ASAS) handbook: a guide to assess spondyloarthritis. *Ann Rheum Dis* 68 Suppl 2, pp. ii1-44.

Smolen, J. S., Aletaha, D., Bijlsma, J. W., Breedveld, F. C., Boumpas, D., Burmester, G., Combe, B., Cutolo, M., de Wit, M., Dougados, M., Emery, P., Gibofsky, A., Gomez-Reino, J. J., Haraoui, B., Kalden, J., Keystone, E. C., Kvien, T. K., McInnes, I., Martin-Mola, E., Montecucco, C., Schoels, M., & van der Heijde, D. (2010). Treating rheumatoid arthritis to target: recommendations of an international task force. *Ann Rheum Dis* 69(4), pp. 631-637.

Taylor, W., Gladman, D., Helliwell, P., Marchesoni, A., Mease, P., & Mielants, H. (2006). Classification criteria for psoriatic arthritis: development of new criteria from a large international study. *Arthritis Rheum* 54(8), pp. 2665-2673.

Taylor, W. J. (2002). Epidemiology of psoriatic arthritis. *Curr Opin Rheumatol* 14(2), pp. 98-103.

Tillett, W., de-Vries, C., & McHugh, N. J. (2011). Work disability in psoriatic arthritis--a systematic review. *Rheumatology (Oxford).*

Tobin, A. M., Veale, D. J., Fitzgerald, O., Rogers, S., Collins, P., O'Shea, D., & Kirby, B. (2010). Cardiovascular disease and risk factors in patients with psoriasis and psoriatic arthritis. *J Rheumatol* 37(7), pp. 1386-1394.

van der Bijl, A. E., Goekoop-Ruiterman, Y. P., de Vries-Bouwstra, J. K., Ten Wolde, S., Han, K. H., van Krugten, M. V., Allaart, C. F., Breedveld, F. C., & Dijkmans, B. A. (2007). Infliximab and methotrexate as induction therapy in patients with early rheumatoid arthritis. *Arthritis Rheum* 56(7), pp. 2129-2134.

van Halm, V. P., Peters, M. J., Voskuyl, A. E., Boers, M., Lems, W. F., Visser, M., Stehouwer, C. D., Spijkerman, A. M., Dekker, J. M., Nijpels, G., Heine, R. J., Bouter, L. M., Smulders, Y. M., Dijkmans, B. A., & Nurmohamed, M. T. (2009). Rheumatoid arthritis versus diabetes as a risk factor for cardiovascular disease: a cross-sectional study, the CARRE Investigation. *Ann Rheum Dis* 68(9), pp. 1395-1400.

Vasey, F. E., L.R. (1984). Psoriatic arthropathy. Orlando, Grune & Stratton.
Verstappen, S. M., Jacobs, J. W., van der Veen, M. J., Heurkens, A. H., Schenk, Y., ter Borg, E. J., Blaauw, A. A., & Bijlsma, J. W. (2007). Intensive treatment with methotrexate in early rheumatoid arthritis: aiming for remission. Computer Assisted Management in Early Rheumatoid Arthritis (CAMERA, an open-label strategy trial). *Ann Rheum Dis* 66(11), pp. 1443-1449.
Verstappen, S. M., Watson, K. D., Lunt, M., McGrother, K., Symmons, D. P., & Hyrich, K. L. (2010). Working status in patients with rheumatoid arthritis, ankylosing spondylitis and psoriatic arthritis: results from the British Society for Rheumatology Biologics Register. *Rheumatology (Oxford)* 49(8), pp. 1570-1577.
Zeidler, H., & Amor, B. (2011). The Assessment in Spondyloarthritis International Society (ASAS) classification criteria for peripheral spondyloarthritis and for spondyloarthritis in general: the spondyloarthritis concept in progress. *Ann Rheum Dis* 70(1), pp. 1-3.
Zink, A., Thiele, K., Huscher, D., Listing, J., Sieper, J., Krause, A., Gromnica-Ihle, E., von Hinueber, U., Wassenberg, S., Genth, E., & Schneider, M. (2006). Healthcare and burden of disease in psoriatic arthritis. A comparison with rheumatoid arthritis and ankylosing spondylitis. *J Rheumatol* 33(1), pp. 86-90.

6

Head and Neck Psoriasis

Sebastiano Bucolo[1], Valerio Torre[2], Giuseppe Romano[3], Carmelo Quattrocchi[4], Maura Filidoro[5] and Claudio Caldarelli[1]
[1]ENT-Maxillofacial Surgery Dept., San Giovanni Bosco Hospital, Turin
[2]Dept. of Pathology, San Donato Hospital, Arezzo
[3]ENT Dept., University of Messina, Messina
[4]ENT Dept., Hospital of Milazzo, Milazzo
[5]ENT Dept, University of Genova, Genova
Italy

1. Introduction

Psoriasis is an immuno-mediated condition whose pathogenesis is still unclear and that in head and neck area presents six specific aspects that justify the title of this chapter: 1) visibility of the lesions and their impact on quality of life (QOL); 2) the very common involvement of the scalp; 3) the difficulty of the treatment; 4) the aberrant epidermal-mesenchymal interactions theory; 5) the rare mucous occurrence and the PPP-tonsil-related disease; 6) the significantly increased risk of head and neck cancer in men with Psoriasis.

2. Visibility and the impact on quality of life

Visibility of head and neck Psoriasis has a considerable impact on patients' QOL. The differential diagnosis for pustular skin disorders is extensive but facial Psoriasis more commonly affects eyebrows, the skin between the nose and the upper lip, the upper forehead and the hairline. Scalp Psoriasis is very common. Multiple instruments have been used to determine the severity of scalp Psoriasis and tools for patient self-assessment have also been developed (Psoriasis Area and Severity Index or PASI, Psoriasis Scalp Severity Index or PSSI, Body Surface Area or BSA, Physicians' Global Assessment or PGA, Lattice Physician Global Assessment or LS-PGA, and Self-assessed Psoriasis Area and Severity Index or SAPASI) but none of the severity scores used for Psoriasis meets all of the validation criteria required for an ideal score. However the PASI score is the most extensively studied (Puzenat & al, 2010).

While head represents only 10% of the whole body's surface, consequences of scalp Psoriasis are disproportionate to its extension as it can be seriously debilitating inducing important social and emotional distress.

Although it is unclear why initial scalp involvement is so common, scalp tissue has unique features that may promote its vulnerability to psoriatic lesions. For example, its high follicular density provides a dark, warm and moist environment that reduces environmental UV exposure which normally would limit lesion development. In addition, inflammation-promoting microorganisms flourish in the sebum-rich setting of the scalp and, as seen in one study, an association with the severity of scalp disease was suggested to be related to isolation of Malassezia globosa yeast from patients scalp (Gupta & al., 2004).

Additional inflammation may be triggered or exacerbated by frequent friction and trauma to the scalp (Koebner phenomenon: psoriatic lesions as consequence of trauma in psoriatic patients) from brushing or use of styling implements.

Psoriasis of the eye is extremely rare. When it does occur, it can cause inflammation, dryness and discomfort. It may cause vision impairment. When Psoriasis affects the eyelids, scales may cover lashes and topical antibiotics may be used to treat infection.

Psoriasis generally affects the external auditory canal without involvement of the ear or behind the eardrum but can cause scale buildup that can block the auditory canal with subsequent temporary hearing loss.

Rarely Psoriasis appears on the gums, the tongue, inside the cheek and the nose or on the lips. The lesions in these areas are usually white or gray and can be relatively uncomfortable as they can cause chewing and swallowing discomfort.

When Psoriasis involves the face, it can be much more disabling and can severily decrease patient's QOL. Facial Psoriasis is difficult to treat and is associated with severe cutaneous disease. In fact, patients who have a long history of Psoriasis or an early age of onset are more likely to suffer from facial involvement. Facial Psoriasis may also be associated with pruritus, psoriatic arthritis, and with a family history of Psoriasis.

Various clinical manifestations of Psoriasis make it more than a dermatological nuisance, as it interferes with many normal daily activities, such as use of hands, walking, sleeping, and sexual activity. At least 30% of patients contemplate suicide, which places Psoriasis on par with other major medical diseases such as depression, heart disease and diabetes (Krueger, 2001).

Alexithymia was originally defined as the inability to recognize and verbalize emotions. It is characterized by an emptiness of feelings, poverty of imagination or of a life fantasy and by difficulties in communicating with other peoples, as well as lack of positive emotions and a high prevalence of negative emotions. Its presence has been incriminated in genesis and maintenance of various psychosomatic pathologies.

As patient's psychological dimension seems to be related to the onset of the illness, to its evolution and to its prognosis, Psoriasis is classified among psychosomatic pathologies too.

In this perspective Alexithymia does not appear to be simply a condition related to Psoriasis, but a worsening of patient's condition, exposing him to other psychosomatic diseases and alcoholism and to a worsening of his global prognosis. That's why psychological approach in treatment favouring expression of patient's emotions and opening a symbolic dimension is as important as the biological approach and is necessary for improvement (Masmoudi, 2009).

A recent cohort study (Gelfand & al., 2011) has also shown that severe Psoriasis (defined as Psoriasis patients with a history of systemic therapy) is associated with an increased risk of mortality as male and female patients in the study died 3.5 and 4.4 years younger respectively than those without Psoriasis (even after adjustment for classical risk factors of mortality). Hence Psoriasis is a major public health problem.

The data analysis suggests that a minimum of two summary scores (one for skin and one for joints), and potentially a third for nails, are required to accurately assess severity across the full spectrum of psoriatic disease. The optimal design of such assessment tools remains the objective of many research projects, with efforts continuing to identify the most meaningful contributing elements that define the full spectrum of the psoriatic disease state (Wittkowski & al., 2011).

2.1 Addictions and Psoriasis

Association between Psoriasis and addictive disorders is a longtime suspect and several studies are supporting association of Psoriasis and alcohol, and of Psoriasis and tobacco. Association between Psoriasis and alcohol seems not to be influenced by gender and shows a dose-effect relation. The most striking link between cigarette smoking and Psoriasis has been established in Palmo-Plantar Pustulosis (PPP). This link also seems to exist for other forms of Psoriasis with a dose-effect relation.

The relationship between cigarette smoking and Psoriasis has been the subject of several studies. It was showed that cigarette smoking represents a significant risk factor for appearance of Psoriasis, especially in women, in a case about five, and it has been pointed out that risk increases with the number of cigarettes consumed per day and increases in those who smoke 20 or more daily. The risk would increase further in those who have a family history of this disease. Also for PPP seems to be a relation to cigarette smoking, with a risk factor 7.2 times higher in smokers than in non smokers. The report is based on leukocyte neutrophil counts: PPP is a neutrophilic dermatosis and cigarette smoke increases peripheral neutrophil counts and alters it in morphological and functional way.

Cigarette smoking may be involved in the high prevalence of lung and oral cancer and cardio-vascular disorders in psoriatic patients. The association between alcohol and development of plaque-type Psoriasis is complex and confusing because many of the initial studies did not control for confounding factors such as tobacco use.

There are a number of difficulties in the assessment of the correlation between Psoriasis, cigarette smoking and alcohol, and even more so in establishing a causal or etiologic relationship between the three because of several confusing factors (Meyer &al., 2008).

Alcohol-controlled studies suggest that women who are smokers have an up to 3.3-fold increased risk of developing plaque-type Psoriasis. Men who are smokers do not exhibit such an increased risk, but studies have shown that smoking more than 10 cigarettes per day by men who are Psoriasis patients may be associated with a more severe expression of disease in their extremities. In addition, smoking among both men and women who are Psoriasis patients has been shown to reduce improvement rates.

Dermatologists are not only the sentinels for early diagnosis of psoriatic arthritis, but also for metabolic complications such as dyslipidemia or diabetes. Moreover, they need to keep in mind interactions between (systemic) anti-psoriatic drugs and the co-medication of their patients as well as possible consequences of these co-medications on the course of Psoriasis (Behnam & al., 2005).

The association between Psoriasis and alcoholism represents one of the major psychodermatological issues where a multidisciplinary approach (including dermatologist, psychiatrist, psychologist and others) is crucial for optimal outcome. Psoriasis is associated with an increased risk of comorbidity and mortality compared to the general population. It appears that patients with Psoriasis have a higher prevalence of metabolic disorders such as diabetes, hypertension, obesity, and hyperlipidemia, as well as a higher frequency of cigarette smoking. These concomitant diseases can complicate the treatment of Psoriasis.

3. The very common involvement of the scalp

The estimated prevalence of Psoriasis worldwide is 0.3-5%, depending on ethnic origin (Naldi, 1994; Valdimarsson, 2007). In a retrospective analysis in children was present scalp involvement in 48% on 125 patients by Stefanaki & al. (2011) and in 50.3% on 137 patients (most common initial site affected) by Wu & al. (2010) .

Psoriasis of the scalp is estimated to occur in 40-90% of patients with Psoriasis. Up to 79% of patients with chronic plaque Psoriasis may have scalp involvement (Farber & Nall, 1992). It can be mild to severe, frequently itchy and so cosmetically embarrassing to affect patient's QOL adversely. Treatment is often prolonged for a long period of time and can be another cause of worsening of patient's QOL because of hair staining, face irritating, messy, time-consuming and cosmetically unacceptable applications prescribed.

As with Psoriasis elsewhere on the body, skin cells grow too quickly on the scalp and cause red lesions to be covered with scales. Scalp Psoriasis can be very mild with slight and fine scaling but can also be severe with thick, crusted plaques covering the entire scalp. Psoriasis can extend beyond the hairline onto the forehead, the back of the neck and around the ears.

The scalp is frequently involved in patients with Psoriasis vulgaris but rarely it is the only site affected. Lesions look like an erythematous crown with net margins covered by dry silvery-white scales. They are located at the hairline in the fronto-temporal, parietal or occipital areas (where, often, the erythematous component is more pronounced) and are associated to scaling-scratching squamous lesions. In the fronto-temporal regions, particularly in young subjects, the spots extend beyond the scalp involving the skin of the forehead and ear. In patients with a long history of scalp Psoriasis the confluence of many spots and the scant evidence of the erythematous component leads to the formation of a real shell that can cover the entire scalp. In other cases, silvery-white scales are seen on a widespread dry pityriasiform furfuracea-like desquamation, sometimes showing follicles. The spots do not produce alopecia and hairs are not incorporated by squamous heaps but in the less restrictive forms the pseudotinea amiantacea can be seen. This lesion, once considered a variant of impetigo, is characterized by the presence of small opaque white adherent scales similar to asbestos, that incorporate the proximal part of the hair shaft.

Psoriasiform lesions localized to the face often represent the extension of scalp lesions to the brow, the temporal regions, the ears and the retroauricular fold where it is observed a tendency to fissures. The involvement of the face in the course of Psoriasis is considered an index of extended or severe disease as in the case of erythrodermic Psoriasis. Rarely small droplike lesion in the face can be seen in case of eruptive Psoriasis; in case of mild forms of Psoriasis Vulgaris (minimal Psoriasis) instead, the eyelid involvement by small patches of whitish scales is characteristic. Psoriasis of the ear is characterized not only by the involvement of the auricle but also by the involvement of external auditory canal by heaps of scales that can stamp it. Diagnosis of SeboPsoriasis, that is characterised by the presence of yellowish-white unctuous scales can be put when psoriasiform lesions are localized exclusively in seborrheic areas of the face (naso-labial fold, glabella and eyebrows, auricle and retroauricular fold) and are associated with similar lesions of the hairline and the presternal area. This clinic form, on the border between Psoriasis Vulgaris and Seborrheic Dermatitis, is considered a Psoriasis arisen on patches of Seborrheic Dermatitis because of the Koebner phenomenon.

Family history may predispose patients to scalp Psoriasis. In an analysis of Psoriasis genes in an Icelandic patient population, 296 of 1,000 Psoriasis patients experienced onset of Psoriasis on the scalp. Cluster analysis (Karason & al., 2005) of this subset of patients determined that 198 patients fit within 79 families and determined a linkage to chromosome 10. The familial nature of Psoriasis has long been recognized with evident intra and interfamilial variability. Thirty nine individual with Psoriasis (25 men and 14 women) from 9 Tunisian unrelated multiplex families (in Tunisian population the estimated prevalence of Psoriasis is of 3%) were investigated during a study period of 1 year (Ammar & al., 2009). The common form of Psoriasis was discovered in 37 cases. The nails, the scalp, the mucous membranes were involved respectively in 21, 12 and 13 cases. The Psoriasis was severe in 11 cases.

Methods used to diagnose scalp Psoriasis vary in sensitivity, reproducibility, and invasiveness. Recently has been introduced a videodermoscopy scalp Psoriasis severity index (VSCAPSI) for evaluation of scalp Psoriasis (Rossi &al., 2011). This index is particularly useful in mild and moderate forms that often are not clinically appreciable. VSCAPSI takes into account extension of the area of the scalp affected, the presence and morphology of vascular patterns, erythema and desquamation. Videodermoscopy images obtained between November 2009 to June 2010 from 900 participants with various scalp and hair disorders were reviewed for distinguishing features. During the 2010 Italian congress on Psoriasis, in order to assess the reproducibility and efficacy of the VSCAPSI, 146 dermatologists were asked to evaluate 16 videodermoscopy images of scalp Psoriasis using the VSCAPSI. Of the 900 patients, 85 new cases of scalp Psoriasis were diagnosed. The other 815 patients were found to be suffering from different scalp and hair diseases. Of 146 dermatologists, 28 did not recognize erythema, 15 desquamation and 7 the vascular patterns. The VSCAPSI provides an important tool for early diagnosis, differential diagnosis and follow-up and screening.

3.1 Histology of head and neck Psoriasis: Gross findings

Head and neck Psoriasis (in the form of the so-called Psoriasis vulgaris or plaque type of Psoriasis and guttate Psoriasis) commonly involves the skin surface of the scalp and the face (eyebrow, nose, upper lip, forehead, and hairline) and presents as papules, well-demarcated erythematous plaques with a scaly surface or as papulo-squamous lesions covered by fine silvery-white and loosely adherent scales. The amount and thickness of the scales is variable such are the plaques, ranging in size from few to several centimeters, with coalescence of smaller plaques into larger and sometimes fissured lesions. On the other hand, less thick plaques and less scaly lesions are commonly encountered in children with face psoriatic localization compared with adults. Pustular forms of Psoriasis are rarely described on the face as annular or circinnate and pustular lesions on an erythematous background with an acute, subacute or chronic clinical course. Pustular eruptions are frequently associated with a classic form of skin Psoriasis, and both hair loss and involvement of tongue mucosal surface may be appreciated. Oral localizations, less commonly observed in children than in adults, appear as pustular and hyperemic lesions within a geographic and fissured tongue. In such a localization, infections, smoking and physical agents all may affect the course and duration of Psoriasis and may cause dysphagia. Unusual mucosal (nose, oral cavity) or ocular localizations are commonly described in patients with otherwise usual skin psoriatic dermatitis. Mucosal lesions show a non-specific macroscopic appearance ranging from erythematous and slightly raised lesions to a white annular, serpiginous and ulcerated pattern that may disappear quickly, with no obvious clinical symptoms, or may have exacerbations and remissions similar to skin lesions. Pustular forms, mixed white and erythematous lesions, ulcerative, vescicular and indurated lesions, multiple annular coin-sized lesions, gray, yellowish, translucent and silvery-white forms are described with macroscopic findings similar to several so-called psoriasiform benign and malignant conditions involving the oral cavity. In this setting, the diagnosis mainly rely on an interdisciplinary clinical and histological approach with a crucial role played by the microscopic findings on mucosal biopsy. Psoriasis vulgaris may also be associated to oral localizations such as the case of geographic tongue and the stomatitis areata migrans. Patients with Psoriasis rarely develop uncommon ocular manifestations such as uveitis, blepharitis and conjunctivitis as a result of changes, alterations and dysfunctions of conjunctival surface, tear film and meibomiam gland changes.

3.2 Microscopic findings

Variabilities in clinical macroscopic findings of Psoriasis reflect different histologic pictures with relation to the stage of the disease. Generally, early stages show more typical and pathognomonic microscopic clues to the diagnosis than that of the advanced and fully developed lesions. Moreover, histologic differences could also be noted in psoriatic lesions affecting mucosal surfaces.

In its classic histologic appearance, cutaneous Psoriasis shows achantosis (thickened of epidermal layers) and parakeratosis (retention of cell nuclei in stratum corneum) of the epidermis, with thin or loss of granular cell layer, downward elongation of rete ridges and thinning of the epidermis overlying the dermal papillae that shows edema and small vessels close to the epidermis. The latter condition underlies the so-called Auspitz sign: when the silvery scales (parakeratotic layers) are removed from the plaque (epidermal achantosis), small pinpoint bleeding (from dermal capillaries) is seen.

The inflammatory cutaneous infiltrate of Psoriasis is characterized by neutrophils and lymphocytes throughout the superficial papillary dermis. Activated CD3+ T cells are mainly observed around small papillary vessels and are admixed with neutrophils and macrophages. Neutrophils and lymphocytes can migrate upwards from the dermis to the epidermis and in parakeratotic layers (exocytosis). Collections of intraepithelial neutrophils (Munro abscesses) and those arranged in the epidermis in a network of degenerated keratinocytes (spongiform pustule of Kogoj) are characteristics of Psoriasis but not always present nor specific to the disease.

In the pustular form of Psoriasis, such a collection of neutrophils occurs as characteristic macropustules (abscesses), while epidermal and dermal changes are similar to those seen in Psoriasis vulgaris. The so-called eruptive or guttate Psoriasis, with small and numerous red papules and an acute onset on clinical examination, shows similar microscopic findings to that of early Psoriasis vulgaris lesions unless the same degree of achantosis.

Mucosal localizations show a more variable histological presentation ranging from classic hyperparakeratotic lesions, with thinning of the suprapapillary plate and mixed inflammatory infiltrate with neutrophils exocytosis to mild and quickly self-limited erythematous inflammatory conditions with capillaries engorgement but without microabscess formation. Similar microscopic characteristic are shared by different inflammatory mucosal diseases generally known as psoriasiform mucositis or psoriasiform lesions. In such instances, histological distinction between Psoriasis and other inflammatory mucosal entities cannot be made with confidence unless mucosal lesions are associated to or are coincident with cutaneous psoriatic dermatitis and additional data (family history, HLA typing) are available.

3.3 Differential diagnosis

Although the diagnosis of Psoriasis mainly rely on clinical settings, histological evaluation should be used to confirm the diagnosis as well as to evaluate unusual clinical lesions and to exclude benign and malignant conditions that may mimic Psoriasis or may be associated to it.

On the other hand, microscopic findings alone should pose problems in differential diagnosis with other inflammatory disorders as well as in the evaluation of the phase of Psoriasis normally evolving through early, advanced and later lesions with a different microscopic variability with lesion's age and activity.

Skin psoriatic manifestations should sometimes require a differential diagnosis from dermatoses such as lichen planopilaris, florid seborrheic dermatitis and discoid lupus erythematosus.

On the other hand, differential diagnosis of oral localization of Psoriasis could also consider Reiter's syndrome, erythema migrans, benign migratory glossitis, oral lichen planus and other inflammatory conditions generally described as psoriasiform lesions.

Clinical data alone may be inadequate such as the case of Koebner phenomenon that could be present in lichen planus.

In this settings, the macroscopic characteristics of cutaneous psoriatic lesions (well defined elevated lesions, with silvery-white or micaceous scale), the clinical data (symmetrical distribution, Auspitz sign, patient's history reporting itchy, skin scaling and peeling, lesions at site of injury or trauma) and the classic histologic findings may all contribute to a definitive diagnosis of Psoriasis.

Oral lichen planus, mainly occurring in adults, appears as bilateral plaques, papules and erythematous-atrophic or ulcerated lesions on the oral mucosa, gingivae (desquamative gingivitis) and tongue. Oral white striations (so-called Wickham striae) may coincide with cutaneous lesions on the scalp, laryngeal and esophageal mucosa or less frequent conjunctival lesions. Skin involvement of the scalp (lichen plano-pilaris) appears as scarring alopecia and violaceous and erythematous papules with hair loss. On histologic examination, more irregular acanthosis, prominent granular cell layer and dense sub-epithelial T-cell CD8+ inflammatory infiltrate along with damage of basal keratinocytes represent clues to the diagnosis in contrast to Psoriasis. Moreover, since patients with oral lichen planus could develop oral squamous cell carcinoma and commonly show a significant local morbidity with negative impact on QOL, a proper diagnosis based on clinical and histological findings is mandatory.

Discoid lupus erythematosus may sometimes be responsible for unusual manifestations in head and neck localizations that can mimic several skin diseases (Psoriasis, acne rosacea, lichen planopilaris) or be associated with liken planus-like lesions and Psoriasis. Nonetheless, clinical findings are usually characteristic as erythematous papules and plaques that progress to scaling lesions with pigmentary changes (central hypopigmentation and peripheral hyperpigmentation) in a centrifugal spread. Cutaneous scalp lesions may result in permanent alopecia with atrophy and scarring (localized form of discoid lupus erythematosus) with histologic picture similar to that of lichen planopilaris. Rare mucosal involvement are described with clinical and microscopic characteristic that may simulate lichen planus lesions. In this setting, laboratory data (hematologic and serologic abnormalities frequently observed in widespread discoid lupus erythematosus) along with meticulous clinical attention and microscopic findings (essentially dependent on familiarity with these lesions) can pose a correct diagnosis.

Psoriatic lesions may also not look much different from those caused by seborrheic dermatitis, a papulo-squamous disease of the scalp, face and trunk. In its facial localization, the disease may be associated with squamous blepharitis, a chronic inflammation of the lid margins with small white scales accumulated among the lashes, or may present as mild scaling to widespread crust adherent to the skin of the scalp, forehead, neck and postauricolar skin. Secondary infections may occur as eczematoid dermatitis. Microscopic picture shows a more irregular acanthosis than that seen in psoriatic lesions along with spongiosis and follicular ostia involvement.

The guttate variety of Psoriasis may appears as an acute exanthema in young adults, often associated to streptococcal pharyngitis, with papules on the face similar to those seen in psoriasiform drug eruption. The latter condition is also known as localized drug reactions related to medications and usually involving the face, chest and back with a papulo-erythematous or vescicular and pustular appearance. Similarly, psychogenic and emotional factors, infections and environmental factors may all contribute to the development of cutaneous lesions similar to those seen in Psoriasis or may be related to increase in Psoriasis activity and severity.

Histologic overlapping in such cases, with lacking of microscopic characteristic features, require a correct clinical evaluation in the differential diagnosis of these conditions.

Differential diagnosis of head and neck Psoriasis, in both cutaneous and mucosal localizations, should also consider preneoplastic and neoplastic conditions. Since head and neck Psoriasis is more often a chronic and long standing process, frequently associated with severe cutaneous disease and difficult treatment, a significant risk of cancer has been noted. Such an association could be related to the reactive epidermal hyperproliferation seen in psoriatic lesions along with keratinocytes activation and expression of molecules involved in cell proliferation. In particular, basal cell and squamous cell carcinomas are frequently reported and should be taken into account when evaluating psoriatic patients.

Moreover, malignant conditions should be ruled out as is the case of the rare acrokeratosis paraneoplastica (Bazex syndrome). The disease can be associated with head and neck and upper aerodigestive tract squamous cell carcinomas and differs from Psoriasis in its localizations (erythematous squamous plaques or scaly patches of earlobes, helices and tip of the nose along with similar lesions in the extremities and nail dystrophy) and lack of histological findings typical of Psoriasis.

Investigators use several physical examination measures to assess clinical features and severity of Psoriasis and psoriatic arthritis (PsA) in clinical trials, clinical registries, and clinical practice; however, no relevant training modules are widely available to teach and standardize the performance of these measures. At a GRAPPA (Group for Research and Assessment of Psoriasis and Psoriatic Arthritis) meeting adjacent to the 2009 International Federation of Psoriasis Associations in Stockholm, members were updated on the development status of online training videos of Psoriasis and PsA examination measures. Dermatology assessment modules include the PASI, the PGA, the BSA, the original and modified Nail Psoriasis Severity Index (NPSI), the Palmar-Plantar Pustular Psoriasis Area and Severity Index (PPP-PASI), and the PSSI. Rheumatology modules include assessment of tender and swollen joint counts used in the American College of Rheumatology criteria, Disease Activity Score, and other composite arthritis scores; enthesitis assessment used in various enthesitis scoring systems; dactylitis; and spine disease. Each module will include background information for each measure, diagrams and photographs to emphasize teaching points, demonstration video of examination where applicable, and an optional examination at the end. Future plans include evaluating the modules for their influence on interrater and intrarater reliability and development of additional modules (Callis Duffin & Mease, 2011).

4. The difficulty of the treatment

Head and neck Psoriasis treatment is still a challenge because its difficult to get topical agents through hair to be absorbed by the scalp. In fact, scalp is not susceptible to many topical Psoriasis treatment or phototherapy because hair prevent adequate contact with the affected tissue. Moreover current therapies can only bring some relief to the symptoms without any cure to the disease and treatments can carry important side effects in face of high therapeutic costs.

Medications for scalp Psoriasis include those to be left on the scalp and wash off products. Left on products are gels, lotions and ointments containing steroids, coal tar, salicylic acid or vitamin D analogs.

Wash off products are shampoos containing coal tar, salicylic acid, sulfur, selenium, ketoconazole or zinc pyrithione. Recently, Handa (2010) proposed a treatment algorithm for scalp Psoriasis (see Tab. 1), dividing a first line and a second line therapies.

In 2009 van de Kerkhof & al. divided treatment of scalp Psoriasis into four phases. First phase involves descaling using salicylic acid or urea preparations. The second phase is the clearing phase in which topical corticosteroids, vitamin D analogs, tar, dithranol, antifungal treatment, ultraviolet B light therapy or systemic treatment are used. The third phase is stabilization using a steroid-sparing vitamin D analog during the week and a super potent topical corticosteroid at weekends. Finally, the fourth phase is maintenance, using a vitamin D analog alone or with a tar shampoo.

First line therapies
Salicylic acid/Urea
Topical corticosteroids (short term use)
Calcipotriol
Dithranol/Anthralin
Coal tar (Shampoo/pomade)
Tazarotene
Combination therapies
Second line therapies (for recalcitrant or severe disease)
Phototherapy
Systemic drugs (Methotrexate, Acitretin, Cyclosporine)
Biologics

Table 1. Treatment algorithm for scalp Psoriasis (from Hanna S., 2010)

4.1 Corticosteroids

Topical corticosteroids are the recommended first-line therapy for short-term use. Response to treatment is quick but high potential for side effects, such as atrophy, striae, telangiectasias and tachyphylaxis, limits the period of use. These side effects are virtually never seen in the scalp. Use of potent steroids (twice a day) should be limited to 4 weeks. The choice of preparation such as ointment, cream, gel, lotion, foam, spray or shampoo should be patient oriented.

In any single patient the lowest strength preparation that allows clinical clearing should be used for the shortest time, in order to minimize side effects and tachyphylaxis. Nevertheless, long-term use of mid-potency preparations or intermittent use of potent steroids is more commonly practiced by physicians. Clobetasol propionate (CP) 0.05% and betamethasone dipropionate 0.05% are the most potent topical corticosteroid preparations currently used. Exceptionally intralesional corticosteroids can be used for one or two localized patches not responding to topical steroids. Foam vehicles are the new alternatives to traditional topical preparations because of the advantage of minimal residue and increased ease of application. They are absorbed more rapidly, have a higher bioavailability, are not associated with suppression of the hypothalamic pituitary adrenal (HPA) axis and once-daily administration has been seen to be as effective as twice daily administration. They are also associated with better patient compliance. CP foam 0.05% is generally as effective as CP solution for scalp Psoriasis and may produce superior results against scaling. Dose is limited to 50 g/week. Mid-potency corticosteroid betamethasone valerate (BMV) has also become available in a new thermolabile, low-residue foam vehicle, BMV 0.12% foam. In a recent study BMV foam produced greater improvement in the primary signs of scalp Psoriasis than BMV lotion, placebo or other standard topical therapies (Stein, 2005). Shampoo preparations are another new development. When clobetasol shampoo 0.05% was tried in a patient experience program, 50% of the patients said that the shampoo was easy to use and did not interfere with their daily routine. Almost 90% of patients found the shampoo better than other prescriptions they had used before for their scalp Psoriasis.

Medication used to treat facial Psoriasis should be applied carefully and sparingly; creams and ointments can irritate eyes. Because facial skin is delicate, prolonged use of steroids may cause it to become thin, shiny and/or prone to enlarged capillaries. Treatment with steroids is safe if a careful treatment schedule is followed.

4.2 Non steroidal topical preparations

This group includes: Calcipotriene/calcipotriol, Anthralin, Coal Tar, Tazarotene.

4.2.1 Calcipotriene/calcipotriol

These are vitamin D 3 derivatives used for chronic, moderately/severe Psoriasis of the scalp. The 0.005% solution is applied to the affected area and rubbed gently onto the scalp twice a day. Response to therapy takes about 8 weeks. It is not recommended in patients with acute psoriatic eruptions on the scalp, those with hypercalcemia or hypervitaminosis D. The main side effects are burning, itching, irritation and dryness. Irritation tends to decrease with time. Clearance has been observed even with 8 weeks of once a day treatment in up to 60% of patients.

4.2.2 Anthralin

Anthralin 0.1-3% cream has been used for long-term treatment of scalp Psoriasis. Concentration should be gradually increased according to body response and tolerance of the patient. Anthralin is applied in a thin layer to the psoriatic area once a day, rubbed in well and left on the scalp for 5-10 minutes before washing with a shampoo and rinsing well. It is not used for acutely inflamed scalp Psoriasis. Redness or irritation of the treated scalp is common. Anthralin may temporarily stain the fingernails, gray/white hair, skin and fabrics. Caution is advised in patients having history of allergy to anthralin or to condoms (e.g., parabens).

4.2.3 Coal tar

Coal tar is an effective and cheap treatment modality for scalp Psoriasis but staining and an acrid smell associated with its use may have an important impact on patients QOL. Topical tar solution (liquor picis carbonis-LPC, or liquor carbonis detergens-LCD) is widely available and commonly used for scalp Psoriasis. Newer preparations specifically meant for scalp include coconut oil compound ointment (coal tar solution with precipitated sulfur, salicylic acid, coconut oil, yellow soft paraffin and emulsifying wax) and tar pomades (contain LCD, Tween 20 and salicylic acid in a hydrophilic ointment). Compound ointment should be applied once at night and washed off the next morning with a coal tar shampoo. Coal tar shampoos contain 1-20% coal tar extract. They are used twice a week. A tar blend 1% shampoo Polytar (Steifel, Johannesburg, South Africa) is made of coal tar, juniper tar (cade oil) and pine tar. In a comparative 4-week study of tar blend 1% shampoo (Polytar) and CP 0.05% shampoo (Clobex, Galderma, Ft. Worth, USA), the corticosteroid shampoo was significantly more effective and showed a better patient's compliance too.

Coal tar has been a very popular traditional treatment for various types of Psoriasis for over a century and still it's the first-line treatment for scalp, hand, and foot Psoriasis. However, application of coal tar on hair invariably causes staining, which results in a high degree of patient non-compliance, especially in patients with non-black hair. Thus, treatment of scalp Psoriasis with a topical coal tar formulation requires that special concern to be paid to product esthetics. A novel lecithinized coal tar (LCT) formulation seems to be less likely to stain hair and thus has excellent potential to be exploited in treatment of scalp Psoriasis (Bhatia & al. 2011).

4.2.4 Tazarotene

There are no controlled studies on the use of tazarotene in scalp Psoriasis. Response to tazarotene (0.1%) compared to topical calcipotriol or steroids is less effective but relapse rates are reported to be minor as well. Dryness and irritation are common side effects.

4.3 Combination therapies

Combining different treatment allows enhanced efficacy and minimizes toxicity. Corticosteroids, when combined with vitamin D analogs, require a minor total amount of dose and induce less skin irritation. In treatment of moderate to severe plaque Psoriasis of the scalp, the fixed-combination suspension containing betamethasone 0.05% and calcipotriene 0.005% is used once a day. In a randomized double-blind controlled trial over 8 weeks, 71.2% patients achieved "absent" or "very mild" disease with the two-compound scalp formulation, compared to 64% treated with betamethasone dipropionate, 36.8% with calcipotriene and only 22.8% with the vehicle alone. Pruritus was the only adverse event reported.

Topical steroids with Puvasol gave better results: 37.3% clearance versus 13.3% with Puvasol alone. LPC 10% along with 2% salicylic acid in a cream base along with Puvasol for 8 weeks gave a much better clearance rate than Puvasol alone. Tazarotene has also been found to be efficacious in combination with topical steroids and calcipotriol.

In a prospective non-interventional trial in German dermatological practices, 721 patients with scalp Psoriasis received Xamiol(®) gel (calcipotriol 50 µg/g, betamethasone 0,5 mg/g) topically for 4 weeks. Severity was assessed by physician's global assessment (PGA) and QOL was assessed by using a scalp-specific questionnaire at the beginning of the study and after 4 weeks treatment. The mean disease severity of scalp Psoriasis (PGA) improved from 4.26 to 2.49 (-41.8 %, $p < 0.0001$) during 4 weeks treatment and QOL improved from 10.57 to 3.22 (-69.5 %, $p < 0.0001$). Among patients with pre-treatment 89.5% of patients and 87.9% of dermatologists judged treatment response to Xamiol(®) gel as better/much better compared to previous therapy. Tolerability of Xamiol(®) gel was rated good/very good by 98 % of dermatologists and patients, respectively. The use of Xamiol(®) gel was found easy/very easy by 90.4 % of the patients (Mrowietz, 2011).

McCormack (2001) reviewed the efficacy and tolerability of calcipotriol/betamethasone dipropionate in patients with Psoriasis vulgaris summarizing its pharmacological properties. Calcipotriol/betamethasone dipropionate showed low systemic absorption and displayed local anti-inflammatory and immunoregulatory properties. It reduced hyperproliferation of keratinocytes and helped normalize keratinocyte differentiation. In large, well designed clinical trials, calcipotriol/betamethasone dipropionate, either as the ointment or the gel formulation, applied once a day for 4-8 weeks, was more effective than placebo, calcipotriol and tacalcitol, as well as betamethasone dipropionate in most instances, for the topical, symptomatic treatment of Psoriasis vulgaris of the trunk/limbs. Likewise, calcipotriol/betamethasone dipropionate gel applied once daily for 8 weeks was more effective than placebo or either component alone in the topical, symptomatic treatment of Psoriasis vulgaris of the scalp. Long-term, once a day, when required therapy with calcipotriol/betamethasone dipropionate for 52 weeks was more effective than calcipotriol alone for the treatment of scalp Psoriasis and was at least as effective as switching to calcipotriol for 48 weeks after 4 weeks of calcipotriol/betamethasone dipropionate or alternating between calcipotriol/betamethasone dipropionate and calcipotriol every 4 weeks for 52 weeks in the treatment of Psoriasis vulgaris of the trunk/limbs. Calcipotriol/betamethasone dipropionate also improved health-related QOL.

Calcipotriol/betamethasone dipropionate was generally well tolerated, with most adverse drug reactions being lesional or perilesional effects of mild or moderate severity (see Fig. 1).

Calcipotriol/betamethasone dipropionate was often associated with fewer lesional/ perilesional adverse reactions than calcipotriol or tacalcitol and did not appear to be

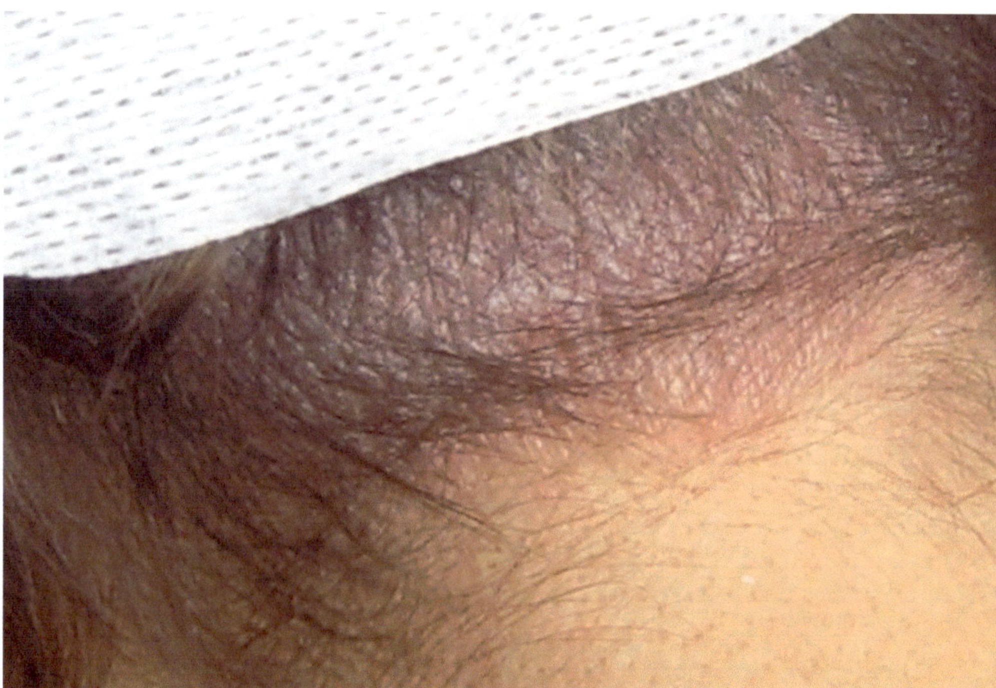

Fig. 1. Scalp Psoriasis after treatment with calcipotriol/betamethasone dipropionate gel formulation , applied once daily for 4 weeks.

associated with a higher incidence of corticosteroid-related adverse events during long-term therapy. Pharmaco-economic analyses predicted calcipotriol/betamethasone dipropionate to be more cost effective than other topical therapies.

Puig & al. (2010) reported the recommendations developed by an expert panel using the Delphi process to reach a consensus and then ratified by the members of the Psoriasis Group of the Spanish Academy of Dermatology and Venereology. The recommended induction therapy for scalp Psoriasis is either a topical corticosteroid or a topical treatment combining calcipotriol and betamethasone. The choice of an appropriate vehicle is crucial in improving effectiveness and patient adherence to treatment. The only formulations that have been studied in long-term treatment of scalp Psoriasis are a combination of calcipotriol and betamethasone in gel and calcipotriol alone in solution.

4.4 Second line treatments for recalcitrant disease

These are used when all topical treatments fail. No controlled studies exist regarding their use and include phototherapy and systemic drugs like methotrexate, retinoids, cyclosporine and biologics. They are used based on physician experience, choice and risk versus benefit ratio.

4.4.1 Phototherapy

Hair blocks adequate penetration of ultraviolet light. Better results are achieved with conventional UV units, if hair is parted in many rows or if the patient has thin hair or if the head is shaved. Hand-held devices (UV combs) deliver a higher intensity of UV light. There are reports of the use of targeted phototherapy with excimer laser which provides narrowband ultraviolet B (NB-UVB) (308 nm) phototherapy with a very high irradiance, allowing for a shorter treatment time.

4.4.2 Biologics

The emergence of biologic therapies as an effective modality for treatment of plaque Psoriasis may provide another option for patients. The biological agents employed in therapy of Psoriasis are classified into three groups (see Tab. 2).

Inhibitors of tumor necrosis factor-α
Adalimumab
Certolizumab
Etanercept
Golimumab
Infliximab
Inhibitors of Interleukin-12 and Interleukin-23
Ustekinumab
Briakinumab
T-cell modulating agents
Alefacept
Efalizumab

Table 2. Biological agents employed in scalp Psoriasis.

Recent findings suggest that Efalizumab may be effective for treatment of head and neck Psoriasis (Krell & al., 2008). Katsambas (2009) recorded a PSSI score for 1150 patients at baseline and by week 12; there had been a median improvement in PSSI score of 73.3% (IQR 33.3–94.3) compared with baseline. At week 12, PSSI 50 and PSSI 75 responses were achieved by 62.4% (718/1150) and 44.7% (514/1150) of patients, respectively. In many cases, a response to Efalizumab was apparent early in treatment, with over half of the patients classified as PSSI 50 responders at week 12 having already achieved this response by week 4 (n = 425).

However, Efalizumab has now been recommended for withdrawal in European market due to adverse effects. European Medicines Agency evaluated all safety data in light of post-marketing surveillance of patients with Psoriasis receiving Efalizumab continuously for more than 3 years that showed opportunistic infections and, in particular, cases of JC virus infection (polyomavirus) resulting in progressive multifocal leucoencephalopathy (PML). It was concluded that the benefits of Efalizumab treatment no longer outweighed the risks associated with the drug and was recommended suspension of marketing authorization on 19 February 2009. The drug has also been voluntarily withdrawn from the US market.

Adalimumab, a monoclonal humanized tumor necrosis factor alpha inhibitor proved to be successful in treatment of severe facial Psoriasis (Noiles & Vender, 2008).

Accumulating evidence supports efficacy and safety of ustekinumab for treatment of moderate to severe Psoriasis. There is some suggestion from head-to-head comparisons that ustekinumab may offer some advantage over TNF-α inhibitors. However, there is a need for larger and longer-term studies to assess the safety profile, cost-effectiveness and advantages of anti-interleukin 12 and 23 activity in the modern era of biological therapy (Garcia-Valladares & al., 2011).

4.5 Miscellaneous agents

Salicylic acid 5-10% is combined with other topical therapies as a keratolytic. Many topical treatments do not work well until thick scales that reduce drug penetration are removed. Urea 10% and lactic acid 10% have been used as scalp moisturizers. In resistant cases topical imidazole derivatives are used to control the overgrowth of Pityrosporum in scalp Psoriasis.

Kircik (2011) stated that Salicylic acid 6% emollient foam provides a useful option that is highly effective, well tolerated and acceptable to patients. Efficacy, tolerability and patient acceptability of salicylic acid 6% emollient foam were assessed in an open-label pilot study of 10 subjects with scalp Psoriasis. All Psoriasis severity parameters were reduced with a significant decrease in PSSI score from 15.3 to 3.0 after four weeks of monotherapy ($P<0.001$). Sixty percent of subjects were either "completely cleared" or "almost cleared" from their Psoriasis. No adverse events were reported.

Psoriasis skin lesions can be secondarily infected with bacteria according with Brook (Brook & al., 1999). In this report the predominant aerobic and facultative bacteria were S. aureus, group D Enterococcus and Escherichia coli while the predominant anaerobes were Peptostreptococcus spp. and Bacteroides spp., Propionibacterium acnes and pigmented Prevotella spp. in two each. Nineteen of the micro-organisms isolated from 78% patients produced lactamase.

The U.S. Food and Drug Administration (FDA) has approved two drugs, Protopic and Elidel, for treatment of eczema which many dermatologists have found to work well in treating Psoriasis of the face or of other sensitive areas.

5. The aberrant epidermal-mesenchymal interactions theory

The normal adult epidermis is a self-renewing tissue consisting of 10 to 20 layers in which cell proliferation is primarily restricted to the basal layer. Orthokeratinized epithelium similar to that in skin is seen in the hard palate, whereas other regions are either parakeratinized (gingiva) or nonkeratinized (buccal mucosa) (Squier & al., 1976). Injury to the epidermis activates a homeostatic response resulting in inflammation, re-epithelialization, followed by tissue remodelling (Martin, 1997). Several studies have suggested release of interleukin-1 from keratinocytes at the wound site as the initial trigger for the inflammatory reaction. This serves as an autocrine signal to surrounding keratinocytes and paracrine signal to other cells, such as fibroblasts, endothelial cells, and lymphocytes resulting in a pleiotropic effect on them (Freedberg & al., 2001). The changes in gene expression that accompany re-epithelialization are similar to those seen in other disorders associated with hyperproliferation such as Psoriasis, contact dermatitis, and squamous cell carcinoma (SCC) suggesting considerable overlap in the signaling cascades. The development of a normal scar is dependent on the reversal of expression of these genes at the wound site. However, in some cases the inflammatory and proliferative signals persist even after wound closure resulting in pathological scars, such as hypertrophic (HTS) and keloid scars. Although most previous studies have considered these scars as dermal phenomena (Akagi & al., 1999), others have identified abnormalities associated with epidermal keratinocytes in HTS perhaps as a result of aberrant epidermal-mesenchymal interaction (Niessen & al., 2001). One of the most sensitive biochemical markers of terminal differentiation in keratinocytes is the keratin protein family that constitutes the major cytoskeletal architecture of all epithelia. In humans, the family consists of 30 polypeptides (including trichocytic keratins of hair and nail) that are divided into two types; type I is acidic and includes K9 to K20; type II is basic/neutral and includes K1 to K8. The normal expression of K2e in the upper spinous and granular layers of interfollicular epidermis is increased in keloid scars but showed distinct down-regulation in Psoriasis and hypertrophic scars where keratinocytes are known to undergo activation. Unlike normal and psoriatic skin, K2e expression in hypertrophic and keloid scars began in the deepest suprabasal layer. In cutaneous basal and squamous cell carcinomas, K2e was absent in most tumor islands but the overlying epidermis showed strong expression. In mild-to-moderate oral dysplasia with orthokeratinization, K2e was highly expressed compared with parakeratinized areas but in severe dysplasia as well as in oral squamous cell carcinoma, K2e expression was undetectable. Taken together, the data suggest that K2e expression in skin is sensitive to keratinocyte activation but its up-regulation in oral lesions is a reflection of the degree of orthokeratinization (Bloor & al., 2003). K 15 protein and mRNA are primarily located in the basal keratinocytes of stratified tissues (Waseem al., 1999) and the k 15 gene is upregulated in human subjects where both alleles for k 14 have beeen inactivated. In hyperproliferating epidermis, such as in Psoriasis, K 15 expression, both protein and mRNA, is downregulated, suggesting that K 15 expression may not be compatible with the activated phenotype.

6. The rare mucous occurrence and the PPP-tonsil-related disease

6.1 Mucous membrane localization

The occurrence of true psoriatic lesions on mucous membranes is disputed. For many years it has been claimed that this disease does not affect oral mucosa. Today it is thought that involvement of the oral cavity is rare but does exist. Oppenheim (1903) was the first to describe oral Psoriasis in a biopsy after histological examination. In a review of English-language and European non-English literature Younai and Phelan (1997) identified only 57 cases of oral Psoriasis. Since then, few new cases have been reported bringing the total to less than 100 cases described. The reports described a number of oral sites affected, such as lips, buccal mucosa, gums, palate, tongue and floor of the mouth. In the cases reviewed by Younai and Phelan, clinical presentation was a white intraoral lesion in 44% of patients, erythematous in 24% and red and white mixed in 13%. The remaining lesions appeared ulcerative, vesicular, pustular, or indurated. The histopathological findings in oral mucous membranes are assumed to be similar to those found in skin lesions. Epithelial parakeratosis, elongated rete ridges and the presence of an inflammatory infiltrate of the upper dermis were described in most cases. Differential diagnosis from other oral diseases such as benign migratory glossitis, fissured tongue, oral candidosis and the oral lesions of Reiter's syndrome may be subtle. The diagnosis is easily made when the clinical features of oral lesions parallels that of skin lesions and it is supported by histological investigation (Weathers et al., 1974; Younai and Phelan, 1997; Bruce and Rogers, 2003).

6.2 Recurrent streptococcal infection theory in pathogenesis of psoriasis

Recent immunological studies have shown that hyperactivation of tonsillar T cells is caused by a hyperimmune response to α-streptococci; recruitment of the T cells to lesions may be involved in the pathogenesis of PPP. ß1 integrin, expressed on T cells, not only provides a co-stimulatory signal for T-cell activation but also facilitates the accumulation of T cells in inflammatory skin lesions. In this study was found that expression of ß1 integrin on both tonsillar and peripheral blood CD4-positive T cells was higher in PPP patients than in non-PPP patients. It was demonstrated that ß1 integrin may play a key role in the pathogenesis of PPP (Ueda & al., 2010).

Psoriasis is a T-cell-mediated disease that can be triggered by group A beta-haemolytic streptococci infection.

The results of many experimental studies provide evidence that Psoriasis is largely a T-cell mediated disorder. It may result from antigen-specific activation of T cells in the skin of genetically predisposed individuals. These T cells apparently have a particular functional differentiation and promote the psoriatic skin changes by secreting a certain set of cytokines. Based on the fact that streptococcal throat infections are a trigger of guttate Psoriasis, the putative psoriatic antigens are assumed to be in keratinocyte proteins that share structural homologies with streptococcal proteins and thus induce cross-reactive responses of antibacterial T cells against skin components. Together with the particular phenotype of psoriatic skin lesions these findings can suggest that Psoriasis represents a sterile antibacterial tissue reaction, which is mediated by streptococci-specific T cells that cross-react against epidermal autoantigens.

Psoriasis is strongly associated with streptococcal throat infection and patients have increased occurrence of such infections. Psoriatic lesional T cells are oligoclonal, and T cells recognizing determinants common to streptococcal M-protein and keratin have been detected in patients' blood. The streptococcal association might reflect the concurrence of superantigen production promoting skin-homing of tonsil T cells, M-protein mimicking keratin determinants, and adjuvant effects of the peptidoglycan. Accordingly, improvement of Psoriasis after tonsillectomy should be associated with fewer T cells that recognize keratin and streptococcal determinants (Valdimarsson & al., 2009).

6.3 Tonsillectomy and antistreptococcal antibiotic therapy

Tonsillectomy may be a successful treatment modality in selected patients with recalcitrant guttate or chronic plaque Psoriasis. In the study of Hone & al. (1996) Psoriasis was cleared completely after tonsillectomy in five out of six patients (83%) with guttate Psoriasis and was improved in one patient. Two out of seven patients with plaque Psoriasis (29%) were cleared, two (29%) were improved and three (42%) were unchanged.

Numerous studies implicate subclinical or recurrent streptococcal infection as a trigger or maintenance factor in the pathogenesis of Psoriasis in children but the study of Wilson & al. (2003) stated that the available evidence does not demonstrate the efficacy of either antibiotic therapy or tonsillectomy in treatment of childhood Psoriasis. Clinical trials assessing the efficacy of antibiotics or tonsillectomy as treatments for childhood Psoriasis were identified with a search of the medical literature and the results were compared. Only one controlled clinical trial was identified and it did not find a significant effect of antibiotic treatment on Psoriasis. In other studies, the percentage of Psoriasis patients who experienced a disease clearance with antibiotic therapy ranged from 0% to 55%, with no patients experiencing disease worsening during treatment. No controlled trials of tonsillectomy for Psoriasis were identified. The percentage of patients who experienced a disease clearance after tonsillectomy in uncontrolled trials ranged from 32% to 53% and a similar percentage reported significant improvement in their Psoriasis, with a maximum of 7% noting worsening of the disease after operation.

Owen & al. (2000) agreed on the previous conclusions. They searched the Cochrane Clinical Trials Register (Cochrane Library, Issue 3, 1999), Medline (1966- September 1999), Embase (1988-September 1999), the Salford Database of Psoriasis Trials (to November 1999) and the European Dermato-Epidemiology Network (EDEN) Psoriasis Trials Database (to November 1999) for terms [STREPTOCOCC* or ANTIBIOTIC* or TONSIL*] and PSORIASIS using the Cochrane Skin Group search strategy. The only one eligible trial identified compared the use of two oral antibiotic schedules in 20 Psoriasis patients, predominantly of guttate type, who had evidence of beta-haemolytic streptococcal colonisation. Either rifampicin or placebo was added to the end of a standard course of antistreptococcal antibiotic (phenoxymethylpenicillin or erythromycin). No patient in either arm of the study improved during the observation period. No randomised trials of tonsillectomy for Psoriasis were identified. Although both antibiotics and tonsillectomy have frequently been advocated for patients with recurrent guttate Psoriasis or chronic plaque Psoriasis, there is no good evidence that either intervention is beneficial to date.

Because these treatments are relatively benign compared to other treatments for severe Psoriasis, the use of antibiotic therapy or tonsillectomy may still be worth considering, especially for those patients with recurrent streptococcal infections that seem to trigger or maintain their skin disease.

6.4 Psoriasis as T cell-mediated disease and correlation with PPP

Another item of correlation between Psoriasis and inflammatory disease of the upper aerodigestive tract is represented by PPP. PPP is a tonsil-related disease and tonsillectomy is somewhat effective in treating the condition. However, aetiological association between tonsils disease and PPP has not been elucidated fully. Recently, some chemokines and chemokine receptors, including CC chemokine receptor (CCR) 4, CCR6 and CX chemokine receptor (CXCR) 3, have been reported to play important roles in the development of Psoriasis, which is related closely to PPP. Chemokines and chemokine receptors have been known to play a crucial role in directing the movement of mononuclear cells throughout the body, contributing to the pathogenesis of several skin diseases. In the skin lesions of PPP and/or Psoriasis, IL-8 and regulated upon activation normal T cell expressed and secreted are reported to be up-regulated on epidermal keratinocytes, suggesting that such chemokines may play an important role for migration of leucocytes and T cells.

Yoshizaki & al.(2009) have demonstrated that: (1) CCR6 expression was up-regulated in both tonsillar and peripheral blood T cells; (2) CCR6 expression on tonsillar T cells was enhanced by in vitro stimulus with a-streptococcal antigens; (3) tonsillar T cells exhibit more intense chemotactic responses to CCL20; (4) the number of CCR6-positive peripheral blood T cells decreased after tonsillectomy and this reduction was correlated with an improvement in skin lesions; and (5) CCR6 expression of T cells and CCL20 expression of epidermal cells were up-regulated in PPP skin lesions.

These results indicate that CCR6 may be induced by a novel immune response to α-streptococci in tonsillar T cells in PPP patients. CCR6-positive tonsillar T cells may be recruited to the skin via peripheral blood circulation and then attracted to keratinocytes expressing CCL20 in the epidermis. Therefore, CCR6 may act as an important factor, bridging the tonsils and PPP. CCR6-positive tonsillar T cells may move and circulate in the peripheral blood, being recruited ultimately to the skin lesions of PPP patients. The mechanism underlying the manner in which CCR6-expressing tonsillar T cells are recruited to the skin lesions of PPP patients remains obscure; the skin-specific homing receptor CLA may play an important role.

The pathogenic role of T lymphocytes and immune cross-reaction between human-HSP60 and bacterial-HSP65 in PPP was also revealed (Hayashi & al. 2009).

The evidence that T lymphocytes play a key role in the pathogenesis of Psoriasis is now compelling. Eruption of psoriatic skin lesions coincides with epidermal infiltration and activation of T cells and spontaneous or treatment-induced resolution of the lesions is preceded by the reduction or disappearance of epidermal T cells. An up-regulation has also been demonstrated for various molecules associated with T-cell mediated inflammation and treatments selectively directed against T cells have proved to be very effective. Infections with group A beta-haemolytic streptococci have been associated with onset of acute Psoriasis and exacerbation of chronic Psoriasis. Such infections are also frequently accompanied by erythematous skin rashes. Also, recent reports indicate that streptococcal superantigens can induce expression of cutaneous lymphocyte antigens (CLA), believed to play a major role in enabling T cells to migrate to the skin. A novel immune response to alpha-streptococci may enhance CLA expression on tonsillar T-cells through TGF-beta production in patients with PPP, resulting in moving of CLA-positive tonsillar T-cells to skin and tissue damages. This may play a key role in pathogenesis of PPP (Nozawa & al., 2005).

Helper T-cells are frequently activated in tonsils from PPP patients and this activation may be related to unresponsiveness of TGF-beta1 by overexpression of Smad7. Such hyper-activation of T-cell may increase the risk of elicitation of self-reactive T-cell, being associated with pathogenesis of PPP (Takahara & al., 2005).

Furthermore, T-cell lines isolated from psoriatic lesions may show strong reactivity to streptococcal antigens. It was demonstrated that active Psoriasis is associated with a Th1 type response to short peptides with epitopes shared by streptococcal M-protein and keratin. This is consistent with the hypothesis that Psoriasis may be induced and exacerbated in susceptible individuals by M-protein-specific Th1-like cells that cross-react with human epidermal keratin (Valdimarsson & al., 1997).

6.5 Interaction between epidermal keratinocytes and the immune system

Psoriasis is associated with an increase of Th17 cytokines, such as IL-17, IL-22, IL-21, and TNF-α, which are produced by Th 17 cells. Adipokines are peptide hormones or cytokines secreted from adipose tissues and involved in the pathogenesis of metabolic syndrome. Psoriasis patients have a high prevalence of metabolic syndrome. Increased serum levels of IL-22 and adiponectin were positively correlated with PASI. In contrast, serum high molecular weight adiponectin levels were decreased in Psoriasis and negatively correlated with PASI (Nakajima & al. 2011).

Th 17 cells have crucial functions in host defense and dysregulated Th17 responses mediate a variety of autoimmune and inflammatory conditions. Th17 cells coexpress interleukin-22 and its receptor is expressed on epidermal keratinocytes. IL-17 and IL-22 cooperatively enhance some immunological responses. A close relationship between IL-17 and the cutaneous milieu has been suggested by a number of observations. IL-17 induces the production of certain cytokines, chemokines and antimicrobial peptides by keratinocytes, and its cooperation with IL-22 has been documented. Recent findings have suggested that Th17 cells profoundly participate in the pathogenesis of certain skin disorders, in particular, Psoriasis. The concept of the subsets of T cells responsible for Psoriasis has been modified in the order of Th1, T cytotoxic 1, and again Thl, and Thl7 cells. IL-22 is the strongest cytokine in the keratinocyte-proliferative ability. Since IL-22 is produced by Th17 cells, they are crucial for the proliferation of keratinocytes. Furthermore, IL-22 with the help of IL-17 can induce the critical events of Psoriasis, including signal transducer and activator of transcription 3 (STAT3) activation, cytokine/chemokine (IL-8 etc.) production, and antimicrobial peptide elaboration. For maintaining Th17 cells, IL-23 is required and is released from tumor necrosis factor-alpha (TNF-alpha) and inducible nitric oxide synthetase (iNOS)-producing dendritic cells (TIP-DCs). TIP-DCs are activated via an autocrine mechanism by virtue of TNF-alpha.

The above cytokine network in the pathogenesis of Psoriasis has been proven by the therapeutic effectiveness of cytokine-blocking biologics. Antibodies against TNF-alpha or its soluble receptor have already been widely used in the treatment of Psoriasis.

The involvement of Th17 cells has also been shown in allergen-specific immune responses. The percentage of Th17 cells is increased in the peripheral blood of patients with atopic dermatitis (AD) and associated with the severity of AD. Drug eruption is another disease where Th17 cells are involved in the pathogenesis. The percentage of circulating Th17 cells are increased in drug-induced hypersensitivity syndrome, etc. Th17 cells and IL-22 are increased in patients with acute generalized exanthematous pustulosis. Since IL-17 and IL-22 cooperatively stimulate keratinocytes to produce IL-8, keratinocyte-derived IL-8 contributes to the accumulation of neutrophils in the lesional epidermis of this drug eruption (Tokura & al., 2010).

In conclusion, more recent data suggest that Psoriasis is caused by an interaction between epidermal keratinocytes and the immune system and that one possible candidate linking the immune system and epidermal keratinocytes is IL-22, a T-cell-derived cytokine that is produced by Th17 polarized T cells that are stimulated by IL-23, but that acts on epidermal keratinocytes to induce acanthosis and differentiation toward a psoriatic phenotype. Regardless of the specific underlying pathogenesis, Psoriasis is characterized by a disregulated epidermal acanthosis, dermal and epidermal leukocytic infiltration, and dilatation of dermal blood vessels—lesions that are maintained by the complex interplay between T cells and their cytokines, other leukocytes, vascular endothelium, and epidermal keratinocytes. As noted above, epidermal keratinocytes as well as vascular endothelial cells are active participants in the psoriatic inflammatory process via secretion of cytokines and growth factors, and the up regulation of signaling and adhesion molecules on their surfaces (Danilenko, 2008).

6.6 SAPHO syndrome and CMRO

SAPHO (synovitis, acne, pustulosis, hyperostosis, osteitis) syndrome and CMRO (chronic recurrent multifocal osteomyelitis) represent pathologic entities related to Psoriasis and PPP in regard to the relationship between infection and autoimmunity. In genetically susceptible individuals, environmental factors (mainly infections) play a critical role in the pathogenesis of autoimmune diseases. Molecular similarity of microbial and host antigens has recently been proposed as a promoting factor for pathogen expansion when microbial agents are not recognized as alien and not completely eliminated (Rozin, 2009).

SAPHO syndrome is now recognized as a distinct medical entity: a reactive infectious osteitis. Infectious agents isolated from SAPHO patients have gained special attention for many years. Their possible etiological role is supported by the pathogen isolation from different sites: anterior chest wall, spine, synovial fluid, bone tissue and skin pustules. A range of pathogens have been found, including Staphylococcus aureus, Hemophilus parainfluenzae, Actinomyces, and even Treponema pallidum (Arnson, 2008). Propionibacterium acnes is a much more frequent pathogen and plays a particular role. Multiple affected members who segregated a SAPHO syndrome-like phenotype had neutrophil dysfunction and reduced internal oxydant production (Ferguson & al., 2008). That may explain the inability of the innate system to eliminate the pathogen from affected sites and justifies long-term or permanent antibiotic therapy (Rozin, 2009; Magrey, 2009). Treatment of SAPHO syndrome remains empirical as the underlying aetiopathogenesis is unclear.

A growing body of literature has identified the association between neutrophilic dermatoses and multifocal, aseptic bone lesions in children, termed chronic recurrent multifocal osteomyelitis (CRMO). Classically, patients present with swelling, pain, and impaired mobility of the affected area, with skin lesions developing concurrently or in the future. Bone biopsy reveals inflammatory changes consistent with infectious osteomyelitis, but cultures and histologic staining invariably fail to identify an infectious source. Patients are refractory to antibiotic therapy, but dramatically respond to systemic steroids and may need to be maintained on low-dose steroids to prevent relapse. Numerous authors have suggested that CRMO and SAPHO syndrome lie along the same clinical spectrum (Tlougan, 2009; Shilling, 2000).

7. Psoriasis and tumours in head and neck area

Overexpression of S100A7 (psoriasin), a small calcium-binding protein, has been associated with the development of Psoriasis and carcinomas in different types of epithelia but its precise functions are still unknown. Using human tissue specimens, cultured cell lines and a mouse model it was found (Zhou & al., 2008) that S100A7 is highly expressed in preinvasive, well-differentiated and early staged human squamous cell carcinoma of the oral cavity (SCCOC), but little or no expression was found in poorly differentiated, later-staged invasive tumors. Interestingly those researchers showed that S100A7 inhibits both SCCOC cell proliferation in vitro and tumor growth/invasion in vivo. Furthermore, they demonstrated that S100A7 is associated with the beta-catenin complex, and inhibits beta-catenin signaling by targeting beta-catenin degradation via a non canonical mechanism that is independent of GSK3beta-mediated phosphorylation. More importantly their studies also indicated that beta-catenin signaling negatively regulates S100A7 expression. Thus, this reciprocal negative regulation between S100A7 and beta-catenin signaling implies their important roles in tumor development and progression. Despite its high levels of expression in early stage of SCCOC tumorigenesis, S100A7 actually inhibits SCCOC tumor growth/invasion as well as tumor progression. Downregulation of S100A7 in later stages of tumorigenesis increases beta-catenin signaling, leading to promotion of tumor growth and tumor progression.

Significantly increased risk of cancer was demonstrated in patients with Psoriasis at an average of 9.3 years after discharge from hospital. This risk, amounting to 1.4 times that in the general population, is mainly relative to skin and lung cancer in both sexes and to pharynx and larynx cancer in men. Still this data are not definitive as no studies have been published with bias correction for smoke and alcohol consumption. Non-melanoma skin cancer is the most common malignancy, occurring in 196 of 795 patients with cancer: standardized incidence ratio 2.4 for men and 2.6 for women. This means an overall lifetime risk (up to the age of 75 years) of 14.1%. Women run the highest risk of basal cell carcinoma in the age range 20-40 years, while men in the age range 30-60 years run a particularly high risk of squamous cell carcinoma (Frentz & Olsen, 1999).

Standardized incidence ratios (SIR) was found to be 2.80 (95% CI 1.96, 3.87) for oral cavity and pharynx cancer in a nationwide series of psoriasis patients from Sweden with a hospital discharge diagnosis of psoriasis made during 1965–83, who were alive and free from malignancy 1 year after first discharge, compared with the national population (Boffetta & al., 2001). Psoriasis was associated with a significantly increased prevalence ratio of lip, oral cavity and pharynx cancer (1.49; [1.22, 1.80]), in a national database in Taiwan (Tsai & al. 2011).

8. Conclusion

Psoriasis is a disease treated near exclusively from dermatologists. Nevertheless some factors indicate the need for a new attention by the head and neck area specialists, especially by the otorhinolaringologists and maxillofacial surgeons.

Recent literature focuses on relationship between autoimmunity and infection, the latter representing the prince environmental factor that could play a critical role in the pathogenesis of autoimmune diseases in susceptible individuals with the production of cross-reacting antibodies and the induction of the inflammatory second hit. When infectious agents are not recognized as alien and not completely eliminated, pathogen expansion could be promoted by molecular similarity of microbial and host antigens.

As above mentioned important relationship has been demonstrated between tonsillar T cells and skin lesion in PPP patients with immune response to α-streptococci.

Further investigations with translation from bench research to clinical knowledge and vice versa and with interrelation between dermatologists and head and neck specialists could result in considerable progress in understanding immunopathogenesis of Psoriasis and other immuno-mediated diseases.

9. References

Akagi, A. ; Tajima, S. ; Ishibashi, A. ; Yamaguchi, N. & Nagai, Y. (1999). Expression of type XVI collagen in human skin fibroblasts: enhanced expression in fibrotic skin diseases, *J Invest Dermatol*, 113:246–250.

Al Robaee, A.A. (2010). Molecular genetics of Psoriasis (Principles, technology, gene location, genetic polymorphism and gene expression), *Int J Health Sci (Qassim)* 4(2):103-27.

Ammar, M. ;Zaraa, I. ; Bouchleka Souissi, C. ; Dhaoui, A. ; Doss, N. ; Ben Osman, A. ; El Gaied, A. & Mokni, M. (2009). Familial Psoriasis : descriptive report of 9 families, *La tunisie Medicale*, 87 (011): 750-754.

Arnson, Y. ; Rubibow, A. ; Amital, H. (2008). Secondary syphilis presenting as SAPHO syndrome features. *Clin Exp Rheumatol*, 26:1119-1121.

Bhatia, A. ; Singh, B. ; Amarji, B. ; Negi, P. ; Shukla, A. & Katare, O.P.(2011). Novel stain-free lecithinized coal tar formulation for Psoriasis, *Int J Dermatol*, 15. doi: 10.1111/j.1365-4632.2011.04913.x. [Epub ahead of print]

Behnam, S.M. ; Behnam, S.E. & Koo, J.Y. (2005). Smoking and Psoriasis, *Skinmed.*,4(3):174-6.

Bloor, B.K. ; Tidman, N ; Leigh, I.M. ; Odell, E. ; Dogan, B. ; Wollina, U. ; Ghali, L. & Waseem, A. (2003). Expression of keratin K2e in cutaneous and oral lesions:

association with keratinocyte activation, proliferation, and keratinization, *Am J Pathol.* 162(3):963-75.

Boffetta, P. ; Gridley, G.; Lindelöf, B. (2001). Cancer Risk in a Population-Based Cohort of Patients Hospitalized for Psoriasis in Sweden, *Journal of Investigative Dermatology,* 117 :1531–1537; doi:10.1046/j.0022-202x.2001.01520.x.

Bolognia, J.L. ; Brewer, Y.P. & Cooper, D.L. (1991) Bazex syndrome (acrokeratosis paraneoplastica). An analytic review, *Medicine* (Baltimore) 70(4): 269-80.

Boralevi, F. ; Marco-Bonnet, J. ; Lepreux, S. ; Buzenet, C. ; Couprie, B. & Taïeb, A. (2006). Hyperkeratotic head and neck Malassezia dermatosis, *Dermatology* 212(1): 36-40.

Bowen, S.L. ; Bloor, B.K. ; Leigh, I.M. & Waseem, A. (2003). Adducin expression in cutaneous and oral lesions: alpha- and beta-adducin transcripts down-regulate with keratinocyte differentiation in stratified epithelia, *J Pathol.* 201(1): 119-26.

Brook, I. ; Frazier, E.H. & Yeager, J.K. (1999). Microbiology of infected pustular Psoriasis lesions. *Int J Dermatol,* 38: 579–581.

Bruce, A.J. & Rogers, 3rd R.S.. (2003). Oral Psoriasis, *Dermatol Clin,* 21:99-104.

Callis Duffin, K. & Mease, P.J. (2011).Psoriasis and Psoriatic Arthritis Video Project 2010: a report from the GRAPPA annual meeting, *J Rheumatol,* 38(3):562-3.

Canto, A.M. ; Müller, H. ; Freitas, R.R. & Santos, P.S. (2010). Oral lichen planus (OLP): clinical and complementary diagnosis, *An Bras Dermatol.* 85(5): 669-75.

Costa, S.C. ; Hirota S.K. ; Takahashi, M.D. ; Andrade, H. Jr. & Migliari, D.A. (2009). Oral lesions in 166 patients with cutaneous Psoriasis: a controlled study, *Med Oral Patol Oral Cir Bucal* 14(8): e371-5.

Daneshpazhooh, M. ; Moslehi, H. ; Akhyani, M. & Etesami, M. (2004). Tongue lesions in Psoriasis: a controlled study, *BMC Dermatol.* 4(1): 16.

Danilenko, D.M. (2008). Review Paper: Preclinical Models of Psoriasis, *Vet Pathol,* 45:563–575.

Farber, E.M. & Nall, L.(1992). Natural history and treatment of scalp Psoriasis, *Cutis,* 49:396-400.

Ferguson, P.J. ; Lokuta, M.A. ; El-Shanti, H.I. ; Muhle, L. ; Bing, X. & Huttenlocher, A. (2008). Neutrophil dysfunction in a family with a SAPHO syndrome-like phenotype, *Arthritis Rheum,* 58:3264-3269.

Freedberg, I.M. ; Tomic-Canic, M. ; Komine, M. & Blumenberg, M. (2001). Keratins and the keratinocyte activation cycle, *J Invest Dermatol,* 116: 633–640.

Frentz, G. & Olsen, J.H. (1999). Malignant tumours and Psoriasis: a follow-up study, *Br J Dermatol.* 140(2): 237-42.

Garcia-Valladares I.; Cuchacovich R.; Espinoza, L.R. (2011). Comparative assessment of biologics in treatment of Psoriasis: drug design and clinical effectiveness of ustekinumab, *Drug Design, Development and Therapy,*5 :41-49.

Gelfand, J.M. ; Mehta, N.N. & Langan, S.M. (2011). Psoriasis and cardiovascular risk: strength in numbers, part II. *J Invest Dermatol,* 131(5):1007-10.

Gonçalves, L.M. ; Bezerra Júnior, J.R. & Cruz, M.C. (2010). Clinical evaluation of oral lesions associated with dermatologic diseases, *An Bras Dermato,.* 85(2): 150-6.

Gupta, A.K. ; Batra, R. ; Bluhm, R. (2004). Skin diseases associated with Malassezia species, *J Am Acad Dermatol,* 51:785-798.

Handa, S. (2010). Newer trends in the management of Psoriasis at difficult to treat locations: Scalp, palmoplantar disease and nails, *Indian J Dermatol Venereol Leprol*,76:634-44.

Hayashi, M. ; Fujihara, K. ; Beder, L.B. ; Yamamoto, Y. ; Hotomi, M. & Yamanaka, N. (2009). Pathogenic role of tonsillar lymphocytes in associated with HSP60/65 in Pustulosis palmaris et plantaris, *Auris Nasus Larynx*, 36(5):578-85. Epub 2009 Mar 5.

Hone, S.W. ; Donnelly, M.J. ; Powell, F. & Blayney, A.W. Clearance of recalcitrant Psoriasis after tonsillectomy, *Clin Otolaryngol Allied Sci*, 21(6):546-7.

Karason, A. ; Gudjonsson, J.E. ; Jonsson, H.H. & (2005). Genetics of Psoriasis in Iceland: Evidence for linkage of subphenotypes to distinct loci, *J Invest Dermatol.*,124:1177-1185.

Katsambas, A. ; Peris, K. ; Vena, G. ; Freidmann, P. ; Wozel, G. ; Daudén, E. ; Licu, D. ; Placchi, M. & De La Brassinne, M. (2009). Assessing the Impact of Efalizumab on Nail, Scalp and Palmoplantar Psoriasis and on Quality of Life: Results from a Multicentre, Open-label, Phase IIIb/IV Trial, *Arch Drug Info*,2:66–70.

Kircik, L. (2011). Salicylic Acid 6% in an ammonium lactate emollient foam vehicle in the treatment of mild-to-moderate scalp Psoriasis, *J Drugs Dermatol*, 10(3):270-3.

Krell, J. ; Chen, Y. & Caro, I. (2008). Response of head and neck Psoriasis to efalizumab: A pooled data analysis. Presented at: *Summer Meeting of the American Academy of Dermatology*, July 30-August 3, 2008, Chicago, IL. Poster 2407.

Krueger, G.G. (1999). New method being developed for assessing Psoriasis, *National Psoriasis Foundation Forum.*,5:4-5.

Magrey, M. & Khan MA. New insights into synovitis, acne, pustulosis, hyperostosis, and osteitis (SAPHO) syndrome, *Curr Rheumatol Rep*, 11(5):329-33.

Martin, P. (1997). Wound healing—aiming for perfect skin regeneration, *Science*, 276:75–81.

Masmoudi,J. ; Maalej, I. ; Masmoudi, A. ; Rached, H. ; Rebai, A.; Turki, H. ; Jaoua, A. (2009). Alexithymia and Psoriasis: a case-control study of 53 patients, *Encephale*, 35(1) :10-7.

McCormack, P.L. (2011). Calcipotriol/betamethasone dipropionate: a review of its use in the treatment of Psoriasis vulgaris of the trunk, limbs and scalp, *Drugs*, 16;71(6):709-30. doi: 10.2165/11207300-000000000-00000.

Mengesha, Y.M. & Bennett, M.L. (2002). Pustular skin disorders: diagnosis and treatment, *Am J Clin Dermatol.* 3(6): 389-400.

Meyer, N. ; Viraben, R. & Paul, C. (2008). Addictions and Psoriasis: an example of the dermatologist's implication in preventive medicine? *Ann Dermatol Venereol*, 2008,135 Suppl 4:S259-62.

Mrowietz, U. ; Macheleidt, O. & Eicke, C. (2011). Effective treatment and improvement of quality of life in patients with scalp Psoriasis by topical use of calcipotriol/betamethasone (Xamiol(®) -gel): results, *J Dtsch Dermatol Ges*, 12. doi: 10.1111/j.1610-0387.2011.07695.x. [Epub ahead of print].

Nakajima, H. ; Nakajima, K. ; Tarutani, M. ; Morishige, R. & Sano S. Kinetics of circulating Th17 cytokines and adipokines in Psoriasis patients, *Arch Dermatol Res*,17. [Epub ahead of print].

Naldi, L. & Rzany, B. (2009). Psoriasis (chronic plaque), *Clin Evid (Online)* 9, pii: 1706.

Naldi, L. ; Tognoni, G. & Cainelli, T. (1994). Analytic epidemiology in Psoriasis, *J Invest Dermatol*, 102: 19s-23s.

Niessen, F.B. ; Andriessen, M.P. ; Schalkwijk, J. ; Visser, L. & Timens, W. (2001). Keratinocyte-derived growth factors play a role in the formation of hypertrophic scars, *J Pathol*, 194:207–216.

Noiles, K. & Vender, R. (2008). Treatment of severe facial Psoriasis with adalimumab, *J Drugs Dermatol*, 7(12):1165-7.

Nozawa, H. ; Kishibe, K. ; Takahara, M. & Harabuchi, Y. (2005). Expression of cutaneous lymphocyte-associated antigen (CLA) in tonsillar T-cells and its induction by in vitro stimulation with alpha-streptococci in patients with pustulosis palmaris et plantaris (PPP), *Clin Immunol*, 116(1):42-53.

Ogunmakin, K.O. ; Rashid, R.M. (2011) Alopecia: the case for medical necessity, *Skinmed*, 9(2): 79-84.

Oppenheim, M. (1903). Psoriasis mucosae oris, *Monatsschr Prakt Dermatol*, 37: 481.

Owen, C.M. ; Chalmers, R.J. ; O'Sullivan, T. & Griffiths, C.E. (2000). Antistreptococcal interventions for guttate and chronic plaque Psoriasis, *Cochrane Database Syst Rev*;(2):CD001976.

Puig, L. ; Ribera, M. ; Hernanz, J.M. ; Belinchón, I. ; Santos-Juanes, J. ; Linares, M. ; Querol, I. ; Colomé, E. & Caballé, G. (2010). Treatment of scalp Psoriasis: review of the evidence and Delphi consensus of the Psoriasis Group of the Spanish Academy of Dermatology and Venereology, *Actas Dermosifiliogr*, 101(10):827-46.

Puzenat E. ; Bronsard, V. ; Prey, S. ; Gourraud, P.A. ; Aractingi, S. ; Bagot, M. ; Cribier, B. ; Joly, P. ; Jullien, D. ; Le Maitre, M. ; Paul, C. ; Richard-Lallemand, M.A. ; Ortonne, J.P. ; Aubin, F. (2010). What are the best outcome measures for assessing plaque Psoriasis severity? A systematic review of the literature, *Eur Acad Dermatol Venereol*, 24 (Suppl 2):10-6.

Rossi, A. ; Mandel, V.D. ; Garelli, V. ; Mari, E. ; Fortuna, M.C. ; Carlesimo, M. ; Richetta, A. ; Scarnò, M. ; Trucchia, A. & Calvieri, S. (2011). Videodermoscopy Scalp Psoriasis Severity Index (VSCAPSI): A useful tool for evaluation of scalp Psoriasis, *Eur J Dermatol* 9. [Epub ahead of print].

Rozin, A.P. (2009). SAPHO syndrome: Is a range of pathogen-associated rheumatic diseases extended? *Arthritis Research & Therapy*, 11:131 (doi:10.1186/ar2837).

Santos-Silva, A.R. ; Correa, M.B. ; Vargas, P.A. ; Almeida, O.P. & Lopes, M.A. (2010). Bazex syndrome (acrokeratosis paraneoplastica) diagnosed in a patient with oral persistent ulcerations, *Head Neck Pathol*. 4(4): 312-7.

Schilling, F. & Kessler S. (2000). SAPHO syndrome : clinico-rheumatologic and radiologic differentiatiation and classification of a patient sample of 86 cases, *Z Rheumatol*, 59 (1) :1-28.

Squier, C.A. ; Johnson, N.W. & Hopps, R.M. (1976). Human Oral Mucosa: Development, Structure and Function. Oxford, *Blackwell Scientific Publications*, pp 7–44.

Stefanaki, C. ; Lagogianni, E.; Kontochristopoulos, G. ; Verra, P.; Barkas, G. ; Katsambas, A. & Katsarou, A. (2011). Psoriasis in children: a retrospective analysis, *J Eur Acad Dermatol Venereol*. 25(4): 417-21.

Stein, L. (2005). Clinical studies of a new vehicle formulation for topical corticosteroids in the treatment of Psoriasis, *J Am Acad Dermatol*. 53(1 Suppl 1):S39-49.

Takahara, M. ; Kishibe, K. ; Nozawa, H. ; Harabuchi, Y. (2005). Increase of activated T-cells and up-regulation of Smad7 without elevation of TGF-beta expression in tonsils from patients with pustulosis palmaris et plantaris, *Clin Immunol*, 115(2):192-9.

Tlougan, B.E. ; Podjasek, J.O. ; O'Haver, J. ; Cordova, K.B. ; Nguyen, X.H. ; Tee, R. ; Pinckard-Hansen, K.C. & Hansen, R.C. Chronic recurrent multifocal osteomyelitis (CRMO) and synovitis, acne, pustulosis, hyperostosis, and osteitis (SAPHO) syndrome with associated neutrophilic dermatoses: a report of seven cases and review of the literature, *Pediatr Dermatol*, 26(5):497-505.

Tokura, Y. ; Mori, T. & Hino, R. (2010). Psoriasis and other Th17-mediated skin diseases, *J UOEH*, 32(4):317-28.

Tsai, T.F. ; Wang, T.S. ; Hung, S.T. ; Tsai, P.I. ; Schenkel, B. ; Zhang, M. ; Tang, C.H. (2011). Epidemiology and comorbidities of psoriasis patients in a national database in Taiwan, *J Dermatol Sci*, 63:40-6.

Ueda, S. ; Takahara, M. ; Tohtani, T. ; Yoshizaki, T. ; Kishibe, K. ; Harabuchi, Y. (2010). Up-regulation of ß1 integrin on tonsillar T cells and its induction by in vitro stimulation with α-streptococci in patients with pustulosis Palmaris et Plantaris, *J Clin Immunol*, 30(6):861-71. Epub 2010 Aug 17.

Valdimarsson, H. (2007).The genetic basis of Psoriasis, *Clin Dermatol*; 25: 563-7.

van de Kerkhof, P.C. ; Kleinpenning, M. & Gerritsen, R. (2009).Scalp Psoriasis. In: Koo J, Lee CS, Lebwohl M, editors. *Mild-To-Moderate Psoriasis*. 2 nd ed. London: Informa Healthcare.

Waseem, A.; Dogan, B. ; Tidman, N. ; Alam, Y. ; Purkis, P. ; Jackson, S. ; Lalli, A. ; Machesney, M. & Leigh, I.M. (1999). Keratin 15 expression in stratified epithelia: downregulation in activated keratinocytes, *J Invest Dermatol*. 112(3): 362-9.

Weathers, D.R. ; Baker, G. ; Archard, H.O.& Burkes, Jr. E.J. (1974). Psoriasiform lesions of the oral mucosa (with emphasis on "ectopic geographictongue"), *Oral Surg Oral Med Oral Pathol*, 37: 872-888.

Wilson, J.K. ; Al-Suwaidan, S.N. ; Krowchuk, D. & Feldman, S.R. (2003). Treatment of Psoriasis in children: is there a role for antibiotic therapy and tonsillectomy? *Pediatr Dermatol*, 20(1):11-5.

Wittkowski, K.M. ; Leonardi, C. ; Gottlieb, A. ; Menter, A. ; Krueger, G.G. ; Tebbey, P.W. ; Belasco, J. ; Soltani-Arabshahi, R. ; Gray, J. ; Horn, L. & Krueger J.G. (2011) Clinical Symptoms of Skin, Nails, and Joints Manifest Independently in Patients with Concomitant Psoriasis and Psoriatic Arthritis, *PLoS ONE* 6(6): e20279. doi:10.1371/journal.pone.0020279.

Wu, Y. ; Lin, Y. ; Liu, H.J. ; Huang, C.Z. ; Feng, A.P. & Li, J.W. (2010). Childhood Psoriasis: a study of 137 cases from central China, *World J Pediatr*,6(3):260-4.

Yaghoobi, R. ; Feily, A. ; Behrooz, B. ; Yaghoobi, E. & Mokhtarzadeh, S. (2010). Palpebral involvement as a presenting and sole manifestation of discoid lupus erythematosus, *ScientificWorldJournal*. 10: 2130-1.

Yoshizaki, T. ; Bandoh, N. ; Ueda, S. ; Nozawa, H.; Goto, T. ; Kishibe, K. ; Takahara, M. & Harabuchi, Y. (2009). Up-regulation of CC chemokine receptor 6 on tonsillar T cells and its induction by in vitro stimulation with α-streptococci in patients with pustulosis palmaris et plantari, *Clinical and Experimental Immunology*, 157: 71–82.

Younai, F.S. & Phelan, J.A. (1997).Oral mucositis with features of Psoriasis: report of a case and review of the literature, *Oral Surg Oral Med Oral Pathol Oral Radiol Endod*,84:61-67.

Young, O. ; Murphy, M. ; Fitzgibbon, J. & O'Sullivan, P. (2009). Koebner phenomenon of the ear canal skin, *Auris Nasus Larynx*, 36(1): 82-4.

Zhu, J.F. ; Kaminski, M.J. ; Pulitzer, D.R. ; Hu, J. & Thomas, H.F. (1996). Psoriasis: pathophysiology and oral manifestations, *Oral Dis*, 2(2): 135-44.

7

Metabolic Features in Psoriasis

Giulia Ganzetti, Anna Campanati, Giulia Liberati and Annamaria Offidani
Dermatologic Clinic, Polythecnic University of Marche Region
Italy

1. Introduction

Psoriasis is a chronic inflammatory disease affecting about 3% of the worldwide population (Gottlieb A et al, 2007).

Recent findings have shown that the previous concept " psoriasis as a disease of healthy people" must be revisited into psoriasis as a complex entity with multisistemic involvement.

Although the overall mortality attributed to psoriasis is about 0.64 deaths per 100 000 psoriatic patients annually in the USA, erythrodermic and generalized pustular soriasis, are associated with a greater risk of mortality and morbidity (Boyd AS et al, 1989; Prystowsky JH et al, 1995).

Psoriasis can be associated with other disease, such as metabolic syndrome, which may have a major impact on quality of life, morbidity and mortality.

The aim of this chapter is to focus on two newly emergent comorbidities in psoriatic patients, the cardiovascular disease (CVD) and the metabolic syndrome (MetS).

2. The metabolic syndrome

The metabolic syndrome (MetS) is a cluster of risk factors including obesity, atherogenic dyslipidaemia, hypertension, glucose intolerance and a proinflammatory and prothrombotic state predisposing the patients to cardiovascular diseases (CVD), type 2 diabetes (DM), renal failure and stroke (Gisondi et al, 2007).

Furthermore, it has recently been suggested that the metabolic syndrome might be a risk factor for cancer, in particular colon cancer (Gottlieb A et al, 2007).

The MetS prevalence in Western Europe population ranges from 15% to 35% and it strictly correlates with age, increasing sharply after the age of 60 (Gisondi et al, 2007).

The National Cholesterol Education Program (NCEP) Adult Treatment Panel III (ATP III) have proposed the criteria for the metabolic syndrome diagnosis; other organizations, such as The World Health Organization (WHO) and the European Group on Insulin resistance, agree with it in the essential components, differing from it in the details and criteria (Chung CP et al, 2005).

According to NCEP ATPIII the diagnosis of MetS requires at least three of these following criteria:

- Abdominal obesity, defined as waist circumference ≥ 102 cm in men and ≥ 88 cm in women
- Tryglicerides plasma levels ≥ 150 mg/dl
- HDL cholesterol plasma levels less than 40 mg/dl in men and 50 mg/dl in women
- Blood pressure more than 130 mmHg (systolic) and 85 mmHg (diastolic)
- Fasting plasma glucose levels more than 100 mg/dL [Grundy et al., 2005]

It is now thought that non-alcoholic fatty liver disease (NAFLD) is a component of metabolic syndrome, that may progress to steatoepatitis (NASH) with complications of fibrosis and cirrhosis (Capeau J, 2008).

Recent study have demonstrated that the prevalence of metabolic syndrome is significantly higher in psoriatic patients compared to controls after the age of 40 years and psoriatic patients have an increased risk for the individual components of MetS (Gisondi et al, 2007).

Moreover, the association between psoriasis and metabolic syndrome is also true for mild severity psoriasis and it is independent from the tendency of psoriatic patients to be obese (Mallbris L et al, 2006; Neimann AL et al, 2006; Sommer DM et al, 2006).

Although the link between psoriasis and metabolic syndrome is not completely elucidated, the pathophysiology of both these entities shows many shared cytokines contributing to the underlying chronic inflammatory status.

It is known that both innate and adaptive immunity are involved in psoriatic pathogenesis and, in particular, NK cells appear crucial in the inflammatory process initiation, with an increased release of proinflammatory cytokines, such as TNF-alpha and IFN-gamma and the subsequent interaction with TH1 and Th17 cells (Teunissen MBM et al , 2007).

Dysregulation of T-cell antigen presenting cell interactions and overexpression of proinflammatory cytokines lead to the hyperproliferation of keratinocytes and the activation of neutrophils and endothelial cells until the development of the characteristic psoriatic skin lesions (Kimball AB et al, 2008).

The molecular mechanisms involved in psoriasis-associated dysregulation of metabolic functions are believed to be due to an underlying low and persistent inflammatory status with increased levels of proinflammatory factors, such as tumor necrosis factor-alpha and IL-6 (Fig.1).

TNF-alpha is a proinflammatory cytokine produced by many cell lines, such as keratinocites, T cells, NK cells, dendritic cells, neutrophils, mast cells and adipocytes (Ronti T et al, 2006).

It is expressed as a 26-kD cell surface trans-membrane protein that undergoes cleavage to produce a 17-kD soluble, biologically active form of TNF-α (Ronti T et al, 2006).

IL-6, a pleiotropic circulating cytokine, shows multiple effects ranging from inflammation to host defence and tissue injury. It is secreted by many cell types, including immune cells, fibroblasts, endothelial cells, skeletal muscle and adipocytes (Ronti T et al, 2006).

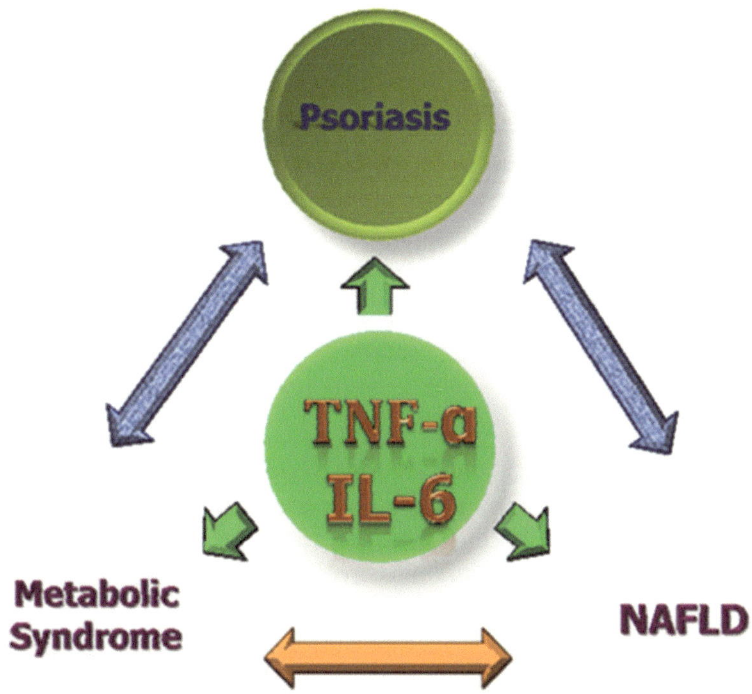

Fig. 1. The molecular mechanisms involved in psoriasis-associated dysregulation of metabolic function.

3. Obesity and psoriasis

Among different MetS components, the association between obesity and psoriasis is the best documented.

Several studies have shown that the severity of PsO may be linked to obesity and a population-based study of mild or severe PsO has demonstrated that the risk of obesity was significantly increased in PsO patients compared with healthy controls. Unlike in other inflammatory diseases, such as rheumatoid arthritis, the risk of obesity is strongly associated with disease severity (Sterry W et al, 2004).

Although it is controversial if psoriasis is the result or the cause of obesity itself , recent data support the obesity is a consequence of psoriasis (Henseler T et al, 1995; Neimann AL et al, 2006; Herron MD et al. 2005).

Obesity is considered the main pathogenic factor in the metabolic syndrome and it is characterized by a low and persistent sistemic inflammatory status, whose mainstay is the adipose tissue (Greenberg et al., 2006).

Adipose tissue is principally divided into two compartments, subcutaneously and centrally: the central one is characterized by omental adipose tissue and other intra-abdominal fat sources such as mesenteric fat. Central adipose tissue, also called visceral fat, is considered more metabolically active than peripheral subcutaneous fat (Kershaw EE et al, 2004; Galic S et al, 2010).

The importance of adipose tissue location in terms of dysmetabolism risk is evident: patients with excess visceral fat (central obesity) show an higher risk of developing insulin resistance and the features of the metabolic syndrome than patients with excess subcutaneous fat (Kissebach AH et al, 1982).

One of the most commonly used antropometric indexes is BMI (Body mass index), which measures adiposity and body composition as weight in kilograms divided by the square ofthe height measurement in metres (kg/m2). BMI have high specificity, but low sensitivity to identify adiposity and excess body fat (Okorodudu DO et al, 2010).

Waist circumference (WC), alone or in combination with BMI, has been shown to be an accurate predictor of visceral fat directly reflecting total abdominal fat mass but failing to quantify the visceral and subcutaneous fat compartments individually (Kashihara H et al, 2009).

The visceral adipose tissue is not only an energy storage organ, but also an important component of the immune system through the adipocytes' expression of toll receptors and a real active endocrine organ producing proinflammatory cytokines (TNF-alpha, IL-6), free fatty acids, procoagulant molecules and bioactive products called adipokines (Ronti et al, 2006).

Many adipokines have been identified, such as leptin, visfatin, resistin and adiponectin; they act in a communications network with other tissues and organs such as the skeletal muscle, adrenal cortex, brain and sympathetic nervous system and participate in appetite and energy balance, immunity, insulin sensitivity, angiogenesis, blood pressure, lipid metabolism and haemostasis (Ronti T et al, 2006).

In particular, leptin and resistin appear to be two proinflammatory cytokines, while adiponectin has anti-inflammatory properties (Ronti T et al, 2006).

Leptin, a 16-kD adipocyte-derived cytokine, is synthesized and released from fat cells in response to changes in body fat. Leptin circulates partially bound to plasma proteins and enters the CNS by diffusion through capillary junctures in the median eminence and by saturable receptor transport in the choroid plexus. In the hypothalamus, leptin binds to receptors that stimulate anorexigenic peptides such as proopiomelanocortin and cocaine- and amphetamine-regulated transcript and inhibit orexigenic peptides, such as neuropeptide Y. Leptin reduces intracellular lipid levels in skeletal muscle, liver and pancreatic beta cells, thereby improving insulin sensitivity. There is strong evidence showing that the dominant action of leptin is to act as a 'starvation signal': leptin declines rapidly during fasting.Therefore, leptin deficiency was perceived as a state of unmitigated starvation, leading to compensatory responses, such as hyperphagia, decreased metabolic rate and changes in hormone levels, designed to restore energy balance. The concept of 'leptin resistance' was introduced when increased adipose leptin production was observed in obese individuals, who were not leptin-deficient. Moreovere, some studies suggest leptin may affect vascular structure with an angiogenic activity and contributes to arterial thrombosis through the platelet leptin receptor. Leptin also stimulates production of reactive oxygen species as a result of monocyte activation. Therefore, in an obese subject leptin may no longer be able to regulate caloric intake and energy balance, but may still exert its angiogenic activity and production of reactive oxigen species, which affect vessel walls (Ronti T et al, 2006).

Resistin is a dimeric protein. In murine models, obesity is associated with rises in circulating resistin concentrations. Resistin increases blood glucose and insulin concentrations and impairs hypoglycaemic response to insulin infusion. In obese mice, antiresistin antibodies decrease blood glucose and improve insulin sensitivity: these data support the hypothesis that in obese rodents, resistin induces insulin resistance and contributes to impaired insulin sensitivity. In humans, the physiological role of resistin must be elucidated and its role in obesity and insulin resistance and/or diabetes is controversial. In humans, as resistin is primarily produced in peripheral blood monocytes and its levels correlate with IL-6 concentrations. the question of its inflammatory role has been raised (Ronti et al, 2006).

Four genes encode for resistin in the mouse and two in humans. Some genetic case control studies demonstrated genetic variations in the resistin gene are associated with insulin resistance and obesity in humans. Others show that the very low resistin mRNA expression in isolated human adipocytes does not correlate consistently with insulin resistance or obesity, making the role of human resistin in insulin resistance unclear. No differences have been observed in resistin expression in adipocytes from normal, insulin-resistant, and type 2 diabetic individuals. Mc Ternan et al. reported greater resistin mRNA expression in fat depots in the abdomen than in the thigh, suggesting human resistin could play a role in obesity-related insulin resistance (McTernan et al, 2002; Ronti et al, 2006).

Adiponectin is almost exclusively expressed in white adipose tissue, whose expression is inhibited by IL- 6 and TNF-α. Unlike most adipokines, adiponectin expression and serum concentrations are reduced in obese and insulin-resistant states and, in vivo, high plasma adiponectin levels are associated with reduced risk of myocardial infarction. Although further studies are needed to clarify whether adiponectin independently predicts coronary heart disease events, in men with type 2 diabetes, increased adiponectin levels are associated with a moderately decreased risk of coronary heart disease. The association seems to be mediated in part by the effects of adiponectin on high-density lipoprotein cholesterol (HDL), through parallel increases in both. Moreover, it has been demonstrated that weight loss, caloric restriction and thiazoladinedione treatment increase adiponectin plasma levels and gene expression in white adipose tissue (Ronti et al, 2006).

Recent studies have evidenced a high leptin levels and decreased serum levels of adiponectin in obesity, insulin-resistent PsO patients and they emphasized an inverse correlation between serum levels of adiponectin and IL-6 (Satapathy SK et al, 2004).

The precise physiological events leading to the initiation of the inflammatory response in obesity remain incompletely understood. One theory underlined that the expansion of adipose tissue leads to adipocyte hypertrophy and hyperplasia with a consequent local oxygen supply, cell hypoxia and the activation of cellular stress pathways releasing proinflammatory cytokines and signals. These proinflammatory chemokines attract pro-inflammatory macrophages into the adipose tissue with the creation of crown-like structures around hypertrophic dead or dying adipocytes. Furthermore, these macrophages release cytokines that stimulate an inflammation in neighboring adipocytes developing a vicious circle (Esposito K et al, 2004; Das UN, 2001).

Thus, excess adipose tissue results in elevated levels of pro-inflammatory adipokines, resulting in an imbalance between increased inflammatory stimuli and decreased anti-inflammatory mechanism leading to persistent low-grade inflammation (Wajchenberg BL et al, 2000; Esposito K et al, 2004; Das UN, 2001).

Among proinflammatory cytokines, TNF-a and IL-6 represent two driving cytokines, which link psoriasis with many MetS components, such as obesity-related insulin-resistance (Ronti T et al, 2006).

In humans TNF-α is synthesized and secreted by adipocytes and stromovascular cells: adipose tissue TNF-α is not secreted in systemic circulation and acts in an autocrine and paracrine pathways. Adipose tissue TNF-α mRNA correlates with body mass index, percentage of body fat and hyperinsulinaemia; weight loss decreases TNF-α levels (Ronti T et al, 2006).

TNF-α modifies the gene expression profile of adipocytes and liver with an increased release and production of FFAs, cholesterol and VLDL; elevated IL-6 levels appears to be associated with decreased levels of HDL cholesterol, which may contribute to a state of chronic inflammation (Gottlieb A et al, 2008).

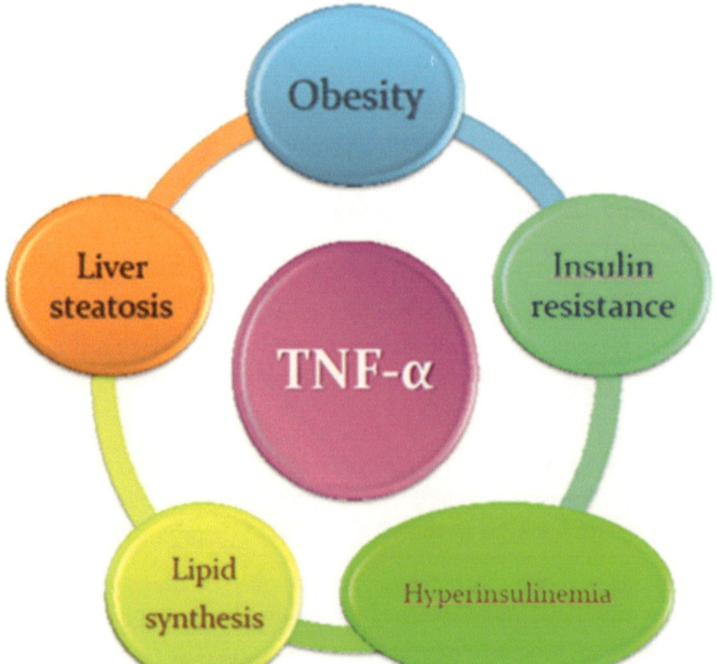

Fig. 2. The vicious circle linking obesity and hyperinsulinemia

Moreover, levels of soluble TNF-α receptors are directly proportional to total and LDL cholesterol concentrations and inversely correlated with certain HDL cholesterol subfraction levels (Gottlieb A et al, 2008).

Obesity-induced chronic inflammation is a key component in the pathogenesis of insulin resistance (Fig.2).

4. Insulin-resistance

Several studies have demonstrated a potential association between PsO and increased serum fasting glucose levels, hyperinsulinemia, insulin-resistance, and type 2 diabetes. However, insulin resistance does not significantly correlate with PsO disease severity and duration (Gottlieb A et al, 2008).

Insulin resistance is a characteristic feature of most patients with Type 2 diabetes mellitus and is one of the MetS clinical features. Insulin is a pleiotropic hormone stimulating nutrient transport into cells, regulating gene expression, modifying enzymatic activity and regulating energy homeostasis (De Luca C et al, 2008).

Insulin exerted to these multiple functions through several intracellular signaling cascades, such as the phosphatidylinositol 3-kinase (PI3K)-AKT (also called protein kinase B (PKB)) pathway and the Ras-mitogen activated protein kinase (MAPK) pathway. PI3K-AKT is largely responsible for insulin action on glucose uptake and in the suppression of gluconeogenesis, while MAPK mediates gene expression and controls cell growth and differentiation, interacting with the first pathway. The insulin action is evidenced on target tissue, such as liver, adipose tissue and skeletal muscle (De Luca C et al, 2008).

In the liver, insulin regulates glucose metabolism depending on the meal or starvation, while in adipose tissue insulin signaling results in decreased hormone sensitive lipase activity and this anti-lipolytic effect inhibits free fatty acid efflux out of adipocytes (De Luca C et al, 2008).

Increased levels of TNF-alpha, IL-6 and FFAs produced by excess visceral adipose tissue can cause insulin resistance in adipose tissue, skeletal muscle and liver by inhibiting insulin signal transduction and they can determine the production of other inflammatory-related factors, such as CRP (Gottlieb A et al, 2008).

TNF-alpha causes a decrease in the autophosphorylation of tyrosine residues of insulin receptor (IR) and phosphorylation of insulin receptor substrate 1 (IRS-1) (Hotamisligil GS, 2003).

Thus, in psoriasis obesity and insulin resistance have a proinflammatory effect perpetuated through a positive feedback loop in PsO patients.

5. NAFLD

The liver plays a central role in lipid metabolism, importing serum free fatty acids and manufacturing, storing and exporting lipids and lipoproteins (Adams LA et al, 2005).

NAFLD is the acronym for nonalcoholic fatty liver disease and it includes a wide spectrum of liver pathology, from hepatocellular steatosis to nonalcoholic steatohepatitis (NASH) (Browning JD et al, 2004).

The prevalence of NAFLD is 10–25% in the western world and it is a an emergent condition now recognized as the most frequent cause of abnormal liver tests, especially in obese individuals (Papatheodoridis GV et al, 2007).

NAFLD is considered the hepatic manifestation of the metabolic syndrome closely associated to visceral obesity and insulin resistance (Marchesini G et al, 2003; Tsochatzis EA et al, 2009).

Adipocytokines, free fatty acids, mitochondrial dysfunction, bacterial endotoxin and vascular disturbance have all been implicated in the development of hepatic inflammation and fibrosis in patients with NAFLD (Adams LA et al, 2005).

The pathogenesis of NAFLD is currently seen as a two steps process, initially characterized by the accumulation of liver fat followed by the development of necroinflammation and fibrosis (Day CP et al,1998).

Insulin resistance results in both increased adipose tissue lipolysis and increased hepatic lipogenesis leading to lipid accumulation in the hepatocytes, mainly in the form of triglycerides and FFAs (Emmanuel A et al, 2009).

The increased liver deposition of TG and FFAs contributes to lipotoxicity and predisposes hepatocytes to the second step: the mythocondrial disfunction and the oxidative stress (Emmanuel A et al, 2009).

A recent study has emphasized that NAFLD is highly prevalent among psoriasis patients and it seems that patients with NAFLD and psoriasis are at higher risk for severe liver fibrosis than their age, sex and BMI-matched counterparts with NAFLD without psoriasis (Marra M et al, 2007).

Psoriasis, metabolic syndrome and NAFLD might share a common underlying mechanism characterized by a low level inflammatory status characterized by a pro-inflammatory cytokines generalized activation (Marra M et al, 2007).

As in obesity and insulin resistance, TNF-alpha seems to have a pivotal role: both serum and hepatic levels of TNF-alpha are elevated in patients with NAFLD and it is directly correlated considering the markers of liver damage (Marra M et al, 2007).

AST, ALT and mostly AST/ALT ratio are considered important parameters of liver damage and they appear correlated to the severity of the hepatic damage to histological disease severity.[Pulzi FBU et al, 2011]

It has already demonstrated that psoriatic patients with NAFLD show a higher mean AST/ALT ratio, a parameter proved to be an independent predictor factor of liver fibrosis in NAFLD patients (Angulo P et al, 2007).

AST serum levels increase more than those of ALT with the progression of the hepatic disease; therefore, an higher than 1 AST/ALT ratio may be one element of more advanced disease (Vanni E et al, 2010).

6. Atherogenic dyslipidemia

Many evidences suggest a strong link between PsO and abnormalities in fatty acid metabolism: psoriatic patients show dyslipidemia with increased plasma cholesterol, triglycerides (TG), low-density lipoprotein (LDL) cholesterol, very low-density lipoprotein (VLDL) cholesterol, and decreased HDL cholesterol and antioxidant capacity. In particular, a recent study has underlined that the dyslipidemic profile could precede the psoriasis manifestations (Gottlieb A et al, 2008).

Studies on lipid profile in psoriatic patients have been conducted since 1994 focusing on the presence of a significant content in total cholesterol and of the cholesterol/protein ratio in low-density lipoproteins (LDL) and in high-density lipoproteins (HDL) of psoriatic children. The compositional changes were associated with alterations of fluidity in LDL and HDL of psoriatic patients (Offidani AM et al, 1994).

In PsO patients, the detection of raised levels of LDL and low levels of HDL cholesterol is associated with coronary artery disease and with accelerated mortality for cardiovascular disease (Jones SM et al, 2000).

7. Hypertension

In PsO patients a higher occurrence of hypertension compared with controls has been reported. The underlying mechanism of hypertension in psoriasis has been discussed and multiple hypothesis have been emerged on this topic (Gottlieb A et al, 2008).

The pathogenesis of hypertension in psoriasis seems to be linked to increased production of angiotensinogen by adipose tissue, subsequently converted to angiotensin II through angiotensin converting enzyme (ACE) (Armstrong AW et al, 2011).

ACE serum levels are increased in psoriasis patients (Gottlieb A et al, 2008).

Angiotensin II not only promotes salt retention by kidney but also it regulates vascular tone, acting a vasoconstrictor and stimulates T-cell proliferation promoting inflammation and the development of atherosclerosis (Armstrong AW et al, 2011).

The association between psoriasis and hypertension may also be attributed to the increased oxidative stress in psoriasis patients. Greater levels of reactive oxygen species can damage endothelium-dependent vasodilation (Armstrong AW et al, 2011).

Other studies emphasized the role of endothelin-1 in hypertension development among PsO patients. Endothelin-1 is a protein produced by several different cell types including keratinocytes; it induces blood vessels vasoconstriction increasing blood pressure. In PsO patients endothelin-1 expression appears to be altered in lesional skin and serum and correlated to psoriasis disease severity (Armstrong AW et al, 2011).

8. Protrombotic state

A proinflammatory and/or prothrombotic state has been associated with MetS and PsO, probably linked to elevated serum levels of PAI-1, fibrinogen and CRP. Elevated CRP levels are induced by IL-6 and they have been shown to be predictive of future CVD in initially healthy individuals, and the risk of CVD in patients with either diabetes or MetS is significantly increased in the presence of elevated CRP levels (Gottlieb A et al, 2008).

9. Anti-TNF-alpha in psoriasis and metabolic syndrome

TNF-alpha is an inflammatory cytokine promoting inflammation via the activation and induction of proinflammatory cytokines (IL-1, IL-6, IL-8) and by the upregulation of adhesion molecules on endothelial cells leading to increased leukocyte extravasation (Channual J et al, 2009).

Given that TNF-a show a pivotal role in many inflammatory conditions and that it represents one of possible link between psoriasis and metabolic syndrome, theoretically the TNF-alpha blockade might have a widespread potential in the treatment of both pathological entities (Channual J et al, 2009).

Although it is well known the TNF-alpha inhibitors efficacy on PsO and Psoriatic arthritis (PsA), little is known about their effects on the MetS components in PsO patients.

Currently, three available in the United States are approved for psoriasis and psoriatic arthritis (PsA): infliximab, etanercept, and adalimumab (Channual J et al, 2009).

Infliximab is a chimeric monoclonal antibody binding the human tumor necrosis factor alpha (Staidle JP et al, 2011).

Actually there are no data in literature about infliximab effect on insulin resistance or sensitivity in PsO patients.

About lipid profiles, studies have shown that infliximab does not significantly modify total cholesterol, triglycerides and, interestingly, the patient's lipid profile reverted to baseline values after infliximab discontinuation (Gisondi P et al, 2008; Antoniou KM et al, 2008).

Studies investigating the effect of infliximab on body weight have reported significant increase in weight gain and in BMI, without differences among males and females (Saraceno R et al, 2009).

Etanercept is a fusion protein consisting of two molecules of extracellular domain of human p75 TNF-alpha receptor attached to the Fc domain of human immunoglobulin G1 (IgG1), that binds to TNF-alpha with greater affinity than natural receptor. The binding makes TNF-alpha biologically inactive, with consequent reduction of inflammation (Weinberg JM, 2003).

Although there are conflicting results on the effect of Etanercept in insulin-resistance, etanercept have shown an interesting action on reducing serum insulin levels and improving insulin sensitivity. Similar to Infliximab, Etanercept does not significantly modify lipid profiles; furthermore, PsO patients treated by etanercept gradually and progressively gain weight, in particular lean ones (Marra M et al, 2007).

Adalimumab is human monoclonal antibody against TNF-alpha (Staidle JP et al, 2011).

Although there are no reports in literature discussing about adalimumab effect on insulin resistance or sensitivity in PsO patients, a recent case revealed episodes of hyperglycemia in a PsO-PsA patient; these increased serum glucose levels resolved after adalimumab discontinuation (Wu JJ et al, 2008).

Similar to Infliximab and Etanercept, Adalimumab does not modify lipid profiles and it increases BMI and weight gain (Saraceno R et al, 2009).

10. Conclusion

Despite further studies on anti-TNF-alpha drug effect on MetS syndrome are required, an examination of literature data suggest that the combined effects of improved insulin resistance and sensitivity and a significant reduction in systemic inflammation may interrupt inflammatory cascade linking PsO and MetS.

Taking into consideration the high potentiality of biological therapies to reduce the metabolic effect of TNF-alpha, the future goal might be to demonstrate a real in vivo preventing effect on development of cardiovascular comorbidities in Pso/PsA patients. For these reason other longitudinal long term clinical studies are needed.

11. References

Adams, LA. & Lindor, KD. (2005). Nonalcoholic fatty liver disease. *CMAJ.*,172,899-905.

Angulo, P.; Hui, JM.; Marchesini, G.& al. (2007). The NAFLD fibrosis score: a non invasive system that identifies liver fibrosis in patients with NAFLD. *Hepatology.*,45(4),846-54.

Antoniou, KM.; Mamoulaki, M.; Malagari, K.; Kritikos, HD.; Bouros, D.; Siafakas, NM. & Boumpas, D. (2007). Infliximab therapy in pulmonary fibrosis associated with collagen vascular disease. *Clin Exp Rheumatol.*,25(1),23-8.

Armstrong, AW.; Lin, SW.; Chambers, CJ.; Sockolov, ME. & Chin, DL. (2011) Psoriasis and Hypertension Severity: Results from a Case-Control Study. *PLoSONE.*,6(3),e18227. doi:10.1371/journal.pone.0018227.

Browning, JD.; Szczepaniak, LS.; Dobbins, R. & al. (2004). Prevalence of hepatic steatosis in an urban population in the United States: impact of ethnicity. *Hepatology,* 40(6),1387-1395.

Capeau, J. (2008). Insulin resistance and steatosis in humans. *Diabet and Metab.*, 34,649-57.

Channual, J.; Wu, JJ. & Dann, FJ. (2009) Effects of tumor necrosis factor-alpha blockade on metabolic syndrome components in psoriasis and psoriatic arthritis and additional lessons learned from rheumatoid arthritis. *Dermatol Ther.*,22(1),61-73.

Chung, CP.; Oeser, A.; Raggi, P.; Gebretsadik, T.; Shintani, AK.; Sokka, T.; Pincus, T.; Avalos, I. & Stein, CM. (2005). Increased coronary-artery atherosclerosis in rheumatoid arthritis: relationship to disease duration and cardiovascular risk factors. *Arthritis Rheum.*, 52(10),3045-53.

Das, UN. (2001). Is obesity an inflammatory condition? *Nutrition.*, 17,953-966.

Day, CP. & James OFW. Steatohepatitis: a tale of two "hits"?. (1998). *Gastroenterology,* 114(4),842-845.

de Luca, C. & Olefsky, JM. (2008). Inflammation and Insulin Resistance. *FEBS Lett.*, 582(1), 97-105.

Esposito, K. & Giugliano, D. (2004). The metabolic syndrome and inflammation: association or causation? *Nutr Metab Cardiovasc Dis.*,14,228-232.

Ferretti, G.; Alleva, R.; Taus, M.; Simonetti, O.; Cinti, B.; Offidani, AM.; Bossi, G. & Curatola, G. (1994). Abnormalities of plasma lipoprotein composition and fluidity in psoriasis. *Acta Derm Venereol.*,74(3),171-5.

Galic, S.; Oakhill, JS. & Steinberg, GR. Adipose tissue as an endocrine organ. (2010). *Mol Cell Endocrinol.*,316,129-139.

Gisondi, P.; Cotena, C.; Tessari, G. & Girolomoni, G. (2008). Anti-tumour necrosis factor-alpha therapy increases body weight in patients with chronic plaque psoriasis: a retrospective cohort study. *J Eur Acad Dermatol Venereol.*,22(3), 341-4.

Gisondi, P.; Tessari, G.; Conti, A.; Piaserico, S.; Schianchi, S.; Peserico, A.; Giannetti, A. & Girolomoni, G. (2007). Prevalence of metabolic syndrome in patients with psoriasis: a hospital-based case-control study. *Br J Dermatol.*, 157(1),68-73.

Henseler, T. & Christophers, E. (1995). Disease concomitance in psoriasis. *J Am Acad Dermatol.*, 32,982–6.

Herron, MD.; Hinckley, M.; Hoffman, MS.; Papenfuss, J.; Hansen, CB., Callis, KP. & al. (2005). Impact of obesity and smoking on psoriasis presentation and management. *Arch Dermatol.*,141,1527–34.

Hotamisligil, GS. (2003). Inflammatory pathways and insulin action. *Int J Obes.*, 27(S), 53.

Jones, SM.; Harris, CPD.; Lloyd,J.; Stirling, CA.; Reckless, JPD & McHugh, NJ. (2000). Lipoproteins and their subfractions in psoriatic arthritis: identification of an atherogenic profile with active joint disease. *Ann Rheum Dis.*,59,904–909

Kashihara, H.; Lee, J.; Kawakubo, K.; Tamura, M. & Akabayashi, A. (2009). Criteria of Waist Circumference According to Computed Tomography-Measured Visceral Fat Area and the Clustering of Cardiovascular Risk Factors. *Circ J.*,73,1881-1886.

Kershaw, EE. & Flier, JS. Adipose tissue as an endocrine organ. (2004). *J Clin Endocrinol Metab*, 89,2548-2556.

Kissebach, AH.; Vydelingum, N.; Murray, R.; Evans, DJ.; Kalkhoff, RK. & Adams PW. (1982). Relation of Body Fat Distribution to Metabolic Complications of Obesity. *J Clin Endocrinol Metab.*,54,254-260.

Mallbris, L.; Ritchlin, CT. & Stahle, M. (2006). Metabolic disorders in patients with psoriasis and psoriatic arthritis. *Curr Rheumatol Rep*,8,355–63.

Marchesini, G.; Bugianesi, E.; Forlani, G. & al. (2003). Nonalcoholic fatty liver, steatohepatitis, and the metabolic syndrome. *Hepatology.*, 37(4),917–923.

Marra, M.; Campanati, A.; Testa, R. & al. (2007). Effect of Etanercept on insulin sensitivity in nine patients with psoriasis. *Int J Physiol Pharmacol*, 20(4),731-36.

McTernan, C.L.; McTernan, P.G.; Harte, A.L.; Levick, P.L.; Barnett,A.H. & Kumar, S. (2002) Resistin, central obesity, and type 2 diabetes. *Lancet*, 359, 46–47.

Neimann, AL.; Shin, DB.; Wang, X.; Margolis, DJ.; Troxel, AB. & Gelfand, JM. (2006). Prevalence of cardiovascular risk factors in patients with psoriasis. *J Am Acad Dermatol.*,55, 829–35.

Okorodudu, DO.; Jumean, MF.; Montori, VH.; Romero-Corral, A.; Somers, VK.; Erwin, PJ. & Lopez-Jimenez, F. (2010). Diagnostic performance of body mass index to identify obesity as defined by body adiposity: a systemic review and meta-analysis. *Internation Journal of Obesity.*,34,791-799.

Papatheodoridis, GV.; Goulis, J.; Christodoulou, D. & al. (2007). High prevalence of elevated liver enzymes in blood donors: associations with male gender and central adiposity. *European Journal of Gastroenterology & Hepatology.*,19,(4), 281–287.

Saraceno, R.; Schipani, C.; Mazzotta, A.; Esposito, M.; Di Renzo, L.; De Lorenzo, A. & Chimenti, S. (2008). Effect of anti-tumor necrosis factor-alpha therapies on body mass index in patients with psoriasis. *Pharmacol Res.*,57(4),290-5.

Satapathy, SK.; Garg, S.; Chauhan, R.; Sakhuja, P.; Malhotra, V.; Sharma, BC. & Sarin, SK. (2004). Beneficial effects of tumor necrosis factor-alpha inhibition by pentoxifylline on clinical, biochemical, and metabolic parameters of patients with nonalcoholic steatohepatitis. *Am J Gastroenterol.*,99(10),1946-52.

Sommer, DM.; Jenisch, S.; Suchan, M; Christophers, E. & Weichenthal, M. (2006). Increased prevalence of the metabolic syndrome in patients with moderate to severe psoriasis. *Arch Dermatol Res*,(298):321–8.

Staidle, JP.; Dabade, TS. & Feldman, SR. (2011). A pharmacoeconomic analysis of severe psoriasis therapy: a review of treatment choices and cost efficiency. Expert Opin Pharmacother., Jul 8.

Sterry, W.; Barker, J.; Boehncke, WH.; Bos, JD.; Chimenti, S.; Christophers, E.; De La Brassinne, M.; Ferrandiz, C.; Griffiths, C.; Katsambas, A.; Kragballe, K.; Lynde, C.; Menter, A.; Ortonne, JP.; Papp, K.; Prinz, J.; Rzany, B.; Ronnevig, J.; Saurat, JH.; Stahle, M.; Stengel, FM.; Van De Kerkhof, P. & Voorhees J. (2004). Biological therapies in the systemic management of psoriasis: International Consensus Conference. *Br J Dermatol.*,151 Suppl 69,3-17.

Teunissen, MBM.; Piskin, G.; Res, PCJM.; De Groot, M.; Picavet, DI.; De Rie, MA. & Bos, JD. (2007). State of the art in the immunopathogenesis of psoriasis. *G Ital Dermatol Venerol.*, 142, 229-42.

Tsochatzis, S.; Manolakopoulos, GV.; Papatheodoridis, A. & Archimandritis,AJ. (2009). Insulin resistance and metabolic syndrome in chronic liver diseases: old entities with new implications. *Scandinavian Journal of Gastroenterology*, 44(1),6–14.

Vanni, E.; Bugianesi, E.; Kotronen, A.; De Minicis, S.; Yki-Jarvinen, H. & Svegliati Baroni, G. (2010). From the metabolic syndrome to NAFLD or vice versa?. *Dig Liver Dis*, 42(5),320-30.

Wajchenberg, BL. (2000). Subcutaneous and visceral adipose tissue: their relation to the metabolic syndrome. *Endocr Rev.*,21,697-738.

Weinberg, JM. (2003). An overview of infliximab, etanercept, efalizumab, and alefacept as biologic therapy for psoriasis. *Clin Ther.*,25(10),2487-505.

Wu, JJ. & Tsai, TF. (2008). Recurrent hyperglycemia during adalimumab treatment in a patient with psoriasis. *Arch Dermatol.*,144(10),1403-4.

8

UVB and Vitamin D in Psoriasis

A. Osmancevic
Dept of Dermatology, Sahlgrenska University Hospital, Gothenburg, Sweden

1. Introduction

Psoriasis is a chronic, inflammatory disease affecting the skin and potentially the joints. Both genetic and environmental factors are important in the etiology of the disease. Psoriasis is characterized by keratinocyte hyperproliferation, abnormal keratinocyte differentiation, and immune-cell infiltration into the epidermis and dermis.

Disease management is dependent on severity, psychosocial effects and the patient's lifestyle. Currently, psoriasis may be treated with phototherapy or by using various topical, systemic, and biologic drug treatments. Topical treatments include creams and ointments containing tar, dithranol, corticosteroids, salicylic acid or vitamin D-related compounds.

Vitamin D3 analogs inhibit proliferation, induce terminal differentiation of human keratinocytes and exhibit immunomodulating properties. Several studies have shown vitamin D analogs to be a safe, efficacious and long-term treatment option for psoriasis. Vitamin D3 analogs are also used in combination with phototherapy.

Phototherapy (broadband UVB, narrowband UVB (NBUVB) and heliotherapy - treatment with natural sunlight) is a commonly used treatment modality for widespread psoriasis. A similar wavelength spectrum of UVB (280-315 nm) is responsible for vitamin D synthesis in the skin. Vitamin D3, or cholecalciferol, is produced from 7-dehydrocholesterol in the basal epidermis when exposed to UVB, and is then hydroxylated in the liver into 25-hydroxyvitamin D [25(OH)D], which is the major circulating metabolite. Further hydroxylation into 1,25-dihydroxyvitamin D [1,25(OH)2D] occurs primarily in the kidneys. Hydroxylation in the kidneys is stimulated by parathyroid hormone (PTH) and suppressed by phosphate. Homeostatic mechanisms include parathyroid activity, serum calcium and serum 1,25(OH)2D3 itself. Vitamin D is an essential steroid not only for calcium homeostasis and skeletal health, but also for regulation of cellular growth, cell proliferation and cell differentiation. Vitamin D is obtained by skin production in response to UVB or by intake of vitamin D rich food or supplements. Vitamin D status is measured by serum/blood concentration of its metabolite 25(OH)D.

The wavelength spectrum of UVB responsible for vitamin D synthesis (broadband UVB, 290-320 nm) has been used successfully for years to treat psoriasis and other chronic inflammatory skin disorders. This chapter aims to increase knowledge about the effects of UVB on vitamin D production during treatment with phototherapy in patients with psoriasis and to investigate the impact of UVB-induced vitamin D on psoriasis, bone, lipid and carbohydrate status in psoriasis patients. A review of the published studies will be used to accomplish this task. In our previously published studies, the serum concentrations of 25(OH)D, 1,25(OH)2D, PTH, calcium and creatinine were measured before and after phototherapy in Caucasian patients with moderate to severe active plaque psoriasis. Bone mineral density (BMD) was examined using dual-energy X-ray absorptiometry (DEXA) at the hip and lumbar spine in a group of postmenopausal women with psoriasis. Lipid and carbohydrate status were assessed in patients treated with heliotherapy.

We found that UVB/heliotherapy improved the psoriasis score and lipid and carbohydrate status of the patients, increased serum 25(OH)D synthesis and reduced serum PTH concentrations. Vitamin D production in psoriasis patients increased less with narrowband UVB than with broadband UVB phototherapy. There was no correlation between the dose of UVB and the increase in 25(OH)D. The ratio of low density lipoprotein (LDL) and high density lipoprotein (HDL) cholesterol decreased, and the levels of glycosylated hemoglobin A1c (HbA1c) also decreased in psoriasis patients during heliotherapy. Postmenopausal women with psoriasis had higher BMD than age-matched controls, a finding that could be related to their higher body weight, levels of physical activity and UVB exposure.

The changes in serum concentrations of vitamin D metabolite 25(OH)D were not related to the degree of improvement in psoriasis severity. This can be explained by the fact that 25(OH)D is biologically inert. It is unclear if the serum 25(OH)D level is linked to the level of the active form of vitamin D3 (1,25(OH)2D) present in the skin. It has been suggested that cutaneous conversion of 25(OH)D to 1,25(OH)2D does not play a role because the amount of free 25(OH)D3 that penetrates the cell membrane of epidermal keratinocytes is too small to produce sufficient amounts of 1,25(OH)2D. Therefore, of great interest will be the study of UVB induced local effects on vitamin D synthesis and metabolism in psoriatic skin.

2. Content

2.1 Vitamin D, skin production and metabolism

Vitamin D or calciferol refers to cholecalciferol or vitamin D3 and ergocalciferol or vitamin D2. D3 is produced in the skin as a result of ultraviolet irradiation of 7-dehydrocholesterol (7-DHC) and D2 is produced by ultraviolet irradiation of the plant sterol ergosterol(1).

Vitamin D was discovered in the 1900's as a result of research efforts geared towards the treatment of the disease, rickets. Within the last decade, vitamin D has become a popular topic in medical research as investigators aim to elucidate the role it plays in both maintaining health and contributing to the onset of disease.

Most people obtain their vitamin D requirement from sunlight exposure (2) in addition to smaller amounts obtained through the diet since very few foods naturally contain vitamin D.

7-DHC absorbs ultraviolet B (UVB) radiation and optimum wavelengths for vitamin D3 production are between 295 nm and 300 nm with a peak at 297 nm(3). Levels of 7-DHC have been observed to decline with age, which might negatively impact vitamin D3 synthesis in the skin (2). Vitamin D3 produced in the skin or ingested from the diet can be stored in body fat and later released into circulation. Vitamin D3 is sequestered deep into body fat, making it less bioavailable in obese individuals(4). Vitamin D is biologically inert and must be hydroxylated in the liver to form 25-hydroxyvitamin D [25(OH)D or calcidiol], which is the major circulating metabolite. Further hydroxylation into 1,25-dihydroxyvitamin D [1,25(OH)2D or calcitriol] occurs primarily in the kidneys (Figure 1). Hydroxylation in the kidneys is stimulated by parathyroid hormone (PTH) and suppressed by phosphate. Homeostatic mechanisms include parathyroid activity, serum calcium and serum 1,25(OH)2D itself. Conversion of vitamin D to 25(OH)D is mediated by the enzyme vitamin D-25-hydroxylase (CYP27A1). The synthesis and degradation of calcitriol are regulated by the enzymes 25(OH)D-1-α-hydroxylase (CYP27B1) and 25(OH)2D-24-hydroxylase (CYP24A1), respectively. The combined activity of these enzymes is an important factor in determining the circulating concentrations of 25(OH)D, and 1,25(OH)2D(1). In addition to the kidney, other tissues and cells, including keratinocytes and immune cells, contain these enzymes and are able to convert 25(OH)D to active 1,25(OH)2D(5).

Besides being an essential steroid for calcium homeostasis and skeletal health, vitamin D also plays a role in regulation of cellular growth, cell proliferation and cell differentiation. Vitamin D also regulates the immune system, controls cancer cell growth and plays a role in the regulation of blood pressure(6). These effects are mediated through the intracellularly located vitamin D receptor (VDR). VDR is a member of the steroid, estrogen and retinoid receptor gene family of proteins that mediate transcriptional activities of the respective ligands. The VDR complex interacts with vitamin D responsive elements on the target gene. Alterations in calcitriol levels and polymorphisms of the VDR gene have been shown to be associated with several malignant and autoimmune diseases including psoriasis vulgaris(7).

25(OH)D is used clinically to measure vitamin D status. The cut-off level for serum 25(OH)D, which is used as a diagnostic marker for vitamin D deficiency, has varied over the years(8-10). The early biochemical changes in vitamin D insufficiency include a rise in serum PTH, which begins to increase as serum 25(OH)D levels fall below 30 ng/ml or 75 nmol/l(9). This level of 25(OH)D has become the suggested cut-off point for vitamin D deficiency or inadequacy(9, 11-13). At the present time, there is no clear consensus regarding levels of 25(OH)D for optimal health but levels of > 50 nmol/l (20 ng/ml)(14) and > 75 nmol/l (30 ng/ml) have been based on considering the outcomes of bone health, fracture prevention and colorectal cancer(15,16). Sun exposure is the strongest factor influencing 25(OH)D. The serum concentrations of 25(OH)D vary seasonally, with maximum and minimum values in the late summer and winter respectively(17). The extent of this seasonal variation depends on factors such as latitude, skin pigmentation, clothing, and the use of sunscreen(18).

Currently, limited data is available on the role of vitamin D deficiency in the pathogenesis or outcomes of psoriasis. The lack of conclusive data combined with vitamin D's immunomodulatory role, warrants further research investigating the role of vitamin D insufficiency in chronic diseases as well as monitoring 25(OH)D levels in children and adults of all ages as a part of routine physical examinations.

2.2 The effects of vitamin D in psoriasis

Vitamin D has pleotropic functions; it acts as a hormone by controlling calcium homeostasis as well as exerting autocrine/paracrine effects on tissues that express CYP27B1 and VDR. Besides its local effects, calcitriol may also act in psoriasis through its immunomodulatory properties by inhibiting T-cell proliferation and Th1 development, modulating antigen-presenting cell (APCs) function, inducing hyporesponsiveness to antigens, inhibiting production of IL-2, IL-17, IL-8 and interferon-γ, increasing the production of IL-10 and regulatory T cells(19, 20). Calcitriol has also been suggested to reduce production of interferon-α in some cells(21). Calcitriol is involved in the regulation of antimicrobial peptides cathelicidin and human β-defensin 2 (HBD2), which both participate in the pathogenesis of psoriasis (22). Vitamin D's role in psoriasis is further supported by studies that confirm the link between VDR polymorphism and psoriasis (23, 24). An association between VDR genotypes (Apa1) and the mean age at onset of psoriasis were previously observed (25). Since VDR gene polymorphisms show ethnic variability, concern arises on how to treat psoriasis patients of different populations according to their potentially varied treatment response (26). Moreover, it has been demonstrated that VDR gene polymorphisms may also play a role in partial resistance to calcipotriol therapy (24).

There are few studies on high-dose vitamin D3 in the treatment of psoriasis while systemic administration of 1,25(OH)2D for the treatment of psoriasis might be limited by its toxicity. A number of small trials show the efficacy and safety of vitamin D metabolites in the treatment of psoriasis and psoriatic arthritis (27-29). Systemic calcitriol treatment had an immunomodulatory effect manifested by a short-term temporary decrease in type 1 immune responses and a decrease in disease activity in patients with psoriatic arthropathy (27). Administration of vitamin D3 could be a better option than calcitriol or alphacalcidol since it is safer and less expensive, although more studies are needed to assess its efficacy (21). However, the use of calcitiol in dermatology is hampered by its hypercalcemic activity. There is limited information on the role of vitamin D deficiency in the pathogenesis of psoriasis or the role of vitamin D deficiency in response to treatments with topical or systemic drugs. There is a report of resolution of anti-TNFα-induced psoriasiform lesions by high doses of vitamin D3, in a patient with rheumatoid arthritis and vitamin D deficiency (21). More studies are needed to assess the possible usefulness of high-dose vitamin D3 in the treatment of psoriasis.

2.3 Effects of vitamin D3 analogues in psoriasis

The observation that keratinocytes and T cells express VDR and that 1,25(OH)2D is a potent stimulator of keratinocyte differentiation provides a potential basis for the clinical use of VDR ligands for the treatment of psoriasis (30, 31). Clinical data that first supported the use of vitamin D analogs was obtained when a patient treated orally with 1-hydroxyvitamin D3 for osteoporosis showed remarkable remission of psoriatic lesions(32). In addition, promising clinical results were obtained in studies using oral 1-hydroxyvitamin D3, oral and topical calcitriol which led to improvement of psoriatic lesions in approximately 70-80% of patients (33). Vitamin D3 analogs (calcipotriol (Dovonex), calcitriol (Silkis) or tacalcitol (Curatoderm)) inhibit proliferation, induce terminal differentiation of human keratinocytes and exhibit immunomodulating properties (33). Differentiation of keratinocytes results in the formation of a cornified envelope (CE) that provides the barrier function of the skin. The expression of involucrin, a component of the CE, and transglutaminase I (TGase I), the enzyme that cross-links the components of CE, was increased by calcitriol and other VDR ligands(35). Treatment of keratinocytes with a medium containing high calcium also stimulated keratinocyte differentiation by increasing the expression of involucrin and TGase I. 1,25(OH)2D also promoted keratinocyte differentiation, at least in part by increasing intracellular calcium and by increased expression of calcium receptors in keratinocytes(36). Calcitriol indirectly induces the expression of keratin 1, involucrin, TGase I, loricrin, and filaggrin, which are required for CE formation. VDR ligands decreased the expression of proinflammatory cytokines IL-2, IFN-γ, IL-6, IL-8 (37-40) and proliferation of T lymphocytes and keratinocytes. Furthermore, topical calcipotriol increased anti-inflammatory cytokine IL-10 in psoriatic lesions(41), and increased the expression of IL-10 receptor in keratinocytes(42).

Antigen presenting cells (APCs), which play an important role in psoriasis, are one of the major targets of calcitriol-mediated immunosuppressive action (43). VDR ligands prevent the activation, differentiation, maturation and survival of APCs, leading to T cell hyporesponsiveness(44). Calcitriol also increased the expression of IL-10 and decreased the expression of IL-12, two major cytokines that are involved in Th1-Th2 balance(45).

Several studies have shown that calcipotriol as well as calcitriol and tacalcitol are efficacious, safe and can be used on a long-term basis for psoriasis (43, 46-49). Vitamin D3 analogs can be used in combination with phototherapy(50).

2.4 Vitamin D status in patients with psoriasis

Few studies on vitamin D status and its role in psoriasis have been performed or published. Low vitamin D status is associated with an increased risk of cancer, autoimmune, infectious, and inflammatory diseases, although the role of vitamin D status in the pathogenesis of psoriasis is unknown.

3. The effects of phototherapy on vitamin D status in patients with psoriasis

A similar wavelength spectrum of UVB is responsible for vitamin D synthesis (280-315 nm), which has been successfully used for years to treat psoriasis and other chronic inflammatory skin disorders.

Phototherapy (broadband UVB, narrowband UVB and heliotherapy - treatment with natural sunlight) is an effective treatment, commonly used for widespread psoriasis. Therefore, phototherapy is an excellent option for patients with generalized psoriasis because of its superior systemic safety profile in comparison to systemic and biologic agents (51).

In addition to standard broadband ultraviolet radiation B (BUVB), (280-315 nm), narrowband phototherapy (NBUVB) (monochromatic UV between 311-312 nm) and heliotherapy (treatment with natural sunlight) have become important treatment modalities for psoriasis. Research suggests that NBUVB is more effective than broadband UVB for reducing PASI scores, as well as being a safer and better tolerated option for patients in comparison to PUVA when taken at suberythemogenic doses (52). Furthermore, these advantages along with the handling ease of the NBUVB lamp led to a reduction in the usage of broadband UVB. However, one drawback of the new lamp is that the radiation times have almost doubled (54). Additionally, several studies indicate that combination therapy using both calcipotriol and UVB radiation illustrate more rapid healing of psoriasis when compared to monotherapy of either treatment (50,55).

Serum levels of 25(OH)D increased during treatment with artificial UV (BUVB and NBUVB) and during heliotherapy(56-59). The increase in 25(OH)D was higher in the BUVB treated patients when compared to the NBUVB ($p=0.008$) and heliotherapy ($p=0.017$) treated groups. Low-dose NBUVB treatment significantly increased vitamin D status in patients with psoriasis, atopic eczema and other skin disorders with low initial levels of 25(OH)D(60, 61). Within the following intervention studies, age showed no correlation with the observed increase in 25(OH)D levels (57, 58, 62). This indicates the skin's capacity to produce vitamin D3 during phototherapy of psoriasis is independent of the patient's age or psoriasis severity. Phototherapy of psoriasis is the time-consuming procedure long enough to provide adequate cutaneous production of vitamin D even in elderly patients. The ability of the skin to produce vitamin D declines with age (63) due to insufficient sunlight exposure (11, 64) and a reduction in the functional production capacity of the skin(63, 65, 66). The increase in 25(OH)D3 was enhanced in patients with low baseline levels of vitamin D.

Vitamin D production in patients with psoriasis increased less with NBUVB than with BUVB phototherapy(58). One explanation might be that the optimal wavelength for initiation of the vitamin D3 pathway was 300±5 nm in vitro and in vivo(67, 68) which is in the BUVB range (280-315 nm). The synthesis of vitamin D was stimulated by wavelengths between 290-315 nm, but not for wavelengths longer than 315 nm. One study (58) reported that a wavelength of 311 nm effectively induced vitamin D synthesis, but not to the same extent as wavelengths in the BUVB range. UVB treatment including NBUVB treatment of psoriasis was a sufficiently time-consuming procedure to increase vitamin D. The time required for NBUVB to have an effect can reduce the difference in the potential of vitamin D production between the two lamps. The treatment time correlated strongly with the type of lamp (patients treated with NBUVB required 4 times the exposure patients treated with BUVB needed). This is consistent with other studies demonstrating that the dose response of the erythemal spectra of NBUVB should be about 4.2 times that of BUVB(69). The dose of UVB also correlated with the type of lamp, but no correlation between the dose of UVB and the increase of 25(OH)D3 levels was found (58). This might be due to the fact that serum concentrations of 25(OH)D3 were measured at different time points and a plateau level was reached after three weeks, which was also seen in a previous study(70). An *in vitro* study demonstrated that the dose-response relationship of UV exposure and cholecalciferol synthesis was nonlinear. It was hypothesized that exposure to additional UV did not result in a proportional increase in vitamin D levels(71). This might be explained by autoregulation of the skin synthesis, storage, and slow, steady release of vitamin D3 from the skin into the circulation(3). Non-linear vitamin D synthesis is easily explained by the photo equilibrium that is set up as a result of continued exposure to ultraviolet radiation as reported by Holick et al(72). Vitamin D production is a unique, autoregulated mechanism which occurs at two levels. Excessive sun exposure does not lead to overdosing of vitamin D3 due to conversion of previtamin D3 to inactive photoproducts (lumisterol 3 and tachisterol 3) as well as conversion of vitamin D3 to its isomers in the skin (5,6-trans vitamin D3, suprasterol I, suprasterol II) which are thought to have a low calcemic effect at physiological concentrations. The synthesis of previtamin D3 reached a plateau at about 10 to 15 percent of the original 7-dehydrocholesterol content(72). Vitamin D3 is synthesized in the skin and released steadily and slowly from the skin into the circulation(3).

In a study by Ryan, the number of exposures to NBUVB was the sole predictor of an increase in serum 25(OH)D level, whereas prior phototherapy was the only predictor of baseline serum 25(OH)D levels in the group of psoriasis patients treated with phototherapy(73).

Patients with lower 25(OH)D levels at baseline responded better to sunlight and phototherapy which is consistent with other studies(3, 6, 57). All patients reached serum levels of 30 ng/ml (75 nmol/l) after two weeks of sun exposure(62). A circulating level of 25(OH)D of >30 ng/ml, or >75 nmol/L, appears to be necessary to maximize the health benefits of vitamin D(6).

Sun exposure is the major source of vitamin D for most humans(6). During the winter months vitamin D production is insufficient to meet the optimal requirements in both younger and older adults at Northern latitudes(74). Psoriasis lesions usually worsen during winter, and many patients are therefore given repeated UVB treatment during this season. In addition to healing psoriatic lesions, UVB therapy also provides these patients with vitamin D during the winter months, when levels of 25(OH)D in Northern countries are generally low. UVB therapy even increased serum 25(OH)D levels in patients taking vitamin D supplements. This is in line with previous studies, which reported that UV-induced vitamin D synthesis had a greater influence on the serum levels of circulating calcidiol than the per oral intake of supplements(75, 76).

Skin pigment, sunscreen use, aging, time of day, season, and latitude all affect previtamin D3 synthesis(18). There was no difference in the increase of 25(OH)D between the different skin types in the present studies(59). This was most likely due to subjects being exposed to individually adjusted doses of UVB depending on skin phototype and erythemal response to therapy. All patients had previously experienced UVB therapy for their psoriasis disease. As expected, fair-skinned patients required lower doses of UVB (broadband and narrowband) than patients with skin type III and IV. This finding is consistent with other studies examining the effect of skin pigmentation on vitamin D synthesis(77). Melanin pigment in human skin competes with, and absorbs UVB photons responsible for the vitamin D synthesis(77).

The increase in 25(OH)D during the first two weeks of heliotherapy was very similar to the increase in 25(OH)D during treatment with BUVB and NBUVB for two to three months. The correlation between sunlight measures and serum 25(OH)D is evidently weak(78). Patients reached their plateau of daily sun exposure after the first week. It is likely that vitamin D production was most prominent during the first week, when the patients experienced redness and some of them even got sunburned(56).

The increase in 25(OH)D during 15 days of climate therapy was significant even though patients used sunscreen on body sites susceptible to sunburn, and though the skin was affected by psoriasis lesions(56, 62). This indicates that short-term therapeutic UVB exposures are sufficient to increase vitamin D synthesis in psoriasis patients. SPF-8 sunscreen has been observed to reduce the skin's production of vitamin D3 by 95%(79). Clothing also completely blocks all solar UVB radiation and thereby prevents vitamin D3 production(79).

Psoriasis improved in all patients, with a reduction in the PASI score of about 75% on all regimens(59, 73). Improvement in psoriasis correlated positively with the increase in 25(OH)D3 levels in one (58) ($p=0.047$; the group of patients treated with BUVB and NBUVB) but not in the other studies (57, 61, 62, 73). There was no correlation between change in serum 25(OH)D levels and change in PASI or change in DLQI in the study of psoriasis patients treated with NBUVB in Ireland(73). No relationship was found between levels of 25(OH)D and psoriasis but a negative correlation was found between the severity of psoriasis and the basal serum level of 1,25(OH)2D(80).

The skin is the only tissue yet known in which the complete UVB-induced pathway from 7-DHC via intermediates (previtamin D3, vitamin D3, 25(OH)D) to the final product 1,25(OH)2D, takes place under physiological conditions(81), (Figure 1). Levels of 1,25(OH)2D tended to increase during phototherapy, but significant increases were noticed only during heliotherapy, and only in women with 25(OH)D3 below 30 ng/ml, and in ages ≥ 70 years. One explanation might be that these patients had lower serum concentrations of 25(OH)D at the start of the treatment.

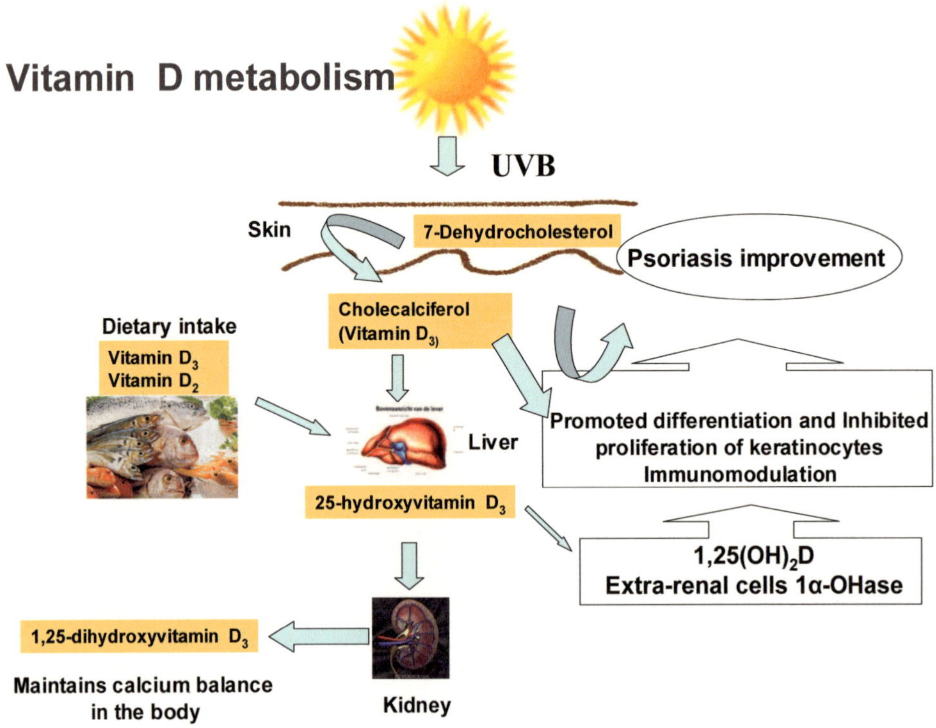

Fig. 1. Schematic outline of vitamin D metabolism and mechanism of action in psoriasis.

It has been postulated that the synthesis of 1,25(OH)2D is tightly regulated, and that increases in 25(OH)D concentrations due to exposure to sunlight have no effect on serum 1,25(OH)2D levels(6, 82). The observation that both 25(OH)D and 1,25(OH)2D increased in vitamin D deficient subjects following UVB exposure(83) or after vitamin D supplementation(84) has been reported previously. The increase of 1,25(OH)2D levels between patients treated with heliotherapy and patients treated with NBUVB differed (p=0.02). This might be explained by lower values of 25(OH)D at baseline in patients treated with heliotherapy(59).

Keratinocytes are capable of producing a variety of vitamin D metabolites, including 1,25(OH)2D, 24,25(OH)2D, 1,24,25(OH)3D(85) from exogenous and endogenous sources of 25(OH)D. Thus, the local UVB-triggered production of calcitriol may primarily regulate epidermal cellular functions in an auto- and paracrine manner, but this should not be crucial for systemic vitamin D effects (5) and systemic vitamin D deficiency does not stimulate epidermal synthesis of 1,25(OH)2D(86).

Cutaneous production of 1,25(OH)2D3 may regulate growth, differentiation, apoptosis and other biological processes in the skin(87, 88). Therefore, topical vitamin D analogs have been used as a safe and effective treatment for psoriasis vulgaris(89, 90). The NBUVB has been shown to have less capacity to induce a local skin production of 1,25(OH)2D3 at 44% of the monochromatic irradiation at 300 ±2.5 nm(68). Nevertheless, the known therapeutic effect of UVB light therapy for the treatment of psoriasis may be mediated via UVB-induced production of 1,25(OH)2D(81). In vitro studies have shown that the substrate concentration of cholecalciferol in keratinocytes mainly determines the synthesis rate of 1,25(OH)2D in these cells(91). Thus, higher synthesis rates of cholecalciferol should result in a faster and more pronounced release of 1,25(OH)2D into the extracellular fluid. UVB-induced membrane damage to epidermal keratinocytes may also increase the outflow of newly synthesized calcitriol(92).

It is not clear if the serum 25(OH)D level is linked to the level of the active form of vitamin D3 present in the skin. It has been suggested that cutaneous conversion of 25(OH)D to 1,25(OH)2D does not play a role because the amount of free 25(OH)D3 that penetrates the cell membrane of epidermal keratinocytes is too small to produce sufficient amounts of 1,25(OH)2D(88). The main form of circulating 25(OH)D is presented in a complex with vitamin D-binding protein (DBP) with only a very small amount (0.03%) available as the free form. Furthermore, the deeper layers of the epidermis are not vascularized, which further impairs the passage of the 25(OH)D3-DBP complex from blood to epidermal keratinocytes(88).

The receptor for calcitriol and the production of 1,25(OH)2D vary with the differentiation in a manner suggesting feedback regulation, and both are reduced in the later stages of differentiation(93). 1,25(OH)2D increases involucrin, transglutaminase activity, and cornified envelope formation in preconfluent keratinocytes(94). NBUVB treatment increases cathelicidin and decreases HBD2 levels in healing skin lesions of psoriasis and atopic dermatitis(61). It has been shown that HBD2 and cathelicidin expression in psoriatic skin are higher in serum vitamin D sufficient patients than in serum vitamin D deficient psoriasis patients(95).

The 1,25(OH)2D molecule and its analogs, as well as UVB phototherapy, exert antiproliferative, prodifferentiative, and immune-modulatory effects on keratinocytes that are of particular importance for the therapy of hyperproliferative skin diseases such as psoriasis vulgaris(5, 96). However, the full range of UVB and vitamin D3 effects is not completely understood.

4. Serum PTH in psoriasis patients during treatment with phototherapy

PTH decreased after the treatment with phototherapy(57). 25(OH)D concentrations below 30 ng/ml (75 nmol/l) resulted in secondary hyperparathyroidism and a decrease in BMD(97). PTH increases with increasing age, possibly due to less sunlight exposure and/or reduced calcium/vitamin D intake(98). The clear concomitant decrease in serum PTH after UVB exposure indicates that the skin's capacity to synthesize vitamin D is maintained even at older ages and with part of the skin covered by psoriatic lesions. Serum concentrations of calcium and creatinine were unaltered after phototherapy(58).

5. Bone status in patients with psoriasis treated with UVB phototherapy

Multiple risk factors that contribute to low serum 25(OH)D and osteoporosis have been identified. They include inadequate sun exposure(99), insufficient intake of fortified foods or vitamin D supplements(100), low body mass index, white ethnicity, lack of exercise, use of medications that accelerate vitamin D metabolism, diseases that alter vitamin D metabolism such as malabsorption syndromes, and chronic liver disease(9, 13, 101).

Information regarding the prevalence of osteoporosis in addition to the epidemiological study of risk factors for developing osteoporosis among psoriasis patients has been sparse and controversial. Psoriasis patients with or without arthritis may suffer from osteoporosis(102). However, a previous study showed that patients with chronic plaque psoriasis had a low BMD despite risk factors, although the subgroup with joint involvement appeared to be at a higher risk of developing osteoporosis and therefore required prevention therapy(103). Reduced BMD has been linked to palmoplantar pustular psoriasis(104). The existence of less severe periarticular osteoporosis has also been reported(105). Psoriasis patients with peripheral arthritis with longer duration of joint disease(106) and patients with a greater number of affected joints are at a higher risk of developing osteoporosis(102).In a study by Pedreira, patients with psoriasis and psoriatic arthritis did not present with a lower BMD, but they had a higher prevalence of osteoporotic fractures and were at a higher risk of developing metabolic syndrome(107).

Postmenopausal women with psoriasis treated with phototherapy had higher BMD of both the hip and lumbar spine compared with age-matched controls (57, 108). In the same study(108), patients with 25(OH)D levels below 30 ng/ml and secondary hyperparathyroidism had lower BMD in terms of both T and Z scores of the hip and the lumbar spine compared with those with higher vitamin D levels, consistent with another study(109). No relationship between psoriasis onset and bone status was found. Higher body weight and BMI are factors, which may have contributed to the higher BMD in patients(108) compared with controls

In general, bone loss increases with age. BMD has been shown to be a predictive indicator for bone fractures in healthy subjects and in patients with osteoporosis(111).

A family history of fractures, physical activity, smoking and estrogen substitution are important factors influencing bone mass(112-114). Low body weight is related to low skeletal muscle mass and an increased risk of fractures(114, 115). Muscle tissue and strength are important for body balance and the prevention of falls(116). Previous studies confirm the protective effect of weight gain against fractures(17).

Physical activity correlated positively with BMD in psoriasis patients(108). Physical activity has been claimed to be beneficial for bone mass and protective against fractures(117). Regular walking in middle-aged and elderly women is associated with a reduced risk of vertebral deformity(118). Subjects who took a daily walk of at least 30 min had a significantly better climbing capacity, higher BMD and lower concentration of serum triglycerides than subjects who walked less(119). Lifetime exercise was also positively associated with BMD of the hip(120).

Vitamin D is important for bone metabolism(121). Vitamin D deficiency thus contributes to the pathogenesis of osteoporosis and hip fractures(122). Supplementation strategies involving calcium and vitamin D supplements are cost-effective for preventing osteoporotic fractures(123).

The same range of UVB (290–315 nm) that induces vitamin D synthesis also improves psoriasis. Treatment with UVB in patients with psoriasis is most common during winter months when UVB is lacking, and levels of vitamin D are low in Northern countries(123). Furthermore, UVB therapy heals psoriasis and supplies these patients with vitamin D at levels similar to those of the general population(123), which might have positive effects on bone status as well.

6. Blood glucose and lipid status in psoriasis patients during treatment with heliotherapy

Psoriasis is considered a chronic and debilitating inflammatory disease associated with serious comorbidities (124, 125). Large epidemiological studies have shown that psoriasis and psoriatic arthritis are associated with metabolic diseases including obesity, dyslipidemia and diabetes(126). The chronic inflammation in psoriasis can predispose patients to other inflammatory conditions. The proinflammatory cytokines, such as tumor necrosis factor-α (TNF-α), and other factors that are overproduced in patients with psoriasis likely contribute to the increased risk for the development of metabolic syndrome(127, 128).

Inflammatory factors have also been associated with insulin resistance and β-cell failure, both of which are key features of type 2 diabetes mellitus (129). There is evidence that vitamin D may stimulate pancreatic insulin secretion directly through nuclear receptors that are found in a wide variety of tissues, including T and B lymphocytes, skeletal muscle, and the pancreatic islet β-cells(130). There is some evidence that suggests increased PTH activity is associated with, and possibly causes, reduced insulin sensitivity(130). The prevalence of impaired glucose tolerance and diabetes mellitus is increased in patients with primary hyperparathyroidism (131, 132).

Vitamin D has a wide range of effects on the immune system: it promotes the differentiation of monocytes into macrophages thus increasing their cytotoxic activity; reduces the antigen-presenting activity of macrophages to lymphocytes; prevents dendritic cell maturation; inhibits T lymphocyte-mediated immunoglobulin synthesis in B cells and inhibits delayed-type hypersensitivity reactions(8, 133, 134). Furthermore vitamin D has been reported to down-regulate the production of several cytokines: IL-2, IL-6 and IL-12, interferon-γ, TNF-α, and TNF-β (134, 135). Alternations in vitamin D status and/or action may affect insulin sensitivity, β-cell function or both. Therefore, vitamin D may be involved in the pathogenesis of type 2 diabetes mellitus at both environmental and genetic levels(129). Psoriasis patients are more likely to be insulin resistant and to have impaired glucose tolerance, higher fasting insulin levels, and impaired β-cell function than non-psoriatic subjects(136).

Heliotherapy improves lipid and carbohydrate status of psoriasis patients(56). Increases in high-density lipoprotein (HDL)-cholesterol and decreases in HbA1c during climate therapy could be explained by several factors. One possible mechanism could be a direct effect of vitamin D on insulin sensitivity(130). Another is that sun exposure usually implies greater outdoor physical activity, leading to beneficial effects on lipids and insulin sensitivity, unrelated to serum 25(OH)D concentrations(130). Diet might also influence glucose and lipid metabolism. Although climate therapy did not change the basal glucose levels of the patients, the HbA1c levels decreased about 10 %, indicating improved insulin sensitivity (56). The observed associations between vitamin D, insulin, and glucose metabolism in humans have not yet been confirmed by intervention studies and, hence, a causal association has not been established(130).

A high prevalence of atherosclerosis is also reported in psoriasis patients. High serum lipid levels have been suggested in the pathogenesis of atherosclerosis. High serum lipid levels are more common in psoriasis and may be responsible for an elevated prevalence of cardiovascular accidents in this group of patients(137). Patients with psoriasis exhibit a dyslipidemic profile, including increased levels of plasma cholesterol, triglycerides (TG), LDL, very low-density lipoprotein (VLDL) cholesterol and decreased levels of HDL cholesterol. Lipid abnormalities in psoriasis patients may be genetically determined(138). The ratio of low-density lipoprotein cholesterol (LDL) and high-density lipoprotein cholesterol (HDL) decreased, and the levels of hemoglobin A1c (HbA1c) also decreased in psoriasis patients during heliotherapy(56). Serum concentrations of 25(OH)D at baseline in psoriasis patients treated with heliotherapy correlated positively with serum HDL at baseline(56), consistent with a previously published study(139).

Psoriasis is associated with obesity, which is a component of metabolic syndrome. Obesity has been shown to be an independent risk factor for the development of psoriasis, and is also associated with more severe psoriasis (140). Abdominal obesity is a proinflammatory state with the visceral adipose tissue providing a rich source of inflammatory molecules known as adipocytokines including leptin, adiponectin, visfatin and resistin. This may explain an important association between obesity, insulin resistance and related inflammatory disorders.

Inflammation plays a key role in the pathogenesis of psoriasis and a number of chronic inflammatory systemic diseases listed above. Activated inflammatory cells and pro-inflammatory cytokines, such as TNF-α and IL-1β, contribute to the development of psoriatic lesions and play an important role in atherosclerosis (141).

7. Conclusion

Recent literature has provided plenty of information concerning the preventive and therapeutic role of vitamin D in many inflammatory diseases including psoriasis. Vitamin D inhibits proinflammatory processes by suppressing the enhanced activity of immune cells that take part in the autoimmune reaction. Phototherapy (UVB and heliotherapy) improved psoriasis and lipid and carbohydrate status of the patients, increased serum 25(OH)D synthesis and reduced serum PTH concentrations. UVB therapy heals psoriasis and supplies these patients with vitamin D, which might have positive effects on bone status as well.

The beneficial role of vitamin D for psoriasis might be due to both a skin and systemic increase in vitamin D metabolism. Cutaneous 1,25(OH)2D generated in psoriatic skin after UVB exposure develops a growth-inhibitory effect on proliferating epidermal keratinocytes similar to topically applicated calcitriol. It is unknown if skin affected by diseases such as psoriasis or eczema differ in vitamin D production compared to normal skin. Further research is needed to achieve a more comprehensive understanding of the synthesis of vitamin D in psoriatic skin and the role of vitamin D status in the prevention and treatment of psoriasis.

8. References

[1] Bikle DD. Vitamin D: Production, metabolism, and mechanisms of action. Diseases of Bone and Calcium Metabolism, Hyperparathyroidism: Endotex.com, 2004. p. 1-27.
[2] Holick MF. McCollum Award Lecture, 1994: vitamin D--new horizons for the 21st century. Am J Clin Nutr. 1994 Oct;60(4):619-30.
[3] Holick MF. The cutaneous photosynthesis of previtamin D3: a unique photoendocrine system. J Invest Dermatol. 1981 Jul;77(1):51-8.
[4] Holick MF. The vitamin D epidemic and its health consequences. J Nutr. 2005 Nov;135(11):2739S-48S.
[5] Bar M, Domaschke D, Meye A, Lehmann B, Meurer M. Wavelength-dependent induction of CYP24A1-mRNA after UVB-triggered calcitriol synthesis in cultured human keratinocytes. J Invest Dermatol. 2007 Jan;127(1):206-13.
[6] Holick MF, Chen TC. Vitamin D deficiency: a worldwide problem with health consequences. Am J Clin Nutr. 2008 Apr;87(4):1080S-6S.
[7] Rucevic I, Barisic-Drusko V, Glavas-Obrovac L, Stefanic M. Vitamin D endocrine system and psoriasis vulgaris--review of the literature. Acta Dermatovenerol Croat. 2009;17(3):187-92.
[8] Zittermann A. Vitamin D in preventive medicine: are we ignoring the evidence? Br J Nutr. 2003 May;89(5):552-72.
[9] Favus MJ. Postmenopausal osteoporosis and the detection of so-called secondary causes of low bone density. J Clin Endocrinol Metab. 2005 Jun;90(6):3800-1.
[10] Grant WB, Holick MF. Benefits and requirements of vitamin D for optimal health: a review. Altern Med Rev. 2005 Jun;10(2):94-111.
[11] Chapuy MC, Preziosi P, Maamer M, Arnaud S, Galan P, Hercberg S, et al. Prevalence of vitamin D insufficiency in an adult normal population. Osteoporos Int. 1997;7(5):439-43.
[12] Holick MF, Siris ES, Binkley N, Beard MK, Khan A, Katzer JT, et al. Prevalence of Vitamin D Inadequacy Among Postmenopausal North American Women Receiving Osteoporosis Therapy. Obstet Gynecol Surv. 2005 Oct;60(10):658-9.
[13] Lips P. Vitamin D deficiency and secondary hyperparathyroidism in the elderly: consequences for bone loss and fractures and therapeutic implications. Endocr Rev. 2001 Aug;22(4):477-501.
[14] Lips P. Which circulating level of 25-hydroxyvitamin D is appropriate? J Steroid Biochem Mol Biol. 2004 May;89-90(1-5):611-4.
[15] Bischoff-Ferrari HA, Giovannucci E, Willett WC, Dietrich T, Dawson-Hughes B. Estimation of optimal serum concentrations of 25-hydroxyvitamin D for multiple health outcomes. Am J Clin Nutr. 2006 Jul;84(1):18-28.
[16] Holick MF. Sunlight and vitamin D for bone health and prevention of autoimmune diseases, cancers, and cardiovascular disease. Am J Clin Nutr. 2004 Dec;80(6 Suppl):1678S-88S.
[17] Landin-Wilhelmsen K, Wilhelmsen L, Wilske J, Lappas G, Rosen T, Lindstedt G, et al. Sunlight increases serum 25(OH) vitamin D concentration whereas 1,25(OH)2D3 is unaffected. Results from a general population study in Goteborg, Sweden (The WHO MONICA Project). Eur J Clin Nutr. 1995 Jun;49(6):400-7.
[18] Holick MF. Sunlight, UV-radiation, vitamin D and skin cancer: how much sunlight do we need? Adv Exp Med Biol. 2008;624:1-15.

[19] Arnson Y, Amital H, Shoenfeld Y. Vitamin D and autoimmunity: new aetiological and therapeutic considerations. Ann Rheum Dis. 2007 Sep;66(9):1137-42.
[20] Adams JS, Hewison M. Update in vitamin D. J Clin Endocrinol Metab. Feb;95(2):471-8.
[21] Werner de Castro GR, Neves FS, Pereira IA, Fialho SC, Ribeiro G, Zimmermann AF. Resolution of adalimumab-induced psoriasis after vitamin D deficiency treatment. Rheumatol Int. Feb 3.
[22] Hollox EJ, Huffmeier U, Zeeuwen PL, Palla R, Lascorz J, Rodijk-Olthuis D, et al. Psoriasis is associated with increased beta-defensin genomic copy number. Nat Genet. 2008 Jan;40(1):23-5.
[23] Okita H, Ohtsuka T, Yamakage A, Yamazaki S. Polymorphism of the vitamin D(3) receptor in patients with psoriasis. Arch Dermatol Res. 2002 Jul;294(4):159-62.
[24] Dayangac-Erden D, Karaduman A, Erdem-Yurter H. Polymorphisms of vitamin D receptor gene in Turkish familial psoriasis patients. Arch Dermatol Res. 2007 Dec;299(10):487-91.
[25] Park BS, Park JS, Lee DY, Youn JI, Kim IG. Vitamin D receptor polymorphism is associated with psoriasis. J Invest Dermatol. 1999 Jan;112(1):113-6.
[26] Zuel-Fakkar NM, Kamel MM, Asaad MK, Mahran MZ, Shehab AA. A study of ApaI and TaqI genotypes of the vitamin D receptor in Egyptian patients with psoriasis. Clin Exp Dermatol. Jun;36(4):355-9.
[27] Gaal J, Lakos G, Szodoray P, Kiss J, Horvath I, Horkay E, et al. Immunological and clinical effects of alphacalcidol in patients with psoriatic arthropathy: results of an open, follow-up pilot study. Acta Derm Venereol. 2009;89(2):140-4.
[28] Perez A, Raab R, Chen TC, Turner A, Holick MF. Safety and efficacy of oral calcitriol (1,25-dihydroxyvitamin D3) for the treatment of psoriasis. Br J Dermatol. 1996 Jun;134(6):1070-8.
[29] Huckins D, Felson DT, Holick M. Treatment of psoriatic arthritis with oral 1,25-dihydroxyvitamin D3: a pilot study. Arthritis Rheum. 1990 Nov;33(11):1723-7.
[30] Feldman D, Chen T, Hirst M, Colston K, Karasek M, Cone C. Demonstration of 1,25-dihydroxyvitamin D3 receptors in human skin biopsies. J Clin Endocrinol Metab. 1980 Dec;51(6):1463-5.
[31] Provvedini DM, Tsoukas CD, Deftos LJ, Manolagas SC. 1,25-dihydroxyvitamin D3 receptors in human leukocytes. Science. 1983 Sep 16;221(4616):1181-3.
[32] Morimoto S, Kumahara Y. A patient with psoriasis cured by 1 alpha-hydroxyvitamin D3. Med J Osaka Univ. 1985 Mar;35(3-4):51-4.
[33] Nagpal S, Lu J, Boehm MF. Vitamin D analogs: mechanism of action and therapeutic applications. Curr Med Chem. 2001 Nov;8(13):1661-79.
[34] van der Vleuten CJ, Gerritsen MJ, Steijlen PM, de Jong EM, van de Kerkhof PC. A therapeutic approach to erythrodermic psoriasis: report of a case and a discussion of therapeutic options. Acta Derm Venereol. 1996 Jan;76(1):65-7.
[35] Pillai S, Bikle DD. Role of intracellular-free calcium in the cornified envelope formation of keratinocytes: differences in the mode of action of extracellular calcium and 1,25 dihydroxyvitamin D3. J Cell Physiol. 1991 Jan;146(1):94-100.
[36] Ratnam AV, Bikle DD, Cho JK. 1,25 dihydroxyvitamin D3 enhances the calcium response of keratinocytes. J Cell Physiol. 1999 Feb;178(2):188-96.
[37] Manolagas SC, Provvedini DM, Tsoukas CD. Interactions of 1,25-dihydroxyvitamin D3 and the immune system. Mol Cell Endocrinol. 1985 Dec;43(2-3):113-22.

[38] Muller K, Bendtzen K. 1,25-Dihydroxyvitamin D3 as a natural regulator of human immune functions. J Investig Dermatol Symp Proc. 1996 Apr;1(1):68-71.
[39] Pinette KV, Yee YK, Amegadzie BY, Nagpal S. Vitamin D receptor as a drug discovery target. Mini Rev Med Chem. 2003 May;3(3):193-204.
[40] Tobler A, Gasson J, Reichel H, Norman AW, Koeffler HP. Granulocyte-macrophage colony-stimulating factor. Sensitive and receptor-mediated regulation by 1,25-dihydroxyvitamin D3 in normal human peripheral blood lymphocytes. J Clin Invest. 1987 Jun;79(6):1700-5.
[41] Kang S, Yi S, Griffiths CE, Fancher L, Hamilton TA, Choi JH. Calcipotriene-induced improvement in psoriasis is associated with reduced interleukin-8 and increased interleukin-10 levels within lesions. Br J Dermatol. 1998 Jan;138(1):77-83.
[42] Michel G, Gailis A, Jarzebska-Deussen B, Muschen A, Mirmohammadsadegh A, Ruzicka T. 1,25-(OH)2-vitamin D3 and calcipotriol induce IL-10 receptor gene expression in human epidermal cells. Inflamm Res. 1997 Jan;46(1):32-4.
[43] Nagpal S, Na S, Rathnachalam R. Noncalcemic actions of vitamin D receptor ligands. Endocr Rev. 2005 Aug;26(5):662-87.
[44] Penna G, Adorini L. 1 Alpha,25-dihydroxyvitamin D3 inhibits differentiation, maturation, activation, and survival of dendritic cells leading to impaired alloreactive T cell activation. J Immunol. 2000 Mar 1;164(5):2405-11.
[45] Adorini L, Penna G, Giarratana N, Uskokovic M. Tolerogenic dendritic cells induced by vitamin D receptor ligands enhance regulatory T cells inhibiting allograft rejection and autoimmune diseases. J Cell Biochem. 2003 Feb 1;88(2):227-33.
[46] Bourke JF, Iqbal SJ, Hutchinson PE. The effects of UVB plus calcipotriol on systemic calcium homeostasis in patients with chronic plaque psoriasis. Clin Exp Dermatol. 1997 Nov;22(6):259-61.
[47] Fogh K, Kragballe K. Recent developments in vitamin D analogs. Curr Pharm Des. 2000 Jun;6(9):961-72.
[48] Langner A, Ashton P, Van De Kerkhof PC, Verjans H. A long-term multicentre assessment of the safety and tolerability of calcitriol ointment in the treatment of chronic plaque psoriasis. Br J Dermatol. 1996 Sep;135(3):385-9.
[49] van de Kerkhof PC, Berth-Jones J, Griffiths CE, Harrison PV, Honigsmann H, Marks R, et al. Long-term efficacy and safety of tacalcitol ointment in patients with chronic plaque psoriasis. Br J Dermatol. 2002 Mar;146(3):414-22.
[50] Kragballe K. Vitamin D and UVB radiation therapy. Cutis. 2002 Nov;70(5 Suppl):9-12.
[51] Nguyen T, Gattu S, Pugashetti R, Koo J. Practice of phototherapy in the treatment of moderate-to-severe psoriasis. Curr Probl Dermatol. 2009;38:59-78.
[52] Barbagallo J, Spann CT, Tutrone WD, Weinberg JM. Narrowband UVB phototherapy for the treatment of psoriasis: a review and update. Cutis. 2001 Nov;68(5):345-7.
[53] Storbeck K, Holzle E, Schurer N, Lehmann P, Plewig G. Narrow-band UVB (311 nm) versus conventional broad-band UVB with and without dithranol in phototherapy for psoriasis. J Am Acad Dermatol. 1993 Feb;28(2 Pt 1):227-31.
[54] Larko O. Treatment of psoriasis with a new UVB-lamp. Acta Derm Venereol. 1989;69(4):357-9.
[55] Schiener R, Behrens-Williams SC, Pillekamp H, Kaskel P, Peter RU, Kerscher M. Calcipotriol vs. tazarotene as combination therapy with narrowband ultraviolet B (311 nm): efficacy in patients with severe psoriasis. Br J Dermatol. 2000 Dec;143(6):1275-8.

[56] Osmancevic A, Nilsen LT, Landin-Wilhelmsen K, Soyland E, Abusdal Torjesen P, Hagve TA, et al. Effect of climate therapy at Gran Canaria on vitamin D production, blood glucose and lipids in patients with psoriasis. J Eur Acad Dermatol Venereol. 2009 Oct;23(10):1133-40.
[57] Osmancevic A, Landin-Wilhelmsen K, Larko O, Mellstrom D, Wennberg AM, Hulthen L, et al. UVB therapy increases 25(OH) vitamin D syntheses in postmenopausal women with psoriasis. Photodermatol Photoimmunol Photomed. 2007 Oct;23(5):172-8.
[58] Osmancevic A, Landin-Wilhelmsen K, Larko O, Wennberg AM, Krogstad AL. Vitamin D production in psoriasis patients increases less with narrowband than with broadband ultraviolet B phototherapy. Photodermatol Photoimmunol Photomed. 2009 Jun;25(3):119-23.
[59] Osmancevic A, Landin-Wilhelmsen K, Larko O, Krogstad AL. Vitamin D status in psoriasis patients during different treatments with phototherapy. J Photochem Photobiol B. Nov 3;101(2):117-23.
[60] Cicarma E, Mork C, Porojnicu AC, Juzeniene A, Tam TT, Dahlback A, et al. Influence of narrowband UVB phototherapy on vitamin D and folate status. Exp Dermatol. 2009 Oct 22.
[61] Vahavihu K, Ala-Houhala M, Peric M, Karisola P, Kautiainen H, Hasan T, et al. Narrowband ultraviolet B treatment improves vitamin D balance and alters antimicrobial peptide expression in skin lesions of psoriasis and atopic dermatitis. Br J Dermatol. Aug;163(2):321-8.
[62] Osmancevic A, Nilsen LT, Landin-Wilhelmsen K, Soyland E, Abusdal Torjesen P, Hagve TA, et al. Effect of climate therapy at Gran Canaria on vitamin D production, blood glucose and lipids in patients with psoriasis. J Eur Acad Dermatol Venereol. 2009 Apr 24.
[63] MacLaughlin J, Holick MF. Aging decreases the capacity of human skin to produce vitamin D3. J Clin Invest. 1985 Oct;76(4):1536-8.
[64] Barth J, Gerlach B, Knuschke P, Lehmann B. Serum 25(OH)D3 and ultraviolet exposure of residents in an old people's home in Germany. Photodermatol Photoimmunol Photomed. 1992 Oct;9(5):229-31.
[65] Holick MF, Matsuoka LY, Wortsman J. Age, vitamin D, and solar ultraviolet. Lancet. 1989 Nov 4;2(8671):1104-5.
[66] Need AG, Morris HA, Horowitz M, Nordin C. Effects of skin thickness, age, body fat, and sunlight on serum 25-hydroxyvitamin D. Am J Clin Nutr. 1993 Dec;58(6):882-5.
[67] MacLaughlin JA, Anderson RR, Holick MF. Spectral character of sunlight modulates photosynthesis of previtamin D3 and its photoisomers in human skin. Science. 1982 May 28;216(4549):1001-3.
[68] Lehmann B, Knuschke P, Meurer M. The UVB-induced synthesis of vitamin D3 and 1alpha,25-dihydroxyvitamin D3 (calcitriol) in organotypic cultures of keratinocytes: effectiveness of the narrowband Philips TL-01 lamp (311 nm). J Steroid Biochem Mol Biol. 2007 Mar;103(3-5):682-5.
[69] Leenutaphong V, Sudtim S. A comparison of erythema efficacy of ultraviolet B irradiation from Philips TL12 and TL01 lamps. Photodermatol Photoimmunol Photomed. 1998 Jun-Aug;14(3-4):112-5.
[70] Porojnicu AC, Bruland OS, Aksnes L, Grant WB, Moan J. Sun beds and cod liver oil as vitamin D sources. J Photochem Photobiol B. 2008 May 29;91(2-3):125-31.

[71] Olds WJ, McKinley AR, Moore MR, Kimlin MG. In vitro model of vitamin D(3) (Cholecalciferol) synthesis by UV radiation: Dose-response relationships. J Photochem Photobiol B. 2008 Nov 13;93(2):88-93.
[72] Holick MF, MacLaughlin JA, Doppelt SH. Regulation of cutaneous previtamin D3 photosynthesis in man: skin pigment is not an essential regulator. Science. 1981 Feb 6;211(4482):590-3.
[73] Ryan C, Moran B, McKenna MJ, Murray BF, Brady J, Collins P, et al. The effect of narrowband UV-B treatment for psoriasis on vitamin D status during wintertime in Ireland. Arch Dermatol. Aug;146(8):836-42.
[74] Devgun MS, Paterson CR, Johnson BE, Cohen C. Vitamin D nutrition in relation to season and occupation. Am J Clin Nutr. 1981 Aug;34(8):1501-4.
[75] Armas LA, Hollis BW, Heaney RP. Vitamin D2 is much less effective than vitamin D3 in humans. J Clin Endocrinol Metab. 2004 Nov;89(11):5387-91.
[76] Holick MF. Vitamin D: A millenium perspective. J Cell Biochem. 2003 Feb 1;88(2):296-307.
[77] Chen TC, Chimeh F, Lu Z, Mathieu J, Person KS, Zhang A, et al. Factors that influence the cutaneous synthesis and dietary sources of vitamin D. Arch Biochem Biophys. 2007 Apr 15;460(2):213-7.
[78] McCarty CA. Sunlight exposure assessment: can we accurately assess vitamin D exposure from sunlight questionnaires? Am J Clin Nutr. 2008 Apr;87(4):1097S-101S.
[79] Matsuoka LY, Wortsman J, Hollis BW. Use of topical sunscreen for the evaluation of regional synthesis of vitamin D3. J Am Acad Dermatol. 1990 May;22(5 Pt 1):772-5.
[80] Morimoto S, Yoshikawa K. Psoriasis and vitamin D3. A review of our experience. Arch Dermatol. 1989 Feb;125(2):231-4.
[81] Lehmann B, Querings K, Reichrath J. Vitamin D and skin: new aspects for dermatology. Exp Dermatol. 2004;13 Suppl 4:11-5.
[82] Chesney RW, Rosen JF, Hamstra AJ, Smith C, Mahaffey K, DeLuca HF. Absence of seasonal variation in serum concentrations of 1,25-dihydroxyvitamin D despite a rise in 25-hydroxyvitamin D in summer. J Clin Endocrinol Metab. 1981 Jul;53(1):139-42.
[83] Adams JS, Clemens TL, Parrish JA, Holick MF. Vitamin-D synthesis and metabolism after ultraviolet irradiation of normal and vitamin-D-deficient subjects. N Engl J Med. 1982 Mar 25;306(12):722-5.
[84] Lips P, Wiersinga A, van Ginkel FC, Jongen MJ, Netelenbos JC, Hackeng WH, et al. The effect of vitamin D supplementation on vitamin D status and parathyroid function in elderly subjects. J Clin Endocrinol Metab. 1988 Oct;67(4):644-50.
[85] Bikle DD, Nemanic MK, Gee E, Elias P. 1,25-Dihydroxyvitamin D3 production by human keratinocytes. Kinetics and regulation. J Clin Invest. 1986 Aug;78(2):557-66.
[86] Vanhooke JL, Prahl JM, Kimmel-Jehan C, Mendelsohn M, Danielson EW, Healy KD, et al. CYP27B1 null mice with LacZreporter gene display no 25-hydroxyvitamin D3-1alpha-hydroxylase promoter activity in the skin. Proc Natl Acad Sci U S A. 2006 Jan 3;103(1):75-80.
[87] Reichrath J. Vitamin D and the skin: an ancient friend, revisited. Exp Dermatol. 2007 Jul;16(7):618-25.
[88] Lehmann B. The vitamin D3 pathway in human skin and its role for regulation of biological processes. Photochem Photobiol. 2005 Nov-Dec;81(6):1246-51.

[89] Sigmon JR, Yentzer BA, Feldman SR. Calcitriol ointment: a review of a topical vitamin D analog for psoriasis. J Dermatolog Treat. 2009;20(4):208-12.
[90] Tanghetti EA. The role of topical vitamin D modulators in psoriasis therapy. J Drugs Dermatol. 2009 Aug;8(8 Suppl):s4-8.
[91] Lehmann B, Knuschke P, Meurer M. UVB-induced conversion of 7-dehydrocholesterol to 1 alpha,25-dihydroxyvitamin D3 (calcitriol) in the human keratinocyte line HaCaT. Photochem Photobiol. 2000 Dec;72(6):803-9.
[92] Lehmann B, Sauter W, Knuschke P, Dressler S, Meurer M. Demonstration of UVB-induced synthesis of 1 alpha,25-dihydroxyvitamin D3 (calcitriol) in human skin by microdialysis. Arch Dermatol Res. 2003 Apr;295(1):24-8.
[93] Merke J, Schwittay D, Furstenberger G, Gross M, Marks F, Ritz E. Demonstration and characterization of 1,25-dihydroxyvitamin D3 receptors in basal cells of epidermis of neonatal and adult mice. Calcif Tissue Int. 1985 May;37(3):257-67.
[94] Hosomi J, Hosoi J, Abe E, Suda T, Kuroki T. Regulation of terminal differentiation of cultured mouse epidermal cells by 1 alpha,25-dihydroxyvitamin D3. Endocrinology. 1983 Dec;113(6):1950-7.
[95] Kim SK, Park S, Lee ES. Toll-like receptors and antimicrobial peptides expressions of psoriasis: correlation with serum vitamin D level. J Korean Med Sci. Oct;25(10):1506-12.
[96] van de Kerkhof PC. Biological activity of vitamin D analogues in the skin, with special reference to antipsoriatic mechanisms. Br J Dermatol. 1995 May;132(5):675-82.
[97] Sahota O, Mundey MK, San P, Godber IM, Lawson N, Hosking DJ. The relationship between vitamin D and parathyroid hormone: calcium homeostasis, bone turnover, and bone mineral density in postmenopausal women with established osteoporosis. Bone. 2004 Jul;35(1):312-9.
[98] Landin-Wilhelmsen K, Wilhelmsen L, Lappas G, Rosen T, Lindstedt G, Lundberg PA, et al. Serum intact parathyroid hormone in a random population sample of men and women: relationship to anthropometry, life-style factors, blood pressure, and vitamin D. Calcif Tissue Int. 1995 Feb;56(2):104-8.
[99] Webb AR, Kline L, Holick MF. Influence of season and latitude on the cutaneous synthesis of vitamin D3: exposure to winter sunlight in Boston and Edmonton will not promote vitamin D3 synthesis in human skin. J Clin Endocrinol Metab. 1988 Aug;67(2):373-8.
[100] Vieth R. Vitamin D supplementation, 25-hydroxyvitamin D concentrations, and safety. Am J Clin Nutr. 1999 May;69(5):842-56.
[101] Landin-Wilhelmsen K, Wilhelmsen L, Bengtsson BA. Postmenopausal osteoporosis is more related to hormonal aberrations than to lifestyle factors. Clin Endocrinol (Oxf). 1999 Oct;51(4):387-94.
[102] Attia EA, Khafagy A, Abdel-Raheem S, Fathi S, Saad AA. Assessment of osteoporosis in psoriasis with and without arthritis: correlation with disease severity. Int J Dermatol. Jan;50(1):30-5.
[103] Millard TP, Antoniades L, Evans AV, Smith HR, Spector TD, Barker JN. Bone mineral density of patients with chronic plaque psoriasis. Clin Exp Dermatol. 2001 Jul;26(5):446-8.
[104] Nymann P, Kollerup G, Jemec GB, Grossmann E. Decreased bone mineral density in patients with pustulosis palmaris et plantaris. Dermatology. 1996;192(4):307-11.

[105] Frediani B, Allegri A, Falsetti P, Storri L, Bisogno S, Baldi F, et al. Bone mineral density in patients with psoriatic arthritis. J Rheumatol. 2001 Jan;28(1):138-43.
[106] Borman P, Babaoglu S, Gur G, Bingol S, Bodur H. Bone mineral density and bone turnover in patients with psoriatic arthritis. Clin Rheumatol. 2008 Apr;27(4):443-7.
[107] Pedreira PG, Pinheiro MM, Szejnfeld VL. Bone mineral density and body composition in postmenopausal women with psoriasis and psoriatic arthritis. Arthritis Res Ther. Feb 7;13(1):R16.
[108] Osmancevic A, Landin-Wilhelmsen K, Larko O, Mellstrom D, Wennberg AM, Hulthen L, et al. Risk factors for osteoporosis and bone status in postmenopausal women with psoriasis treated with UVB therapy. Acta Derm Venereol. 2008;88(3):240-6.
[109] Tangpricha V, Turner A, Spina C, Decastro S, Chen TC, Holick MF. Tanning is associated with optimal vitamin D status (serum 25-hydroxyvitamin D concentration) and higher bone mineral density. Am J Clin Nutr. 2004 Dec;80(6):1645-9.
[110] Naldi L, Chatenoud L, Linder D, Belloni Fortina A, Peserico A, Virgili AR, et al. Cigarette smoking, body mass index, and stressful life events as risk factors for psoriasis: results from an Italian case-control study. J Invest Dermatol. 2005 Jul;125(1):61-7.
[111] Fogelman I, Blake GM. Different approaches to bone densitometry. J Nucl Med. 2000 Dec;41(12):2015-25.
[112] Riggs BL. Pathogenesis of osteoporosis. Am J Obstet Gynecol. 1987 May;156(5):1342-6.
[113] Cummings SR, Nevitt MC, Browner WS, Stone K, Fox KM, Ensrud KE, et al. Risk factors for hip fracture in white women. Study of Osteoporotic Fractures Research Group. N Engl J Med. 1995 Mar 23;332(12):767-73.
[114] Johnell O, Gullberg B, Kanis JA, Allander E, Elffors L, Dequeker J, et al. Risk factors for hip fracture in European women: the MEDOS Study. Mediterranean Osteoporosis Study. J Bone Miner Res. 1995 Nov;10(11):1802-15.
[115] Cummings SR, Melton LJ. Epidemiology and outcomes of osteoporotic fractures. Lancet. 2002 May 18;359(9319):1761-7.
[116] Aniansson A, Zetterberg C, Hedberg M, Henriksson KG. Impaired muscle function with aging. A background factor in the incidence of fractures of the proximal end of the femur. Clin Orthop Relat Res. 1984 Dec(191):193-201.
[117] Cooper C, Barker DJ, Wickham C. Physical activity, muscle strength, and calcium intake in fracture of the proximal femur in Britain. Bmj. 1988 Dec 3;297(6661):1443-6.
[118] Silman AJ, O'Neill TW, Cooper C, Kanis J, Felsenberg D. Influence of physical activity on vertebral deformity in men and women: results from the European Vertebral Osteoporosis Study. J Bone Miner Res. 1997 May;12(5):813-9.
[119] Frandin K, Grimby G, Mellstrom D, Svanborg A. Walking habits and health-related factors in a 70-year-old population. Gerontology. 1991;37(5):281-8.
[120] Greendale GA, Barrett-Connor E, Edelstein S, Ingles S, Haile R. Lifetime leisure exercise and osteoporosis. The Rancho Bernardo study. Am J Epidemiol. 1995 May 15;141(10):951-9.
[121] Chapuy MC, Arlot ME, Duboeuf F, Brun J, Crouzet B, Arnaud S, et al. Vitamin D3 and calcium to prevent hip fractures in the elderly women. N Engl J Med. 1992 Dec 3;327(23):1637-42.

[122] Chel VG, Ooms ME, Popp-Snijders C, Pavel S, Schothorst AA, Meulemans CC, et al. Ultraviolet irradiation corrects vitamin D deficiency and suppresses secondary hyperparathyroidism in the elderly. J Bone Miner Res. 1998 Aug;13(8):1238-42.
[123] Lilliu H, Pamphile R, Chapuy MC, Schulten J, Arlot M, Meunier PJ. Calcium-vitamin D3 supplementation is cost-effective in hip fractures prevention. Maturitas. 2003 Apr 25;44(4):299-305.
[124] Gottlieb AB, Chao C, Dann F. Psoriasis comorbidities. J Dermatolog Treat. 2008;19(1):5-21.
[125] Christophers E. Comorbidities in psoriasis. Clin Dermatol. 2007 Nov-Dec;25(6):529-34.
[126] Girolomoni G, Gisondi P. Psoriasis and metabolic comorbidities: the importance of well-designed prospective studies. Commentary. Dermatology. 2008;217(3):222-4.
[127] Gottlieb AB, Dann F, Menter A. Psoriasis and the metabolic syndrome. J Drugs Dermatol. 2008 Jun;7(6):563-72.
[128] Sommer DM, Jenisch S, Suchan M, Christophers E, Weichenthal M. Increased prevalence of the metabolic syndrome in patients with moderate to severe psoriasis. Arch Dermatol Res. 2006 Dec;298(7):321-8.
[129] Palomer X, Gonzalez-Clemente JM, Blanco-Vaca F, Mauricio D. Role of vitamin D in the pathogenesis of type 2 diabetes mellitus. Diabetes Obes Metab. 2008 Mar;10(3):185-97.
[130] Tai K, Need AG, Horowitz M, Chapman IM. Vitamin D, glucose, insulin, and insulin sensitivity. Nutrition. 2008 Mar;24(3):279-85.
[131] Procopio M, Magro G, Cesario F, Piovesan A, Pia A, Molineri N, et al. The oral glucose tolerance test reveals a high frequency of both impaired glucose tolerance and undiagnosed Type 2 diabetes mellitus in primary hyperparathyroidism. Diabet Med. 2002 Nov;19(11):958-61.
[132] Taylor WH, Khaleeli AA. Prevalence of primary hyperparathyroidism in patients with diabetes mellitus. Diabet Med. 1997 May;14(5):386-9.
[133] Luong K, Nguyen LT, Nguyen DN. The role of vitamin D in protecting type 1 diabetes mellitus. Diabetes Metab Res Rev. 2005 Jul-Aug;21(4):338-46.
[134] Mauricio D, Mandrup-Poulsen T, Nerup J. Vitamin D analogues in insulin-dependent diabetes mellitus and other autoimmune diseases: a therapeutic perspective. Diabetes Metab Rev. 1996 Apr;12(1):57-68.
[135] Lemire JM. Immunomodulatory actions of 1,25-dihydroxyvitamin D3. J Steroid Biochem Mol Biol. 1995 Jun;53(1-6):599-602.
[136] Ucak S, Ekmekci TR, Basat O, Koslu A, Altuntas Y. Comparison of various insulin sensitivity indices in psoriatic patients and their relationship with type of psoriasis. J Eur Acad Dermatol Venereol. 2006 May;20(5):517-22.
[137] Akhyani M, Ehsani AH, Robati RM, Robati AM. The lipid profile in psoriasis: a controlled study. J Eur Acad Dermatol Venereol. 2007 Nov;21(10):1330-2.
[138] Mallbris L, Granath F, Hamsten A, Stahle M. Psoriasis is associated with lipid abnormalities at the onset of skin disease. J Am Acad Dermatol. 2006 Apr;54(4):614-21.
[139] Carbone LD, Rosenberg EW, Tolley EA, Holick MF, Hughes TA, Watsky MA, et al. 25-Hydroxyvitamin D, cholesterol, and ultraviolet irradiation. Metabolism. 2008 Jun;57(6):741-8.
[140] Azfar RS, Gelfand JM. Psoriasis and metabolic disease: epidemiology and pathophysiology. Curr Opin Rheumatol. 2008 Jul;20(4):416-22.
[141] Libby P. Inflammation and cardiovascular disease mechanisms. Am J Clin Nutr. 2006 Feb;83(2):456S-60S.

9

Nail Psoriasis

Eckart Haneke
[1]Dept Dermatol, Inselspital, Univ Bern, Bern,
[2]Practice of Dermatology Dermaticum, Freiburg,
[3]Centro de Dermatología Epidermis, Instituto CUF, Porto,
[4]Dept Dermatol, Acad Hosp, Univ Gent, Gent,
[1]Switzerland
[2]Germany
[3]Portugal
[4]Belgium

1. Introduction

During the 8th gestational week, a condensation of cells develops on the distal dorsal aspect of the digital tip. At week 9, this migrates proximally to form a flat groove, the nail field. At week 11, an invagination develops from the proximal groove, which later forms the nail pocket or cul-de-sac, with the matrix at its bottom. Nail production starts around week 13. At the age of 20 weeks, the nail production is similar to that of an adult. From week 32 on, all nail components can be recognized (Lewis, 1954, Zaias, 1963).

The nail apparatus consists of epithelial and connective tissue components and covers the tip of the fingers and toes (Figure 1) (Lewin, 1965, Morgan et al, 2001, Zook et al, 1980). Its functions are support, protection and maintenance of the digital tips as well as enhancement of the sensory functions of the digital pulps, and the nail is a tool for scratching, defense, fine manual work, etc. The cosmetic-aesthetic and social functions of the nail have attained a lot of attention in recent years.

The nail has four epithelial components:

- The matrix epithelium is the sole structure to produce the nail plate. It is commonly divided into the proximal, medial and distal matrix (Figure 2). The existence of a so-called dorsal matrix is controversial. Most of the matrix is covered by the proximal nail fold. Under normal circumstances, its distal portion, the whitish lunula, is only seen in the thumb, index and middle finger as well as the great toe; however, manicure with pushing the free margin of the proximal nail fold back makes more of the matrix visible through the nail and lets the nail plate appear longer.

The matrix epithelium consists of a basal compartment seen as cuboid basophilic cells that migrate up to form the more eosinophilic superficial compartment (Perrin et al, 2004). Whenever a nail is avulsed the superficial compartment remains attached to it. During onychotisation, the superficial cells undergo nuclear fragmentation. Under normal circumstances, there is no granular layer.

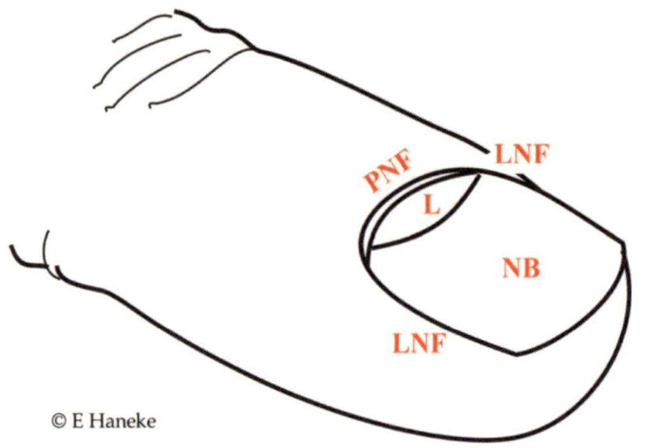

a)

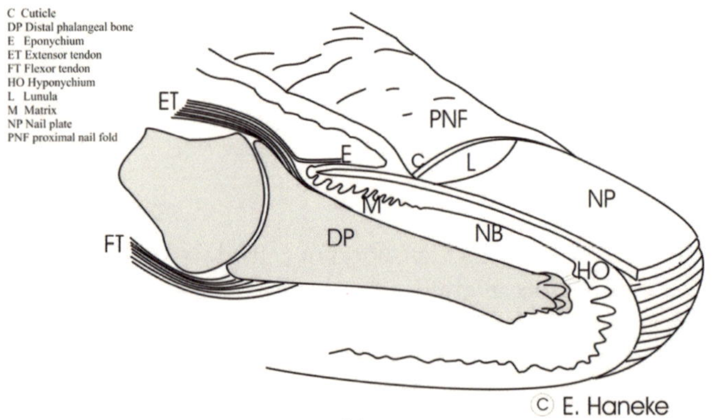

b)

Fig. 1. Anatomy of the nail apparatus. Oblique view (A) and sagittal section (B) through the distal phalanx.

The matrix contains melanocytes most of which are located suprabasally. In light-skinned individuals, they remain functionally inactive. Independent from the skin type, the distal matrix contains more melanocytes than the proximal one (Tosti et al, 1994, Perrin et al, 1997).

The matrix connective tissue is relatively loose containing blood vessels and a considerable number of glomus bodies. Recent studies have found that matrix fibroblasts are CD 10+ similar to perifollicular fibroblasts (Lee et al, 2007- 2010). The matrix dermis has an important morphogenetic capacity allowing it to reproduce matrix epithelium when enough of it is left after trauma or superficial surgical removal. The distance from the most proximal matrix epithelium to the bone of the terminal phalanx is about 0.8 – 1 mm (Haneke, 2006, Kim et al, 2011).

- The nail bed epithelium is a relatively thin layer of keratinocytes structurally similar to tricholemmal cells. It firmly attaches the nail to the underlying distal phalanx and produces a tiny amount of nail bed keratin, which allows the nail plate to virtually slide over the nail bed without being detached from it. The nail bed keratin is structurally different from the nail plate keratin. The nail bed does not produce nail plate (de Berker and Angus, 1996, Nishi et al, 1996, Zaias and Alvarez, 1968) although this is also controversial (Johnson et al, 1991). A normal nail bed does not form a granular layer.

The nail bed epithelium-connective tissue interface is characterized by unique longitudinal rete ridges, in which 3 to 6 layers of longitudinally running capillaries are arranged one above the other. Trauma to these capillaries may produce the characteristic splinter haemorrhages, which in nail psoriasis are equivalent to Auspitz' phenomenon of the skin. The connective tissue of the nail bed is a firm layer directly attached to the bone without any subdermal fat. This and the abundance of nervous structures in the nail bed and matrix are probably the reason for the extraordinary pain elicited by trauma to the nail apparatus.

- The hyponychium is localized at the distal end of the nail bed and forms a particular structure allowing the plate to get detached from the bed without injury. It seals the virtual space between the nail and the nail bed. The normal hyponychium shows a broad granular layer (Hanno et al, 1986, Perrin, 2008). Distal to it, digital pulp skin is present.
- The eponychium is a thin layer of keratin produced by the undersurface of the proximal nail fold (PNF). Approximately halfway it divides into the true eponychium remaining firmly attached to the dorsal surface of the nail plate and the false eponychium attached to the epidermis of the PNF's ventral surface. It forms the bulk of the cuticle, the function of which is to seal the cul-de-sac or nail pocket.

Proximally and laterally, the nail is ensheathed by the proximal and two lateral nail folds, which form a frame leaving the distal margin of the nail plate free. This allows the nail plate to grow out and not up. The proximal nail fold is a continuation of the dorsal aspect of the skin of the tip of the digit, which folds on itself thereby producing a cover for most of the matrix. Its free margin forms an acute angle, which bears the cuticle. This is the most distal portion of the false eponychium. When the distal free margin of the proximal nail fold rounds up it loses its ability to form a cuticle, and within usually a relatively short period of time the undersurface of the proximal nailfold detaches from the underlying nail plate.

The lateral nail folds are rolls of connective tissue covered with normal epithelium. Their border to the nail bed is the lateral nail groove. This is firmly attached to the nail plate preventing foreign substances from getting under the nail plate. The lateral grooves are important to guide the nails during their forward growth.

The nail plate – commonly called "the nail" - is the product of the matrix. It is made up of keratin which is a sulfur-rich fibrous keratin embedded in a sulfur-rich amorphous matrix. The fibrous protein structure is seen clearly under polarized light. In contrast to hair, which is made up of exactly the same material, it has no special outer structure like a cuticle of scales and the nail grows continuously from birth to death without a cyclical pattern. The plate exhibits a slight longitudinal and a more pronounced transverse curvature, the degree of which varies between different fingers and toes, during age and some diseases, and has a concave border proximally and a convex free margin. The lunula border reflects the shape of the matrix as it runs parallel to the proximal border of the nail. Usually three layers of the nail plate are distinguished (Figure 2): dorsal (superficial), middle, and deep (ventral). The dorsal nail plate layer is produced by the proximal matrix. Its cells are considerably flatter and thus, despite its lesser thickness, it has approximately as many cell layers as the considerably thicker middle nail plate layer with its higher cells. The dorsal nail plate is responsible for the nail shine. The ventral layer is not true nail but keratin derived from the nail bed. Histologically, it is easily distinguished from nail plate.

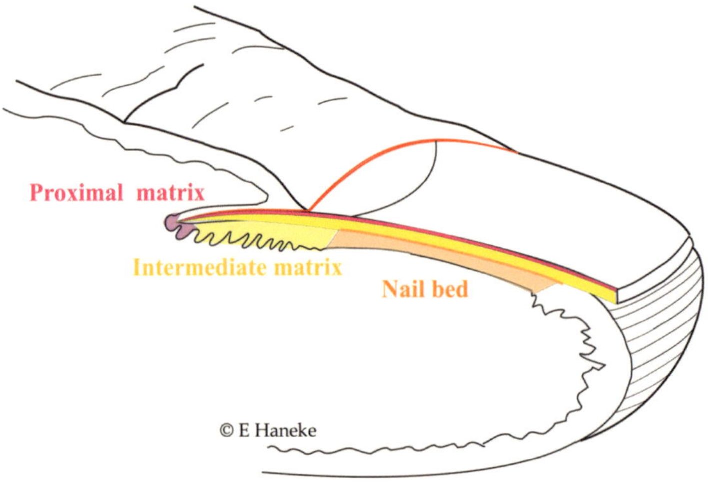

Fig. 2. Origin of the nail plate layers: The dorsal layer is produced by the proximal matrix (pink), the main intermediate and deep nail layer by the intermediate matrix (yellow) and the so-called ventral nail layer is the keratin produced by the nail bed (orange).

The nail organ is an integral part of the functional and sensory finger tip unit (Morgan et al, 2001). This is formed by the nail apparatus itself, all constituents of the finger tip, the distal interphalangeal joints with their capsule, tendons and ligaments. The entheses, insertion structures of bone with ligaments and tendons, play an important role for the functional and aesthetic integrity of the nail and have recently been found to be of utmost importance in psoriatic arthritis and nail psoriasis (McGonagle et al, 2010, 2011). The proximal tip of the matrix is just 0.8 to 1 mm from the bone of the terminal phalanx and also very close to the distal interphalangeal joint (Haneke, 2006). The joint capsule is enforced by the flexor and extensor tendons which form the dorsal and volar aponeuroses. They insert mostly at the base of the distal phalanx, but there are also fibers radiating to the more distal dorsal surface of the bone and into the connective tissue of the proximal nail fold (Frentz et al, 2000). This led some authors to call the nail a musculo-skeletal appendage (McGonagle et al, 2009a, b). Thus not only do the complex blood supply of the distal joint and nail, but also the anatomic vicinity of matrix and joint give a possible explanation why nail involvement is so frequent in psoriatic arthritis patients.

Nails grow continuously, finger nails about 3 times faster than those of the toes. The middle finger of the dominant hand has the fastest growing nail, growing between 3 to 5 mm per month. A big toenail grows about 1 mm per month. In summer and at daytime, the nails grow faster, during winter, at night, in high altitude slower. In psoriatic subjects, the nail growth rate is slightly increased. Some drugs also enhance nail growth, such as high-dose itraconazole and fluconazole, possibly also cyclosporine. Most cytostatic drugs including methotrexate, which is often used as a systemic drug for psoriasis treatment, slow down the nail growth rate. Fast growing nails are more prone to develop psoriatic pits.

2. Histopathologic nail reactions

In contrast to skin, the nail demonstrates a variety of specific reactions that are sometimes opposite to the rest of the skin. Whereas irritation and a number of inflammatory reactions cause parakeratosis in skin they may induce a granular layer in the nail, some psoriatic reactions included. Several dermatoses that are not characterized by spongiosis, may exhibit marked intercellular oedema of matrix and nail bed epithelium, e.g. in ungual lichen planus and psoriasis.

As the dorsal layer of the nail plate is produced by the most proximal portion of the matrix any alterations of the proximal matrix will translate into changes of the nail surface and uppermost layers. The bulk of the nail is produced by the middle matrix portion; alterations here will modify the nail plate both in its thickness as well as optical coherence. When the distal matrix is involved the resulting nail alterations will appear at the undersurface of the nail (Figure 2). All matrix-derived alterations will grow out with the nail. In contrast, nail bed alterations will be seen through the nail, but will not be integrated into the nail. As the nail bed keratin moves slower than the nail plate nail bed alterations remain longer or may even appear non-migratory.

Psoriasis of the nails induces characteristic histopathological changes that are pathognomonic in the vast majority of cases; however, in the beginning and with less pronounced changes it may mimic a spongiotic dermatitis or may be indistinguishable from onychomycosis if there is no proof of fungal invasion.

3. Histopathology of nail psoriasis

Whereas the main criteria for psoriasis of the skin also apply for ungual psoriasis there are some differences and, above all, there are signs not seen in the rest of the skin.

Pits are the most frequent lesions in nail psoriasis (Figs. 3, 4) with roughly 70% of the patients presenting at least some of these characteristic tiny depressions (Zaias, 1969, Tham et al, 1988). Histologically, their appearance varies slightly. In the distal nail plate, they are seen as a depression in the nail plate surface that may be lined by some parakeratotic nail cells. The more proximal the biopsy is taken, the more parakeratosis is left. Under the proximal nail fold there are not yet pits but saucer-shaped small areas of parakeratosis. When these do not break out as it most commonly happens tiny white spots remain visible giving rise to spotted nails. Usually the rest of the nail organ appears normal and only in rare circumstances is a tiny inflammatory psoriatic lesion seen at the proximal tip of the matrix. Whether or not the pits may also originate from the most proximal portion of the ventral surface of the proximal nail fold (Zaias, 1990) remains a matter of dispute. Anyhow, it is surprising how rarely the original inflammatory matrix lesions giving rise to spots and pits are seen in histopathological slides.

Nail bed changes are the second most common ungual sign of psoriasis. They may present as salmon or oil spots, which represent a small psoriatic plaque of the nailbed entirely covered by the nail plate, as onycholysis when the psoriatic plaque extends to the hyponychium, or as subungual hyperkeratosis representing a hyperkeratotic psoriatic plaque. A typical salmon spot shows slight acanthosis of the nail bed epithelium, an inflammatory infiltrate mainly made up of lymphocytes that tend to migrate into the epithelium and cause spongiosis, as well as parakeratosis on top of the epithelium, which

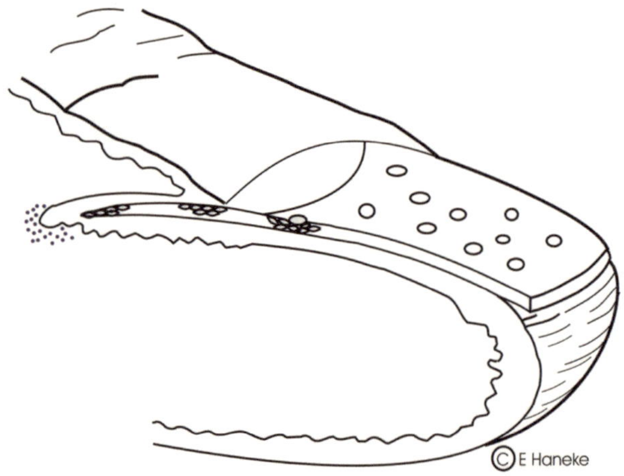

Fig. 3. Formation of psoriatic pits from a tiny inflammatory focus at the most proximal matrix.

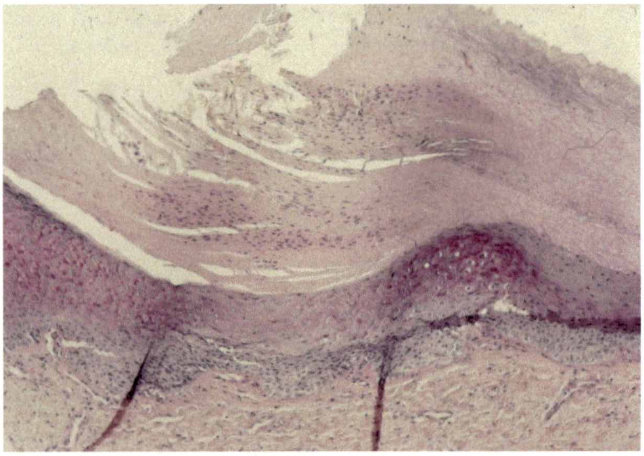

Fig. 4. Histological picture of an incipient pit, which is seen as a saucer-shaped mass of parakeratosis on the matrix epithelium.

often contains neutrophils. In more pronounced acute lesions, Munro's microabscesses may be seen. Typical for psoriasis is the arrangement of parakeratosis in obliquely ascending columns. This and the lack of fungal elements in PAS stained slides helps to distinguish this pattern from onychomycosis, which also often exhibits neutrophil collections as seen in Munro's microabscesses. Psoriatic onycholysis is located more distally in the nail bed, but principally very similar to oil spots. The neutrophil exocytosis may be less pronounced, and in old lesions it may be difficult to make the diagnosis of nail psoriasis at all as the nailbed may develop a granular layer and layered orthokeratotic hyperkeratosis. Subungual hyperkeratosis in psoriasis may sometimes be extreme mimicking even pachyonychia congenita. Huge thickening of the keratosis with parakeratosis both in horizontal layers and oblique columns may be present along with serum inclusions. The latter may form large round to oval globules, but also present as very small longitudinal structures. These serum inclusions are PAS positive and may be difficult to be dífferentiated by the non-experienced;

however, in contrast to fungal elements they are homogeneously positive and have no membrane staining like fungi.

At the hyponychium, the normal granular layer is lost and the tight connection of the nail plate with the most distal portion of the nail bed is loosened. Parakeratosis develops without attachment with the nail plate.

Both the matrix and nail bed may transform to an epidermis-like pattern of differentiation in old lesions with development of a granular layer and some orthokeratosis.

Isolated involvement of the middle matrix appears to be less frequent. It leads to nail plate changes clinically often seen as psoriatic leukonychia. Histopathologically, the matrix shows acanthosis and spongiosis, a dense subepithelial inflammatory infiltrate mainly of lymphocytes that also migrate into the matrix epithelium. Neutrophils may be present and sometimes concentrate under the nail plate to form spongiform pustule-like collections. There may also be parakeratotic layers in the nail plate; these "paronychotic" cell layers are distinct from areas of incomplete nuclear disintegration, which are not infrequently seen in avulsed nail strips of ingrown nails. These inclusions of parakeratosis in the nail plate give rise to the clinical picture of leukonychia (Fig. 5, 6, 7).

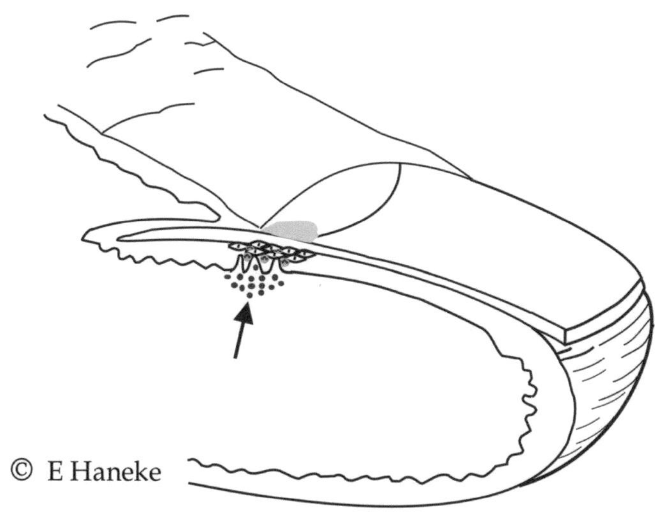

Fig. 5. Psoriatic leukonychia is seen when there is a psoriatic lesion in the middle or distal matrix

Splinter haemorrhages are a characteristic of nail psoriasis not seen in onychomycosis. They are analogous to Auspitz' phenomenon of the skin. When the fragile thinned suprapapillary epithelial plate of a psoriasis lesion is traumatized a minute droplet of blood is seen to appear in a skin lesion because the epidermis has rete pegs and finger like dermal papillae. In contrast, the nail bed is unique to have rete ridges in parallel arrangement; when a microbleeding develops it forms a narrow stripe of haemorrhage, about 0.5 - 1mm wide and 3 - maximally 10 mm long (Fig. 8, 9). They are soon included by newly produced nail bed keratin and seen as small blood lakes between the papillomatous appearing keratosis of the nail bed and the undersurface of the nail plate.

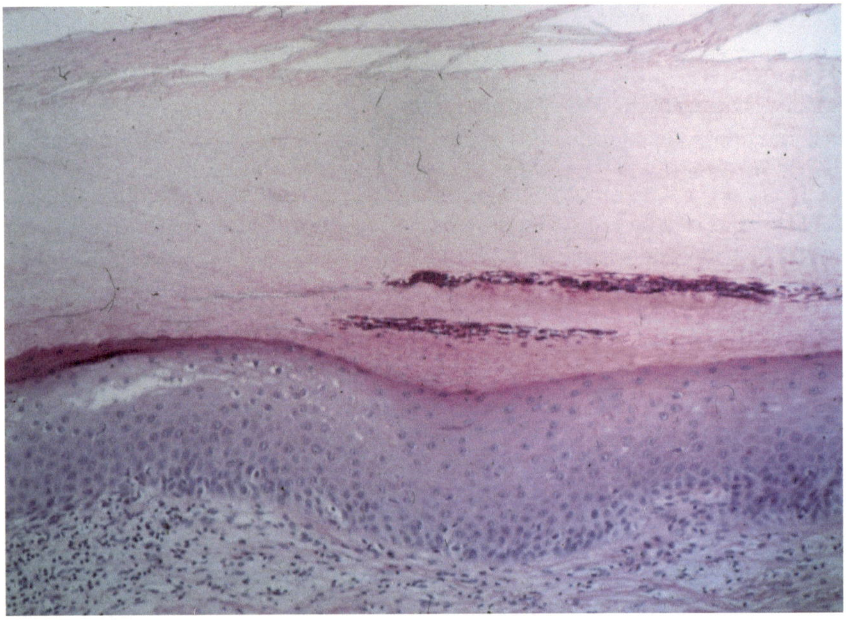

Fig. 6. Munro's microabscesses in the deep nail plate appear as leukonychic spots in the nail

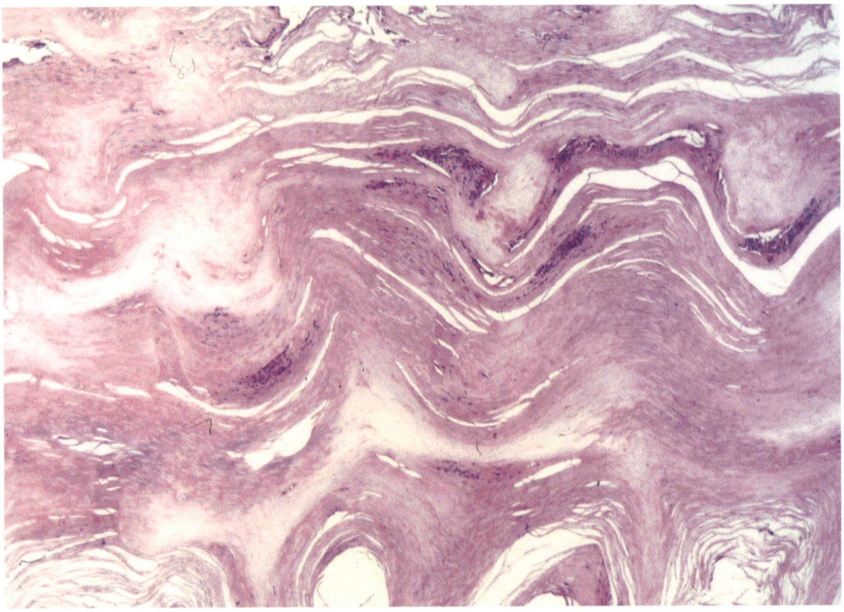

Fig. 7. This nail plate is irregular in its structure and contains many Munro's microabscesses making it appear intransparent and grayish-white

Acrodermatitis continua suppurativa is a particular form of pustular psoriasis; however, histopathologically three forms exist: with characteristic spongiform pustules, with marked spongiosis and even spongiotic vesicles, and a mixed form with spongiform pustules and spongiosis.

In pustular psoriasis, spongiform pustule formation is usually seen with collection of neutrophils gradually increasing in density toward the superficial layers of both the matrix and nail bed epithelium (Fig. 10).

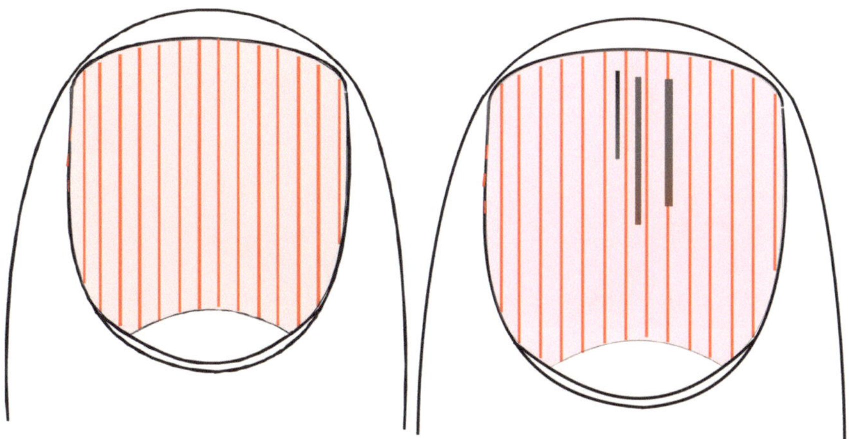

Fig. 8. Splinter haemorrhages develop when there is haemorrhage in the papillary rete ridges or when the horizontally running capillaries thrombose.

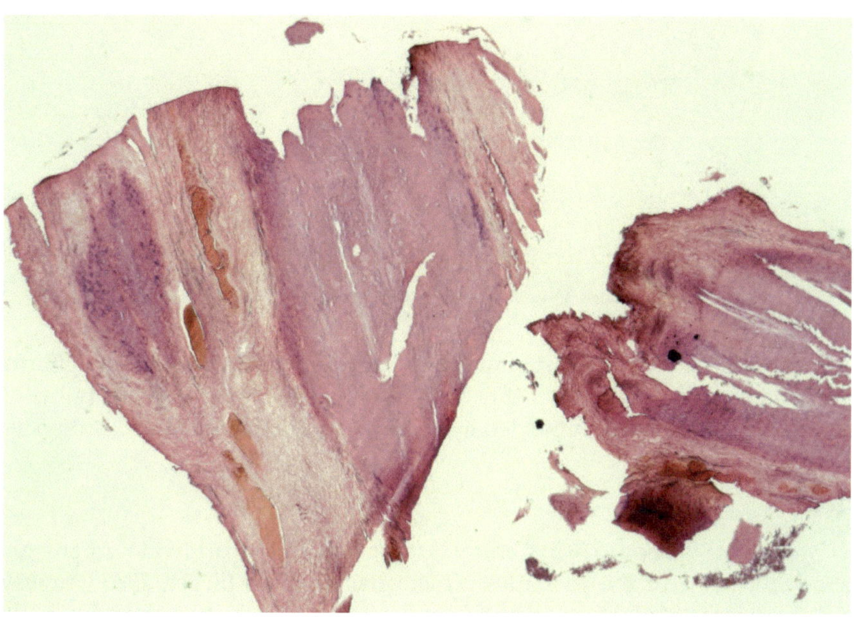

Fig. 9. Longitudinal section of a nail bed biopsy showing oval lakes of blood as sign of splinter haemorrhages.

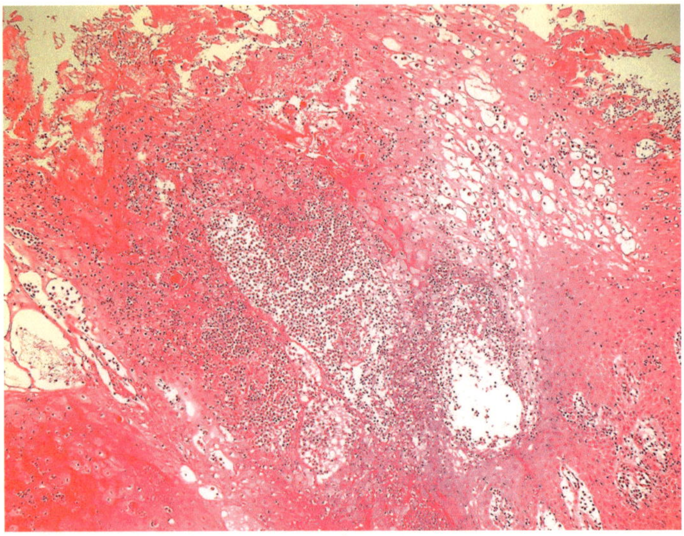

a)

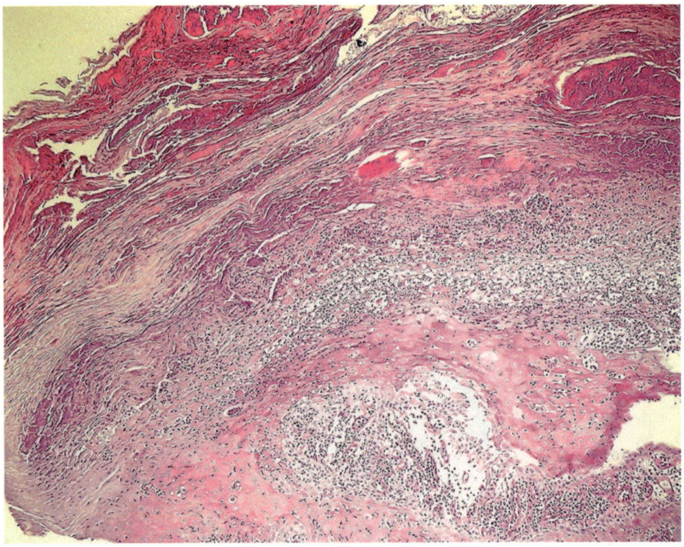

b)

Fig. 10. Acrodermatitis continua suppurativa of Hallopeau with massive spongiform pustule formation; a. Huge amounts of neutrophils are seen in the nail bed epithelium, b. Collections of neutrophils are embedded in a matrix of cornified nail bed keratinocytes.

4. Frequency

Psoriasis prevalence is about 2% in Central Europe and 1-3% worldwide. At any given time point, about 10 - 50% of the psoriatics present nail changes (Scher, 1985, Augustin et al, 2010), but approximately 90% of all psoriatic subjects will have developed nail alterations during life time. The prevalence of nail psoriasis in men is about 11% higher than in women (Augustin et al, 2010). Isolated nail psoriasis is seen in 1 - 5% (Lavaroni et al, 1994).

In a Swiss cohort of 1222 psoriasis patients, 9.4% suffered from nail involvement (Ruprecht et al, 2011).

Whereas there is a striking difference in the frequency of familiar cases between psoriasis in Caucasian children (83%) as compared to Asian children (13.4%)) nail psoriasis is insignificantly more frequent in Singaporean (35.8%) than in Dutch children (22.2%). Pitting is the most common nail sign (Chiam et al, 2011). The frequency of nail psoriasis appears to be similar in Indian children (Nanda et al, 1990).

Nail psoriasis is more common in psoriatic arthritis, the prevalence is usually greater than 80%.

It appears that nail disease is relatively more frequent in males than in females (Wittkowski et al, 2011).

5. Immunogenetics

Psoriasis is a multifactorial disorder with a strong genetic background. Environmental co-factors play an important role in its manifestation. Various psoriasis susceptibility (PSORS) factors have been identified, of which PSORS1 on chromosome 6p21 has been reproduced in all studies.

Nail psoriasis has more frequently a positive family history as compared to psoriasis of the skin (52.7% vs. 43.8%), is more often associated with psoriatic arthritis (29.7% vs. 11.5%), is more often linked to early onset psoriasis (74.1% vs. 65.5%) and is fewer positive for the HLA allele Cw*0602 (33% vs. 50.3%) (Armesto et al, 2011, Gudjonsson et al, 2006). It may also be speculated that the IL23R polymorphism that is a common susceptibility factor for psoriasis (Cargill et al, 2007) and is not or only rarely found in Han Chinese may account for the higher rate of familiarity of psoriasis in Caucasians as compared to Asians (Chiam et al, 2011).

Nail psoriasis is associated with a higher frequency of psoriatic arthritis and a more progressive form of the disease (Williamson et al, 2004, Serarslan et al, 2007). The skin and nail lesion usually manifest before the arthritis (Mease , 2002).

6. Clinical lesions of nail psoriasis

Psoriasis patients with nail involvement have a longer disease duration, higher disease severity, more than double the frequency of psoriatic arthritis, more pronounced impairment of disease related quality of life, they were statistically significantly longer off work, and had a 2.5 fold higher rate of in-hospital treatments (Augustin et al, 2010).

Nail psoriasis is characterized by pits, salmon spots, onycholysis, subungual hyperkeratosis and some more signs that are less frequent. The psoriatic nail changes may be classified according to their origin: Pitting, leukonychia, nail plate thickening, crumbling and red spots in the lunula originate in the matrix whereas oil drop discoloration (salmon spots), nail bed hyperkeratosis, onycholysis and splinter haemorrhages derive from the nail bed. Swelling of the proximal nail fold reflects paronychia and swelling of the distal interphalangeal joint is suggestive of psoriatic arthritis. Psoriatic pachydermoperiostosis leads to enlargement of the entire distal phalanx.

Pits are generally said to be the most frequent signs. They are small, well delimited depressions on the surface of the nail plate with usually equal size and depth (Figs 11-12).

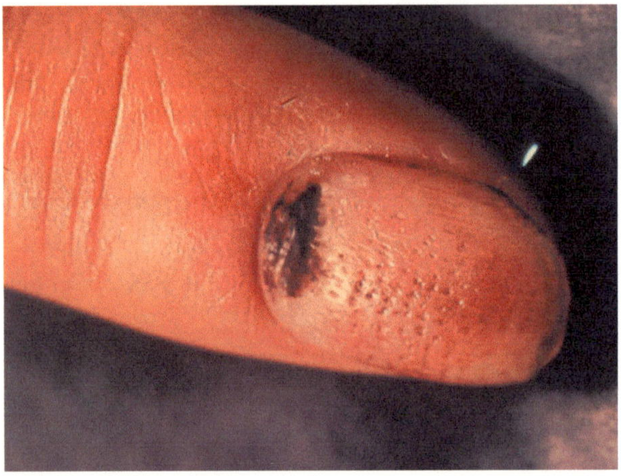

a)

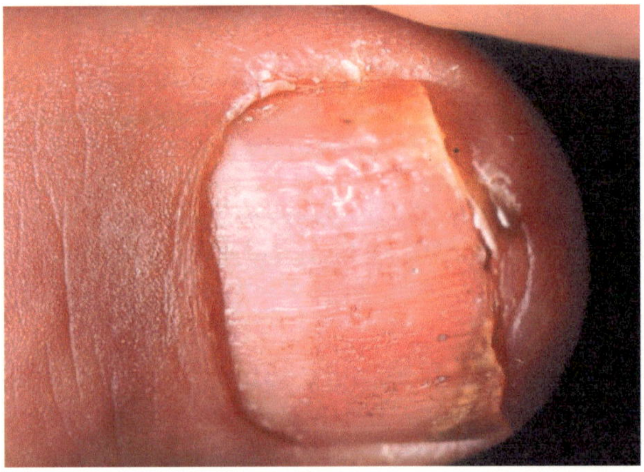

b)

Fig. 11. Psoriatic pits are small depressions of the nail surface of equal size and depth. The pits in a are artificially stained by dithranol treatment, b shows distal onycholysis in addition.

Analogous lesions are small white to yellowish spots that are mainly seen in the proximal nail plate when the parakeratosis does not break off the plate. This is called spotted nails (Tüpfelnägel in German), a term not commonly used in the Anglo-American literature. A number of ten or more pits per nail or more than 60 pits in all nails is commonly seen as proof of psoriasis (Baran & Haneke, 2007). Both pits and spots derive from tiny lesions in the most proximal matrix and possibly the most proximal part of the ventral surface of the proximal nail fold (Zaias, 1990). The length of a pit represents the length of time of the psoriatic matrix lesion, its width is indicative of the width of the lesions and the depth either of the severity of the lesion or a lesion that extends a bit into the intermediate matrix. Pits are usually arranged irregularly but sometimes they form longitudinal or even

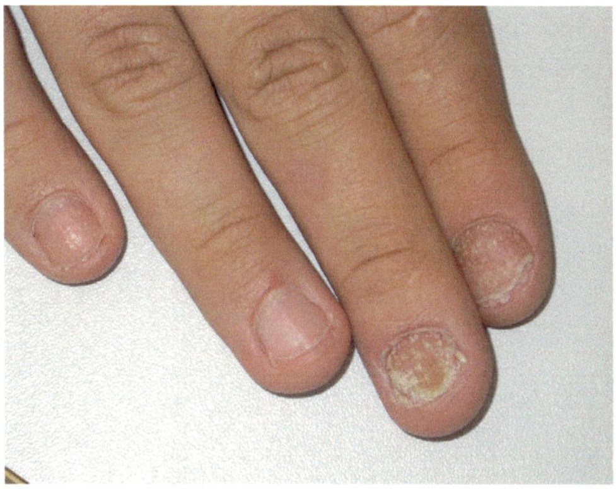

a)

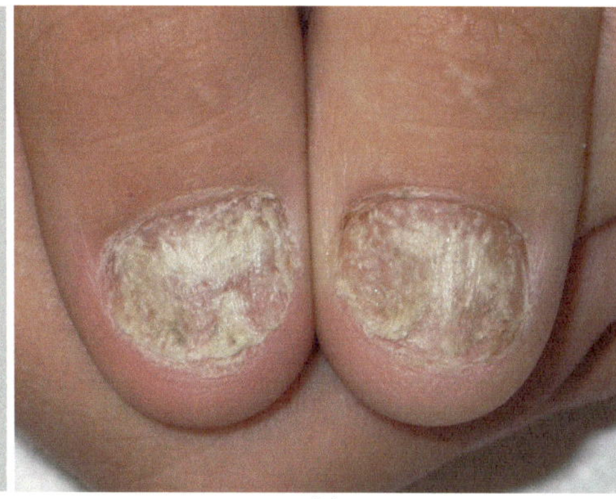

b)

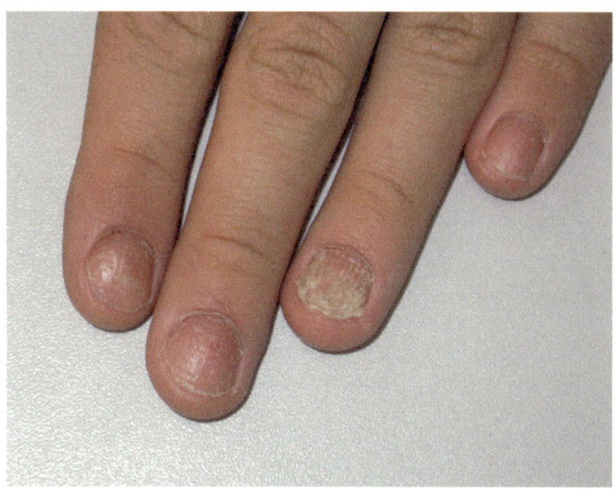

b)

Fig. 12. a - c. 16-year-old boy with marked nail psoriasis. Note that some nails are almost destroyed, other are much less involved.

transverse rows. Longitudinal rows of pits are due to repeated minor trauma at exactly the same location of the proximal matrix whereas transverse ones may reflect a trauma that elicited a Köbner phenomenon at many spots at the same time. Rarely, shallow transverse lines are seen indicating a microtrauma to the entire width of the matrix. The variable arrangement of the pits may cause a clinical picture that varies within a relatively short period of time. It is now thought that pits may be due to microtrauma of the proximal matrix, which is the closest to the articulation, from the distal interphalangeal joint. Pits in horizontal rows are equivalent to Beau's lines (Fig. 13).

In pustular psoriasis, pits may occur that are much larger than usual pits (Fig. 14); they are also called elkonyxis.

Salmon or oil spots represent circumscribed psoriasis plaques of the nail bed. Their specific colour is due to the fact that the psoriatic scales are compressed under the nail plate and imbibed with serum that makes them appear yellowish-reddish mimicking a drop of oil on a sheet of paper. Once a psoriatic plaque has reached the hyponychium or when it started at the hyponychium the scales are not or no longer compressed by the overlying nail plate and may break out giving rise to onycholysis (Fig 15).

Small lesions in the intermediate and distal matrix may appear as red spots whereas extensive lesions may cause a red lunula before the resultant nail plate changes obscure these alterations.

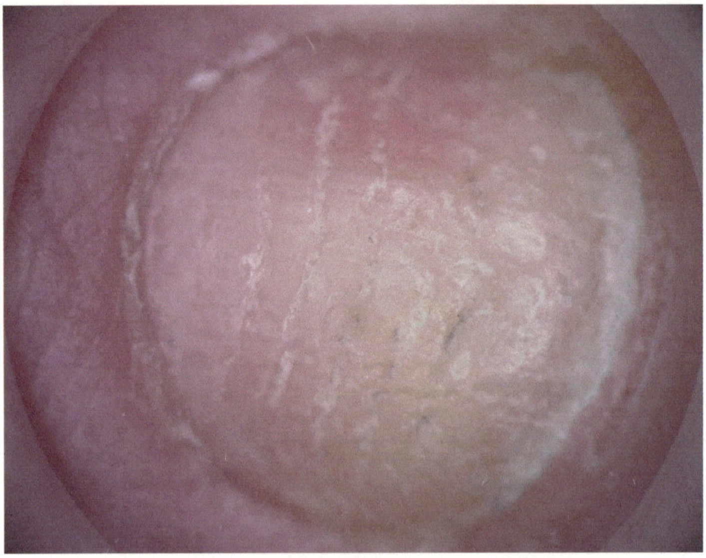

a)

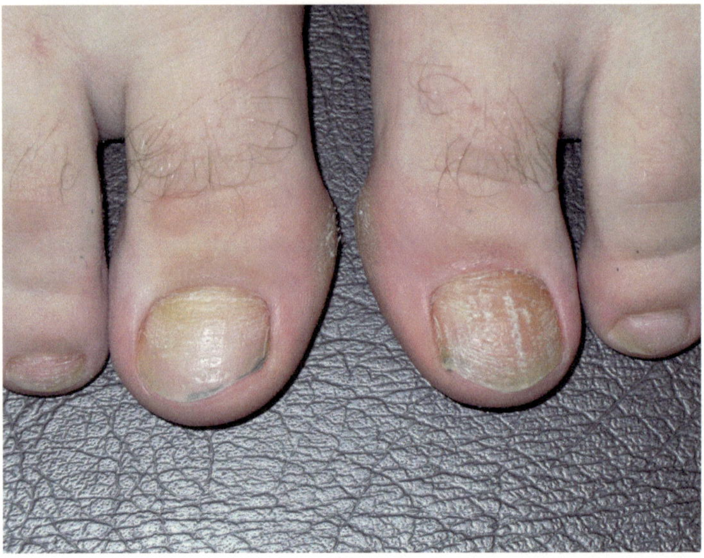

b)

Fig. 13. Pits arranged in horizontal rows. On finger nails, which grow faster they are still identifiable as single pits (A) whereas on toenails, due to their slow growth rate they appear as transverse furrows and lines (B).

Sometimes, psoriasis of the nail bed may cause important hyperkeratosis that may in extreme cases resemble pachyonychia congenita. In addition to subungual hyperkeratosis there may also be a thickening of the nail plate itself. Clinically this looks like a rough nail with irregular surface and loss of transparency, which is mainly due to wavy arrangement of the nail lamellae as well as inclusion of serum and neutrophilic abscesses.

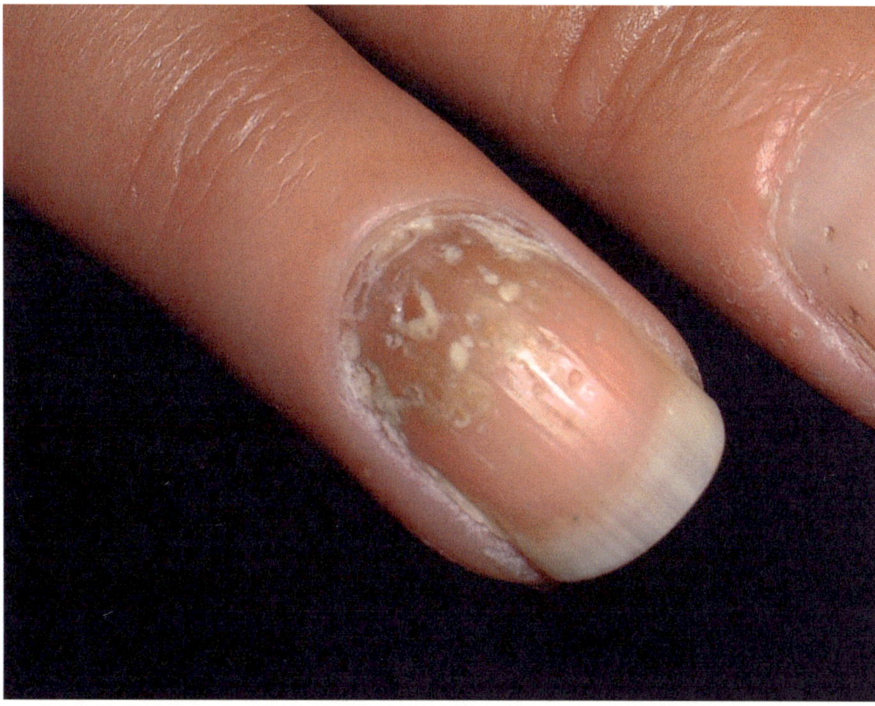

Fig. 14. Nail involvement in pustular psoriasis of the palms and soles (Barber-Königsbeck type). Note the relatively large pits and some ivory-coloured spots. These large surface depressions are called elkonyxis.

Small dark-brown to black longitudinal streaks in the nail bed, mainly in distal location, are called splinter haemorrages (Fig 16). They are due to thromboses of the dilated capillaries of the nail bed papillary ridges, which run all along the nail bed with 3 to 5 layers of capillaries one above the other.

Psoriatic leukonychia is relatively rare. It usually represents a focus of parakeratosis in the intermediate nail layers. It is often associated with other signs of nail psoriasis and may be seen as an advancing edge in acute-onset nail psoriasis.

Larger psoriatic lesions of the nail matrix cause crumbly nails, even complete nail destruction. They are often associated with psoriatic arthritis.

Pustular psoriasis of the nails is seen in palmar plantar pustular psoriasis of Barber-Königsbeck (Figures 14, 17), in generalized pustular psoriasis of von Zumbusch and in Hallopeau's acrodermatitis continua suppurativa. In palmar plantar pustular psoriasis, nail involvement is commonly seen as yellow lakes of pus under the nail plate. This is often associated with elkonyxis. In generalized pustular psoriasis, nail involvement usually leads to nail dystrophy.

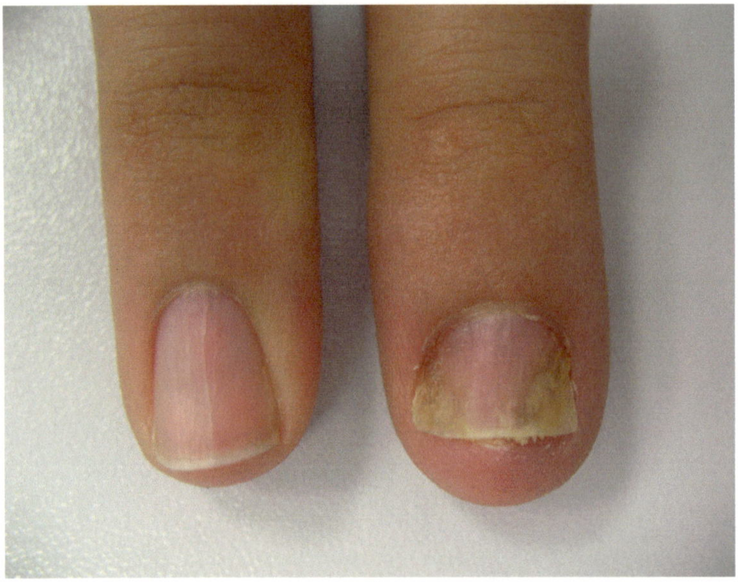

a)

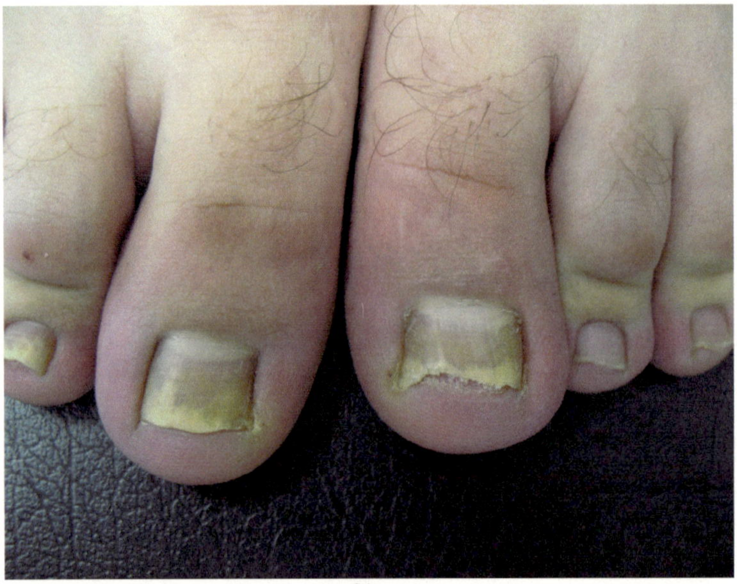

b)

Fig. 15. Subungual hyperkeratosis in distal nail bed psoriasis. A. Fingernails, B toe nails.

Acrodermatitis continua suppurativa of Hallopeau is an insidiously developing disease of the tip of the finger commonly commencing dorsally and slowly involving the nail apparatus (Figs. 18, 19 a, b). The diagnosis is often only made late when there is already a certain degree of nail dystrophy. In very typical cases, the finger or toe tip rounds up, loses its nail, the skin is fiercely red with some tiny pustules. Radiographically, resorption of the corona unguicularis becomes evident. In acute cases, the skin may appear superficially necrotic.

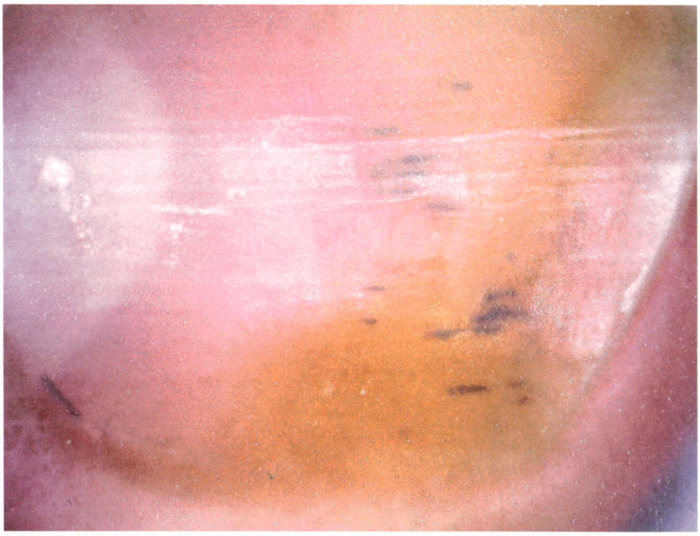

Fig. 16. Splinter haemorrhages in a nail with salmon spot

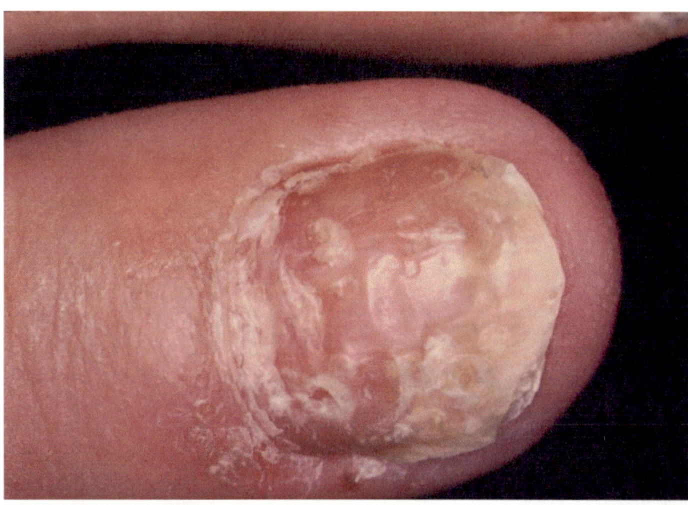

Fig. 17. Psoriasis pustulosa of Barber-Königsbeck

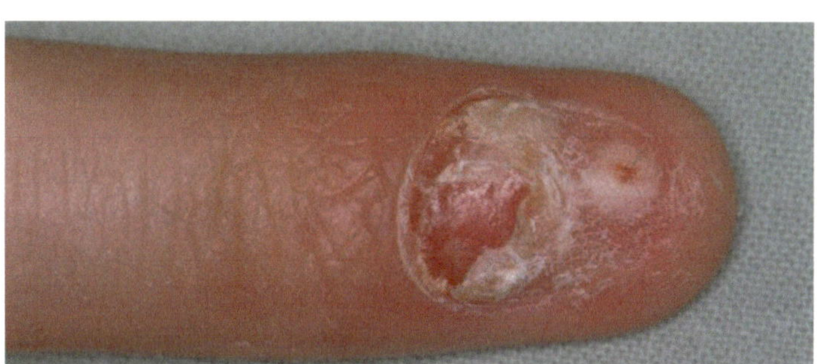

Fig. 18. Early acrodermatitis continua suppurativa

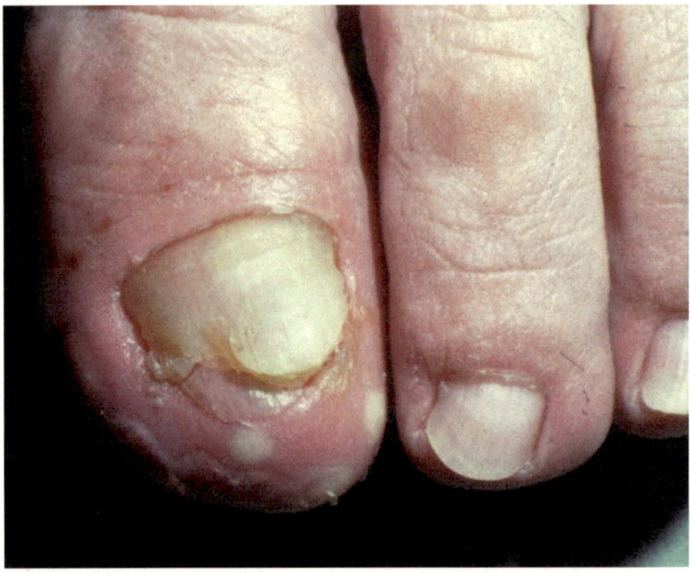

a)

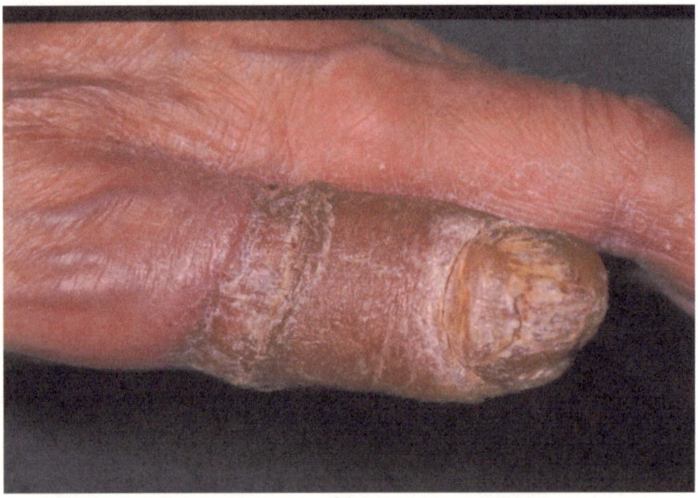

b)

Fig. 19. Acrodermatitis continua suppurativa. A. Pustules have been present for more than 12 years in this elderly lady. B. Relatively acute onset of acrodermatitis continua suppurativa in a patient with bronchial carcinoma; whether this is a causal or accidental association is not clear.

Psoriatic paronychia develops when the periungual skin is affected by psoriasis, but it is also commonly seen in psoriatic arthritis with nail involvement (Fig. 20). The chronic inflammation causes thickening of the free edge of the proximal nail fold with consecutive loss of the cuticle and later loss of attachment of the nail fold's ventral surface to the underlying nail plate. This allows foreign material such as dirt, microorganisms or allergenic substances to enter the space under the nail fold where they may aggravate the inflammation.

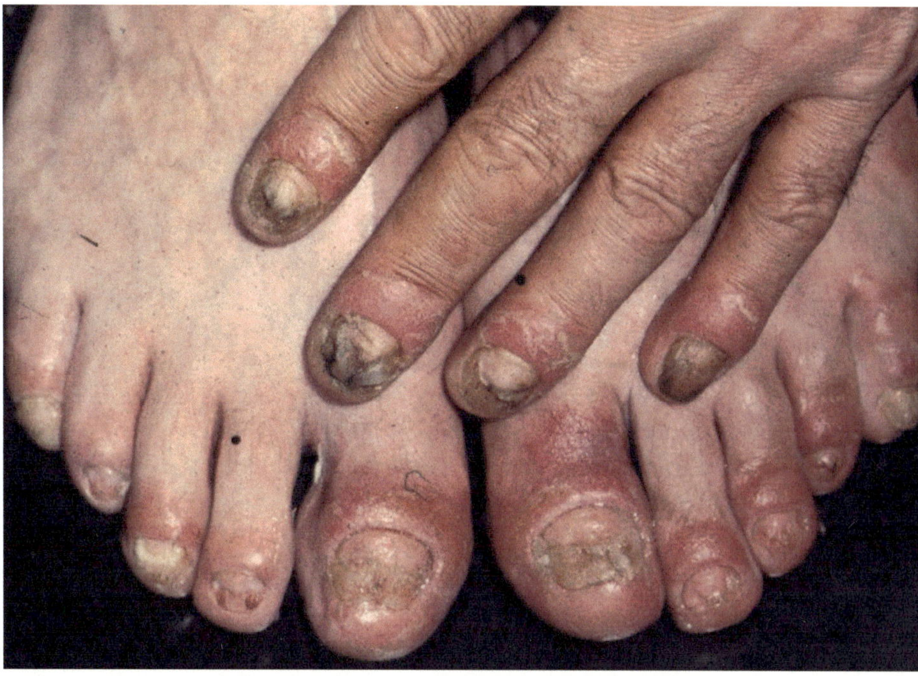

Fig. 20. Psoriatic paronychia in a patient with psoriasis arthropathy.

Psoriatic enthesitis of the distal interphalangeal joint is a painful inflammation of the insertions of tendons and ligaments mainly at the base of the distal phalanx. This may cause swelling of the distal joint with stiffness and loss of the dorsal creases of the distal interphalangeal joint and a shiny skin.

Psoriatic pachydermoperiostosis is a rare event. It is associated with bone appositions which also lead to a widening of the base of the distal phalanx with consecutive widening of the nail plate.

In almost a quarter of the patients with latent psoriatic arthritis, radiological assessment will detect changes not seen clinically (Khan et al, 2003).

7. Quality of life

Nail psoriasis has been shown to severely impair quality of life (see Scoring of nail psoriasis). Pain, cosmetic embarrassment, impaired function, loss of dexterity are just some of the complaints brought forward by the patients (De Jong et al, 1996). More than 90% of the patients consider their nail psoriasis to be a significant social problem affecting their professional work, and more than half of them experienced pain (de Berker, 2009, Gupta and Cooper, 2009).

7.1 Scoring of nail psoriasis

To score the extent and severity of nail psoriasis the **nail psoriasis severity index** (NAPSI) was developed (Rich and Scher, 2003). Each nail is divided into 4 quadrants by a horizontal and a vertical line. Nail matrix and nail bed are scored independently. Any of the matrix signs - pitting, leukonychia, red lunula spots and crumbling - as well as the nail bed signs - onycholysis, salmon or oil spots, subungual hyperkeratosis, splinter hemorrhage - are counted. Absence is given 0, presence in one quadrant 1, presence in two quadrants 2 etc up to 4 quadrants receiving 4. Matrix and nail bed signs are added resulting in a maximum score of 8 per nail. All finger nails can have a maximum NAPSI score of 80, finger and toenails of 160. All of the 8 individual features of matrix and nail bed psoriasis are just given one score independent from their number per quadrant. For a target nail, the same technique can be used to evaluate all 8 parameters (pitting, leukonychia, red spots in lunula, crumbling, oil drop, onycholysis, hyperkeratosis, and splinter hemorrhages) in each quadrant of the nail, giving that one nail a score of 0-32. The NAPSI is a useful tool for nail evaluation in the course of therapeutic studies, both for the effect on all nails as well as for the judgment of a target nail (Rich and Scher, 2003). Interobserver reliability for the total NAPSI score is good whereas the nail score only shows moderate agreement (Aktan et al, 2006).

The NAPSI has some limitations. It does not consider the number of pits or red spots of the lunula per quadrant nor the size of an oil spot or the thickness of subungual hyperkeratosis. This limits its use to assess improvement in the course of a treatment (Parrish et al, 2004). Therefore, an additional gradation was proposed for each sign from absent (= 0), mild (= 1), moderate (= 2) and severe (=3) as a qualitative scale similar to that used in the Psoriasis Area and Severity Index (PASI). Nail crumbling is given the same score like a pit, but is considerably more severe. Pustular psoriasis and psoriatic arthritis are not included in the NAPSI.

A **modified NAPSI** was developed for patients with psoriatic arthritis (Maejima et al, 2010). This modified NAPSI is higher in patients with psoriasis of the proximal nail fold, distal interphalangeal (DIP) joint arthritis whereas there was no correlation with the modified NAPSI and other systemic signs. Nail psoriasis was assumed to be related to the Koebner phenomenon and local inflammatory DIP joint arthritis in PsA patients, and nail involvement in PsA was suggested to be among the disorders indicative of distal phalanx enthesitis (Tan et al, 2007, Elder et al,2010).

Nail psoriasis has both a physical and psychological impact on the patients negatively influencing their quality of life (QoL). A **nail psoriasis quality of life index** (NPQ10) was developed to measure life quality impairment due to nail psoriasis and its modification in the course of treatment (Ortonne et al, 2010). Again, psoriatic arthritis patients are not included in the NPQ10. Of the 17000 members of the French Association pour la lutte contre le psoriasis, 4000 were asked to fill in a questionnaire regarding the physical aspects of nail psoriasis. Roughly one third responded and 795 of them had nail psoriasis. The items were elaborated by physicians and patients alike. The patients rated their nail psoriasis as bothersome in 86%, as unsightly in 87%, and as painful in 59%. The number of nails involved significantly affected the pain, aesthetic and functional impairment. Whereas 86% received therapy, 72% were dissatisfied with their treatment. From these facts, 10 questions were created, only one of which concerned pain, the other 9 were related to functional handicaps in daily life. Answers are scored from 0 to 2 with 0 being 'no without hesitation' (absent) or 'not painful', 1 not for 'yes sometimes' or 'not very painful', and 2 for 'yes without hesitation' or 'very painful'. Item 2 and 6 are specific for toe and finger nail psoriasis, respectively. Item 7 relates only to patients driving a car. Scores are transferred into percentages in order to be able to compare them always resulting in a maximum of 100. A test-retest questionnaire was sent out to a few patients yielding a very good reproducibility. NPQ10 scores are significantly higher in patients having both finger and toe nail psoriasis, in female psoriatics, and in patients with a shorter history of psoriasis (Ortonne et al, 2010). The NPQ10 score shows good correlation with the dermatology life quality index (DLQI) (Finlay and Khan, 1994).

State the location of your psoriasis of the nails 1. Fingernails 2. Toenails 3. Both			
1. Would you say that your psoriasis of the nails is mostly:	1. Very painful	2. Not very painful	3. Not painful
2. Because of my psoriasis of the nails, I have difficulty putting my shoes on:	1. Always	2. Sometimes	3. Never
3. Because of my psoriasis of the nails, I don't do any of the jobs I usually do around the house:	1. Always	2. Sometimes	3. Never
4. Because of my psoriasis of the nails, I get dressed more slowly than usual:	1. Always	2. Sometimes	3. Never
5. Because of my psoriasis of the nails, I have trouble putting on my socks (or stockings or tights):	1. Always	2. Sometimes	3. Never
6. Because of my psoriasis of the nails, I have trouble turning my door key:	1. Always	2. Sometimes	3. Never
7. Because of my psoriasis of the nails, I have trouble driving my car:	1. Always	2. Sometimes	3. Never
8. Because of my psoriasis of the nails, someone helps me to get dressed:	1. Always	2. Sometimes	3. Never
9. Because of my psoriasis of the nails, I avoid doing big jobs around the house:	1. Always	2. Sometimes	3. Never
10. Because of my psoriasis of the nails, I am more irritable than usual, and bad-tempered with people:	1. Always	2. Sometimes	3. Never

Table 1. Questionnaire of the NPQ10 (Ortonne et al, 2010)

The **psoriasis weighted extent and severity index** (PWESI) evaluates the skin disease on a scale from 0 (none) to 4 (extensive) and severity of skin disease on a scale of 0 to 4 (intensely inflamed). Ten areas are assessed, among them hands/fingers/fingernails (Wittkowski et al, 2011).

The **extended 10-area linear psoriasis area and severity index (XL-PASI)** combines the PASI and PWESI scoring methods (Feldman and Krueger, 2005) and includes the assessment of surface area involved as well as dimension for scaling, erythema, thickness and joint involvement for specific areas of psoriatic involvement. As with the PASI, severity is graded from 0 to 4 and body surface is divided into ten areas and each is quantified. The XL-PASI scale ranges from 0 to 148 (Wittkowski et al, 2011).

8. Differential diagnosis of nail psoriasis

There is a wide range of potential differential diagnoses, the most important of which are onychomycoses (Table 2) and nail dystrophies after minor trauma, in chronic venous insufficiency and impairment of the peripheral circulation.

Onychomycoses are the most frequent nail disorders. Distal and distal-lateral subungual onychomycosis (DLSO) are mainly due to dermatophytes with *Trichophyton rubrum* being the most frequent pathogen although T mentagrophytes (interdigitale) also plays an important role. All other dermatophytes are rather rare and the role of most yeasts and non-dermatophyte moulds as primary nail pathogens remains disputed. DLSO begins at the hyponychium from where the fungus slowly invades the nail bed in the direction toward the matrix. The infection apparently irritates the nail bed epithelium that produces a reactive hyperkeratosis, which harbours most of the fungal elements whereas the nail plate rather acts as a barrier. In contrast to psoriatic onycholysis that exhibits the classical salmon spot colour at its proximal margin, mycotic onycholysis has no reddish-brown margin (Fig 21 a&b). Nail psoriasis and onychomycosis may coexist (Natarajan et al, 2010).

	Onychomycosis	**Psoriasis**
Pits	Rare	Very frequent
Onycholysis	Frequent	Frequent
Discoloration	Yellow - brown	None - yellow
Loss of nail transparency	Frequent	Less frequent
Fungi	Very frequent, depends on type of OM	rare
Transverse ridges	Rare	Rare
Splinter haemorrhages	Almost never	Rare
Leuconychia	Depends on onychomycosis type: Superficial white OM Proximal white subungual OM	Rare
Paronychia	In onychomycoses due to moulds	In psoriatic arthritis and periungual psoriasis
Finger vs. toe involvement	Toe nails 7 to 10 times more often infected	Finger nails more often affected by psoriatic alterations
Other skin lesions	Tinea pedum and/or manuum	Psoriasis elsewhere
Heredity	Autosomal dominant susceptibility to get a dermatophyte nail infection	Frequent familiarity, particularly in early onset psoriasis and HLA-Cw6 positive subjects

Table 2. Differential diagnostic clinical signs in onychomycosis (OM) and nail psoriasis

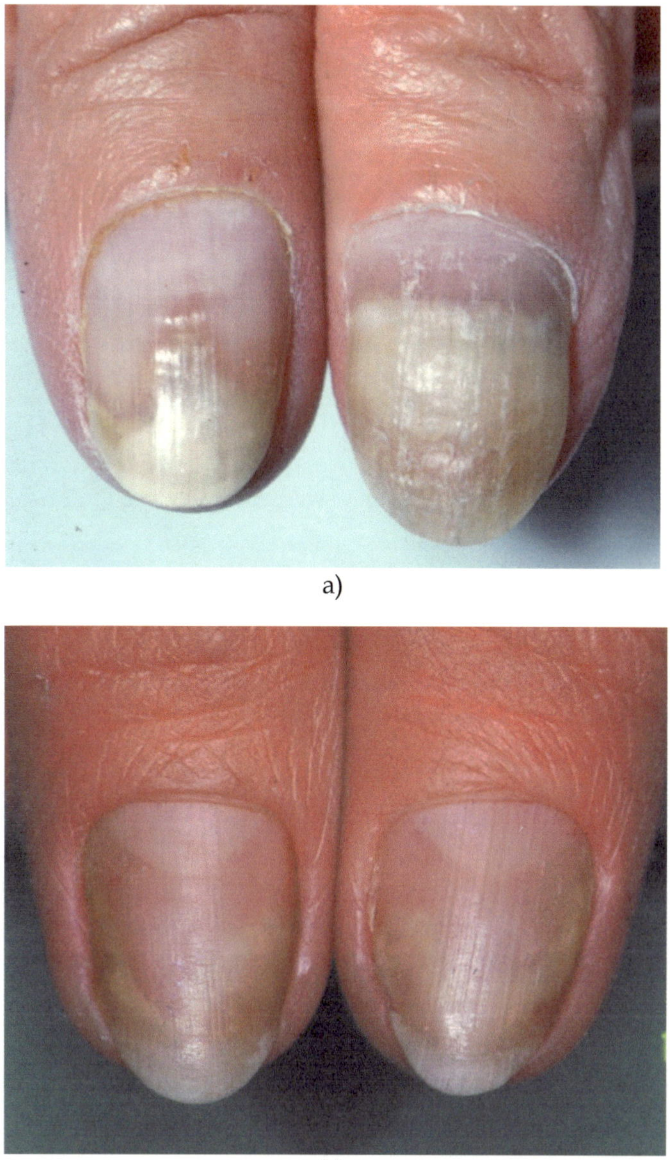

a)

b)

Fig. 21. Psoriatic onycholysis demonstrates a livid-red proximal margin (A), which is not seen in mycotic onycholysis (B).

There are also many histopathological signs in common of onychomycosis and nail psoriasis (Table 3). This may render the differential diagnosis between these two frequent nail conditions very difficult if not impossible. Furthermore, it is possible that both onychomycosis and psoriasis are present in the same subject in different digits as well as in the same nail (Fig.22). It is therefore self-evident that a specimen sent for histopathological diagnosis of nail psoriasis is also stained with periodic acid-Schiff (PAS) or another fungal stain like silver-methene amine (Grocott).

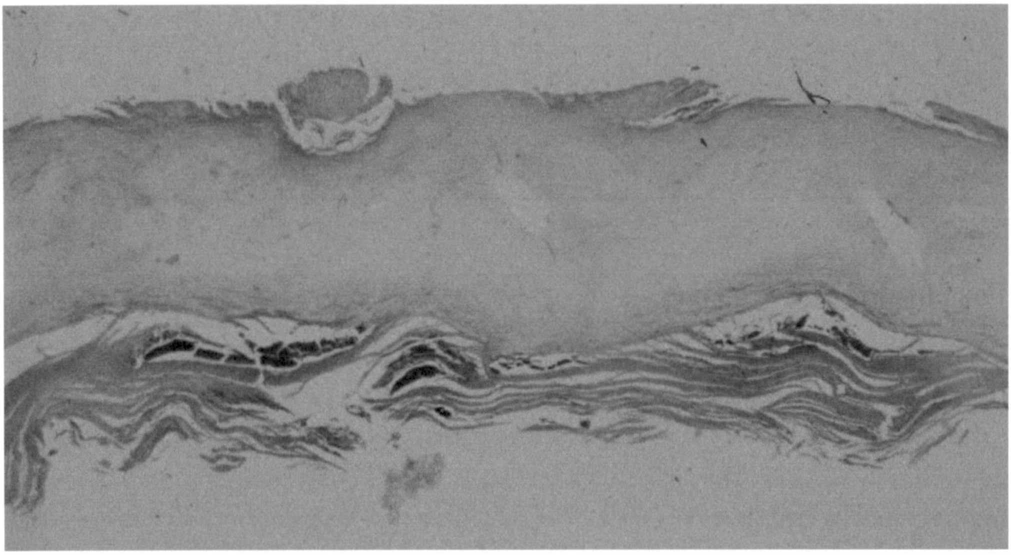

Fig. 22. This nail histopathology shows both psoriasis and onychomycosis: on the surface, 2 pits are seen; the nail itself is a bit wavy and displays fungal hyphae seen as fine eosinophilic lines in the deep layer of the nail in this haematoxylin & eosin stain section; at the undersurface of the nail there is loose keratin, which is mostly parakeratotic and contains several Munro's microabscesses.

	Onychomycosis	**Psoriasis**
Subungual hyperkeratosis	Marked hyperkeratosis with accumulation of neutrophils and serum globules	Marked hyperkeratosis with accumulation of neutrophils and serum globules
Nail bed and matrix granulosis	Patchy hypergranulosis	Patchy hypergranulosis
Nail bed hyperplasia	Papillomatous hyperplasia of nail bed	Papillomatous hyperplasia of nail bed
Spongiosis and exocytosis	Spongiosis and mononuclear exocytosis	Spongiosis and mononuclear exocytosis
Surface alterations	Usually not present	Cup-shaped depression of nail plate surface with parakeratosis: psoriatic pit
Demonstration of fungi	Hyphae and spores in subungual hyperkeratosis and undersurface of nail plate	May be present in double pathology

Table 3. Histopathological differential diagnosis of nail psoriasis and onychomycosis

Reiter's disease is an infrequent reactive arthritis with changes of the ocular, genital and oral mucosae such as conjunctivitis, blepharitis, scleritis or iridocyclitis, balanitis, vulvitis or stomatitis circinata, which are virtually indistinguishable from lingua geographica and its very rare extralingual analogues, and painful inflammation of joints and the vertebral column. Many patients are HLA-B27 positive. Nail changes often start with pits and salmon patches remaining indistinguishable for a long time from nail psoriasis (Pajarre et al, 1977, Lovy et al, 1980) before the nails become destroyed (Fig. 23) (Table 4).

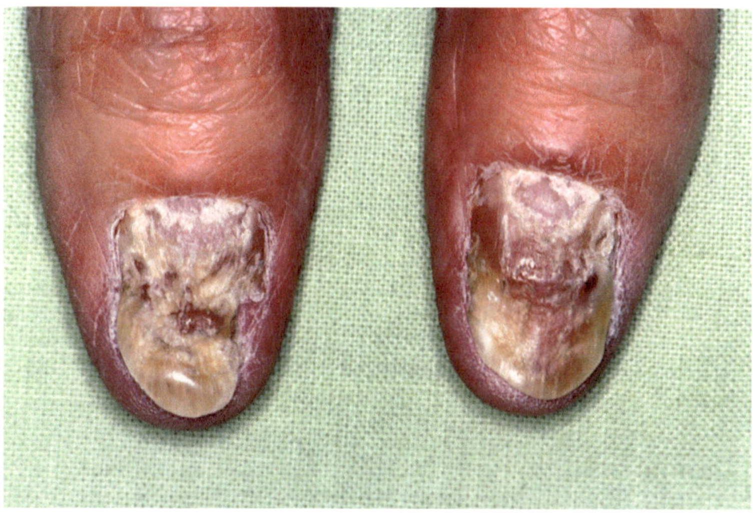

Fig. 23. Reiter's disease of the nails (Courtesy T Ruzicka, Munich)

	Psoriasis	Reiter's disease
Pitting	Very frequent	Less frequent
Onycholysis	Frequent	Frequent
Subungual keratosis	Variable	Pronounced
Salmon patch	Reddish	More brown
Nail destruction	Rare	Marked
Skin lesions elsewhere	Frequent	Palmar and plantar lesions, joint changes, mucosal lesions

Table 4. Differential diagnosis of nail psoriasis and nail changes in Reiter's disease

Onycholysis is often due to overzealous manicure, but psoriasis of the nails renders them more susceptible to develop onycholysis due to minor trauma. Again, psoriatic onycholysis has usually a reddish proximal margin, which is lacking in onycholysis semilunaris (Fig. 24).

Eczema involving the nail apparatus usually causes pit-like depressions leading to a rough nail surface called trachyonychia as well as to irregular transverse lines. The depressions are commonly less deep and less regular in size than in psoriasis. Although these depressions are more common in allergic contact dermatitis and nummular eczema they are also seen in atopic eczema (Nnoruka et al, 2004). Despite the trachyonychia, the nail may still retain its shine. In contrast, subungual contact dermatitis, e.g. as seen in acrylate allergy, causes subungual hyperkeratosis and later onycholysis as well as loss of nail transparency and shine (Hemmer et al, 1996).

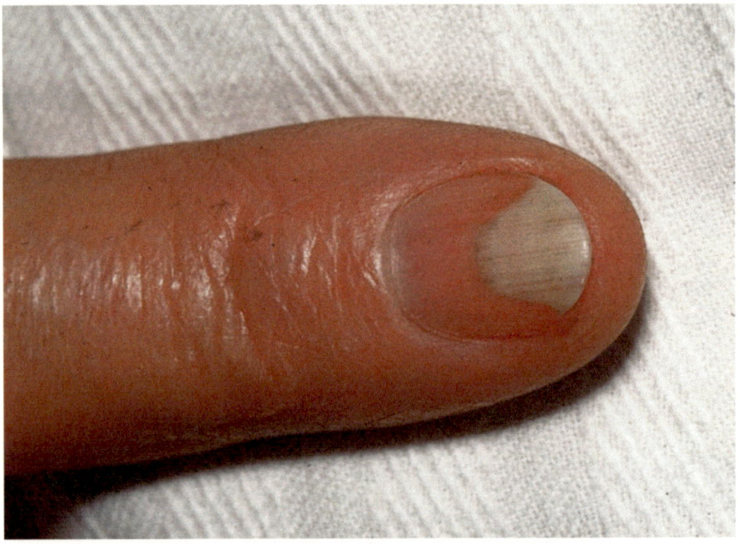

a)

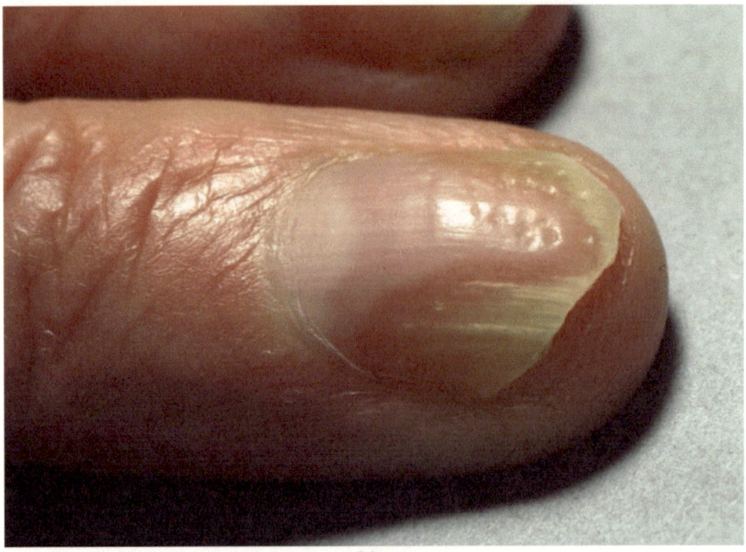

b)

Fig. 24. Onycholysis semilunaris (A) is characterized by its half-moon shape and clear border whereas psoriatic onycholysis has the typical appearance of an oil spot at its proximal margin (B).

When many or even all nails are affected the condition is called twenty nail dystrophy; this may, however, be a manifestation of ungual lichen planus, alopecia areata, eczema or psoriasis and the exact diagnosis often requires a histopathological examination of a nail biopsy.

Irritant contact dermatitis was also estimated to mimic nail psoriasis (Takeuchi et al, 2010).

Alopecia areata is known to be associated with rough nails. The more extensive the alopecia areata is the more likely the patients also get nail changes. Most probably, isolated alopecia areata of the nails does exist (Tan et al, 2002, Nanda et al. 2002). Alopecia areata nails grow slower than psoriatic nails. They are often indistinguishable from eczema nails, and in fact, both have a microscopical spongiotic dermatitis in common. Serum is in the spongiotic vesicles and becomes included into the nail; when it is very superficial it may break out and leave a depression, but when the origin is in the intermediate matrix the dried serum will remain in the nail and be the reason for the loss of nail transparence, nail thickening and brittleness.

When almost all nails are affected the so-called twenty-nail dystrophy is diagnosed (Samman, 1979). Even though this term does note denote a specific condition it is still widely used, particularly for 20-nail dystrophy of children (Horn and Odom, 1980, Baran and Dawber, 1987).

9. Treatment of nail psoriasis

Psoriasis of the nails is an often neglected or overlooked disease as is evidenced by the most recent 100-page strong guidelines on psoriasis treatment (Nast et al, 2011), and it has a serious impact on the individual's daily life.

The therapy of nail psoriasis is difficult, particularly that of isolated nail psoriasis as one usually hesitates to treat it systemically. In general, systemic treatment regimens that are effective in cutaneous psoriasis also improve nail lesions. There is a general lack of well-documented studies and they are often not or difficult to compare (Jiaravuthisan et al, 2007) and few evidence-based treatments exist (Cassell and Kavanaugh, 2006). A standardized therapeutic approach does therefore not exist and preferred treatment regimens also differ between various countries. The treatment also depends on the nail structure involved, how severe the nail dystrophy is, whether there are extraungual lesions, the time needed for applying a specific therapy, and not the least also on its cost.

9.1 Topical therapy

Topical treatments are generally held not to be very effective. This has several simple reasons: Pits come from the depth of the nail pocket where the lesions are protected by the overlying proximal nail fold from being treated; lesions in the intermediate matrix are both hidden by the proximal nail fold and the nail plate; nail bed lesions are under the nail plate, which is a considerable obstacle to penetration of drugs. Ointments applied on finger nails may interfere with paper work. There are very few controlled studies on topical therapies.

Urea (carbamide) is known for its keratolytic property. A paste containing 40% urea (Onyster®) softens fungus infected nails to a degree that it can be atraumatically removed; this may be a starting point for topical teatment. A 10% urea nail varnish was shown to improve the biophysical properties of the nail (Krüger et al, 2006). A 15% stable urea nail lacquer (Onypso®) is advertised as "the only specific topical treatment for nail psoriasis" as it is claimed to reduce subungual hyperkeratosis. No controlled studies are available.

Anthralin (dithranol, cignoline) suppresses cell proliferation, inhibits neutrophils and monocytes, neutrophile migration and lymphocyte proliferation. It exerts a strong antiproliferative action on keratinocytes (Schröder et al, 1985). It is an old, extremely safe and very effective psoriasis remedy. Anthraline 0.4 to 2% in petrolatum was used in a study of 20 patients over a period of approximately 5 months (Yamamoto et al, 1998). There was no response in 8 and little to fair response on onycholysis, subungual hyperkeratosis and pitting in 12 individuals. Anthraline is not popular because it stains skin and clothes. Therefore the patients washed the anthraline ointment off after 30 minutes and applied 10% triethanol amine. However, nail staining cannot be completely avoided making the lesions even more obvious and embarrassing.

There are no studies on anthralin in combination with ultraviolet (Ingram regimen) or coal tar without or with UV (Goeckerman regimen) in nail psoriasis.

5-Fluorouracil (5-FU) is a cytostatic agent inhibiting nucleic acid synthesis and thus reducing cellular renewal. It was mainly used for the treatment of actinic keratoses and superficial basal carcinomas, but the application under occlusion or twice daily until an erosive reaction was achieved did not make it popular amongst the patients. A prospective study on 20 patients with very long-standing psoriatic pitting, hyperkeratosis or onycholysis was conducted with 1% 5-FU solution twice daily. This had to be massaged into the skin immediately adjacent to the nail for 6 months. Seventeen of the 20 subjects experienced marked improvement in pitting and subungual hyperkeratosis (Fredriksson, 1974). One patient with onycholysis lost all affected nails that finally regrew but with the same onycholysis as before.

In a double blind controlled study, 5-FU in a penetration enhancer consisting of urea and propylene glycol was compared to the penetration enhancer solution alone. The preparation was applied once daily over a period of 12 weeks. There was a statistically significant improvement of the total nail area severity (NAS) score comprised of the number of pits, degree of pitting, subungual hyperkeratosis, onycholysis and salmon spots, for both preparations with no superior results seen in the 5-FU group (de Jong et al, 1999). Six subjects in the 5-FU group experienced side effects such as pain, swelling, inflammation, discoloration, onycholysis, and nail perforations. 5-FU is not widely used anymore.

Topical steroids have been and continue to be the most commonly used therapeutic agents for local treatment of nail psoriasis. They exert an anti-inflammatory and immunosuppressive action, inhibit leukocyte migration into the skin, decrease vascular permeability, reduce the effect of pro-inflammatory cytokines, and have an antiproliferative action. All these effects taken together make them a good treatment of nail psoriasis provided they can reach the psoriatic lesion of the nail. However, no standard therapeutic regimes exist for topical steroid therapy of nail psoriasis (Jiaravuthisan et al, 2007) as there are very few controlled studies with their use in nail psoriasis. Generally, high-potency topical steroids are prescribed that are applied once or even twice daily to the nail folds and nail bed either as a cream, ointment or solution. Once an effect has been achieved the frequency of application is reduced until about twice weekly. A proactive treatment approach may be superior although there are no controlled studies in nail psoriasis. Side effects of long-term potent topical steroid use are hypopigmentation and skin atrophy with development of telangiectasiae. It may be wise to have the patient apply antiseptics once daily during this treatment as the risk of microbial growth, particularly of *Candida spp*, may be considerable. Topical corticosteroid application has even been linked to tapering of the digits and to phalangeal bone resorption (Wolf et al, 1990).

A study on 10 nail psoriasis patients with 8% clobetasol nail lacquer resulted in reduced pitting, onycholysis and salmon spots after only 3 months of treatment. The treatment was found to be safe, effective and cosmetically acceptable (Sanchéz Regaña et al, 2005).

Betamethasone diproprionate - salicylic acid ointment over 3 to 9 months reduced the nail bed hyperkeratosis by about one half (Tosti et al, 1996), which was virtually identical to the effect of **calcipotriol**. The authors' conclusion was that calcipotriol is a safe alternative to topical steroids in nail bed psoriasis.

A combination treatment with calcipotriol cream and clobetasol cream was shown to reduce subungual keratosis by 72% after 6 months and 81% after 12 months in finger nails whereas the improvement was 70 and 72.5% in toe nails, respectively (Rigopoulos et al, 2002). For the first 6 months, calcipotriol cream was applied on weekday evenings and clobetasol cream on weekend evenings, the next 6 months only clobetasol cream was used. Side effects of calcipotriol in the treatment of nail psoriasis are rare and mild, they mainly consist of irritation, burning, erythema and diffuse urticaria (Tosti et al, 1996, Rigopoulos et al, 2002).

Cyclosporine is an immunosuppressive calcineurin inhibitor ultimately decreasing T cell growth and migration (Baker et al, 1987). A 10% formulation in maize oil was used in three fingers of a patient (Tosti et al, 1990) with marked improvement after 2 months and almost complete clearing after 3 months. No adverse effects were observed. Cyclosporine is a hydrophobic, large molecule of 1.5 kD and difficult to incorporate into a topical preparation, but the newer calcineurin inhibitors tacrolimus and pimecrolimus are available as ointment or cream, respectively. Curiously, no controlled study with any of these two potent drugs has been conducted in nail psoriasis. Tacrolimus was found to be ineffective in plaque psoriasis, most probably due to insufficient penetration because of its large molecular weight of 802 Da, and this might have discouraged investigators to try it in nail psoriasis.

Tazarotene is a third-generation topical retinoid for the treatment of acne and psoriasis. It binds to the nuclear retin acid receptors RAR-β and RAR-γ exerting an effect on epidermal proliferation and differentiation. Its action in psoriasis is mainly normalization of abnormal keratinocyte proliferation and control of inflammation (Kang et al, 1996). In addition to some case reports on tazarotene use in periungual psoriasis, a double-blind controlled study was performed with the vehicle as the control. Both tazarotene 0.1% under occlusion as well as without occlusion yielded a statistically significant better reduction in onycholysis and pitting (Scher et al, 2001). Erythema, peeling of the paronychia, irritation of the finger skin and paronychia were the side effects seen in the tazarotene group whereas the vehicle was tolerated without adverse effects.

Indigo naturalis is a dark-blue powder from the leaves of indigo-bearing plants. It inhibits proliferation, promotes differentiation of epidermal keratinocytes, inhibits neutrophil proinflammatory responses and suppresses TNF-α induced vascular cell adhesion molecule 1 expression in endothelial cells thereby exerting an antipsoriatic effect (Lin et al, 2009). Six patients with psoriasis who had been treated for 4 years with indigo naturalis ointment or systemic Chinese herbs and whose skin lesions had responded well whereas the nails remained unchanged were treated twice daily with 1 to 2 drops of indigo naturalis oil extract onto the nail plate, fold and hyponychium. After three months, the mean reduction in PASI was 51%, and two patients had even PASI reductions of 89 and 82%, respectively. No adverse side effects were noted (Lin, 2011).

9.2 Intralesional treatments

Intralesional injections of **corticosteroids** are widely used, either with an injection needle or by a high-pressure injector (Dermojet®, Port-O-Jet®). In most cases, crystal suspensions of triamcinolone acetonide are used with variable concentrations of 1 mg/mL (Zaias,1990) to 10 mg/mL (Scher and Daniels, 2003, de Berker and Lawrence 1998). Injections ranged from a single one (Gerstein, 1962) to once every 3 to 4 weeks for 4 to 6 months (Abell and Samman, 1973, Zaias, 1990) or monthly for the first 6 months and then 4 injections over the next 6 months followed by once every two months for the next 6 to 12 months (Norton, 1982). It appears that the number of affected nails may be a limiting factor as many patients complain of discomfort and pain. In our experience, even though most patients prefer the needle-less high pressure air gun they admitted that injection with a 30-gauge needle is less painful (unpubl. observation). The sort of high pressure injector appears to be important as there are good results with some devices and disappointing ones with others. Side effects of high pressure devices are subungual haematomas, short-term paraesthesias, atrophy at the injection site, epidermoid inclusion cysts (de Berker, 2000), tattooing with minute rubber particles and blood splash back on the instrument and the physician.

Most intralesional injections are given into the proximal nail fold, best one each into each side of it with sparing the central area where the extensor tendon inserts in order to avoid steroid-induced tendolysis. These injection sites are good for lesions originating from the matrix, i.e. pits, ridges and severe nail plate dystrophy whereas nail bed-derived lesions such as subungual hyperkeratosis and salmon spots profit from sub-nailbed injections. These are, however, even more painful and usually require an anaesthesia to be applied.

The concentration of triamcinolon per mL does not appear to be critical as there are variations from 1mg/mL to 10 mg/mL in the literature. Higher concentrations allow smaller volumes to be injected, which then is less painful. It is still a matter of debate whether lidocaine or another local anaesthetic should be used to dilute the triamcinolone solution. In our opinion, it is both the needle prick and the pressure from the injection that are felt as uncomfortable to painful and no local anaesthetic can prevent this. Topical anaesthesia may be used, for instance with lidocaine-prilocain mixture (EMLA®), to alleviate the needle prick.

Intralesional methotrexate (MTX) has recently been used in a single patient (Sarıcaoglu et al, 2011). MTX is a folic acid analogue irreversibly binding to dehydrofolate reductase thus blocking deoxyribonucleic acid synthesis. In addition, it was shown to exhibit an anti-inflammatory effect by inhibiting the polyamine pathway in autoimmune diseases. Intralesional MTX has been shown to be effective and safe in a variety of conditions (Agostini et al, 2007). This was the rationale to use it in a psoriatic patient with pitting and subungual hyperkeratosis of only one nail. MTX 2.5 mg was injected into each side of the proximal nail fold once weekly for 6 weeks. Pain was tolerable. During the 4-month follow-up, the psoriatic nail alterations improved and no clinical or laboratory side effects were noted. No recurrence of the nail lesions was observed in the following two years.

Although **intralesional cyclosporine** has shown good effects in cutaneous psoriasis there are no reports on intralesional cyclosporine in nail psoriasis.

9.3 Physical treatment modalities

9.3.1 Phototherapy and photochemotherapy

Phototherapy has been used for psoriasis for more than 100 years. Ultraviolet (UV) is known to exert an immunosuppressive effect through an effect on local and circulating immune cells, particularly on dendritic cells. Narrow band UV B of 311 nm has been shown to be most effective. Photochemotherapy combines the use of UV, usually UV A, with the topical or systemic administration of a photosensitizing agent, most commonly a psoralen. In contrast to skin psoriasis, nail psoriasis barely responds. In a study with oral PUVA on 10 patients, the skin of the proximal nail fold improved, but pitting did not improve. Nail plate crumbling cleared in three out of 4 individuals whereas onycholysis and oil drops improved slightly by approximately 50% (Marx and Scher, 1980). In contrast, in a retrospective study on the effect of different systemic treatments, PUVA improved the NAPSI score after 12, 24 and 48 weeks by 21%, 51% and 69%, Re-PUVA (combination of a retinoid with PUVA) by 27%, 65%, and 85%, ReNUVB (retinoid plus narrow-band UV B) by 21%, 48% and 64%, respectively, whereas narrow-band UV B alone had no beneficial effect (Regana et al, 2011). Topical PUVA resulted in clearing of 2 subjects with pitting and 2 with onycholysis improved substantially (Handfield-Jones et al, 1987). Even these results are surprising as the nail is a very efficient UV shield (Stern et al, 2011).

9.3.2 Laser treatment

Various studies have shown efficacy of laser treatments on cutaneous psoriasis. As angiogenesis was found to be one of the driving factors in psoriasis pathogenesis (Heidenreich et al, 2009) most studies were performed with the pulsed dye laser, which specifically targets blood vessels (Taibjee et al, 2005, Bovenschen et al, 2006). Two recent studies used the pulsed dye laser for nail psoriasis, one in comparison with photodynamic treatment (Fernández-Guarino et al, 2009), the other evaluated the effect of PDL on nail psoriasis (Oram et al, 2010). A third study not yet published (Treewittayapoom et al, in press) used two different pulse widths. All studies used a 595-nm pulsed dye laser with a spot size of 7 mm. The pulse duration in the Spanish study was 6 ms, in the Turkish one 1.5, and the Thai one compared the efficacy of 6 ms with 0.45 ms pulse width, fluences were 9, 8 - 10, and 9 and 6 J/cm^2, respectively. Both the PDT and the PDL group showed a decrease in the NAPSI score with no difference between the two groups (Fernández-Guarino et al, 2009). The Turkish study showed an improvement mainly of the nail bed NAPSI (Oram et al, 2010). The Thai study did not demonstrate a difference in treatment outcome between the long 6 ms pulse with 9 J/cm^2 group and the short 0.45 ms pulse duration with 6 J/cm^2 group; however, the pain was statistically significantly more intense in the longer pulse group (Treewittayapoom et al, in press).

9.3.3 Ionising radiation

Superficial radiotherapy delivers the radiation energy mainly to the skin surface. Three patients were treated with 400 to 600 cGy. Although no changes were noted during the 4-

month treatment interval the nails regrew normally in the following 8 to 14 months, and one patient had disease-free nails even 20 years after cessation of the irradiation (Finnerty, 1979). Another ten patients were treated in a randomized prospective double-blind study with twice fractioned doses of 150 cGy superficial radiotherapy each a week apart. One hand was treated and the other left for comparison. After 10 and 15 weeks posttreatment, the irradiated hand was significantly better concerning pitting, subungual hyperkeratosis, onycholysis, total nail destruction and nail thickness, but afte 20 weeks no difference was seen anymore between the treated and untreated hands (Yu and King, 1992).

Grenz rays are very soft X-rays not penetrating the skin. In a randomized, double-blind study of 22 patients, 5 Gy of Grenz rays were applied in ten weekly courses to one hand only. Only 1 patient showed complete clearance, 7 mild improvement and 14 remained unchanged. Only non-hyperkeratotic lesions responded, which might have to be expected as Grenz rays do not penetrate the skin and hyperkeratosis. Six months after the irradiation, 2 patients were improved, two had worsened, and 18 remained unchanged. Slight nail fold pigmentation was the only adverse effect (Lindelöf, 1989).

Electron beam therapy was chosen by another group as the electrons are able to penetrate the nail bed (Kwang et al, 1995). Twelve patients were treated on one hand with a weekly dose of 750 cGy for a period of 8 weeks. Assessment at 3, 6 and 12 months showed improvement in 3 patients, slight improvement in 6 subjects, and a complete failure in 3 individuals after 3 months. At 6 and 12 months, only one patient continued to improve, 9 regressed to pretreatment conditions. A temporary deep brown-black discoloration of the treated nails was observed in some subjects.

All ionizing treatments have to be used with utmost care as long-term side effects may occur, often so late that the patient does not remember to have been treated with this modality.

9.3.4 Climatotherapy

Climatotherapy, in particular balneotherapy in sunny regions, is very popular in countries with little sunshine. It often has a positive effect on the skin and the emotional aspect of the patients. Although some patients claim that also their nails improve there are no systematic evaluations of the treatment modality on psoriatic nails.

9.4 Systemic therapies

Systemic treatments are indicated when there is wide-spread skin involvement. Isolated nail psoriasis is rarely seen as an indication for systemic therapy. All systemic treatments known to reduce skin lesions will also have a beneficial effect on nail lesions. Controlled studies are as a whole rather rare.

9.4.1 Immunosupressive treatments

Corticosteroids have for a long time given to psoriatics although their disadvantages such as general steroid adverse effects, tachyphylaxis and rebound phenomenon have been known for decades. There are no controlled trials of systemic steroids in nail psoriasis.

Cyclosporine is a powerful immunosuppressive agent used successfully in wide-spread psoriasis. Nail lesions usually also respond favorably. In a median dose of 2.5 mg/kg bodyweight daily, cyclosporine effectively reduces skin and nail psoriasis. In a comparative trial, cyclosporine versus etretinate were given to 210 patients two thirds of whom had nail involvement. At the end of 10 weeks, both groups showed slight improvement of their nails which continued in the group that continued with tapered cyclosporine (Mahrle et al, 1995). Another patient was treated for her severe nail psoriasis with cyclosporine 3mg/kg/d, and the dose was increased twice by one mg after 4 weeks each. After 16 weeks, both skin and nails had improved with the nail improvement having been considerably faster. "Proximal nail clearing" was observed to be 45 to 60%. The patient stopped cyclosporine on her own because of drug-induced hypertrichosis (Arnold et al, 1993). In a retrospective evaluation, cyclosporine was found to improve the NAPSI score after 12, 24 and 48 weeks by 40%, 72%, and 89%, respectively (Sánchez-Regaña et al, 2011).

Cyclosporine adverse effects, such as gastrointestinal symptoms, fatigue, leg cramps, diastolic blood pressure increase, and peripheral oedema were more common than in the etretinate group that suffered more skin symptoms like dry skin, cheilitis, and dry mouth (Mahrle et al, 1995).

Even though there are many reports on treatment of moderate to severe skin psoriasis with methotrexate, tacrolimus, mycophenolate mofetil, hydroxyurea, 6-thioguanine, sulfasalazine, fumaric esters, azathioprine, carbamazepine, calcitriol, and propylthiouracil, controlled studies concerning nail lesions in these patient cohorts are lacking. However, one may assume that they might also improve nail lesions when they are able to improve the skin.

Methotrexate is still often administered for wide-spread skin psoriasis although lung, liver and kidney fibrosis are well documented adverse effects of long-term treatment. There is only one report specificially relating to MTX low dose therapy for 20-nail psoriasis (Lee, 2009). In an evaluation of patients with nail psoriasis treated systemically, MTX produced NAPSI score improvements of 7%, 31%, and 35%, respectively, after 12, 24 and 48 weeks (Sánchez-Regaña et al, 2011). MTX as a classical cytostatic drug not only inhibits the inflammatory and hyperproliferative processes of psoriasis but may also slow down nail growth speed making it difficult to observe a positive effect in a reasonable time period.

9.4.2 Retinoids

Retinoids are vitamin A derivatives that are used for disorders of keratinisation. Their use in skin psoriasis is well documented with a number of studies. However, their potentials in nail psoriasis have not independently and systematically be studied (Tosti et al, 2009). In a comparative evaluation, acitretin was found to reduce the NAPSI score after 12, 24 and 48 weeks by 19%, 41%, and 52%, respectively during the treatment of moderate to severe skin psoriasis (Sánchez-Regaña et al, 2011). Acitretin is a first-line drug in pustular psoriasis, reduces subungual hyperkeratosis and improves symptoms in severe nail psoriasis (Duhard-Brohan, 1999, Piraccini et al, 2001, Tosti et al, 2009). Apart from the many potential side effects of retinoids, they may be onychodestructive in high doses as is high-dose vitamin A (Baran 1986).

9.4.3 Nimesulide

Nimesulide is a non-steroidal anti-inflammatory agent. After first positive experience (Piraccini e al 1994) it was given to 13 patients with pustular nail psoriasis of whom 4 responded well to twice daily 100 mg. All these 4 responders relapsed after withdrawal of the drug (Piraccini et al 2001). It was judged as not being superior to other drugs.

9.4.4 Biologics

An increasing number of "biologics" have been developed in the last decade. They counteract extremely potent immunological targets such as tumor necrosis factor-α (TNF-α), T cells, B cells, various cytokines, some immunoglobulins and key enzymes. A variety of them has been used in psoriasis, often with astonishing success (Lawry, 2007). Also nail psoriasis was the object of some studies. This chapter is, however, not suited to discuss all as this will be discussed in the psoriasis treatment chapters.

9.4.4.1 TNF- α inhibitors

TNF- α promotes cytokine secretion, such as interleukin (IL)-1, IL-6, IL-8, by macrophages and other inflammatory cells, activates T cells and induces adhesion molecule expression by vascular endothelial cells which in turn promote angiogenesis and keratinocyte proliferation, both key events in the pathogenesis of psoriasis (Smolen and Emery, 2011).

	Infliximab Remicade®	**Adalimumab** Humira®	**Etanercept** Enbrel®
Structure	Chimaeric antibody	Human monoclonal antibody	Human fusion protein
Application	Intravenous infusion	Subcutaneous	Subcutaneous
Dosage	5 mg/kg at weeks 0, 2, 6, then every 8 weeks	Loading dose: week 0 2x40 mg, week 1 40 mg, then 40 mg every 2 weeks	50 mg/week, or 2x50mg/week for 12 weeks
Indications	Psoriasis, psoriatic arthritis	Psoriasis, psoriatic arthritis	Psoriasis, psoriatic arthritis

Table 5. Application, dosage and indications of the commonly used TNF-α antagonists

Infliximab (Remicade®) is an inhibitor of TNF-α, which is a proinflammatory cytokine in psoriasis, psoriatic arthritis, ankylosing spondylitis, Reiter's disease and several more chronic inflammatory diseases. Given as an intravenous infusion of 5 mg/kg at weeks 0, 2, 6, and then every 8 weeks, infliximab, a chimeric monoclonal antibody, is effective in psoriasis, psoriatic nail lesions (Reich et al, 2005), psoriatic arthritis and Reiter's disease including its nail changes (Gaylis, 2003). Many reports have described the dramatic infliximab-induced improvement of both psoriatic skin and nail lesions (Antoni et al, 2005a, 2005b, Rich et al, 2008, Hussain et al, 2008, Reich, 2009). Another study showed a reduction of the mean NAPSI of 55.8 at baseline to 29.8 at week 14 and 3.3 at 38 (Rigopoulos et al, 2008). In the evaluation mentioned above, NAPSI improvement after 12,

24 and 48 weeks was 50%, 81%, and 92%, respectively (Sánchez-Regaña et al 2011). There appears to be general agreement that infliximab is the most potent antipsoriatic biologic (Noiles and Vender, 2009).

Adalimumab (Humira®) is a human antibody. In an open study, significant NAPSI reductions were obtained for finger and toe nails both in patients with cutaneous psoriasis as well as with psoriatic arthritis (Rigopoulos et al, 2010). In a large cohort of 442 patients with psoriatic arthritis, the mean NAPSI was reduced by 44% (Van den Bosch et al, 2010). Nail psoriasis response may be rapid (Irla and Yawalkar, 2009) although some authors found skin lesions to respond less than articular inflammation (Otten et al, 2011). In a group of ankylosing spondylitis and psoriatic arthritis patients, the NAPSI score was demonstrated to be reduced by 6 points (Rudwaleit et al, 2010). Adalimumab-induced improvement in nail psoriasis correlated with a good response in palmar plantar psoriasis (Langley et al, 2011). In the Spanish study, NAPSI improvement after 12, 24 and 48 weeks was 37%, 73%, 84%, respectively. Adalimumab was also beneficial for nail psoriasis after etanercept treatment (Puig et al, 2010).

Etanercept, a fully human TNF-α receptor fusion protein, binds TNF-α with greater affinity than natural receptors. The bound TNF-α is biologically inactive and many of the proinflammatory pathways responsible for initiation, maintenance, and recurrence of skin lesions in psoriasis are inhibited (Weinberg, 2003). The starting dose is twice weekly 50 mg subcutaneously, which may be reduced to once weekly 50 mg or twice weekly 25 mg. In a comparison of systemic nail psoriasis treatments, NAPSI improvement after 12, 24 and 48 weeks was 24%, 68%, and 87%, respectively (Sánchez-Regaña et al, 2011). The commonest adverse effect is an irritation reaction at the injection site. Infections and reactivations may occur as in infliximab treatment though probably less commonly. It should not be combined with systemic corticosteroids (Sanchez et al, 2006, Scheinfeld, 2004). There are some otherwise rare skin diseases that have been observed during etanercept treatment, such as lupus erythematosus, vasculitis, eosinophilic cellulitis like inflammation and interstitial granulomatous dermatitis (Scheinfeld, 2004, Winfield et al, 2006, Deng et al, 2006).

Golimumab (Simponi®) is a new human monoclonal antibody against TNF-α binding with high affinity and specificity to soluble and transmembrane TNF-α. It was studied once in psoriasis and nail psoriasis and showed an improvement in the NAPSI score of 25% and 43% after 14 weeks and 33% and 54% after 24 weeks in a dose of 50mg or 100 mg subcutaneously, respectively, at weeks 0, 4, 8, 12, 16, and 20 (Kavanaugh et al, 2009).

Certulizumab (Cimzia®) has not been used in nail psoriasis (Gartlehner et al, 2009).

All TNF-α inhibitors were reported to have induced psoriasis or psoriasiform skin and nail lesions (Sfikakis et al, 2005, Wollina et al, 2010). The spectrum of conditions induced by TNF-α is very wide and it apparently does not depend on the specific disease treated nor on the anti-TNF-α agent used (Pine et al, 2010, Conrad et al, 2011; Lee et al 2011). In more than half of the cases, the TNF-α induced skin lesions were successfully suppressed despite continuation of the drug. It is speculated that as TNF-α blockade is one of the strongest inducers of interferon-α production an unabated IFN-α production by plasmocytoid dendritic cells might result in these paradoxical psoriasis flares under anti-TNF-α treatment (Conrad et al, 2011).

Serious adverse events of all TNF- α inhibitors include the development of viral, bacterial, mycobacterial, and fungal infections (Lowther et al, 2007), reactivation of tuberculosis, hepatitis B and C, allergic infusion reactions, malignancies, autoantibody formation with lupus erythematosus, pancytopenia and aplastic anaemia, neurological disorders and worsening of congestive heart failure (Smolen and Emery, 2011). Experience in pregnancy is lacking. Further, infliximab comes with an information what to look for before starting a treatment. Paradoxical sarcoidosis while on anti-TNF-α treatment was also reported (Pine et al, 2010)

9.4.4.2 T cell inhibitors

Alefacept (Amevive®) is a human recombinant fusion protein composed of LFA-3 with the Fc portion of human IgG. In psoriasis, the inflammatory response is amplified when LFA-3 molecule-containing antigen presenting cells bind to the CD2+ receptor of T cells, the result being T cell activation and the release of proinflammatory cytokines. Alefacept binds to the CD2+ receptor of T cells via its LFA-3, thus blocking this interaction with antigen-presenting cells. Furthermore, alefacept triggers apoptosis of memory T cells. Through these two mechanisms, alefacept decreases the number of pathogenic T cells in psoriasis (Weinberg, 2003, Lawry 2007).

Alefacet is usually given in a dose of 15 mg per week for a period of 12 weeks; intravenous administration is also possible. At baseline, the CD4+ T cells should be monitored and then every 2 weeks. A CD4+ count below 250/µl should prompt to withhold the treatment until it has recovered. As alefacept has proven to be very safe the 2-weekly CD4 cell count may be delayed. Side effects include pruritus, headache, fatigue, nausea, viral upper respiratory infections, and arthralgias. Malignancy and serious infections do not appear to occur more frequently with alefacept use (Scheinfeld, 2005).

There are few studies and reports on alefacept use in nail psoriasis (Körver et al, 2006, Parrish et al, 2006). In moderate nail psoriasis, 2 patients improved, 2 remained unchanged and one worsened (Körver et al, 2006).

Efalizumab (Raptiva®) is a humanized monoclonal antibody against the CD11 portion of the LFA-1 molecule on lymphocytes. LFA-1 usually binds to intercellular adhesion molecule and promotes lymphocyte migration. The binding of efalizumab to CD11a cells is reversible and does not deplete T cells, but it prevents them from migrating into the skin (Weinberg, 2003). It has shown efficacy in the treatment of cutaneous and nail psoriasis but the European Medicines Agency (EMA) recommended its suspension of the marketing authorization after the occurrence of cases of progressive multifocal leukoencephalopathy (19 February 2009 Doc. Ref. EMEA/CHMP/20857/2009).

Cytokine inhibitors

Ustekinumab (Stelara®) is a new human IgG1k monoclonal antibody to the p40 epitope common to both IL-12 and IL-23. It blocks the differentiation and expansion of T helper cells 1 and 17 (Leonardi et al, 2008). It is indicated in moderate-to-severe psoriasis resistant to other therapies or with contraindications or intolerance to other systemic treatments. Ustekinumab is given in a dose of 45 mg for individuals under 100 kg body weight. In a patient who had earlier etanercept and failed to respond later ustekinumab was given and a marked improvement of his nail signs was noted after 4 weeks. A complete cure was achieved 4 weeks later after the second injection (Rallis et al, 2010).

Tocilizumab (Actemra®) is an IL-6 receptor inhibitor. No reports on nail psoriasis treatment have been published hitherto.

T cell inhibitors

Abatacept (Orencia®) is a soluble chimeric protein consisting of the extracellular domain of human CD152 linked to the modified Fc portion of human IgG1. By binding to B7-1 (CD80) and B7-2 (CD86) molecules on antigen presenting cells, CTLA4Ig blocks the CD28-mediated costimulatory signal for T cell activation. Success with abatacept has been noted in psoriasis. Abatacept was administered to two patients with refractory psoriasis and psoriatic arthritis after the patients had failed all conventional treatment methods. Both patients experienced very brief improvement in disease (Altmeyer et al, 2011).

Rituximab, a B cell depleting chimeric antibody has no place in the treatment of nail psoriasis.

9.5 Combined treatments

In clinical routine, different treatments are often combined as one is either insufficient or too slow. The combination should always consist of drugs with different mechanisms of action. In contrast to skin psoriasis, there are almost no studies on the effect of combination therapy on nail psoriasis (Jiaravuthisan et al 2007). A single-blinded study on 54 patients with nail psoriasis examined the effects of cyclosporine monotherapy versus cyclosporine systemically plus calcipotiriol cream topically (Feliciani et al 2004). The cyclosporine dose was 3.5 to 4.5 mg/d, calcipotriol was applied twice daily. After 3 months, the combined treatment showed significant improvement of pitting, subungual hyperkeratosis and onycholysis in 79%, whereas the cyclosporine monotherapy group showed 48% marked improvement. Six months after treatment, the cyclosporine monotherapy group showed a relapse rate of 52.9% (9/17), whereas only 37% (10/27) of patients in the combined therapy group had any signs of recurrence.

10. Conclusion

Nail psoriasis is frequent in psoriatic subjects with about 50% of psoriasis patients presenting with nail changes at any time and a life-time prevalence of up to 90%. Nail psoriasis has a strong genetic background and a frequent association with psoriatic arthritis. The most frequent signs of nail matrix involvement are pitting, leukonychia, crumbling and red spots in the lunula, whereas salmon or oil spots, subungual hyperkeratosis, onycholysis and splinter haemorrages represent changes of nail bed involvement. Understanding the mechanism of psoriatic nail sign development requires some basic knowledge of the nail organ, its specific reaction patterns and of nail histopathology. Nail psoriasis has a serious impact on the quality of life interfering particularly with manual work but also being cosmetically embarrassing. Treatment of nail psoriasis is difficult as the matrix pathology is hidden by the proximal nail fold and the nail bed changes are protected against treatment by the overlying nail plate and nail bed hyperkeratosis. Progress has been made with the new biologic drugs, which are however, usually only administered for skin plus nail involvement.

11. References

[1] Agostini A, De Lapparent T, Collette E, Capelle M, Cravello L, Blanc B. In situ methotrexate injection for treatment of recurrent endometriotic cysts. Gynecol Reprod Biol 2007;130:129-131

[2] Aktan Ş, İlknur T, Akin Ç, Özkan Ş. Interobserver reliability of the Nail Psoriasis Severity Index. Clin Exp Dermatol 2006;32:141-144

[3] Armesto S, Esteve A, Coto-Segura P, Drake M, Galache C, Martínez-Borra J, Santos-Juanes J. Nail psoriasis in individuals with psoriasis vulgaris: A study of 661 patients. Actas Dermosifiliogr 2011 2011;102:365-372

[4] Augustin M, Reich K, Blome C, Schäfer I, Laass A, Radtke MA. Nail psoriasis in Germany: epidemiology and burden of disease. Br J Dermatol 2010;163:580-585

[5] Baker BS, Griffiths CE, Lambert S, Powles AV, Leonard JN, Valdimarsson H, Fry L. The effects of cyclosporine A on lymphocyte and dendritic cell sub-populations in psoriasis. Br J Dermatol 1987;116:503-510

[6] Baran R. Etretinate and the nails (study of 130 cases): possible mechanisms of some side-effects. Clin Exp Dermatol 1986;11:148-152

[7] Baran R, Dawber R.Twenty-nail dystrophy of childhood: a misnamed syndrome. Cutis 1987; 39:481–2.

[8] Baran R, Haneke E. The Nail in Differential Diagnosis. Informa Healthcare, Abingdon, Oxon 2007

[9] Bovenschen HJ, Erceg A, Vlijmen-Willems I, van de Kerkhof PC, Seyger MM. Pulsed dye laser versus treatment with calcipotriol/betamethasone dipropionate for localized refractory plaque psoriasis: effects on T-cell infiltration, epidermal proliferation and keratinization. J Dermatol Treat 2007; 18:32-39

[10] Cargill M, Schrodi SJ, Chang M, Garcia VE, Brandon R, Callis KP, Matsunami N, Ardlie KG, Civello D, Catanese JJ, Leong DU, Panko JM, McAllister LB, Hansen CB, Papenfuss J, Prescott SM, White TJ, Leppert MF, Krueger GG, Begovich AB. A large-scale genetic association study confirms IL12B and leads to the identification of IL23R as psoriasis-risk genes. Am J Hum Genet 2007; 80:273–290

[11] Cassell S, Kavanaugh A. Therapies for psoriatic nail disease. A systematic review. J Rheumatol 2006:33: 1452–1456

[12] Cassetty CT, Alexis AF, Shupack JL, Strober BE. Alefacept in the treatment of psoriatic nail disease: a small case series. J Am Acad Dermatol 2005; 52: 1101–1102

[13] Chan ES, Cronstein BN. Methotrexate – how does it really work? Nat Rev Rheumatol 2010;6:175-178

[14] Chiam LYT, de Jager MEA. Giam YC, de Jong EMGJ, van de Kerkhof PCM, Seyger MMB. Juvenile psoriasis in European and Asian children: similarities and differences. Br J Dermatol 2011; 164, 1101–1103

[15] Coelho JD, Diamantino F, Lestre S, Ferreira AM. Treatment of severe nail psoriasis with etanercept. Indian J Dermatol Venereol Leprol 2011;77:72-74

[16] Conrad C, Lapointe AK, Gilliet M. Paradoxic psoriasis induced by anti-TNF treatment – A report of 8 cases and evidence for a new pathogenic mechanism. 93rd Ann Meet Swiss Soc Dermatol Venereol, Geneva, 2011, FC 11, Dermatol Helv 2011;6:30

[17] Davidson SI, Wu X, Liu Y, Wei M, Danoy PA, Thomas G, Cai Q, Sun L, Duncan E, Wang N, Yu Q, Xu A, Fu Y, Brown MA, Xu H. Association of ERAP1, but not

IL23R, with ankylosing spondylitis in a Han Chinese population. Arthritis Rheum 2009; 60:3263-3268

[18] De Berker D. Management of psoriatic nail disease. Sem Cut Med Surg 2009;28:39-43

[19] de Berker DAR, Lawrence CM. A simplified protocol of steroid injection for psoriatic nail dystrophy. Br J Dermatol 1998;138:90-95

[20] De Jong EM, Seegers BA, Gulinck MK, Boezeman JB, van de Kerkhof PC.. Psoriasis of the nails associated with disability in a large number of patients: results of a recent interview with 1,728 patients. Dermatology 1996;193:300-303

[21] Deng A, Harvey V, Sina B, Strobel D, Badros A, Junkins-Hopkins JM, Samuels A, Oghilikhan M, Gaspari A. Interstitial granulomatous dermatitis associated with the use of tumor necrosis factor alpha inhibitors. Arch Dermatol 2006:142: 198-202

[22] Duhard-Brohan E. Psoriasis unguéal. Ann Dermatol Vénéréol 1999;126:445-449

[23] Elder JT, Bruce AT, Gudjonsson JE, Jonstohn A, Stuart PE, Tejasvi T, Voorhees JJ, Molecular Dissection of Psoriasis: Integrating Genetics and biology. Consistent spelling: Molecular dissection of psoriasis: Integrating genetics and biology. J Invest Dermatol 2010;130:1213-1226

[24] European Medicines Agency. European Medicines Agency recommends suspension of the marketing authorisation of Raptiva (efalizumab). http://de.wikipedia.org/wiki/Efalizumab assessed 10 July 2011

[25] Feldman SR, Krueger GG. Psoriasis assessment tools in clinical trials. Ann Rheum Dis 2005;64:ii65-68

[26] Feliciani C, Zampetti A, Forleo P, Cerritelli L, Amerio P, Proietto G, Tulli A, Amerio P. Nail psoriasis: combined therapy with systemic cyclosporine and topical calcipotriol. J Cutan Med Surg 2004;8:122-5.

[27] Fernández-Guarino M, Harto A, Sánchez-Ronco M, García-Morales I, Jaén P. Pulsed dye laser vs photodynamic therapy in the treatment of refractory nail psoriasis: a comparative pilot study. J Eur Acad Dermatol Venereol 2009;23:891-895

[28] Finlay AY, Khan GK. Dermatology Life Quality Index (DLQI) - a simple practical measure for routine clinical use. Clin Exp Dermatol 1994; 19: 210-216

[29] Finnerty EF. Successful treatment of psoriasis of the nails. Cutis 1979;23:43-44

[30] Frenz C, Fritsch H, Hoch J: Plastination histologic investigations on the inserting pars terminalis aponeurosis dorsalis of three-sectioned fingers (in German). Ann Anat 2000;182: 69-73

[31] Gartlehner G, Thieda P, Morgan LC, Thaler K, Hansen RA, Jonas B. Drug Class Review; Targeted Immune Modulators. Update 2 final report. http;//www.ohsu.edu/drugeffectiveness/reports/final.cfm, assessed 8 July 2011

[32] Gaylis N. Infliximab in the treatment of an HIV positive patient with Reiter's syndrome. J Rheumatol 2003;30:407-411

[33] Gregoriou S, Kalogeromitros D, Kosionis N, Gkouvi A, Rigopoulos D. Treatment options for nail psoriasis. Exp Rev Dermatol 2008; 3: 339-344

[34] Gudjonsson JE Karason A, Runarsdottir EH, Antonsdottir AA, Hauksson VB, Jónsson HH, Gulcher J, Stefansson K, Valdimarsson H. Distinct clinical differences between HLA-Cw*0602 positive and negative psoriasis patients - an analysis of 1019 HLA-C and HLA-B typed patients. J Invest Dermatol 2006:126: 740-745

[35] Gümüşel M, Ozdemir M, Mevlitoğlu I, Bodur S. Evaluation of the efficacy of methotrexate and cyclosporine therapies on psoriatic nails: a one-blind,

randomized study. J Eur Acad Dermatol Venereol. 2011;25:1080-1084 [Epub ahead of print]
[36] Gupta AK, Cooper EA. Psoriatic nail disease: quality of life and treatment. J Cutan Med Surg 2009;13 Suppl 2:S102-106
[37] Handfield-Jones SE, Boyle J, Harman RRM. Local PUVA treatment for nail psoriasis. Br J Dermatol 1987;116:280-281
[38] Haneke E. Surgical anatomy of the nail apparatus. Dermatol Clin 2006;24:291-296
[39] Hanno R, Mathes BM, Krull EA. Longitudinal nail biopsy in evaluation of acquired nail dystrophies. J Am Acad Dermatol 1986;14:803-809
[40] Heidenreich R, Röcken M, Ghoreschi K. Angiogenesis drives psoriasis pathogenesis Int J Exp Path 2009;232-248
[41] Hemmer W, Focke M, Wantke F, Götz M, Jarisch R. Allergic contact dermatitis to artificial fingernails prepared from UV light-cured acrylates. J Am Acad Dermatol 1996; 35: 377–380
[42] Higashi N. Melanocytes of nail matrix and nail pigmentation. Arch Dermatol 1968;97:570-574
[43] Horn RT Jr, Odom RB. Twenty nail dystrophy of alopecia areata. Arch Dermatol 1981; 116:573-574
[44] Hussain W, Coulson I, Owen C. Severe recalcitrant nail psoriasis responding dramatically to infliximab: report of two patients. Clin Exp Dermatol 2008;33:520-520
[45] Kang S, Li SY, Voorhees JJ. Pharmacology and molecular action of retinoids and vitamin D in skin. J Invest Dermatol Symposium Proc 1996;1:15-21
[46] Khan M, Schentag C, Gladman DD. Clinical and radiological changes during psoriatic arthritis disease progression. J Rheumatol 2003:30:1022–1026
[47] Kim JY, Jung HJ, Lee WJ, Kim DW, Yoon GS, Kim DS, Park MJ, Lee SJ. Is the distance enough to eradicate in situ or early invasive subungual melanoma by wide local excision from the point of view of matrix-to-bone distance for safe inferior surgical margin in Koreans. Dermatology 2011 Aug 16. [Epub ahead of print]
[48] Körver JE, van de Kerkhof PC, Pasch MC. Alefacept treatment of psoriatic nail disease: how severe should nail psoriasis be? J Am Acad Dermatol 2006; 54: 742–743
[49] Körver J, Langewouters A, van de Kerkhof P, Pasch M. Therapeutic effects of a 12-week course of alefacept on nail psoriasis. J Eur Acad Dermatol Venerol 2006:20:1252–1255
[50] Krüger N, Reuther T, Williams S, Kerscher M. Einfluss eines ureahaltigen Lackes auf die Nagelqualitat: Evaluation mittels klinischer Scores und biophysikalischer Parameter. Hautarzt 2006;57:1089-1094
[51] Kwang TY, Nee TS, Seng KTH. A therapeutic study of nail psoriasis using electron beams. Acta Dermatol Venereol 1995;75:90
[52] Jiaravuthisan MM, Sasseville D, Vender RB, Murphy F, Muhn CY. Psoriasis of the nail: Anatomy, pathology, clinical presentation, and a review of the literature on therapy. J Am Acad Dermatol 2007;57:1-27
[53] Johnson M, Comaish JS, Shuster S. Nail is produced by the normal nail bed: a controversy resolved. Br J Dermatol 1991;125:27-29
[54] Lamerson C, Stevens G, Sax K. Treatment of nail psoriasis with efalizumab: a preliminary study. Cutis 2008; 82: 217–220

[55] Langley R, Crowley J, Unnebrink K, Goldblum O. Improvement in nail psoriasis is associated with improved outcomes in hand and/or foot psoriasis in adalimumab-treated patients: subanalysis of REACH. J Am Acad Dermatol 2011;64 Supp 1:AB7
[56] Lavaroni G, Kokelj F, Pauluzzi P, Trevisan G. The nails in psoriatic arthritis. Acta Derm Venereol (Suppl) (Stockh) 1994; 186:113
[57] Lawry M. Biological therapy and nail psoriasis. Dermatol Ther 2007;20:60-67
[58] Lee DY. Severe 20-nail psoriasis successfully treated by low dose methotrexate. Dermatol Online J 2009;15:8
[59] Lee KJ, Kim WS, Lee JH, Yang JM, Lee ES, Mun GH, Jang KT, Lee DY. CD10, a marker for specialized mesenchymal cells (onychofibroblasts) in the nail unit. J Dermatol Sci 2006;42:65-67
[60] Lee DY, Lee KJ, Kim WS, Yang JM. Presence of specialized mesenchymal cells (onychofibroblasts) in the nail unit: implications for ingrown nail surgery. J Eur Acad Dermatol Venereol 2007;21:575-576
[61] Lee DY, Lee JH, Yang JM, Lee ES, Mun GH, Jang KT. Versican is localized to nail mesenchyme containing onychofibroblasts. J Eur Acad Dermatol Venereol 2009;23:1328-1329
[62] Lee DY, Yang JM, Mun GH. Onychofibroblasts induce hard keratin in skin keratinocytes in vitro. Br J Dermatol 2009;161:960-962
[63] Lee DY, Yang JM, Mun GH, Jang KT, Cho KH. Immunohistochemical study of specialized nail mesenchyme containing onychofibroblasts in transverse sections of the nail unit. Am J Dermatopathol 2011;33:266-270
[64] Lee YH, Pelivani N, Beltraminelli H, Hegyi I, Yawalkar N, Borradori L. Antimicrobial pustulosis-like rash in a patient with Crohn's disease under anti-TNF-alpha blocker. Dermatology 2011 DOI10.1159/000329428
[65] Leonardi CL, Kimball AB, Papp KA, Yeilding N, Guzzo C, Wang Y, Li S, Dooley LT, Gordon KB, PHOENIX 1 study investigators. Efficacy and safety of ustekinumab, a human interleukin-12/23 monoclonal antibody, in patients with psoriasis: 76-week results from a randomised, double-blind, placebo-controlled trial (PHOENIX 1). Lancet. 2008;371:1665-1674.
[66] Lewin K. The normal finger nail. Br J Dermatol 1965;77:421-430
[67] Lewis BL. Microscopic studies of fetal and mature nail and surrounding soft tissue. Arch Dermatol Syph 1954;70:732-734
[68] Lin YK. Indigo naturalis oil extract drops in the treatment of moderate to severe nail psoriasis: a small case series. Arch Dermatol 2011;147:627-629
[69] Lin YK, Leu YL, Yang SH, Chen HW, Wang CT, Pang JH. Antipsoriatic effects of indigo naturalis on the proliferation and differentiation of keratinocytes with indirubin as the active component. J Dermatol Sci 2009;54:168-174
[70] Lindelöf B. Psoriasis of the nails treated with Grenz rays: a double-blind bilateral trial. Acta Dermatol Venereol 1989;69:80-82
[71] Lovy M, Bluhm G, Morales A. The occurrence of pitting in Reiter's syndrome. J Am Acad Dermatol 1980; 2: 66–68
[72] Lowther AL, Somani AK, Camouse M, Florentino FT, Somach SC. Invasive Trichophyton rubrum infection occurring with infliximab and long-term prednisone treatment. J Cutan Med Surg 2007;11:84-88

[73] Maejima H, Taniguchi T, Watarai A, Katsuoka K. Evaluation of nail disease in psoriatic arthritis by using a modified nail psoriasis severity score index. Int J Dermatol. 2010;49:901-906
[74] Mahrle G, Schulze HJ, Färber L, Weidinger G, Steigleder GK. Low dose short term cyclosporin versus etretinate in psoriasis: improvement of skin, nail and joint involvement. J Am Acad Dermatol 1995;32:78-88
[75] Marx JL, Scher RK. Response of psoriatic nails to oral photochemotherapy. Arch Dermatol 1980;116:1023-1024
[76] McGonagle D, Tan AL, Benjamin M. The nail as a musculoskeletal appendage - implications for an improved understanding of the link between psoriasis and arthritis Dermatology 2009;218:97-102
[77] McGonagle D. Enthesitis: an autoinflammatory lesion linking nail and joint involvement in psoriatic disease. J Eur Acad Dermatol Venereol 2009;23 (Suppl 1):9-13
[78] McGonagle D, Ash Z, Dickie L, McDermott M, Aydin S Z. The early phase of psoriatic arthritis. Ann Rheum Dis. 2011 Mar;70 Suppl 1:i71-6
[79] McGonagle D, Palmou Fontana N, Tan AL, Benjamin M. Nailing down the genetic and immunological basis for psoriatic disease. Dermatology. 2010;221 Suppl 1:15-22
[80] Morgan AM, Baran R, Haneke E. Anatomy of the nail unit in relation to the distal digit. In Krull EA, Zook EG, Baran R, Haneke E. Nail Surgery. A Text and Atlas. Lippincott Williams & Wilkins, Philadelphia 2001:1-28
[81] Nanda A, Kaur S, Kaur I, Kumar B. Childhood psoriasis: an epidemiologic survey of 112 patients. Pediatr Dermatol 1990; 7:19–21
[82] Nanda A, Al-Fouzan AS, Al-Hasawi F. Alopecia areata in children: a clinical profile. Pediatr Dermatol 2002; 19:482–485
[83] Nast A, Boehncke W-H, Mrowietz U, Ockenfels H-M, Philipp S, Reich K, Rosenbach T, Sammain A, Schlaeger M, Sebastian M, Sterry W, Streit V, Augustin M, Erdmann R, Klaus J, Koza J, Müller S, Orzechowski H-D, Rosumeck S, SChmd-Ott G, Weberschock T, Rzany B. S3-Leitlinie zur Therapie der Psoriasis vulgaris. Update 2011. J Dtsch Ges Dermatol 2011;) Suppl 2:1-104
[84] Natarajan V, Nath AK, Thappa DM, Singh R, Verma SK. Coexistence of onychomycosis in psoriatic nails: a descriptive study. Indian J Dermatol Venereol Leprol 2010;76:723.
[85] Nishi G, Shibata Y, Tago K, Kubota M, Suzuki M. Nail regeneration in digits replanted after amputation through the distal phalanx. J Hand Surg Am 1996;21:229-233
[86] Nnoruka EN. Current epidemiology of atopic dermatitis in south-eastern Nigeria. Int J Dermatol 2004; 43: 739–744
[87] Noiles K, Vender R. Nail psoriasis and biologics. J Cutan Med Surg 2009;13:1-5
[88] Norton LA. Disease of the nails. In: Conn HF, editor. Current therapy. Philadelphia: WB Saunders; 1982: 664-668.
[89] Oram Y, Karincaoğlu Y, Koyuncu E, Kaharaman F. Pulsed dye laser in the treatment of nail psoriasis. Dermatol Surg 2010; 36:377-381
[90] Ortonne JP, Baran R, Corvest M, Schmitt C, Voisard JJ, Taieb C. Development and validation of nail psoriasis quality of life scale (NPQ10). J Eur Acad Dermatol Venereol 2010; 24: 22–27

[91] Otten MH, Prince FH, Ten Cate R, van Rossum MA, Twilt M, Hoppenreijs EP, Koopman-Keemink Y, Oranje AP, de Waard-van der Spek FB, Gorter SL, Armbrust W, Dolman KM, Wulffraat NM, van Suijlekom-Smit LW. Tumour necrosis factor (TNF)-blocking agents in juvenile psoriatic arthritis: are they effective? Ann Rheum Dis 2011;70:337-340

[92] Pajarre R, Kero M. Nail changes as the first manifestation of the HLA-B27 inheritance. A case report. Dermatologica 1977; 154: 350–354

[93] Parrish, CA, Sobera JO,Elewski BE. Modification of the nail psoriasis severity index. J Am Acad Dermatol 2004;53:745-746

[94] Parrish CA, Sobera JO, Robbins CM, Cantrell WC, Desmond RA, Elewski BE. Alefacept in the treatment of psoriatic nail disease: a proof of concept study. J Drugs Dermatol 2006:5:339-340

[95] Perrin C. The 2 clinical subbands of the distal nail unit and the nail isthmus. Anatomical explanation and new physiological observations in relation to the nail growth. Am J Dermatopathol 2008;30:216-221

[96] Perrin C, Michiels JF, Pisani A, Ortonne JP. Anatomic distribution of melanocytes in normal nail unit: an immunohistochemical investigation. Am J Dermatopathol 1997;19:462-467

[97] Perrin C, Langbein L, Schweizer J. Expression of hair keratins in the adult nail unit: an immunohistochemical analysis of the onychogenesis in the proximal nail fold, matrix and nail bed. Br J Dermatol. 2004;151(2):362-371

[98] Pink AE, Foni A, Smith CH, Barker JNWN. The development of sarcoidosis on antitumour necrosis factor therapy: a paradox. Br J of Dermatol 2010; 163,:641–666

[99] Piraccini BM, Fanti PA, Morelli R, Tosti A. Hallopeau's acrodermatitis continua of the nail apparatus: a clinical and pathological study of 20 patients. Acta Derm Venereol 1994;74:65-67

[100] Piraccini BM, Tosti A, Jorizzo M, Misciali C. Pustular psoriasis of the nails: treatment and long-term follow-up of 46 patients. Br J Dermatol 2001;144:1000-1005

[101] Puig L, Barco D, Vilarrasa E, Alomar A. Treatment of acrodermatitis continua of Hallopeau with TNF-blocking agents: case report and review. Dermatology 2010;220:154-158

[102] Rallis E, Kintzoglu S, Verros C. Ustekinumab for rapid treatment of nail psoriasis. Arch Dermatol 2010;146:1315-1316

[103] Reich K. Approach to managing patients with nail psoriasis. J Eur Acad Dermatol Venereol 2009;23 Suppl 1:15-21

[104] Reich K, Nestle FO, Papp K, Ortonne JP, Evans R, Guzzo C, Li S, Dooley LT, Griffiths CE, EXPRES study investigators. Infliximab induction and maintenance therapy for moderate-to-severe psoriasis: a phase III, multicentre, double-blind trial. Lancet 2005;366:1367-1374

[105] Rich P, Scher R. Nail psoriasis severity index: a useful tool for evaluation of nail psoriasis. J Am Acad Dermatol 2003;49:206-212

[106] Rigopoulos D, Ioannides D, Prastitis N, Katsambas A. Nail psoriasis: a combined treatment using calcipotriol cream and clobetasol propionate cream. Acta Derm Venereol 2002;82:140

[107] Rigopoulos D, Gregoriou S, Stratigos A, Larios G, Kortitis C, Papaioannou D, Antoniou C, Ioannides D. Evaluation of the efficacy and safety of infliximab on psoriatic

nails: an unblinded, nonrandomized, open-label study. Br J Dermatol 2008; 159: 453–456

[108] Rigopoulos D, Gregoriou S, Lazaridou E, Belyayeva E, Apalla Z, Makris M, Katsambas A, Ioannides D. Treatment of nail psoriasis with adalimumab: an open label unblinded study J Eur Acad Dermatol Venereol 2010;24:530-534

[109] Rudwaleit M, Van den Bosch F, Kron M, Kary S, Kupper H. Effectiveness and safety of adalimumab in patients with ankylosing spondylitis or psoriatic arthritis and history of anti-tumor necrosis factor therapy. Arthritis Res Ther 2010;12(3):R117

[110] Ruprecht M, French LE, Navarini AA, Swiss Dermatol Network Targeted Ther. Psoriasis patient population and biologic treatment outcome at one Swiss department of dermatology. 93rd Ann Meet Swiss Soc Dermatol Venereol, Geneva, 2011: P40. Dermatol Helv 2011;6:40

[111] Safa G, Darrieux l: Dramatic response of nail psoriasis to infliximab. Case Rep Med 2011:107928

[112] Samman PD. Trachyonychia (rough nails). Br J Dermatol 1979; 101: 701–705

[113] Sanchez CJL, Mahiques SL, Oliver MV. Safety of etanercept in psoriasis: a critical review. Drug Saf 2006:29: 675–685

[114] Sánchez-Regaña M, Martin Ezquerra G, Umbert Millet P, Llambí Mateos F. Treatment of nail psoriasis with 8% clobetasol lacquer: positive experience in 10 patients. J Eur Acad Dermatol Venereol 2005;19:573-577

[115] Sánchez-Regaña M, Sola-Ortigosa J, Alsina-Gibert M, Vidal-Fernández M, Umbert-Millet P. Nail psoriasis: a retrospective study on the effectiveness of systemic treatments (classical and biological therapy). J Eur Acad Dermatol Venereol 2011;25:579-586

[116] Sarıcaoglu H, Oz A, Turan H. Nail psoriasis successfully treated with intralesional methotrexate: case report. Dermatology 2011;222:5-7

[117] Scheinfeld N. The medical uses and side effects of etanercept with a focus on cutaneous disease. J Drugs Dermatol 2004:3: 653–659

[118] Scher RK. Psoriasis of the nail. Dermatol Clin 1985;3:387-394

[119] Scher RK, Daniel CR III. Nails: therapy, diagnosis, surgery. Philadelphia: WB Saunders Company; 2003

[120] Scher RK, Stiller M, Zhu YI. Tazarotene 0.1% gel in the treatment of fingernail psoriasis: a double-blind, randomized, vehicle-controlled study. Cutis 2001;68:355-358

[121] Schröder JM, Kosfeld U, Christophers E. Multifunctional inhibition by anthralin in nonstimulated and chemotactic factor stimulated human neutrophils. J Invest Dermatol 1985;85:30-34

[122] Sfikakis PP, Iliopoulos A, Elezoglou A, Kittas C, Stratigos A. Psoriasis induced by anti-tumor necrosis factor therapy: a paradoxical adverse reaction. Arthritis Rheum 2005;52:2513-2518

[123] Smolen JS, Emery P. Infliximab: 12 years of experience. Arthritis Res Ther 2011;13 Suppl 1:S2

[124] Stern DK, Creasey AA, Quijije J, Lebwohl MG. UV-A and UV-B penetration of normal human cadaveric fingernail plate. Arch Dermatol 2011;147:439-441

[125] Taibjee SM, Cheung ST, Laube S, Lanigan SW. Controlled study of excimer and pulsed dye lasers in the treatment of psoriasis. Br J Dermatol 2005; 153:960-966

[126] Takahashi MD, Chouela EN, Dorantes GL, Roselino AM, Santamaria J, Allevato MA, Cestari T, de Allaud ME, Stengel FM, Licu D. Efalizumab in the treatment of scalp, palmoplantar and nail psoriasis: Results of a 24-week Latin American study. Arch Drug Inf 2010;3:1-8

[127] Takeuchi S, Matsuzaki Y, Ikenaga S, Nishikawa Y, Kimura K, Nakano H, Sawamura D. Garlic-induced irritant contact dermatitis mimicking nail psoriasis. J Dermatol 2011;38:280-282

[128] Tan AL, Benjamin M, Toumi H, Grainger AJ, Tanner SF, Emery P et al. (2007) The relationship between the extensor tendon enthesis and the nail in distal interphalangeal joint disease in psoriatic arthritis - a highresolution MRI and histological study. Rheumatology (Oxford) 46:253

[129] Tan E, Tay YK, Goh CL, Chin Giam Y. The pattern and profile of alopecia areata in Singapore - a study of 219 Asians. Int J Dermatol 2002; 41: 748–51.

[130] Tham SN, Lim JJ, Tay SH, Chiew YF, Chua TN, Tan E, Tan T. Clinical observations on nail changes in psoriasis. Ann Acad Med Singapore 1988;17:482-485

[131] Tosti A, Cameli N, Piraccini BM, Fanti PA, Ortonne JP. Characterization of nail matrix melanocytes with anti-PEP1, anti-PEP8, TMH-1, and HMB-45 antibodies. J Am Acad Dermatol. 1994;31:193-196

[132] Tosti A, Ricotti C, Romanelli P, Cameli N, Piraccini BM. Evaluation of the efficacy of acitretin therapy for nail psoriasis. Arch Dermatol 2009;145:269-271

[133] Treewittayapoom C, Singvahanont P, Prabudhanitsarn K, Haneke E. The effect of different pulse duration in the treatment of nail psoriasis with 595-nm pulsed dye laser: A randomized, double-blind, intra-patient left-to-right study. J Am Acad Dermatol, accepted

[134] Van den Bosch F, Manger B, Goupille P, McHugh N, Rødevand E, Holck P, van Vollenhoven RF, Leirisalo-Repo M, Fitzgerald O, Kron M, Frank M, Kary S, Kupper H. Effectiveness of adalimumab in treating patients with active psoriatic arthritis and predictors of good clinical responses for arthritis, skin and nail lesions. Ann Rheum Dis 2010;69:394-399

[135] Weinberg JM. An overview of infliximab, etanercept, efalizumab, and alefacept as biological therapy for psoriasis. Clin Therapeutics 2003:25: 2487–2505

[136] Williamson L, Dalbeth N, Dockerty JL, Gee BC, Weatherall R, Wordsworth BP. Extended report: nail disease in psoriatic arthritis-clinically important, potentially treatable and often overlooked. Rheumatology 2004:43:790–794

[137] Winfield H, Lain E, Horn T, Hoskyn J. Eosinophilic cellulitis like reaction to subcutaneous etanercept injection. Arch Dermatol 2006:142: 218–220

[138] Wittkowski KM, Leonardi C, Gottlieb A, Menter A, Krueger GG, Tebbey PW, Belasco J, Soltani-Arabshahi R, Gray J, Horn L, Krueger JG; for the International Psoriasis Council. Clinical symptoms of skin, nails and joints manifest independently in patients with concomitant psoriasis and psoriatic arthritis. PLoS ONE 2011;6(6):e20279

[139] Wolf R, Tur E, Brenner S. Corticosteroid-induced 'disappearing digit'. J Am Acad Dermatol 1990;23:755-756

[140] Wollina U, Hansel G, Koch A, Schönlebe J, Köstler E, Haroske G. Tumor necrosis factor-a inhibitor-induced psoriasis or psoriasiform exanthemata. First 120 cases

from the literature including a series of 6 new cases. Am J Clin Dermatol 2008;9:1-14
[141] Yamamoto T, Katayama I, Nishioka K. Topical anthralin therapy for refractory nail psoriasis. J Dermatol 1998;25:231-233
[142] Yu RCH, King CM. A double-blind study of superficial radiotherapy in psoriatic nail dystrophy. Acta Derm Venereol (Stockh) 1992;72:124-136
[143] Zaias N. The embryology of the human nail. Arch Dermatol 1963;87:37-53.
[144] Zaias N. Psoriasis of the nail: a clinical-pathologic study. Arch Dermatol 1969;99:567-579
[145] Zaias N. The Nail in Health and Disease, 2nd ed. Norwalk: Appleton & Lange; 1990
[146] Zaias N, Alvarez J. The formation of theprimate nail plate. An autoradiographic study in the squirrel monkey. J Invest Dermatol 1968, 51:120-136
[147] Zook EG, Van Beek AL, Russell RC, Beatty ME. Anatomy and physiology of the perionychium: a review of the literature and anatomic study. J Hand Surg 1980;5:528-536

10

Psoriasis and Stress – Psoriasis Aspect of Psychoneuroendocrinology

F.Z. Zangeneh, A. Fazeli and F.S. Shooshtary
Vali-e-Asr, Reproductive Health Research Center, Tehran University of Medical Sciences, Tehran, Iran

1. Introduction

Nowadays stress is a normal part of everyday living and the physiological and behavioral consequences of exposure to stressful situations have been extensively studied for decades. The neuroendocrine stress response is a necessary mechanism but disrupts homeostatic process and it is subserved by a complex system located in both the central nervous system (CNS) and the periphery. Stressor-induced activation of the hypothalamus-pituitary-adrenal (HPA) axis and the sympathetic nervous system (SNS) results in a series of neural and endocrine adaptations known as the "stress response" or "stress cascade." The stress cascade is responsible for allowing the body to make the necessary physiological and metabolic changes required to cope with the demands of a homeostatic challenge. In recent years, evidence has suggested that stress responses are not only under control of the CNS but are influenced by peripheral tissue, outside of the classical HPA axis. Corticotrophin-releasing hormone (CRH) is a central component of the HPA axis and is an important coordinator of the systemic stress response with subsequent modulation of the inflammatory response. In peripheral sites, cutaneous CRH and CRH-receptor1 (CRH-R1) is believed to regulate various functions of the skin that are important for local homeostasis. Common inflammatory skin disorders such as atopic dermatitis and psoriasis exhibit decreased barrier function and recent studies suggest that the complex response of epidermal cells to barrier disruption may aggravate, maintain, or even initiate such conditions.

2. Overview of the stress system

2.1 Historical context

The concept of stress is as old as medical history itself, dating back at least to the time of Hippocrates who referred both to the suffering associated with disease (pathos) and to the toil (ponos) – the fight of the body to restore itself to normalcy (Hippocrates, 1923) . In more recent history, both Walter Cannon (Cannon, 1939) and Claude Bernard (Bernard, 1949) described the ability of all organisms to maintain a constancy of their internal milieu or homeostasis. 70 years ago Hans Selye, the pioneer of contemporary stress research, first described the General Adaptation Syndrome (GAS) as a chronological development of the response to stressors when their action is prolonged (Selye, 1936). Therefore as pointed out for the first time by Hans Selye in Nature in 1936, stress or 'noxious agents' initiate a reaction in the body, which he called the 'general adaptation syndrome' (GAS). Selye distinguished three stages that the body passes when responding to stress in the GAS: 1) the first stage is an 'alarm reaction', in which the body prepares itself for 'fight or flight'; 2) the second stage of adaptation (provided the organism survives the first stage), is one in which a resistance to the stress is built; and 3) finally, if the duration of the stress is sufficiently long, the body enters a stage of exhaustion, a sort of aging, due to 'wear and tear'.

2.2 Stress system & homeostasis

Life exists by maintaining a complex dynamic equilibrium or *homeostasis* that is constantly challenged by intrinsic or extrinsic adverse forces, the *stressors* (Chrousos et al., 1992). Stress has been defined in many ways. To the physicist, the term refers to a force, strain or pressure applied to a system. However, when the stress response is excessive or in appropriate, it disrupts physiological homeostasis and body function and contributes to disease production (Burchfield, 1979). Although the stress response of the body is meant to maintain stability or *homeostasis,* long-term activation of the stress system can have a hazardous or even lethal effect on the body. For example it increases the risk of obesity, heart disease, depression, and a variety of other illnesses (Selye, 1998). According to Hans Sely, mental, psychologic or sociologic and metabolic stressors (Kvetnansky et al., 2009) tall the stable internal environment of the body, that may contribute directly to the production of disease or it can contribute to the development of certain behaviors that increases the risk of disease. The process that counteracts this disruption and maintains homeostasis is termed allostasis. Allostasis activates a wide range of both general and specific physiological systems and behavioral coping mechanisms. The amount of work carried out during allostasis is termed the allostatic load and represents the cost(s) to the animal of responding to the stimulus. Over the past decade, these terms have been introduced to human stress research to differentiate between adaptation, allostasis and the end result, homeostasis, with the aim of producing a measurement of allostatic load that can be used to compare the effects of a wide range of stimuli. Beyond the "flight-or-fight" response to acute stress, there are events in daily life that produce a type of chronic stress and lead over time to wear and tear on the body ("allostatic load"). Yet, hormones associated with stress protect the body in the short-run and promote adaptation ("allostasis").

2.3 Stress system: Response & adaptation

2.3.1 Transient adaptation: Allostasis

Physiologic systems operate within a dynamic range of steady states and maintain internal balance, or homeostasis, in terms of blood pH and electrolyte concentration. When physical or psychologic stressors challenge the body, there is activation of sympathoadrenal and adrenocortical responses that promote adaptation and survival in the short term. This has been referred to as **allostasis**. For example, during exercise or emotional responses, there is transient activation of the hypothalamic-pituitary-adrenocortical (HPA) and sympathoadernomedulary (SAM) systems, resulting in the elevation of blood pressure, heart rate, and circulating catecholamines and glucocorticoids. The patterns of autonomic, neuroendocrine, and behavioral responses vary with the type of stress, the different perceptions of stress by the subject, the extent of control on the stressful stimulus, and the active or passive coping mechanisms in response stress (Benarroch 2006). Stressor-induced activation of the HPA axis and the SAM results in a series of neural and endocrine adaptations known as the "stress response" or "stress cascade." The stress cascade is responsible for allowing the body to make the necessary physiological and metabolic changes required to cope with the demands of a homeostatic challenge (Miller et al., 2002). The strongest stressors produce specific and nonspecific responses. The specific stress responses alter an individual to the presence of the stressors, which involve neuroendocrine responses such as increased autonomic nervous system activity (Tsigos et al., 2005) (Gold et al., 1998). When faced with excessive stress, whether physical or emotional, a subject's adaptive responses attain a relatively stereotypic nonspecific nature, referred to by Selye as "the general adaptation syndrome." We now know that the adaptive responses have some specificity toward the stressor that generates them, which, however, is progressively lost as the severity of the stressor increases. The adaptive response of an individual to stress is determined by a multiplicity of genetic, environmental and developmental factors (Chrousos et al., 1992) and prenatal life, infancy, childhood and adolescence are critical periods characterized by increased vulnerability to stressors (Charmandari et al., 2005).

2.3.2 Regulation of the stress response

The orchestrated interplay of several neurotransmitter systems in the brain underlies the characteristic phenomenology of behavioral, endocrine, autonomic and immune responses to stress (Chrousos, 1998). Stress mediators such as adrenocorticotropic hormone, adrenaline and noradrenaline are subsequently released in specific patterns, reflecting the degree of HPA, adrenomedullary, and sympathetic nervous system activation (Goldstein et al., 2008). All stress responses are centrally integrated in the paraventricular nucleus (PVN) of the hypothalamus (Herman et al., 1997 and 2008) and the adrenal glands are their major peripheral effectors (Goldstein et al., 2008). Hypophysiotropic CRH neurons of the PVN are well known to serve as the origin of the final common pathway of glucocorticoid secretion. The powerful and far reaching action of these steroids (including effects upon metabolic, inflammatory, immune functions and on mood and behavior) has led to intensive investigation into regulatory mechanisms controlling glucocorticoid secretion (Cullinan et al., 2000). This hypothalamic neurohormone (CRH) plays a central role in the regulation of the HPA-axis, i.e., the final common pathway in the stress response. The activation of CRH neurons, increasing both adrenocorticotropic hormone (ACTH) biosynthesis and the best marker in ACTH which reaches a maximum in the first hour, which cortisol is highest during the second hour of stress (Dobson et al., 2000). ACTH may play a crucial, perhaps direct, role in the regulation of catecholamine biosynthetic enzymes in sympathetic nervous system, especially during stress. CRH-R1 is the most abundant subtype found in the anterior pituitary and is also widely distributed in the brain (Wong et al., 1994). Other possible factors that may regulate CRH1 receptor mRNA expression in the PVN of rats are catecholamine and glucocorticoids. Regarding catecholaminergic regulation, studies show that brainstem hemi section, which damaged the ascending noradrenergic bundle at least, attenuated the immobilization stress-induced increase in CRH1 receptor mRNA ipsilaterally in the PVN. This previous finding may reflect up-regulation of CRH1 receptor mRNA in the PVN by noradrenergic input from brainstem nuclei, such as the locus coerulus (LC), during stress (Fig.1)(Makino et al., 2002).

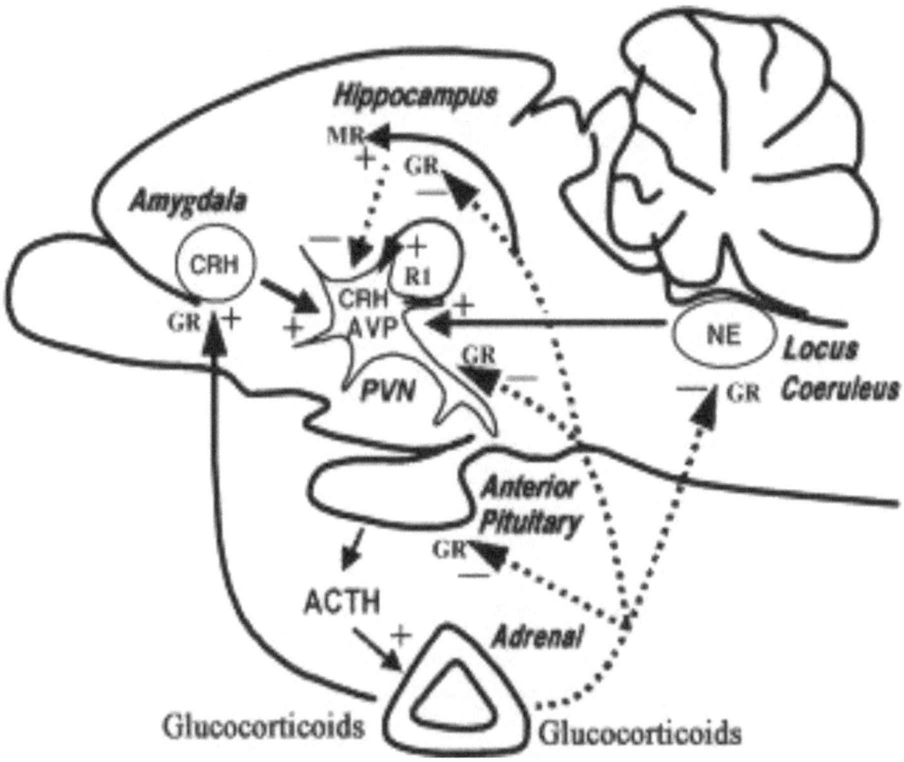

Fig. 1. Multiple feedback loops activating CRH systems during chronic stress. Stress initially activates the hypothalamic CRH system (i.e., CRH in the PVN), resulting in the hyper secretion of glucocorticoids from the adrenal gland. In addition, the psychological component of the stressor stimulates the amygdaloid CRH system (i.e., CRH in the central nucleus of the amygdala). Glucocorticoids exert GR-mediated negative feedback effects on the biosynthesis and release of CRH in the PVN and ACTH in the anterior pituitary (AP) directly or indirectly through the brainstem catecholaminergic nuclei such as the LC, resulting in the termination of stress-induced HPA axis activation. In the chronic phase of stress, down-regulation of GR in the PVN and other brain structures such as the LC fails to restrain hyper function of the HPA axis. Increased CRH in the PVN also induces a putative ultra short positive feedback effects on its own biosynthesis through up-regulation of PVN CRHr-1. The persistent activation of the HPA axis further up-regulates the amygdaloid CRH system involved in the expression of fear and anxiety, and the amygdala may have stimulatory effects on the HPA axis. Thus, the hypothalamic and the amygdaloid CRH systems cooperatively constitute stress-responsive, anxiety-producing neurocircuitry during chronic stress (Makino et al., 2002).

3. Overview of the HPA axis

3.1 Historical context of HPAC

In 1936, Hans Selye reported a historic series of studies on severe stress in rats. Exposure to bacterial infection, toxic chemicals, and other life threatening insults consistently caused adrenal gland enlargement with high levels of corticosterone secretion, atrophy of the immune organs, and gastric ulcers. All three components of this nonspecific stress response are caused by prolonged activation of corticosteroids in the hypothalamic-pituitary-adrenal axis (HPAC), resulting in secretion of stress levels of ACTH and glucocorticoids. In spite of these harmful effects, glucocorticoids in normal levels are necessary for sustaining life (Munck et al., 1984). Here we discuss the key elements of the HPA axis and the neuroendocrine response to systemic and local stress.

3.2 HPA axis-CRH (homeostatic balance)

CRH, synthesized in the PVN of the hypothalamus, represents the main driving force controlling HPA axis activation, the major hormone system responsible to maintain homeostatic balance in response to stressful stimuli (Tsigos et al., 1994).

3.2.1 HPA axis & CRH: Response to systemic stress

The HPA axis originates from the CRH neurons in the parvocellular subdivision of the PVN of hypothalamus, while the sympathetic nervous system is under the regulation of brainstem locus coeruleus (LC), clustered with noradrenaline neurons. Morphological and immunocytochemical studies have demonstrated that reciprocal projections exist between PVN-CRH neurons and LC-NE neurons, forming a CRH-NE-CRH loop, which plays an important role in the stressful responses (Maier, 2003) (Pacak et al., 1998) (Pacak et al., 1995). Central CRH, via glucocorticoids and catecholamines, inhibits the inflammatory reaction, while directly secreted by peripheral nerves CRH stimulates local inflammation (immune CRH) (Tsigos et al., 2002). The gene for CRH is expressed, not only in the brain, but also in extracranial tissues, (Orth, 1992) (Owens et al., 1991) including normal mammalian skin (Slominski et al., 1995) (aSlominski et al., 1993) (bSlominski et al., 1993) (Ermak et al., 1997) (Slominski et al., 1998). It has been proposed that an equivalent to the hypothalamic-pituitary-adrenal axis functions in mammalian skin, in response to local stress (aSlominski et al., 1996).

3.2.2 HPA axis & CRH: Response to local stress

It has been known for several years that the CRH/ POMC skin system fulfils analogous (pro-opiomelanocortin) functions to the HPA stress axis. CRH is the central trigger of HPA axis, and together with related peptides urocortin I-III that are the most important elements of the body response to stress. These elements regulate behavioral, autonomic, endocrine, reproductive, cardiovascular, gastro-intestinal, metabolic and immune systemic functions (Aguilera et al., 2001) (Grammatopoulos et al., 2002). Other actions of CRH include local immunomodulatory (predominantly proinflammatory) effects (Karalis et al., 1991) (Slominski et al., 2003), differing from a central immunosuppressive activity (through the HPA axis) (Chrousos 1995). Moreover, expression of CRH and regulated activity of CRH receptor type 1 (CRH1) can also play an important role in regulation of local stress response in peripheral tissues including skin, gastrointestinal tract or reproductive system. In humans, expression of at least eight variants of CRH1 mRNA (α, β, c, d, e, f, g and h) was detected and alternative splicing was found to be regulated by diverse physiological and pathological factors including: growth conditions, onset of labor during pregnancy or exposure to ultraviolet irradiation (Michal et al., 2010). Of note, locally produced CRH can directly regulate steroid hormone production by adrenals and gonads. Furthermore, CRH in the immune cells can induce production and release of POMC derived ACTH and beta-endorphin peptides. In vertebrates these peptides interact with membrane-bound CRH-R1 and CRH-R2 (Grammatopoulos et al., 2002) (Hillhouse et al., 2002). Both receptor types belong to the group II subfamily of G protein-coupled receptors (GPCRs). In human skin, CRH-R1 is the major receptor, expressed in both epidermal, dermal and subcutis with CRH-R1α being the most prevalent isoform. The CRH-R2 gene was expressed solely in hair follicle keratinocytes and papilla fibroblasts, whereas CRH-R2 antigen was localized predominantly in hair follicles, sebaceous and eccrine glands, muscle and blood vessels (aSlominski et al., 2004). A hair follicle is a typical stress-responding mini organ with a peculiar immune system. The proximal epithelium of an anagen hair follicle is known to be an area of immune privilege within the hair follicle immune system, whose collapse may be crucial for the pathogenesis of alopecia areata (Christoph et al., 2000).

3.3 HPA axis–immune system interactions

It has been known for several decades that stress, whether inflammatory, traumatic or psychological, is associated with concurrent activation of the HPA axis. In the early 1990s, it also became apparent that cytokines and other humoral mediators of inflammation are potent activators of the central stress response, constituting the afferent limb of a feedback loop through which the immune/inflammatory system and the CNS communicate (Chrousos 1995). All three inflammatory cytokines, tumor necrosis factor-(TNF), interleukin-1β and interleukin-6 (IL-6) can cause stimulation of the HPA axis alone, or in synergy with each other (Chrousos, 1995) (Tsigos et al., 1997). There is evidence to suggest that IL-6, the main endocrine cytokine, plays the major role in the immune stimulation of the axis, especially in chronic inflammatory stress. Some of the activating effects of cytokines on the HPA axis may be exerted indirectly by stimulation of the central catecholaminergic pathways. Conversely, activation of the HPA axis has profound inhibitory effects on the inflammatory/immune response because virtually all the components of the immune response are inhibited by cortisol. Alterations of leukocyte traffic and function, decreases in production of cytokines and mediators of inflammation, and inhibition of the latter's effects on target tissues are among the main immunosuppressive effects of glucocorticoids (Chrousos, 1995) (Elenkov, 1999).

3.4 HPA: The field of psychoneuroimmunology

Studies on stress-associated immune dysregulation have interested scientists and clinicians in the field of psychoneuroimmunology (PNI). This field focuses on the interactions among the central nervous system (CNS), the endocrine system and the immune system, and the impact these interactions have on health. Modulation of the immune response by the CNS is mediated by a complex network of signals that function in bi-directional communication among the nervous, endocrine and immune systems. HPA and SAM axes are the two major pathways through which immune function can be altered. The efferent sympathetic/adrenomedullary system apparently participates in a major fashion in the interactions of the HPA axis and the immune/inflammatory reaction by being reciprocally connected with the CRH system, by receiving and transmitting humoral and nervous immune signals from the periphery, by densely innervating both primary and secondary lymphoid organs, and by reaching all sites of inflammation via the postganglionic sympathetic neurons. When activated during stress, the autonomic system exerts its own direct effects on immune organs, which can be immunosuppressive, or both immunopotentiating and antiinflammatory. CRH secreted by postganglionic sympathetic neurons at inflammatory sites has proinflammatory properties (immune *CRH*); one of its key actions is to degranulate mast cells (Elenkov, 1999).

4. Overview of skin

4.1 Skin (epidermal barrier homeostasis)

The epidermis and its array of appendages undergo ongoing renewal by a process called homeostasis. Stem cells in the epidermis have a crucial role in maintaining tissue homeostasis by providing new cells to replace those that are constantly lost during tissue turnover or following injury (Blanpain et al., 2009). A homeostatic process involved in the maintenance of an internal steady state within a defined tissue of an organism, including control of cellular proliferation and death(apoptosis) and control of metabolic function. Mammalian epidermis is a stratified epithelium that retains the ability to self renews under both homeostatic and injury conditions by maintaining a population of mitotically active cells in the hair follicles and innermost basal layer (Niemann et al., 2002) (Ito et al., 2005). The basic mechanisms and signalling pathways that orchestrate epithelial morphogenesis in the skin have been designed for protective effect of this organ. The stratum corneum is the outermost of the 5 layers of the epidermis and is largely responsible for the vital barrier function of the skin. The physical barrier localized primarily in the stratum corneum and consists of protein-enriched cells (corneocytes with cornified envelope and cytoskeletal elements, as well as corneodesmosomes) and lipid-enriched intercellular domains. The nucleated epidermis, with its tight, gap and adherens junctions, additional desmosomes and cytoskeletal elements, also contributes to the barrier. Lipids are synthesized in the keratinocytes during epidermal differentiation and are then extruded into the extracellular domains, where they form lipid-enriched extracellular layers (Jensen et al., 2009). Activation of HPA axis with release of stress neuropeptides is essential for biological homeostasis and responses to external and internal challenges (Lotti et al., 1999) (**b**Slominski et al., 1996).

4.2 Skin – Neuroendocrine organ

More than ten years ago a comprehensive model of the skin acting as neuroendocrine organ has been proposed (Milstone et al., 1988) (**a**Slominski et al., 2000). For example, the skin synthesizes vitamin D, which enters the circulation and, upon activation, exerts profound metabolic and endocrine effects (Kragballe et al., 1996). Although the concept is still evolving, it relies on the skin capacity to communicate with the central system and to regulate global homeostasis through local production and/or systemic release of classical hormones, neuropeptides, neurotransmitters and biological regulators (**b**Slominski et al., 2000).

4.3 Skin – Local stress (neuroendocrine activity)

Skin as a neuroendocrine organ, is a relatively new addition to the field of cutaneous biology; it combines concepts from immunology, endocrinology, and neurobiology to unravel the multidirectional communications between brain, the endocrine and immune systems, and peripheral organs (Blalock, 1989) (Pennisi, 1997) (Turnbull et al., 1999). In this regard, the skin has a unique role because of its location, size, and relative functional diversity. Moreover, cutaneous signals sent to neuroendocrine centers may play modulatory roles, although peripheral intraorgan or inter systemic communications are also necessary to maintain global and local homeostasis. Thus precise stress-response coordination is an additional cutaneous function that appears to be served by locally expressed neuroendocrine activities (**a**Slominski et al., 2000) (**b**Slominski et al., 2000) (Slominski et al., 2001).

4.4 Skin – Stress neuropeptides

CRH/CRH-R1 system: Is it a cutaneous HPA system?

Slominski and colleagues have extensively documented the nature of peripheral CRH, its receptors and their distribution in human and murine skin. They confirmed that skin stress-response system was coordinated by a local cutaneous HPA axis-like system. They demonstrated that CRH, its receptors, the related neuropeptide urocortin and pro-opiomelanocortin-derived peptides are expressed locally in normal skin, normal cycling hair follicle epithelium, benign and malignant melanocytic lesions and non-melanoma skin cancer (**b**Slominski et al., 2004). Corresponding functional receptors (CRH-R) in the same cells confirm paracrine or autocrine modes of action. In human skin, CRH-R1 mediates most phenotypic effects of CRH (Slominski et al., 2001) while the main adnexal location of CRH-R2 indicates a role for this receptor in hair cycling (Kauser et al., 2006). Then a localized circuit regulates the peripheral functions of cutaneous CRH/CRH-R1, and the aberrant expression of CRH/CRH-R1 in the skin disturbs the local homeostasis and leads to abnormal differentiation and proliferation in keratinocytes. Because of the aberrant terminal differentiation of keratinocytes, psoriatic plaques have scale on the surface, which breaks in the protective barrier (Bowcock et al., 2005). However, dysfunction of keratinocytes may decrease CRH/CRH-R1 expression because of disharmony in differentiation and proliferation of keratinocytes. Zhou et al., in 2009 found a significant detuning CRH/CRH-R1 system in psoriatic lesions, which suggests that an aberrant cutaneous HPA system might take part in the pathogenesis of psoriasis, especially the formation of plaque. Thus, they hypothesize that a cutaneous CRH/CRH-R1 system might be aberrant in lesions of psoriasis. The detuning of CRH/CRH-R1 regulation might contribute to the formation of plaque in psoriasis (zhou et al., 2009) (Slominski et al., 2005) (Fig. 2).

POMC is a prohormone that produces various bioactive peptides via a series of enzymatic steps in a tissue-specific manner, including ACTH, α-melanocyte stimulating hormone (α-MSH), and β-endorphin. POMC is expressed not only in the pituitary gland, but also in a variety of non-pituitary organs, including the skin (Millington 2006). The production of POMC peptides in keratinocytes and melanocytes was found to be under regulatory control (Schauer et al., 1994) being stimulated by UVB, selected cytokines, and by disease processes(Slominski et al., 1996**c**, 1998, 1993**a**, 1993**b**)(Chakraborty et al., 1996) (Winzen et al. 1996)(Wakamatsu et al., 1997).

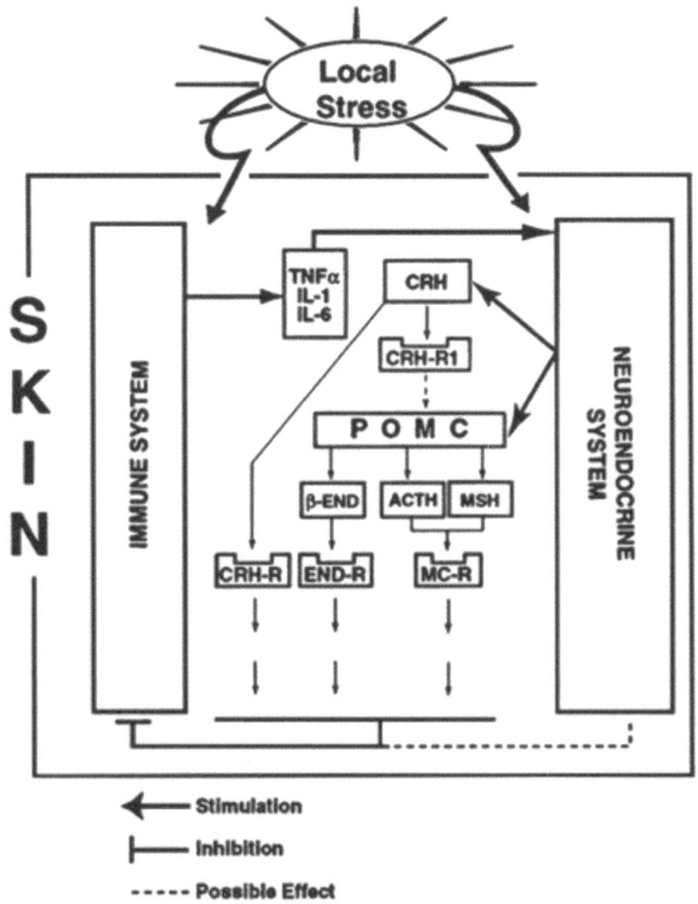

Fig. 2. The skin SNS are mediated via production of CRH and POMC peptides, and modulated by the local skin immune system (SIS). Signals originating in the latter and represented by proinflammatory cytokines perhaps stimulate production of CRH and POMC peptides. In turn, the signals generated by the interaction of CRH, ACTH, MSH, and β-endorphin, with their corresponding receptors, counteract the effect of local stress (Slominski et al., 2006).

4.5 Skin – The field of psychoneuroimmunology

Studies have shown that stress diminishes vaccine responses, exacerbates viral and bacterial pathogenesis, slows wound healing and alters autoimmune diseases (McCabe et al., 2000) (Padgett et al., 1998) (Teunis et al., 2002) (Dowdell et al., 1999). Because lymphocytes, monocytes or macrophages and granulocytes, exhibit receptors for many neuroendocrine products of the HPA and SAM axes, such as cortisol and catecholamines, which can cause changes in cellular trafficking, proliferation, cytokine secretion, antibody production and cytolytic activity .These studies have demonstrated that stress hormones inhibit the trafficking of neutrophils, macrophages, antigen-presenting cells, natural killer (NK) cells and T and B lymphocytes, suppress the production of proinflammatory cytokines and chemokines, downregulate the production of cytokines necessary for the generation of adaptive immune responses and impair effector functions of macrophages, NK cells and lymphocytes. For example, treatment of peripheral blood leukocytes (PBLs) with catecholamines *in vitro* results in the suppression of interleukin-12 (IL-12) synthesis and an increase in IL-10 production (Elenkove et al., 1996). Data from both human and animal studies show that the connections between the neuroendocrine system and immune system provide a finely tuned regulatory system required for health. However, the immune cells and cytokines influencing keratinocyte function play a major role in the development and pathogenesis of psoriasis.

5. Overview of psoriasis

5.1 Psoriasis – Genetic

It is generally accepted that the genetic background for psoriasis susceptibility is pivotal for the appearance of the symptoms. Intensive family studies since the early 1950s and linkage analysis studies pointed out several genetic loci that play a role in psoriasis (Bhalerao et al., 1998). In the last decade, a molecular biology approach emerged to identify abnormally expressed genes and proteins contributing to psoriasis (Jackson et al., 1999) (Chen et al., 2000). Two major genes under investigation are IL12B on chromosome 5q, which expresses interleukin-12B; and IL23R on chromosome 1p, which expresses the interleukin-23 receptor, and is involved in T cell differentiation. T cells are involved in the inflammatory process that leads to psoriasis. These genes are on the pathway that ends up upregulating tumor necrosis factor-α and nuclear factor κB, two genes that are involved in inflammation (Nestle et al., 2009). Genome-wide association studies have also identified several new genomic loci, and compelling evidence has shown an interaction between the HLA-C and ERAP 1 loci, implicating pathways that integrate epidermal barrier dysfunction with innate and adaptive immune dysregulation in psoriasis (Strange et al., 2010).

5.2 Psoriasis – Keratinocytes

Psoriasis is a chronic inflammatory disease characterized by epidermal keratinocytic hyper proliferation and abnormal differentiation (Abdou et al., 2008). The upper most layer of skin, the epidermis, consists primarily of keratinocytes (>90% of all epidermal cells) (Sun et al., 1979). The keratin intermediate filament network is responsible for the extremely high keratinocyte stiffness and resilience. This could manifest into the rugged protective nature of the human epidermis (Lulevich et al., 2010). Therefore, keratinocytes form an effective barrier to the entry of protein antigens, chemical irritants, and infectious agents in to the body (Fuchs 1995), all while resisting environment stress, external pressure, and sheer force. The trigger of the keratinocyte response is thought to be activation of the cellular immune system, with T cells, dendritic cells and various immune-related cytokines and chemokines implicated in pathogenesis (Lowes et al., 2007).

5.2.1 Keratinocytes – Dendritic & T cells

Researchers have identified many of the immune cells involved in psoriasis, and the chemical signals they send to each other to coordinate inflammation. The immune system consists of an innate immune system, and an adaptive immune system. In the innate system, immune cells have receptors that have evolved to target specific proteins and other antigens which are commonly found on pathogens. In the adaptive immune system, immune cells respond to proteins and other antigens that they may never have seen before, which are presented to them by other cells. The immune cells, such as dendritic cells (Dendritic cells are present in tissues in contact with the external environment, such as the skin: Once activated, they migrate to the lymph nodes where they interact with T cells and B cells to initiate and shape the adaptive immune response) and T cells, move from the dermis to the epidermis, secreting chemical signals, such as tumor necrosis factor-α, interleukin-1β, and interleukin-6, which cause inflammation, and interleukin18, 22 which causes keratinocytes to proliferate (Banchereau et al., 1998) (Nestle et al., 2009). Recent studies indicate that various cytokines play an essential role in the induction and maintenance of psoriatic lesion.

5.2.2 Keratinocytes – Cytokines

Various inflammatory cytokines and growth factors have been shown to be strongly induced in keratinocytes in psoriatic lesion. Although it is thought that the induction of cytokine production is the consequence of the activation of infiltrating immune cells rather than a triggering factor for the inflammatory process (Lowes et al., 2007). Three types of cytokines elaborated by keratinocytes are of particular interest in this context: growth factors for keratinocytes, endothelial cells and neutrophil-attracting chemokines. Several growth factors are able to induce keratinocyte proliferation and have been found to be highly expressed in lesional psoriatic epidermis. Transforming growth factor *a* (Elder et al., 1989) (Addison et al., 2010) and amphiregulin-epidermal growth factor (Cook et al., 1992) have been shown to induce epidermal proliferation and reproduce some aspects of the psoriatic phenotype when expressed in epidermal keratinocytes in transgenic animals (Cook et al., 1999) (Vassar et al., 1991). The epidermal growth factor (EGF) receptor ligand amphiregulin (AREG) has been implicated as an important autocrine growth factor in several epithelial malignancies and in psoriasis, a hyperproliferative skin disorder. In vitro, in vivo and clinical studies are well established the role of growth factors and neuropeptides in cutaneous innervation and there is substantial evidence that sensory neuropeptides contribute to the development of psoriasis (Saraceno et al., 2006).

5.2.3 Keratinocytes & peripheral CRH/CRH-R1

CRH is a central component of the local HPA axis, which has a functional equivalent in the skin. The ability of CRH to activate mast cells may explain its proinflammatory actions and the pathophysiology of certain skin conditions, which are precipitated or exacerbated by stress, such as atopic dermatitis, eczema, psoriasis, and urticaria (Theoharides et al., 1998). Mast cells are derived from stem cells in the bone marrow and migrate into tissues where they are prominently located just below the dermal–epidermal junction; they mature, depending on the tissue, under the influence of stem cell factor (SCF), interleukin 3 (IL-3), IL-4 and IL-9 (Wedemeyer et al., 2000). Mast cell infiltration and/or proliferation in the skin can be triggered by SCF released from fibroblasts and other immune cells, nerve growth factor (NGF) released from nerve endings, or RANTES (regulated on activation, normal T cells, expressed and secreted) (Conti et al., 1998) . Mast cells can also secrete SCF (de Paulis et al., 1999) and NGF (Xiang et al., 2000), thus affecting their own growth and activation (Gagari et al., 1997). The cytokines expressed by mast cells are primarily pro-inflammatory or are necessary for innate immunity [e.g. IL-1, IL-6, IL-8 and tumor necrosis factor α (TNF-α) (Wedemeyer et al., 2000). Human mast cells were recently shown to be particularly rich in both CRH and the structurally related peptide urocortin (Ucn) (Kempuraj et al., 2004) and express multiple CRH receptor isoforms which suggests autocrine actions of CRH(Cao et al., 2003).

5.2.4 Keratinocytes – CRH & Mast cells

Skin and hypothalamic mast cells appear to have important physiological functions as sensors of stressful events with bidirectional regulation of the HPA axis; a local increase of the levels of CRH or Ucn in extracranial tissues under stress could adversely affect different disease states (Theoharides et al., 1998). Hypothalamic mast cells are located close to nerve endings that contain CRH and can be activated by acute stress (Rozniecki et al., 1999). Acute stress can trigger mast cell degranulation (Singh et al., 1999) and increased the number of skin mast cells and also can worsened delayed hypersensitivity, effects blocked by pretreatment with a CRH receptor antagonist (Kaneko et al., 2003). Neuropeptides can also activate mast cells in a receptor-independent manner by activating G proteins directly. Regardless of the mechanism of activation, mast cell-derived vasoactive, pro-inflammatory and neurosensitizing molecules could act on keratinocytes, endothelial cells or nerve endings to liberate additional molecules and lead to chronic inflammation and neuropathic hypersensitivity or pain. The Kempuraj et al., findings indicate that mast cells are not only the target, but also a potential source of CRH and Ucn that could have both autocrine and paracrine functions, especially in allergic inflammatory disorders (Kempuraj et al., 2004), atopic dermatitis and psoriasis exacerbated by stress (Theoharides et al., 2004).

5.2.5 Keratinocytes – CRH & Stress

The study of Mitsuma et al., in 2001 showed that CRH induces the proliferation of keratinocytes via interaction with CRH receptors (Mitsuma et al, 2001) and it may indicate the possible correlation of the proliferation of keratinocytes and the degree of stress. Therefore, activation of the stress system, via the direct and indirect effects of CRH, might affect the susceptibility of an individual to certain autoimmune, allergic, infectious, inflammatory or neoplastic diseases (Arbiser et al, 1999). The biological effects of CRH have been shown to include the inhibition of keratinocyte proliferation and regulation of adhesion molecules and cytokines (cSlominski et al, 2000)(Pisarchik et al., 2001)(Quevedo et al, 2001)(Zbytek et al, 2002). Dysregulation of the HPA and SAM systems has been proposed as one possible underlying cause of stress-induced flares of psoriasis (Heller et al., 2011).

5.3 Psoriasis & stress

Generally, in normal individuals, stress elevates stress hormones (i.e., increases cortisol levels). However, according to available studies, exposure to stress in psoriatic patients has been associated with diminished HPA responses and upregulated sympathic adernomedullary (SAM) responses (Richards et al., 2005). Evers et al., found psoriasis patients had significantly lower cortisol levels at moments when daily stressors are at peak levels. The study also reported that psoriasis patients with overall high levels of daily stressors exhibited lower mean cortisol levels, as compared to psoriatics with overall low levels of daily stressors (Evers et al., 2010) (Zangeneh et al., 2008). These blunted HPA axis and elevated SAM system responses to stress may be crucial in better understanding the inflammatory characteristics of psoriasis, particularly in stress-responders. For instance, decreased secretion of cortisol and increased levels of epinephrine (Zangeneh et al., 2008) and norepinephrine may stimulate the release of mast cells, affect skin barrier function, and upregulate proinflammatory cytokines, which could thereby maintain or exacerbate psoriasis severity (Evers et al., 2010). Some authors have commented that this decreased cortisol response may be similar to how psoriasis flares with steroid withdrawal, as evidenced by the well known phenomena of steroid-induced psoriasis rebound (Richards et al., 2005).

5.3.1 Psoriasis & steroidogenic capabilities of keratinocytes

Glucocorticoids are essential for maintaining barrier competency, as exemplified in $GR^{-/-}$ mouse, where loss of GR function led to incomplete epidermal stratification, hyperproliferation and abnormal differentiation (Bayo et al., 2008). In addition, the cortisol analogue dexamethasone has been shown to acutely influence expression of genes regulating cell proliferation, differentiation, apoptosis and inflammation in primary human keratinocytes (PHK) (Elias 2005) (Stojadinovic et al., 2007). Accordingly, cortisol (hydrocortisone) is regarded as the most potent therapy for many inflammatory skin conditions including psoriasis and atopic dermatitis. Keratinocytes contain an abundance of cholesterol, the precursor to all steroids, as they are capable of synthesizing cholesterol de novo (Menon et al., 1985). Additionally, the cholesterol transporter, steroidogenic acute regulatory (StAR) protein has been identified in human epidermis by immunofluorescence histochemistry (**b**Slominski, et al., 2004) (Tuckey 2005). Evers's study in 2010 is the first longitudinal study of patients with psoriasis to show a relationship between cortisol levels and daily stressors, these results suggest that patients who continuously experience higher levels of daily stressors are characterized by persistently lower cortisol levels and might thus be more vulnerable to the effects of stress on their disease (Everse et al., 2010). Hannen et al., in 2011 demonstrated that primary human Keratinocytes (PHK) express all the elements required for cortisol steroidogenesis and metabolite pregnenolone through each intermediate steroid to cortisol. They showed that normal epidermis and cultured PHK express each of the enzymes (CYP11A1, CYP17A1, 3βHSD1, CYP21 and CYP11B1) that are required for cortisol synthesis. Collectively these data show that PHK are capable of extra-adrenal cortisol synthesis, which could be a fundamental pathway in skin biology with implications in psoriasis and atopic dermatitis (Hannen et al., 2011).

5.3.2 Psoriasis & stress axis

HPA axis is a critical adaptive system that maximizes survival potential in the face of physical or psychological challenge. The principal end products of the HPA axis, glucocorticoid hormones, act on multiple organ systems, including the brain, to maintain homeostatic balance. The brain is a target of stress, and the hippocampus is the first brain region, besides the hypothalamus, to be recognized as a target of glucocorticoids (Zangeneh et al., 2009). There is increasing evidence that the experience of stressful events is associated with the course of chronic inflammatory skin diseases. Buske-Kirschbaum et al., reported attenuated responsiveness of the HPA axis and further, an increased reactivity of the SAM system to stress in patients suffering from atopic dermatitis (AD) (Buske-Kirschbaum et al.,

2006) and psoriasis (Buske-Kirschbaum et al., 2010). It has been indicated that the redistribution of leukocytes in response to acute stress is mediated by the SAM, since adrenalectomy or blockade of β-adrenergic receptors has been found to mitigate this effect (Dhabhar et al., 1995) (Engler et al., 2004). It is widely accepted that the SAM system represents a major immunoregulatory system that controls various aspects of immunity (Sanders et al., 2002).

5.3.3 Psoriasis & SAM system: Aspect of psychoneuroimmunology

It has been suggested that a dysfunctional sympathoadernomedulatory (SAM) system may increase the risk of an aberrant immune response, especially under stressful conditions when the system is activated. In fact, altered leukocyte distribution to acute stress, for example, increased numbers of NK cells, monocytes, $CD4^+$ and $CD8^+$ cells have been reported in psoriasis patients (Schmid-Ott et al., 2001). Under non-pathological conditions, this process may optimize immunoprotection in the case of wounding or infection. However, in the psoriatic patient, leukocyte trafficking to the (chronically inflamed) skin has been found to be a major step in the development of psoriatic eruption (Mehlis et al., 2003). Thus, the finding of a stress-induced increase of leukocyte trafficking with a potentially increased influx of leukocytes into the skin could be of clinical significance, and could at least partly explain the often observed stress-induced exacerbation of psoriatic lesions. However, there is growing evidence that T cell mediated autoimmune processes and action of proinflammatory cytokines cause hyperproliferation of keratinocytes and assume the psoriatic phenotype (Krueger et al., 2005). When exposed to psychosocial stress, psoriasis patients showed increased monocyte and (activated) T cell number when compared to healthy controls. Further, a shift towards a TH_1-derived cytokine profile could be identified. These findings suggest that in psoriasis patient's stress may change immune functions towards a pathological relevant immune profile which could explain the often observed aggravation of psoriatic plaques in psoriasis patients under stressful conditions. Just as in many dermatologic conditions, psoriasis appears to worsen with stress in a significant segment of patients. For example, more than half of patients with psoriasis retrospectively report having experienced stressful life events before an exacerbation of the disease (Gupta et al., 1989) (Fortune et al., 1998). Studies report that the proportion of psoriasis patients who are "stress responders" ranges from 37% to 78% (Picardi et al., 2001).

5.3.4 Psoriasis & "stress responders"

Does stress cause or exacerbate psoriasis?

The answer is both, because the stress response disrupts physiological homeostasis and body function and contributes to disease production (Burchfield, 1979). This disruption of physiological homeostasis in the skin barrier is the trigger and stressors may contribute directly to the production of psoriasis disease or it contributes to the development of stress behavior, which increases the risk of disease. Stress has been indicated as a trigger in many dermatologic conditions and with each of these conditions, one encounters both patients who experience a close chronologic association between stress and exacerbation of their skin disease, and patients for whom their emotional states seem to be unrelated to the natural course of their cutaneous disorder. These two groups are considered "stress responders" and "non-stress responders," respectively (Koo 1995). Psoriasis itself can serve as a stressor for patients. Psoriasis can be a disfiguring skin disease causing social stigma. Accordingly, patients often suffer significant interpersonal and psychological distress. Patients commonly experience difficulties in social interactions, especially in meeting new individuals and forming romantic relationships. In general, most patients demonstrate adverse psychological consequences, including poor self-esteem, anxiety, depression, and for some, even develop suicidal ideation (Russo et al 2004). As psoriasis can cause considerable stress for patients and increased levels of stress are likely to exacerbate psoriasis, the disease process, thus, becomes a self-perpetuating, vicious cycle (Kimball et al., 2005). Therefore, treatment considerations for psoriasis stress responders should integrate methods of psychotherapy and pharmacotherapy that can decrease stress.

6. References

Abdou AG, Hanout HM. Evaluation of survivin and NF-kappaB in psoriasis, an immunohistochemical study. J Cutan Pathol 2008; 35: 445–451.

Arbiser JL, Karalis K, Viswanathan A, Koike C, Anand-Apte B, Flynn E, Zetter B, Majzoub JA. Corticotropin-releasing hormone stimulates angiogenesis and epithelial tumor growth in the skin. J Invest Dermatol. 1999; 113: 838-42.

Aguilera G, Rabadan-Diehl C, Nikodemova M. Regulation of pituitary corticotropin releasing hormone receptors. Peptides. 2001; 22: 769–74.

Banchereau J, Steinman RM. Dendritic cells and the control of immunity. Nature 1998; 392: 245–52.

Bayo P, Sanchis A, Bravo A, Cascallana JL, Buder K, Tuckermann J, Schütz G, Pérez P. Glucocorticoid receptor is required for skin barrier competence. Endocrinology. 2008;149: 1377-88.

Benarroch EE. (2006). Basic Neurosciences with Clinical Applications. Mayo Foundation for Medical Education and research. United States of America, Chap: Central control of homeostasis and adaptation, pp:761and 769.

Bhalerao J, Bowcock AM. The genetics of psoriasis: A complex disorder of the skin and immune system. Hum Mol Genet. 1998; 7: 1537-1545.

Blalock JE. Molecular basis for bidirectional communication between the immune and the neuroendocrine systems. Physiol Rev. 1989; 69:1–32.

Blanpain C, Fuchs E. Epidermal homeostasis: a balancing act of stem cells in the skin. Nat Rev Mol Cell Biol. 2009; 10: 207–217.

Bernard C. (1927). An introduction to the study of experimental medicine.1949, (2nd Ed.). New York: H.C. Greene.

Bowcock AM, KruegerJG. Getting under the skin: the immunogenetics of psoriasis. Nature Rev. 2005; 5: 699–711.

Burchfield SR. The evolution of the stress response: A new perspective. Psychosom-Med. 1979; 41,661.

Buske-Kirschbaum A, Ebrecht M, Kern S, et al. Endocrine stress responses in TH1-mediated chronic inflammatory skin disease (psoriasis vulgaris)--do they parallel stress-induced endocrine changes in TH2-mediated inflammatory dermatoses (atopic dermatitis)? Psychoneuroendocrinology 2006; 3: 439-46.

Buske-Kirschbaum A, Kern S, Ebrecht M, Hellhammer DHAltered distribution of leukocyte subsets and cytokine production in response to acute psychosocial stress in patients with psoriasis vulgaris. Brain, Behavior, and Immunity 2007; 21: 92-99

Buske-Kirschbaum A, Ebrecht M, Hellhammer DH. Blunted HPA axis responsiveness to stress in atopic patients is associated with the acuity and severeness of allergic inflammation Brain, Behavior, and Immunity 2010; 24: 1347-1353.

Cannon W B. (1939). The Wisdom of the Body. New York: W.W. Nortyon and Co.

Cao J, Zhao P, Zhao LJ, Wu SM, Zhu SY, Qi ZT. Identification of functional corticotropin-releasing hormone (CRH) receptor isoforms in human leukemic mast cells (HMC-1), Mol. Biol. Cell 2003; 14: L212.

Chakraborty AK, Funasaka Y, Slominski A, Ermak G, Hwang J, Pawelek JM, Ichihashi M. Production an release of proopiomelanocortin (POMC)-derived peptides by human melanocytes and keratinocytes in culture: Regulation by UVB. Biochim. Biophys. Acta 1996; 1313: 130–138.

Charmandari E, Tsigos C, Chrousos G. Endocrinology of stress response. Annual Review of Physiology 2005; 67: 259-284.

Chen SH, Arany I, Apisarnthanarax N, Rajaraman S, Tyring SK, Horikoshi T, Brysk H, Brysk MM. Response of keratinocytes from normal and psoriatic epidermis to interferon-gamma differs in the expression of zinc-alpha (2)-glycoprotein and cathepsin D. Faseb J. 2000 ; 14: 565-71.

Christoph T, Müller-Röver S, Audring H, Tobin DJ, Hermes B, Cotsarelis G, Rückert R, Paus R.The human hair follicle immune system: cellular composition and immune privilege. Br J Dermatol. 2000; 142: 862-73.

Chrousos G.P., Gold P.W. The concepts of stress system disorders: overview of behavioral and physical homeostasis. JAMA, J Am Med Assoc. 1992; 267:1244–1252.

Chrousos GP. The hypothalamic– pituitary– adrenal axis and immune mediated inflammation. N Engl J Med. 1995; 332: 1351– 63.

Chrousos G P. Stressors, stress, and neuroendocrine integration of the adaptive response. The 1997 Hans Selye Memorial Lecture. Ann NY Acad Sc. 1998; 851: 311–335.

Conti P, Reale M, Barbacane RC, Letourneau R, Theoharides TC. Intramuscular injection of hrRANTES causes mast cell recruitment and increased transcription of histidine decarboxylase in mice: lack of effects in genetically mast cell-deficient W/WV mice. ASEB J. 1998; 12: 1693-700.

Cook PW, Pittelkow MR, Keeble WW, Graves-Deal R, Coffey Jr RJ, Shipley GD. Amphiregulin messenger RNA is elevated in psoriatic epidermis and gastrointestinal carcinomas. Cancer Res. 1992; 52: 3224–3227.

Cook PW, Pittelkow MR, Piepkorn M. Overexpression of amphiregulin in the epidermis of transgenic mice induces a psoriasis-like cutaneous phenotype. J Invest Dermatol. 1999; 113: 860.

Cullinan WE, Wolfe TJ. Chronic stress regulates levels of mRNA transcripts encoding beta subunits of the GABA(A) receptor in the rat stress axis. Brain Res. 2000; 887: 118-24.

Dhabhar FS, Miller AH, McEwen BS, Spencer RL. Effects of stress on immune cell distribution. Dynamics and hormonal mechanisms. J Immunol. 1995 ;154(10) :5511-27.

de Paulis A, Minopoli G, Arbustini E, de Crescenzo G, Dal Piaz F, Pucci P, Russo T, Marone G. Stem cell factor is localized in, released from, and cleaved by human mast cells. J Immunol. 1999; 163:2799-808.

Devrimci-Ozguven H, Kundakci TN, Kumbasar H, et al. The depression, anxiety, life satisfaction and affective expression levels in psoriasis patients. J Eur Acad Dermatol Venereol 2000; 14: 267-71.

Dobson H, Smith RF. What is stress, and how does it affect reproduction. Anim Reprod Sci., 2000; 60-61: 743-52.

Dowdell KC, Gienapp IE, Stuckman S, Wardrop RM, Whitacre CC.Neuroendocrine modulation of chronic relapsing experimental autoimmune encephalomyelitis: a critical role for the hypothalamic-pituitary-adrenal axis. J Neuroimmunol. 1999; 100: 243-51.

Elder JT, Fisher GJ, Lindquist PB. Overexpression of transforming growth factor alpha in psoriatic epidermis. Science 1989; 243: 811–814.

Elenkov IJ, Papanicolaou DA, Wilder RL, Chrousos GP. Modulatory effects of glucocorticoids and catecholamines on human interleukin-12 and interleukin-10 production: clinical implications. Proc Assoc Am Physicians. 1996; 108: 374-81.

Elenkov IJ, Webster EL, Torpy DJ, Chrousos GP. Stress, corticotropin-releasing hormone, glucocorticoids, and the immune/inflammatory response: acute and chronic effects. Ann NY Acad Sci. 1999; 876; 1- 11 (discussion 11-3).

Elias PM. Stratum corneum defensive functions: an integrated view. J. Invest. Dermatol. 2005; 125: 183–200.

Engler H, Dawils L, Hoves S, Kurth S, Stevenson JR, Schauenstein K, Stefanski V. Effects of social stress on blood leukocyte distribution: the role of alpha- and beta-adrenergic mechanisms. J Neuroimmunol. 2004 ;156(1-2):153-62.

Ermak G, Slominski A. Production of POMC, CRH-R1, MC1, and MC2 receptor mRNA and expression of tyrosinase gene in relation to hair cycle and dexamethasone treatment in the C57BL/6 mouse skin. J Invest Dermatol. 1997; 108: 160-5.

Evers AW, Verhoeven EW, Kraaimaat FW, de Jong EM, de Brouwer SJ, Schalkwijk J, Sweep FC, van de Kerkhof PC. How stress gets under the skin: cortisol and stress reactivity in psoriasis. Br J Dermatol. 2010; 163: 986-91.

Fortune DG, Richards HL, Main CJ, Griffiths CE. What patients with psoriasis believe about their condition? J Am Acad Dermatol. 1998; 39:196–201.

Fuchs E. Keratins and the skin. Annu Rev Cell Dev Biol. 1995; 11: 123-53.

Gagari E, Tsai M, Lantz CS, Fox LG, Galli SJ. Differential release of mast cell interleukin-6 via c-kit. Blood 1997; 89: 2654-63.

Gold PW, Chrousos GP. The endocrinology of melancholic and atypical depression: relation to neurocircuitry and somatic consequences. Proc Assoc Am Physicians. 1998; 111: 22–34.

Goldstein DS, Kopin IJ. Adrenomedullary, adrenocortical, and sympathoneural responses to stressors: a meta-analysis. Endocr Regul. 2008; 42: 111-9.

Grammatopoulos DK, Chrousos GP. Functional characteristics of CRH receptors and potential clinical applications of CRH-receptor antagonists. Trends Endocrinol Metab. 2002;13:436–44.

Gupta MA, Gupta AK, Kirkby S, et al. A psychocutaneous profile of psoriasis patients who are stress reactors. A study of 127 patients. Gen Hosp Psychiatry 1989; 11:166-73.

Hannen RF, Michael AE, Jaulim A, Bhogal R, Burrin JM, Philpott MP. Steroid synthesis by primary human keratinocytes; implications for skin disease. Biochem Biophys Res Commun. 2011;404: 62-7.

Heller MM, Lee ES, Koo JY. Stress as an influencing factor in psoriasis. Skin Therapy Lett. 2011 ; 16: 1-4.

Herman JP, Cullinan WE. Neurocircuitry of stress: central control of the hypothalamo-pituitary-adrenocortical axis. Trends Neurosci. 1997; 20: 78-84.

Herman JP, Flak J, Jankord R. Chronic stress plasticity in the hypothalamic paraventricular nucleus. Prog Brain Res. 2008; 170: 353-64.

Hillhouse EW, Randeva H, Ladds G, Grammatopoulos D. Corticotropin-releasing hormone receptors. Biochem Soc Trans. 2002 Aug;30(4):428-32.

Hippocrates. On airs, waters, and places. (1923); (translated by WHS Jones, New York). New York: W. Heinmann.

Ito M., et al. Stem cells in the hair follicle bulge contribute to wound repair but not to homeostasis of the epidermis. Nat. Med. 2005; 11: 1351–1354.

Jackson M, Howie SE, Weller R, Sabin E, Hunter JA, McKenzie RC. Psoriatic keratinocytes show reduced IRF-1 and STAT-1alpha activation in response to gamma-IFN. Faseb J. 1999; 13: 495-502

Jensen JM, Proksch E. The skin's barrier. Ital G.Dermatol Venereol. 2009; 144: 689-700.

Kaneko K, Kawana S, Arai K, Shibasaki T. Corticotropin-releasing factor receptor type 1 is involved in the stress-induced exacerbation of chronic contact dermatitis in rats. Exp Dermatol. 2003; 12: 47–52.

Karalis K, Sano H, Redwine J, Listwak S, Wilder RL, Chrousos GP. Autocrine or paracrine inflammatory actions of corticotropin-releasing hormone in vivo. *Science.* 1991; 254: 421–3.

Kastelan M, Massari LP, Brajac I. Apoptosis mediated by cytolytic molecules might be responsible for maintenance of psoriatic plaques. Med Hypotheses. 2006; 67: 336-7.

Kastelan M, Prpić-Massari L, Brajac I. Apoptosis in psoriasis. Acta Dermatovenerol Croat. 2009; 17: 182-6.

Kauser S, Slominski A, Wei ET, Tobin DJ. Modulation of the human hair follicle pigmentary unit by corticotropin-releasing hormone and urocortin peptides. Faseb J. 2006; 20: 882-95.

Kempuraj D, Papadopoulou NG, Lytinas M, Huang M, Kandere-Grzybowska K, Madhappan B, Boucher W, Christodoulou S, Athanassiou A, Theoharides TC. Corticotropin-releasing hormone and its structurally related urocortin are synthesized and secreted by human mast cells. Endocrinology 2004; 145: 43–48.

Kimball AB, Jacobson C, Weiss S, Vreeland MG, Wu Y. The psychosocial burden of psoriasis. Am J Clin Dermatol. 2005; 6: 383-92.

Koo JY. Psychodermatology: a practical manual for clinicians. Cur Prob Dermatol. 1995; 6: 204-32.

Kragballe K, Fogh K, Larsen CG. Vitamin D: actions and applications in dermatology. J Invest Dermatol Symp Proc. 1996; 1:1–114.

Krueger GG, Langley RG, Finlay AY, Griffiths CE, Woolley JM, Lalla D, Jahreis A. Patient-reported outcomes of psoriasis improvement with etanercept therapy: results of a randomized phase III trial. Br J Dermatol. 2005 ; 153: 1192-9

Kvetnansky R, Sabban EL, Palkovits M. Catecholaminergic systems in stress: structural and molecular genetics approaches. Physiol Rev. 2009; 89: 535-606.

Lebwolhl M. Psoriasis. Lancet. 2003; 361:1197–1204.

Lotti T, Bianchi B, Panconesi E. Neuropeptides and skin disorders. The new frontiers of neuro-endocrine-cutaneous immunology. International J Dermatol. 1999; 38: 673–675.

Lowes MA, Bowcock AM, Krueger JG. Pathogenesis and therapy of psoriasis. Nature. 2007;445: 866-73.

Lulevich V, Yang HY, Isseroff RR, Liu GY.Single cell mechanics of keratinocyte cells. Ultramicroscopy. 2010: 110: 1435-42.

McCabe PM, Sheridan JF, Weiss JM, Kaplan JP, Natelson BH, Pare WP. Animal models of disease. Physiol Behav. 2000; 68: 501-7.

Maier S F. Bi-directional immune-brain communication: Implications for understanding stress, pain, and cognition. Brain Behav. Immun. 2003; 17: 69–85

Makino S, Hashimoto K, Gold P W. Multiple feedback mechanisms activating corticotropin-releasing hormone system in the brain during stress. Pharmacol Biochem Behav. 2002; 73: 147-58.

Mehlis SL, Gordon KB. The immunology of psoriasis and biologic immunotherapy. J Am Acad Dermatol. 2003 ;49(2 Suppl): S44-50

Menon GK, Feingold KR, Moser AH, Brown BE, Elias PM. De novo sterologenesis in the skin. II. Regulation by cutaneous barrier requirements. J. Lipid Res.1985; 26: 418–427.

Michal A. Zmijewski and Andrzej T. Slominski. Emerging role of alternative splicing of CRF1 receptor in CRF signaling. Acta Biochim Pol. 2010; 57(1): 1–13.

Miller DB, O'Callaghan JP. Neuroendocrine aspects of the response to stress. Metabolism 2002; 51(6 Suppl 1): 5-10.

Millington GW, Proopiomelanocortin (POMC): the cutaneous roles of its melanocortin products and receptors. Clin Exp Dermatol. 2006; 31: 407–412.

Milstone LM, Edelson RL. Endocrine, metabolic and immunologic functions of keratinocytes. Ann NY Acad Sci 1988; 548:1–366.

Mitsuma T, Matsumoto Y, Tomita Y. Corticotropin releasing hormone stimulates proliferation of keratinocytes. Life Sci. 2001; 69: 1991-8.

Munck A, Guyre PM, Holbrook NJ. Physiological functions of glucocorticoids in stress and their relation to pharmacological actions. Endocr Rev. 1984; 5: 25-44.

Naldi L, Gambini D. The clinical spectrum of psoriasis. Clin Dermatol. 2007;25:510–518.

Nestle FO, Kaplan DH, Barker J. Psoriasis. N. Engl. J. Med.2009; 361: 496–509.

Niemann C, Watt FM. Designer skin: lineage commitment in postnatal epidermis. Trends Cell Biol. 2002;12:185–192.

Orth, DN. Corticotropin-releasing hormone in humans. Endocrine Rev. 1992; 13: 164–191.

Owens, MJ, Nemeroff CB. Physiology and pharmacology of corticotropin releasing factor. Pharmacol. 1991; 43: 425–473.

Pacak K, Palkovits M, Kopin IJ, Goldstein DS. Stress-induced norepinephrine release in the hypothalamic paraventricular nucleus and pituitary-adrenocortical and sympathoadrenal activity: in vivo microdialysis studies. Front. Neuroendocrinol. 1995; 16: 89–150.

Pacak K, Palkovits M, Yadid G, Kvetnansky R, Kopin IJ, Goldstein DS. Heterogeneous neurochemical responses to different stressors: a test of Selye's doctrine of nonspecificity. Am. J. Physiol. 1998; 275: R1247–R1255.

Padgett DA, Marucha PT, Sheridan JF. Restraint stress slows cutaneous wound healing in mice. Brain Behav Immun. 1998 Mar;12(1):64-73.

Pennisi E. Tracing molecules that make the brain-body connection. Science 1997; 275:930–931.

Picardi A, Abeni D. Stressful life events and skin diseases: disentangling evidence from myth. Psychother Psychosom 2001; 70:118-36.

Pisarchik A, Slominski, A: Alternative splicing of CRH-R1 receptors in human and mouse skin: Identification of new variants and their differential expression. Faseb J. 2001; 15: 2754-2756

Quevedo ME, Slominski A, Pinto W, Wei E, Wortsman J. Pleiotropic effects of corticotropin releasing hormone on normal human skin keratinocytes. In Vitro Cell Dev Biol Anim. 2001; 37: 50-4.

Richards HL, Ray DW, Kirby B, Mason D, Plant D, Main CJ, Fortune DG, Griffiths CE.Response of the hypothalamic-pituitary-adrenal axis to psychological stress in patients with psoriasis. Br J Dermatol. 2005; 153: 1114-20.

Rozniecki JJ, Dimitriadou V, Lambracht-Hall M, Pang X, Theoharides TC. Morphological and functional demonstration of rat dura mast cell-neuron interactions in vitro and in vivo, Brain Res. 849 (1999), pp. 1–15.

Russo PA, Ilchef R, Cooper AJ. Psychiatric morbidity in psoriasis: a review. Australas J Dermatol. 2004; 45:155-9.

Sanders VM, Kohm AP. Sympathetic nervous system interaction with the immune system. Int Rev Neurobiol. 2002 ;52 :17-41.

Saraceno R, Kleyn CE, Terenghi G, Griffiths CE. The role of neuropeptides in psoriasis. Br J Dermatol. 2006 ;155: 876-82.

Schauer E, Trautinger F, Köck A, Schwarz A, Bhardwaj R, Simon M, Ansel JC, Schwarz T, Luger TA. Proopiomelanocortin-derived peptides are synthesized and released by human keratinocytes. J. Clin. Invest. 1994; 93: 2258–2262.

Schmid-Ott G, Jaeger B, Adamek C, Koch H, Lamprecht F, Kapp A, Werfel T. Levels of circulating CD8(+) T lymphocytes, natural killer cells, and eosinophils increase upon acute psychosocial stress in patients with atopic dermatitis. J Allergy Clin Immunol. 2001; 107: 171-7.

Selye H. A syndrome produced by diverse nocuous agents. Nature 1936; 138: 230−231.

Selye H. A syndrome produced by diverse nocuous agents. 1936, J. Neuropsychiatry Clin. Neurosci. 1998; 10: 230–231.

Singh LK, Pang X, Alexacos N, Letourneau R, Theoharides TC. Acute immobilization stress triggers skin mast cell degranulation via corticotropin releasing hormone, neurotensin and substance P: A link to neurogenic skin disorders, Brain Behav. Immun. 1999;13: 225–239.

aSlominski, A, Paus R, Wortsman J. On the potential role of proopiomelanocortin in skin physiology and pathology. Mol. Cell. Endocrinol. 1993; 93: C1–C6.

bSlominski A, Wortsman J, Mazurkiewicz JE, Matsuoka L, Dietrich J, Lawrence K, Gorbani A, Paus R. Detection of the proopiomelanocortin-derived antigens in normal and pathologic human skin. J. Lab. Clin. Med.1993; 122: 658–666.

aSlominski, A. Ermak G, Hwang J, Mazurkiewicz J, Corliss D, Eastman A . The expression of proopiomelanocortin (POMC) and of corticotropin releasing hormone receptor (CRH-R) genes in mouse skin. Biochim. Biophys. Acta 1996; 1289: 247–251.

bSlominski A, Mihm MC. Potential mechanism of skin response to stress. Int J Dermatol. 1996 ; 35: 849-51.

Slominski, A, Pawelek J. Animals under the sun: effects of ultraviolet radiation on mammalian skin. Clin. Dermatol.1998; 16: 503–515.

aSlominski A, Wortsman J. Neuroendocrinology of the skin. Endocr Rev. 2000; 21:457-87.

bSlominski A, Wortsman J, Luger T, Paus R, Solomon S. Corticotropin releasing hormone and proopiomelanocortin involvement in the cutaneous response to stress. Physiol Rev. 2000; 80: 979-1020.

cSlominski A, Szczesniewski A, Wortsman J. Liquid chromatography-mass spectrometry detection of corticotropin-releasing hormone and proopiomelanocortin-derived peptides in human skin, J Clin Endocrinol Metab. 2000; 85: 3582–3588.

Slominski A, Wortsman J, Pisarchik A, Zbytek B, Linton EA, Mazurkiewicz JE, and Wei ET. Cutaneous expression of corticotropin-releasing hormone (CRH), urocortin, and CRH receptors. Faseb J. 2001; 15: 1678–1693.

Slominski A, Wortsman J, Linton E, Pisarchik A, Zbytek B. The skin as a model for the immunodulatory effects of corticotropin-releasing hormone. In: Schäfer M, Stein C, editors. Mind over Matter - Regulation of Peripheral Inflammation by the CNS. Birkhäuser Verlag; Basel: 2003.

aSlominski A, Pisarchik A, Tobin DJ, Mazurkiewicz JE, Wortsman J. Differential expression of a cutaneous corticotropin-releasing hormone system. Endocrinology 2004; 145: 941–50.

bSlominski A, Zjawiony J, Wortsman J, Semak I, Stewart J, Pisarchik A, Sweatman T, Marcos J, Dunbar C, Tuckey RT. A novel pathway for sequential transformation of 7-dehydrocholesterol and expression of the P450scc system in mammalian skin. Eur. J. Biochem. 2004; 271: 4178–4188.

Slominski A, Zbytek B, Semak I, Sweatman T, Wortsman J. CRH stimulates POMC activity and corticosterone production in dermal fibroblasts. J Neuroimmunol. 2005: 162: 97–102.

Stojadinovic OP, Lee b, Vouthounis C, Vukelic S, Pastar I, Blumenberg M, Brem H, Tomic-Canic M. Novel genomic effects of glucocorticoids in epidermal keratinocytes: inhibition of apoptosis, interferon-gamma pathway, and wound healing along with promotion of terminal differentiation. J. Biol. Chem. 2007; 282: 4021–4034.

Strange A, Capon F, Spencer CC, et al. A genome-wide association study identifies new psoriasis susceptibility loci and an interaction between HLA-C and ERAP1. Nat Genet. 2010; 42: 985–990.

Sun TT, Shih C, Green H. Keratin cytoskeletons in epithelial cells of internal organs. Proc Natl Acad Sci U S A. 1979; 76: 2813-7.

Theoharides TC, Singh LK, Boucher W, Pang X, Letourneau R, Webster E, Chrousos G. Corticotropin-releasing hormone induces skin mast cell degranulation and increased vascular permeability, a possible explanation for its proinflammatory effects. Endocrinology 1998 ;139: 403-13.

Theoharides TC, Donelan JM, Papadopoulou N, Cao J, Kempuraj D, Conti P. Mast cells as targets of corticotropin-releasing factor and related peptides. Trends Pharmacol Sci. 2004; 25: 563-8.

Tsigos C, Chrousos G P. Physiology of the hypothalamic–pituitary–adrenal axis in health and dysregulation in psychiatric and autoimmune disorders. Endocrinol Metab Clin North Am.1994; 23:451–466.

Tsigos C, Papanicolaou DA, Kyrou I, Defensor R, Mitsiadis CS, Chrousos GP. Dose-dependent effects of recombinant human interleukin-6 on glucose regulation. J Clin Endocrinol Metab. 1997; 82: 4167–70.

Tsigos C, Kyrou I, Chrousos GP. (2005) Stress, endocrine manifestations, and diseases. In: Cooper CL. (ed.) Handbook of Stress, Medicine, and Health. 2nd Edition. Boca Raton FL: CRC Press.pp: 101 - 131.

Tsigos C, Chrousos GP. Hypothalamic-pituitary-adrenal axis, neuroendocrine factors and stress. J Psychosom Res. 2002; 53: 865-71.

Teunis MA, Heijnen CJ, Sluyter F, Bakker JM, Van Dam AM, Hof M, Cools AR, Kavelaars A. Maternal deprivation of rat pups increases clinical symptoms of experimental autoimmune encephalomyelitis at adult age. J Neuroimmunol. 2002; 133: 30-8.

Tuckey RC. Progesterone synthesis by the human placenta, Placenta 2005; 26: 273–281. Vassar R, Fuchs E. Transgenic mice provide new insights into the role of TGF-alpha during epidermal development and differentiation. Genes Dev. 1991; 5: 714–727.

Turnbull AV, Rivier CL. Regulation of the hypothalamic-pituitary-adrenal axis by cytokines: actions and mechanisms of action. Physiol Rev. 1999; 79:1–71.

Verhoeven EW, Kraaimaat FW, de Jong EM, Schalkwijk J, van de Kerkhof PC, Evers AW. Individual differences in the effect of daily stressors on psoriasis: a prospective study. J Invest Dermatol. 2009; 129: 2075–7.

Wakamatsu K, Graham A, Cook D, Thody AJ. Characterization of ACTH peptides in human skin and their activation of the melanocortin-1 receptor. Pigment Cell Res. 1997; 10: 288–297.

Weatherhead SC, Farr PM, Jamieson D, Hallinan JS, Lloyd JJ, Wipat A, Reynolds NJ. Keratinocyte Apoptosis in Epidermal Remodeling and Clearance of Psoriasis Induced by UV Radiation. Invest Dermatol. 2011 May 26. [Epub ahead of print]

Wedemeyer J, Tsai M, Galli SJ. Roles of mast cells and basophils in innate and acquired immunity. Curr Opin Immunol. 2000; 12: 624-31.

Wintzen M, Yaar M, Burbach JP, Gilchrest BA. Proopiomelanocortin gene product regulation in keratinocytes. J. Invest. Dermatol. 1996; 106: 673–678.

Wong M, Licinio J, Pasternak K I, Gold P W. Localization of corticotropin- releasing hormone (CRH) receptor mRNA in adult rat brain by in situ hybridization histochemistry. Endocrinology 1994; 135: 2275– 8.

Xiang Z, Nilsson G. IgE receptor-mediated release of nerve growth factor by mast cells. Clin Exp Allergy. 2000; 30: 1379-86.

Zangeneh FZ, Fazeli A. The significance of stress hormones in psoriasis. Acta Medica Iranica 2008; 46: 485-488.

Zangeneh FZ، Shooshtary FS. Chronic Stress and Limbic-Hypothalamopituitary-Adrenal Axis (LHPA) Response in Female Reproductive system. Journal of Family and Reproductive Health 2009 ;3: 101-108.

Zbytek B, Mysliwski A, Slominski A, Wortsman J, Wei ET, Mysliwska J. Corticotropin-releasing hormone affects cytokine production in human HaCaT keratinocytes. Life Sci. 2002;70: 1013-21.

Zhou C, Yu X, Cai D, Liu C, Li C. Role of corticotropin-releasing hormone and receptor in the pathogenesis of psoriasis. Medical Hypotheses 2009; 73: 513-515.

11

Personality in Patients with Psoriasis

Ramón Martín-Brufau[1], Jorge C. Ulnik[2],
Carmen Brufau Redondo[1] and Francisco-Javier Corbalán Berná[1]
[1]Universidad de Murcia
[2]Universidad de Buenos Aires
[1]Spain
[2]República Argentina

1. Introduction

1.1 Skin diseases and psychological factors

It has been known since antiquity that a connection exists between the skin and the mind. In fact, the first documented case of psychodermatosis dates to 1700 BC, when the physician to the prince of Persia speculated that the prince's psoriasis was caused by anxiety over succeeding his father to the throne (Shafii & Shafii, 1979). However, it was not until 1891 that Brocq and Jacquet coined the term neurodermatitis and hypothesised that there was a pathological association between the skin and the autonomic nervous system, given that itching precipitates the appearance of lesions (Braun-Falco, Plewig, Wolff, & Winkelmann). A further 62 years passed before "Emotional Factors in Skin Disease" (Wittkower & Russell, 1953) was published. Since then, physicians, and dermatologists in particular, have been steadily becoming aware of the impact of an individual's emotional state on skin disease and how this organ can reflect, like a mirror, their psychological state. It should come as no surprise that these two structures have a common origin in the ectoderm.

Psychological factors have traditionally been associated with the onset, development, and persistence of skin disease (Alexander, 1951) and there is evidence to suggest an association between stress and the exacerbation of skin lesions (Kimyai-Asadi & Usman, 2001; Robles, 2007; Vileikyte, 2007). Recent longitudinal studies of a general hospital population show the involvement of psychological factors, such as stress, depression, and anxiety, in individuals who present skin disease (Magin, Sibbritt, & Bailey, 2009). In addition to depression or anxiety (da Silva, Müller, & Bonamigo, 2006; Fried, Gupta, & Gupta, 2005; Lotti, Buggiani et al., 2008; Morell-Dubois et al., 2008; Radmanesh & Shafiei, 2001; Richards & Fortune, 2006), higher rates of dissociative disorders (Konuk, 2007; Gupta, 2006), sexual dysfunction (Mercan, 2008) or problems of excessive alcohol consumption attributed to psychological distress (Kirby et al., 2008) have been found in this group than in the healthy population. Psoriasis has been associated with psychological distress, such as feelings of shame, shyness, low self-esteem, and stigmatization (Magin, Adams, Heading, Pond, & Smith, 2009).

Psychological stress occupies a special place among the factors that trigger psoriasis, of which patients are very aware. They openly identify it as underlying many of their outbreaks of psoriasis. In 1998, the National Psoriasis Foundation (NPF) published the preliminary results of a survey that had been answered by 18,000 psoriasis patients who were members of the NPF. When they were asked to identify the factors that aggravate psoriasis, 52% answered that emotional stress was the most frequent trigger. Some 41% attributed outbreaks to seasonal changes, 9% to chemical substances, 8% to medications, 8% to certain food or diets, 7% to alcohol, and 29% did not know (Annual Report, 1998). Thus, emotional stress was considered the most important factor by more of half of the sample. Subsequently, their findings were published in a scientific journal (Krueger et al., 2001).

The high percentage of dermatological patients who need psychiatric care is also striking. This ranges from 25.2% reported in a sample of 2579 patients attending a dermatology unit (Picardi, Abeni, Melchi, Puddu, & Pasquini, 2000) to 95% of the dermatological patients who fulfilled the criteria for a psychiatric disorder and were referred to a psychosomatic medicine specialist (Woodruff, Higgins, Du Vivier, & Wessely, 1997). A study that reviewed the prevalence of psychiatric symptoms in psoriasis patients found a higher rate of psychiatric disorders than in the healthy population (Russo, Ilchef, & Cooper, 2004). Similarly, another study found that the prevalence of psychiatric disease among psoriasis patients was less than in psychiatric patients but higher than in healthy controls (Chaudhury, Das, John, & Ramadasan, 1998). Psoriasis patients experience a greater number of stressful events (Jankovic et al., 2009; Malhotra & Mehta, 2008; Picardi et al., 2003). A prospective study which measured daily stressors in psoriasis patients found a direct association between disease severity and increased itching on days perceived as more stressful, but not on days of medium or low stress (Verhoeven et al., 2009).

It is generally accepted that psoriasis patients experience reduced quality of life (Hong, Koo, & Koo, 2008). Compared to healthy subjects, psoriasis patients experience greater physical discomfort, mood swings, poor body image and self image, and restricted daily and social activities due to their lesions (De Korte, Sprangers, Mombers, & Bos, 2004). Other authors have found a stronger association between quality of life and psychological variables and fear of rejection than with the physical characteristics of the disease, such as the extent of the lesions and their visibility (Kimball, Jacobson, Weiss, Vreeland, & Wu, 2005). In an intermediate position, some authors suggest that the relationship between psoriasis and psychiatric symptoms could be reciprocal (Devrimci Ozguven, Kundakci, Kumbasar, & Boyvat, 2000).

1.2 Personality, stress, and skin

Given the role of the skin as the interface between the external and internal environment, the personality would be the psychological construct fulfilling the same role between the internal and external environment. That is, the personality would be the psychological analogue of the skin.

The term personality represents the different behavioural styles that individuals present in their habitual habitats or environments (Davis, 1999). In other words, the personality would be the means of responding to the environment. According to Darwinian theory, individuals behave in the way that is most conducive to reproductive success. Millon selected several characteristics present in all living beings and, based on these, generated a dimensional system to classify the way individuals adapt to their environment, thus matching the personality categories presented in DSM-IV (American Psychiatric Association [*DSM-IV-TR*], 2000).

The healthy personality, conceived of in this way, would reflect the specific adaptation modes that individuals find effective in their environment. In turn, personality disorders would be represented by the various maladaptive response styles that can be attributed to deficiencies, imbalances, or conflicts in an individual's capacity to relate to his or her environment (Millon, 2001). In the context of Millon's evolutionary theory, strategies that favour individual survival and reproductive are equivalent to the personality (Million, 1990).

Million compared the personality to the immune system. According to this perspective, the personality can be studied as an interface between the outer and inner world, as described by Freud (Quiroga, 2003), and between the social and biological levels. Just as in the biological perspective the skin or immune system protects the individual from external attacks and maintains the internal environment in homeostasis, similarly, Million suggested that within the framework of the DSM-IV, axis I (clinical disorders due to anxiety or depression, etc), would be equivalent to cough or fever, axis II (personality disorders) would represent a coping style equivalent to the immune system, and axis IV (psychological and social stressors, such as marital or economic conflict) would be analogous to infectious agents.

Personality would be a complex behavioural system that evolved due to the need to deal with a threatening environment undergoing constant change (Million, 1990; Millon, 1999). Million suggested that the different ways of dealing with the environment may be more or less adaptative. It is of interest to apply these ideas to dermatology. Adaptive personality styles could modulate external events and ensure, with increased likelihood, the maintenance of physiological states that may allow the skin to function in a healthy way. However, individuals who experience difficulty in adaptation can be more vulnerable to stressful events and their impact on health. That is, biological differences may not only be due to genetic factors but to an entire group of environmental factors (Davidson, 2001).

Studies have shown how certain personality variables can modulate response to stress. Associations have been found between the tendency to experience positive or negative emotions and extraversion or neuroticism (personality variables), respectively (Ng, 2009). These tendencies may modulate the effect that emotional responses to stressful events have on the physiology of the skin (Mardaga Solange, 2006).

In general, psychological stress has been frequently described as a variable that triggers skin disease, and has been commonly associated with high levels of sympathetic activation and difficulties in regulating emotions (Arck & Paus, 2006; Berg, Svensson, Brandberg, & Nordlind, 2008; Gupta, 2008; Gupta & Gupta, 2004; Mastrolonardo, Alicino, Zefferino, Pasquini, & Picardi, 2007; Arck, 2006; Picardi, Pasquini, Cattaruzza, Gaetano, Melchi, et al., 2003; Wright, Cohen, & Cohen, 2005).

It has also been proposed that patients with skin disease usually present psychological traits that would make them vulnerable to stress (Cordan Yazici et al., 2006; Kim et al., 2006; Papadopoulos, 2003). In fact, psoriasis-associated psychological vulnerability has been described (Valverde, Mestanza, & Asenjo, 2005) and increased reactivity of the hypothalamic-pituitary-adrenal axis has been found in patients with this disease (Richards, Ray, et al., 2005); thus, the link between stressful events and psychological vulnerability may play an important role in the development of skin disease (Laguna, Pena Payero, & Marquez, 2006).

Higher levels of alexithymia have been found among psoriasis patients and other skin diseases than in control groups (Gupta, 2006). One study assessed alexithymia before and after patients received PUVA therapy which led to lesion regression. The level of alexithymia did not vary and thus this disorder could not be a response to the severity of the lesions or the degree of discomfort occasioned by them (Richards, Fortune, Griffiths, & Main, 2005). The authors suggested that alexithymia could be understood as a stable internal psychological trait more than as a strategy to cope with the lesions. Other researchers have not found higher levels of alexithymia in patients with skin disease (Picardi, Pasquini, Cattaruzza, Gaetano, Baliva, et al., 2003).

Taking this into account, it is not surprising that some authors have proposed psoriasis as a psychosomatic disease due to the close link between stress and the exacerbation of psoriasis lesions (Ginsburg, 1995; Kilic, Gulec, Gul, & Gulec, 2008). One of the most valuable, rigorous, and exhaustive studies of psoriasis concluded that the disease is caused by genetic and environmental factors, influenced by psychological stress, and where the patients' attitudes, knowledge of, and behavior towards their disease have a profound effect on its course and severity (Ginsburg, 1995). The author suggested that psoriasis, by attacking the skin, attacks the individual's sense of identity. Thus, the relationship between skin and identity is implicit. In a survey of NPF members conducted by Jobling, 84% of respondents stated that the worst aspect of having psoriasis was the difficulty involved in establishing relationships. What is striking is that few respondents had experienced avoidance or exclusion, such that the problem was more related to their constant anticipation of this occurring rather than it being a real event (Jobling, 1976).

Doodley and Finlay attempted to define social adjustment in psoriasis patients by examining the relationship between subjective experience and various social situations, such as wearing a swimming suit (Dooley & Finlay, 1990). They found no correlation between chronicity, the natural course of the disease, visibility, and the various measures of social adjustment taken by the experimental group compared to the control group.

In an attempt to provide an in-depth account of the patients' subjective experience, Ginsburg and Link assessed 100 patients using the concept of stigma defined as a negative social or biological mark that sets a person off from others and changes how they interact with other people due to the anticipation of rejection, among other reasons. Although bleeding is not one of the main symptom of psoriasis, it is strongly correlated with stigma. This may be caused by scratching scales or their removal that leads to punctate bleeding spots known as Auspitz's sign. Regarding all the aspects of the disease, bleeding lesions was the strongest predictor of feelings of being stigmatized and despair. Thus, feelings of despair and stigmatization may lead to non-compliance with treatment, possibly aggravating the disease (Ginsburg & Link, 1989).

In relation to feelings of stigmatization, evidence suggests that psoriasis patients fear being rejected or negatively labelled, regardless of physical lesions (Richards, Fortune, Griffiths, & Main, 2001). This could be modulated by personality variables (Schmid-Ott et al., 2005), as is the case among patients with other skin diseases such as acne (Krejci-Manwaring, Kerchner, Feldman, Rapp, & Rapp, 2006). All the evidence suggests that the patients themselves are one of the main sources of stigmatization and despair and that these feelings are not caused by the disease.

It has been suggested that psoriasis patients have a particular way of reacting to feelings of stigmatization and that their feelings are divided and denied, to the point that the fact of being rejected due to psoriasis significantly predicted alcohol consumption, without the patient being consciously aware of feeling stigmatized because of the disease. Thus, the patients act out their feelings without being aware of their relationship to behaviour (Ginsburg & Link, 1993).

To sum up, psoriasis, as well as other skin diseases, has frequently been associated with emotional disturbances, vulnerability to stress, and difficulty in expressing emotions. However, up to the present, no personality differences between psoriasis patients and the healthy population have been found. Matussek, Agerer & Seibt reported differences in personality traits between healthy individuals and those with psoriasis (Matussek, Agerer, & Seibt, 1985), but this was not corroborated in later studies conducted by Doodley and Finlay (Dooley & Finlay, 1990), Ginsburg et al. (Ginsburg & Link, 1993) and Gupta et al. (Gupta et al., 1989). Although some studies have identified personality traits associated with the development or exacerbation of skin disease, including psoriasis (Magin, Pond, Smith, Watson, & Goode, 2008), no differences have been found between the healthy population and the psoriatic population or the findings have not been conclusive (Pérez et al., 2000; Willemsen, Roseeuw, & Vanderlinden, 2008). Therefore, more research is required on the way personality traits modulate the course of skin disease (Verhoeven et al., 2008). For example, the hypothesis that individuals with psoriasis share common personality traits that are related to the exacerbation of symptoms has only been partially upheld.

Despite some evidence suggesting that psoriasis patients have poor quality of life, experience emotional disturbances, are vulnerable to stressful events, suffer feelings of stigmatization that are independent of lesion severity, and possibly share nonfunctional personality traits, it cannot be asserted beyond doubt that these patients have personality traits that differ from the healthy population.

2. Is there a different personality profile in psoriasis?

To test this hypothesis a study including 36 psoriasis patients attending the Reina Sofía University Hospital (Murcia, Spain) was conducted. The inclusion criterion was the presence of psoriasis as diagnosed by a dermatologist who agreed to participate in the study. Patients were recruited between October 2005 and June 2009.

The exclusion criteria were as follows: severe psychological disorders such as psychosis, factitious or simulation disorders, neurological disorders, etc. Given that the Million Index of Personality Styles (MIPS) is designed to evaluate the personality of individuals more than 18 years old, younger patients were excluded.

Regarding comorbidity, high levels of depression and anxiety are often observed in populations with skin disease (Konuk, 2007); however, the study participants did not have a clinical diagnosis of depression or anxiety. They had never been admitted to a psychiatric unit due to either of these disorders, and therefore the results obtained are unlikely to be attributable to psychiatric syndromes.

The Spanish version of the MIPS was used to evaluate the participants' personality styles (Millon, 2001). This index measures the healthy personality and analyzes 24 personality dimensions, including a clinical index that measures an individual's level of adaptation to their environment. This instrument has been previously used with dermatological patients and has demonstrated sensitivity to differences with a non-dermatological sample (Martín-Brufau, Corbalán Berná, Ramirez Aandreo, Brufau Redondo, & Limiñana Gras, 2010). The instrument consists of different bipolar scales divided into three dimensions: motivating, thinking, and behaving styles.

For details of the participants and the selection procedure, see above. The questionnaires were given to the participants by the dermatologist who explained the purpose of the research, the requirements for participation and any consequences for the patients. The dermatologist obtained prior consent from the participants.

The Spanish version of the MIPS was validated using a normative sample of 1184 individuals (643 women and 541 men) who were used as the control group. The test showed good psychometric properties.

The control group did not present chronic, severe or disfiguring skin disease. It was assumed that the sociocultural characteristics of both populations were similar. This methodology has been previously used to evaluate personality styles in patients with other disorders (Limiñana Gras, Corbalán Berná, & Sánchez López, 2009) and skin diseases (Martín-Brufau et al., 2010).

The Student t-test was used to analyse mean differences between groups and each personality scale was compared individually. Those items that did not fulfil the reliability index or that the participants did not fill in properly were excluded for the analysis. Mean t values were obtained for the 24 personality scales of the MIPS. The SPSS version 17.0 software package for Mac was used for data analysis.

The social and demographic data for both groups are shown in Table 1.

Characteristics	**Mean/percentage psoriasis N=36**	**Mean/percentage healthy group N=1184**
Female gender, n (%)	22 (59.5%)	634 (54.31%)
Mean age/range (y)	42.59/(24-86)	37.60/(18-65)

Table 1. Sociodemographic Data.

Differences in personality were found between the two groups in the following variables: Self-indulging, Other-nurturing, Intuition, Innovation-seeking, Dissenting, Dominating, and Acquiescent. The results are shown in Table 2.

Personality trait	Psoriasis Mean	Healthy Mean	Student t-test	*P*
1. (1A) - Pleasure-Enhancing	57.67	62.05	-1.155	.256
2. (1B) - Pain-Avoiding	43.75	39.86	0.981	.333
3. (2A) - Actively Modifying	44.56	50.52	-1.371	.179
4. (2B) - Passively Accommodating	55.89	51.63	0.980	.334
5. (3A) - Self-Indulging*	41.72	52.14	-2.390	.022
6. (3B) - Other-Nurturing	60.19	51.64	1.916	.064
7. (4A) - Externally Focused	46.41	48.59	-0.482	.633
8. (4B) - Internally Focused	48.67	51.45	-0.570	.572
9. (5A) - Realistic/Sensing	61.42	58.39	0.859	.396
10. (5B) - Imaginative/Intuiting*	35.22	42.82	-2.529	.016
11. (6A) - Thought-Guided	44.25	49.46	-1.251	.219
12. (6B) - Feeling-Guided	57.83	51.36	1.486	.146
13. (7A) - Conservation-Seeking	49.67	50.30	-0.155	.878
14. (7B) - Innovation-Seeking*	33.22	42.67	-2.396	.022
15. (8A) - Asocial/Withdrawing	55.83	50.60	1.379	.177
16. (8B) - Gregarious/Outgoing	44.36	51.04	-1.680	.102
17. (9A) - Anxious/Hesitating	49.47	46.32	0.672	.506
18. (9B) - Confident/Asserting	44.44	50.89	-1.554	.129
19. (10A) - Unconventional/Dissenting*	36.97	43.62	-2.170	.037
20. (10B) - Dutiful/Conforming	59.31	51.93	1.739	.091
21. (11A) - Submissive/Yielding	45.92	45.33	0.162	.872
22. (11B) - Dominant/Controlling*	34.47	44.65	-2.436	.020
23. (12A) - Dissatisfied/Complaining	39.50	44.62	-1.06	.296
24. (12B) - Cooperative/Agreeing***	77.58	59.18	5.269	.000
Clinical Index**	43.13	50.69	3.111	.004

*p> .05; ** p>.01; ***p>.000.

Table 2. Differences Between Psoriasis Patients and the Healthy Sample.

3. And if so, how do they differ from the normal population?

Individuals with psoriasis have a tendency towards complying with the wishes of other individuals as a motivating style. This tendency is reinforced by the fact that their self-motivation or self-drive is low.

Regarding thinking styles, psoriasis patients had lower scores on the intuition scale than the healthy population, suggesting that they are more oriented toward practical thinking rather than abstract thinking. In addition, they had a tendency not to employ innovative or creative ways of thinking.

In relation to behaving styles, psoriasis patients are more conventional than the reference group. They were less dominating and more acquiescent. Overall, they tend to seek cooperation and agreement and avoid disagreement as a way of bonding with others. They may be dependent, submissive, and lack initiative or their own opinion. In general, the results indicate a personality profile which is not well adjusted, and this has been associated with lower satisfaction with life (Díaz Morales & Sánchez López, 2002). The graph in Figure 1 depicts these differences.

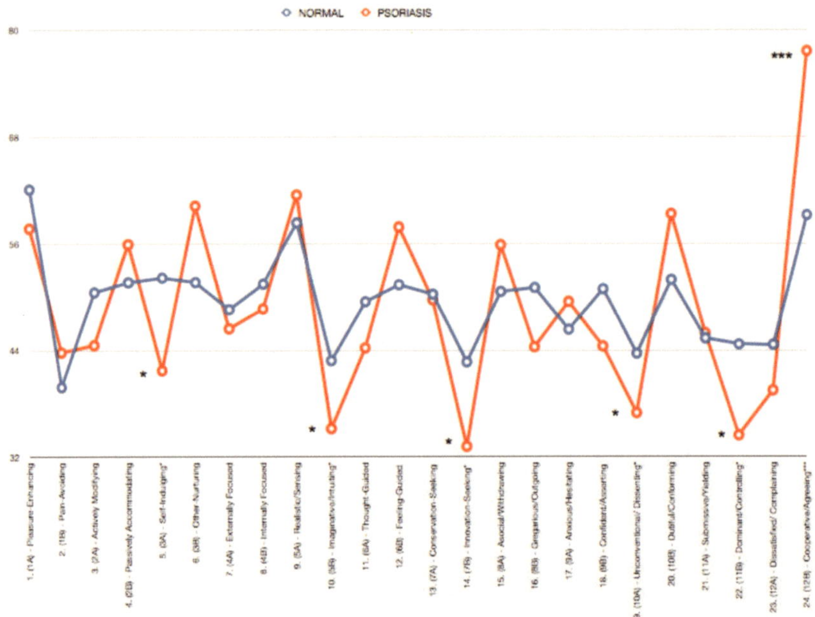

Fig. 1. Graphical representation of psoriasis (red) and non-dermatological (blue) profiles. *p> .05; ** p>.01; ***p>.000.

The results of our study indicate that individuals with psoriasis tend to avoid distancing themselves from others or disagreeing with them. This is suggested by their high scores on acquiescence, low dissatisfaction and low dominance, which could be interpreted as a protective mechanism used by psoriasis patients due to their fear of being rejected or discriminated against (Ulnik, 2007; Ginsburg & Link, 1989; Lu, Duller, van der Valk, & Evers, 2003; Schmid-Ott et al., 2005). This is reflected in an increased tendency to be externally focussed, as shown by other studies: psoriasis patients have low scores on narcissistic traits, are more altruistic and more orientated towards others, and are less aggressive in the face of criticism (Bahmer, 2007). Whereas Matussek et al. (Matussek et al., 1985) found that psoriasis patients presented greater aggressivity toward others compared to the healthy population, the findings in our study are compatible with later studies which reported a decreased ability to express anger toward others (Ginsburg & Link, 1993) and a greater tendency among psoriasis patients who were more sensitive to stress to seek approval, to avoid expressing negative emotions and to avoid being rejected (Gupta et al., 1989). Other studies have also reported that these patients show difficulties in expressing feelings of anger and being assertive, which may be a factor making them vulnerable to stress (Devrimci Ozguven et al., 2000), and could explain the higher level of acquiescence observed in the psoriasis sample. The most relevant aspect of this is that, in contrast to the healthy population, individuals with psoriasis change the way they present themselves in relation to others, and this may correspond to a given personality profile. Patients may behave in this manner to reduce emotional and behavioural conflicts that could damage their relationship with others. It has been found that these patients present attentional bias and are more responsive to subtle signs of rejection (Fortune et al., 2003). The tendency to avoid rejection is compatible with other findings which suggest that the only association with decreased quality of life in psoriasis patients was due to the fear of being rejected rather than to the physical characteristics of the lesions, their localization, or severity (Fortune, Main, O'Sullivan, & Griffiths, 1997).

The available data also shows that psoriasis patients have lower scores in self-directedness, which reinforces the tendency to be non-dominant and suggests that they are dependent, sociable and easily influenced, as reported by other authors (Kilic et al., 2008). However, our results indicate that individuals with psoriasis do not have a greater tendency to avoid pain, unlike the findings of Kilic who reported that psoriasis patients had higher scores on the harm-avoidance item. The high vulnerability to stress found in these patients (Valverde et al., 2005) may reinforce their tendency to avoid conflict with others, and may be related to the avoidance behavior reported in other studies (da Silva et al., 2006; Magin, Adams, et al., 2009). Some authors have explained these differences as being a way to compensate for poorly regulated emotions that may modulate outbreaks of psoriasis plaques (Picardi et al., 2005) and which has been confirmed by other studies (Richards, Fortune, et al., 2005). These personality traits suggest that, regardless of stressful events or lesion severity, psoriasis may be negatively affected by difficulties in managing emotions.

Concerning the clinical index, psoriasis patients as a group have lower scores than the healthy population. This decreased level of adjustment has also been found in other studies (Dooley & Finlay, 1990). Given that a low clinical index has been associated with lower life satisfaction in general (Díaz Morales & Sánchez López, 2002), this could indicate why psoriasis patients have less quality of life than the healthy population (Van Voorhees & Fried, 2009), as well as accounting for the psychological disturbances, such as anxiety, depression and sexual problems, that have been reported in other studies (eg, Mercan, 2008). The foregoing suggests that the personality variables measured by MIPS are poorly adjusted in the psoriasis population, which probably underlies the psychiatric vulnerability reported by other studies (Mastrolonardo et al., 2007; Picardi et al., 2005; Richards, Ray, et al., 2005; Valverde et al., 2005). Therefore, as suggested by other authors (Gieler, Niemeier, Brosig, & Kupfer, 2002; Melamed & Yosipovitch, 2004), psychological variables should be assessed in these patients, who should be referred to mental health specialists (Ginsburg, Prystowsky, Kornfeld, & Wolland, 1993; Schneider et al., 2006; Woodruff et al., 1997; Yosipovitch & Samuel, 2008).

4. Controversy

No consensus exists on the personality of dermatological patients. Buske-Kirschbaum suggests that these patients have a common psychological profile (Buske-Kirschbaum et al., 2004). Despite the existence of features found in such patients, other authors do not accept the existence of a profile that differentiates them from the healthy population (Verhoeven et al., 2008). Similarly, research on personality variables in a Spanish dermatological population (Antuña-Bernardo, 2000), who were assessed using the Eysenck Personality Questionnaire, found that there were no differences between the healthy population and patients with various skin diseases, including psoriasis. However, they were found to have lower quality of life and above-average neuroticism scores.

There may be several reasons why no personality differences have been found between the healthy population and psoriasis patients. Firstly, by including all skin diseases, those less associated with psychological variables may have obscured the influence of distinctive personality patterns, thus hindering the detection of differences between the 2 populations. Second, few studies have analyzed the strategies used or differences in the way psoriasis patients manage their emotions compared to the healthy population (Fortune, Richards, Main, & Griffiths, 2002), whereas, in comparison, psychological research on dermatologic patients has mainly focussed on variables such as stress, anxiety and depression. By placing too much emphasis on variables such as depression and anxiety, or on psychopathological abnormalities based on diagnostic categories, there is an increased risk of losing specificity in the search for potential differences between the healthy population and psoriasis patients. An increase in psychiatric disorders can be observed in the latter group, but it would be more useful to know how these abnormalities arise, how are they qualitatively different, and what characterizes this group of patients. The relevance of personality may have become lost as a research aim, leading to a reduction in the number of empirical studies investigating personality in this group of patients. Finally, another possibility is that instruments used in the past to assess personality were not designed to measure specific personality variables in this group or were not sufficiently sensitive to detect subtle differences. This could explain why some studies have failed to find any differences; questionnaires were used that were not designed to assess profound personality structures. According to some authors, sensitive instruments are now available for assessing the association between personality and disease (Friedman, 1990).

5. Conclusions

The most important conclusion is that personality differences were found between the healthy population and psoriasis patients. These differences suggest that there is a greater tendency among psoriasis patients to be acquiescent and to restrain the expression of negative emotions in order to bond with others. The literature and the results from the study presented here shows a decreased capacity to adjust to the environment, which could, due to poor stress management, increase the risk of suffering psoriasis in susceptible individuals.

The number of subjects in the study presented here was sufficient to establish differences between psoriasis patients and healthy participants and the results are consistent with those obtained by other authors; however, further studies are needed that include a greater number of psoriasis patients, thereby providing stronger support to the results obtained here, as well as a greater degree of generalizability.

If we wish to understand the psychological characteristics of psoriasis patients and their characteristic personality styles, future studies should compare the personality of psoriasis patients to that of patients with other skin diseases associated with psychological traits in order to identify the different adaptation styles, if any.

Finally, the relevance of these findings lies in their deepening our understanding of the psychological problems of psoriasis patients.

If psychopathological abnormalities, such as depression and anxiety, are observed in dermatological patients as a group, then this should lead to investigating potential differences between specific subgroups of dermatological patients, particularly in relation to what qualitatively characterizes psoriasis patients as one such subgroup.

There are few personality studies on dermatological patients, and on psoriasis patients in particular, indicating a need for further research in personality psychology and psycho-dermatology. Such studies would lead to a better understanding of this group of patients and to help them better manage stress and the impact this has on their disease, quality of life, and their relationships with others.

6. References

Alexander, E. J. (1951). Psychosomatic Medicine-Its Principles and Applications. *American Journal of Psychiatry, 108*(4), 318-318. ISSN: 1535-7228.

Aller, M. A. & Lorente, L. (1996). The psycho-neuro-immune endocrine response a physiological and pathological way of life. *Psicothema, 8*(2), 375-381. ISSN: 0214-9915.

American Psychiatric Association. (2000). *Diagnostic and statistical manual of mental disorders* (Revised 4th ed.). Washington, DC. American Psychiatric Association. ISBN: 9781557987914.

Annual Report. (1998). *National Psoriasis Foundation Bulletin, 29*(6). ISSN: 1040-0060.

Antuña-Bernardo, S., García-Vega, E., González menéndez, A., Secades villa, R., Errasti Pérez, J. & Curto Iglesias, J.R. (2000). Perfil Psicológico y calidad de vida en pacientes con enfermedades dermatológicas. *Psichothema, 12*(2), 30-34. ISSN: 0214-9915.

Arck, P., & Paus, R. (2006). From the brain-skin connection: the neuroendocrine-immune misalliance of stress and itch. *Neuroimmunomodulation, 13*(5-6), 347-356. ISSN: 1423-0216.

Arck, P.C., Slominski, A., Theoharides, T. C., Peters, E. M. J. & Paus, R. (2006). Neuroimmunology of stress: skin takes center stage. *J Invest Dermatol, 126*(8), 1697-1704. ISSN: 0022-202X.

Berg, M., Svensson, M., Brandberg, M., & Nordlind, K. (2008). Psoriasis and stress: a prospective study. *J Eur Acad Dermatol Venereol, 22*(6), 670-674. ISSN: 1468-3083.

Braun-Falco, O., Plewig, G., Wolff, H., & Winkelmann, R. Dermatology, 1991: Springer-Verlag Berlin Heidelberg. ISBN: 978-3-540-29312-5.

Brown, R. (2004). Psychological mechanisms of medically unexplained symptoms: an integrative conceptual model. *Sychol Bull, 130*, 793-812. ISSN: 0146-1672.

Buske-Kirschbaum, A., Ebrecht, M., Kern, S., Hollig, H., Gierens, A., & Hellhammer, D. (2004). Personality characteristics and their association with biological stress responses in patients with atopic dermatitis. *Dermatol Psychosom, 5*(1), 12-16. ISSN: 1422-9196.

Camelo-Roa, S. M. (2005). Psiconeuroinmunología: breve panorámica. *Diversitas, 1*(2). ISSN: 1794-9998.

Campos Roldan, M. (2007). La relación psiconeural en el estrés o de las neuronas a la cogniciñon social: una revisión empírica. *Rev. investig. psicol., 10*(1), 125-143. ISSN 1609-7475.

Chaudhury, S., Das, A., John, R. T., & Ramadasan, P. (1998). Psychological factors in psoriasis. *Indian Journal of Psychiatry, 40*(3), 295. ISSN: 0019-5545.

Critchley, H. D. (2002). Electrodermal responses: What happens in the brain. . *Neuroscientists, 8*, 132-142. ISSN: 1073-8584.

da Silva, J., Müller, M., & Bonamigo, R. (2006). Coping strategies and stress levels in patients with psoriasis. *An Bras Dermatol, 81*(2), 143-149. ISSN: 0365-0596.

Davidson, R. J. (2001). Toward a Biology of Personality and Emotion. *Annals New York Academy of Science*, 191-207. ISSN: 00778923.

Davis, R. D. (1999). Millon: Essentials of His Science, Theory, Classification, Assessment, and Therapy. *Journal of Personality Assessment, 72*(3), 330-352. ISSN: 1532-7752.

De Korte, J., Sprangers, M. A. G., Mombers, F. M. C., & Bos, J. D. (2004). *Quality of life in patients with psoriasis: a systematic literature review*. ISSN: 1087-0024.

Devrimci Ozguven, H., Kundakci, N., Kumbasar, H., & Boyvat, A. (2000). The depression, anxiety, life satisfaction and affective expression levels in psoriasis patients. *Journal of the European Academy of Dermatology and Venereology, 14*(4), 267-271. ISSN: 1468-3083.

Díaz Morales, J. F., & Sánchez López, P. (2002). Relaciones entre estilos de personalidad y satisfacción autopercibida en diferentes áreas vitales. *Psicothema, 14*(1), 100. ISSN: 0214-9915.

Dooley, G., & Finlay, A. (1990). Personal construct systems of psoriatic patients. *Clinical and Experimental Dermatology, 15*(6), 401-405. ISSN: 1365-2230.

Eung-Ho Choi, Brown. B. E., Crumrine, D., Chang, S., Man, M-Q., Elias, P. M., & Feingold, K. R. (2005). Mechanisms by wich psychologic stres alters cutaneous permeability barrier homeostasis and stratum corneum integrity. *J Invest Dermatol, 124*, 587-595. ISSN: 0022-202X.

Fortune, D., Main, C., O'sullivan, T., & Griffiths, C. (1997). Quality of life in patients with psoriasis: the contribution of clinical variables and psoriasis specific stress. *British Journal of Dermatology, 137*(5), 755-760. ISSN: 1365-2133.

Fortune, D., Richards, H., Corrin, A., Taylor, R., Griffiths, C., & Main, C. (2003). Attentional Bias for Psoriasis-Specific and Psychosocial Threat in Patients with Psoriasis. *Journal of Behavioral Medicine, 26*(3), 211-224. ISSN: *1573-3521.*

Fortune, D. G., Richards, H. L., Main, C. J., & Griffiths, C. E. (2002). Patients' strategies for coping with psoriasis. *Clin Exp Dermatol, 27*(3), 177-184. ISSN: 1365-2230.

Fried, R. G., Gupta, M. A., & Gupta, A. K. (2005). Depression and skin disease. *Dermatol Clin, 23*(4), 657-664. ISSN: 0733-8635.

Friedman, H. (1990). *Personality and disease*: Wiley. ISBN: 0471-618055.

Gieler, U., Niemeier, V., Brosig, B., & Kupfer, J. (2002). Psychosomatic aspects of pruritus. *Dermatology and Psychosomatics, 3*, 6-13. ISSN: 1424-0564.

Ginsburg, I., Prystowsky, J., Kornfeld, D., & Wolland, H. (1993). Role of emotional factors in adults with atopic dermatitis. *International Journal of Dermatology, 32*(9), 656-660. ISSN: *0011-9059.*

Ginsburg, I. H. (1995). Psychological and psychophysiological aspects of psoriasis. *Dermatologic clinics, 13*(4), 793. ISSN: 1558-0520.

Ginsburg, I. H., & Link, B. G. (1989). Feelings of stigmatization in patients with psoriasis. *Journal of the American Academy of Dermatology, 20*(1), 53-63. ISSN: *0190-9622.*

Ginsburg, I. H., & Link, B. G. (1993). Psychosocial consequences of rejection and stigma feelings in psoriasis patients. *International Journal of Dermatology, 32*(8), 587-591. ISSN: *0011-9059.*

Grimalt, F., & Cotterill, J. A. (2002). Dermatología y Psiquiatría. *Grupo Aula Médica, S.A*, 329. ISBN: 84-7885-282-4.

Gupta, M. (2008). Stress and Urticaria. In: *Neuroimmunology of the Skin: Basic Science to Clinical Practice.* Springer, 209. ISBN: 978-3540359869.

Gupta, M., & Gupta, A. (2004). Stressful major life events are associated with a higher frequency of cutaneous sensory symptoms: an empirical study of non-clinical subjects. *J Eur Acad Dermatol Venereol, 18*, 560-565. ISSN: 1468-3083.

Gupta, M. A., Gupta, A. K., Kirkby, S., Schork, N. J., Gorr, S. K., Ellis, C. N., et al. (1989). A psychocutaneous profile of psoriasis patients who are stress reactors: A study of 127 patients. *General hospital psychiatry, 11*(3), 166-173. ISSN: 0163-8343.

Hong, J., Koo, B., & Koo, J. (2008). The psychosocial and occupational impact of chronic skin disease. *Dermatol Ther, 21*(1), 54-59. ISSN: 1396-0296.

Jankovic, S., Raznatovic, M., Marinkovic, J., Maksimovic, N., Jankovic, J., & Djikanovic, B. (2009). Relevance of psychosomatic factors in psoriasis: a case-control study. *Acta Dermato-Venereologica, 89*(4), 364-368. ISSN: 0001-5555.

Jobling, R. (1976). Psoriasisóa preliminary questionnaire study of sufferers' subjective experience. *Clinical and Experimental Dermatology, 1*(3), 233-236. ISSN: 1365-2230.

Judith A. Bahmer, J. K., Friedrich A. Bahmer. (2007). How Do Personality Systems Interact in Patients With Psoriasis, Atopic Dermatitis and Urticaria? *Acta Derm Venereol, 87*, 317-324. ISSN: 0001-5555.

Kilic, A., Gulec, M. Y., Gul, U., & Gulec, H. (2008). Temperament and character profile of patients with psoriasis. *Journal of the European Academy of Dermatology and Venereology, 22*(5), 537-542. ISSN: 1468-3083.

Kim, T. S., Pae, C. U., Jeong, J. T., Kim, S. D., Chung, K. I., & Lee, C. (2006). Temperament and character dimensions in patients with atopic dermatitis. *J Dermatol, 33*(1), 10-15. ISSN: 1346-8138.

Kimball, A. B., Jacobson, C., Weiss, S., Vreeland, M. G., & Wu, Y. (2005). The psychosocial burden of psoriasis. *American journal of clinical dermatology, 6*(6), 383-392. ISSN: 1175-0561.

Kimyai-Asadi, A., & Usman, A. (2001). The role of psychological stress in skin disease. *Journal of Cutaneous Medicine and Surgery: Incorporating Medical and Surgical Dermatology, 5*(2), 140-145. ISSN: 1615-7109.

Kirby, B., Richards, H., Mason, D., Fortune, D., Main, C., & Griffiths, C. (2008). Alcohol consumption and psychological distress in patients with psoriasis. *British Journal of Dermatology, 158*(1), 138-140. ISSN: 1365-2133.

Konuk N., K. R., Atik L., Muhtar S., Atasoy N., Bostanci B. (2007). Psychopathology, depression and dissociative experiences in patients with lichen simplex chronicus. *General Hospital Psychiatry, 29*(3), 232-235. ISSN: 0163-8343.

Krejci-Manwaring, J., Kerchner, K., Feldman, S. R., Rapp, D. A., & Rapp, S. R. (2006). Social Sensitivity and Acne: The Role of Personality in the Integrative Social Consecuences and Quality of Life. *The International Journal of Psychiatry in Medicine, 36*(1), 121-130. ISSN: 0091-2174.

Krueger, G., Koo, J., Lebwohl, M., Menter, A., Stern, R. S., & Rolstad, T. (2001). The impact of psoriasis on quality of life: results of a 1998 National Psoriasis Foundation patient-membership survey. *Archives of Dermatology. Chicago. 137*(3), 280-286. ISSN: 0096-5359.

Laguna, E. V., Pena Payero, M. L., & Marquez, A. V. (2006). Influencia de la ansiedad en diversas patologías dermatológicas. *Actas dermo-sifiliográficas, 97*(10), 637-643. (ISSN: 1138-8196).

Limiñana Gras, R. M., Corbalán Berná, J., & Sánchez López, P. (2009). Thinking Styles and Coping when Caring for a Child with Severe Spina Bifida. *J Dev Phys Disabil, 21,* 169-183. ISSN: 1573-3580.

Lotti T., Buggiani G., & F., P. (2008). Prurigo nodularis and lichen simplex chronicus. *Dermatologic Therapy, 21*(1), 42-46. ISSN: 1529-8019.

Lu, Y., Duller, P., van der Valk, P., & Evers, A. (2003). Helplessness as predictor of perceived stigmatization in patients with psoriasis and atopic dermatitis. *Dermatol Psychosom, 4*(3), 146-150. ISSN: 1424-0564

Madhulika A. Gupta. (2006). Somatization disorders in dermatology. *International Review of Psychiatry, 18*(1), 41-47. ISSN: 1369-1627.

Madhulika A. Gupta, A. K. G. (2006). Medically unexplained cutaneous sensory symptoms may represent somatoform dissociation: an empirical study. *Journal of Psychosomatic Research, 60,* 131-136. ISSN: 0022-3999.

Magin, P., Adams, J., Heading, G., Pond, D., & Smith, W. (2009). The psychological sequelae of psoriasis: results of a qualitative study. *Psychology, Health and Medicine, 14*(2), 150-161. ISSN:1354-8506.

Magin, P., Pond, C., Smith, W., Watson, A., & Goode, S. (2008). A cross-sectional study of psychological morbidity in patients with acne, psoriasis and atopic dermatitis in specialist dermatology and general practices. *J Eur Acad Dermatol Venereol. ISSN*: 1468-3083.

Magin, P., Sibbritt, D., & Bailey, K. (2009). The Relationship Between Psychiatric Illnesses and Skin Disease: A Longitudinal Analysis of Young Australian Women. *Archives of Dermatology, 145*(8), 896. ISSN: 0096-5359.

Malhotra, S., & Mehta, V. (2008). Role of stressful life events in induction or exacerbation of psoriasis and chronic urticaria. *Indian Journal of Dermatology, Venereology, and Leprology, 74*(6), 594. ISSN: 0973-3922.

Mardaga Solange, L. O., Hansenne Michel. (2006). Personality traits modulate skin conductance response to emotional pictures : An investigation with Cloninger's model of personality. *Personality and individual differences, 40*(8), 1603-1614. ISSN: 0191-8869.

Martín-Brufau, R., Corbalán Berná, J., Ramirez Aandreo, A., Brufau Redondo, C., & Limiñana Gras, R. (2010). Personality differences between patients with lichen simplex chronicus and normal population: A study of pruritus. *European Journal of Dermatology, 1*(1). ISSN: 1167-1122.

Mastrolonardo, M., Alicino, D., Zefferino, R., Pasquini, P., & Picardi, A. (2007). Effect of psychological stress on salivary interleukin-1beta in psoriasis. *Arch Med Res, 38*(2), 206-211. ISSN: 0188-0128.

Matusushima, H., Hayashi, S. & Shimada, S. (2003). Skin scratching switches immune responses from Th2 to Th1 type in epicutaneously immunizd mice. *Journal of Dermatological Science, 32*, 223-230. ISSN: 0923-1811.

Matussek, P., Agerer, D., & Seibt, G. (1985). Aggression in depressives and psoriatics. *Psychotherapy and psychosomatics, 43*(3), 120-125. ISSN: 1423-0348.

Melamed, Y., & Yosipovitch, G. (2004). Itching as a focus of mental disturbance. In: *Itch. Basic Mechanisms and Therapy*, 369–375. Informa Healthcare. ISBN-10: 9780824747473.

Mercan, S., Altunay, Ilknur Kivanc, Demir, Basaran, AkpInar, Abdullah and Kayaoglu, Semra. (2008). Sexual Dysfunctions in Patients with Neurodermatitis and Psoriasis. *Journal of Sex & Marital Therapy, 34*(2), 160-168. ISSN: 1521-0715.

Michael G Griffin, P. A. R., Mindy B Mechanic. (1997). Objective Assesment of Peritraumatic Dissociation: Psychophysiological Indicators. *Am J Psychiatry, 154*(8). ISSN: 1535-7228.

Millon, T. (1990). *Toward a new personology: An evolutionary model*. John Wiley & Sons. ISBN-10: 0471515736.

Millon, T. (1999). Reflections on Psychosynergy: A Model for Integratin Science, Theory, Classification, Assesment, and Therapy. *Journal of Personality Assessment, 72*(3), 437-456. ISSN: 1532-7752.

Millon, T. (2001). Mips, inventario de Estilos de Personalidad de Millon, Manual. *Tea Ediciones. ISBN: 8471749939.*

Mine Ozmen, M. O., Ayten Erdogan, Ertugrul H. Aydemir, Oya Oguz. (2006). Dissociative idntity disorder presenting as dermatitis artefacta. *International Journal of Dermatology, 45*, 770-771. *ISSN: 0011-9059.*

Denda, M., Tsychiya, T., Elias, P. M. & Feingold, K. R.. (2000). Stress alters cutaneous permeability barrier homeostasis. *Am J Physiol Regulatory Integrative comp. Physiol, 278*, 367-372. ISSN: 1522-1490.

Morell-Dubois, S., Carpentier, O., Cottencin, O., Queyrel, V., Hachulla, E., Hatron, P.-Y. & Delaporte, E. (2008). Stressful life events and pemphigus. *Dermatology, 216*(2), 104-108.

Nakano, Y. (2004). Stress-induced modulation of skin immune function: to types of antigen-presenting cells in the epidermis are differentially regulated by chronic stress. *British Journal of Dermatology, 151*, 50-64. *ISSN*: 1365-2133.

Ng, W. (2009). Clarifying the relation between neuroticism and positive emotions. *Personality and Individual Differences*. 47(1), 69-72. ISSN 0191-8869.

Niemeier, V., Kupfer, J., Al-Abesie, S., Schill, W. B., & Gieler, U. (1999). From neuropeptides and cytokines to psychotherapy. Skin diseases between psychoneuroimmunology research and psychosomatic treatment. *Forsch Komplementarmed, 6 Suppl 2*, 14-18. ISSN: 1021-7096.

Nijenhuis, E. (2004). Somatoform dissociation: phenomena, measurement and theoretical issues. *New York: WW Norton & Company*. ISBN: 0393704602.

Nijenhuis E.R., Spinhoven, P., Vanderlinden, J., van Dyck, R. & Van der Hart, O. (1998). Somatoform dissociative symptoms as related to animal defensive reactions to predatory imminence and injury. *Journal of Abnormal Psycology, 107*(1), 63-73. ISSN: 0021-843X.

Papadopoulos L. & Walker, C. (2003). Personality, Coping and Sex as Psychosocial Aspects of Psoriatic Arthropathy. *Dermatol Psychosom, 4*(1), 27-32. *ISSN*: 1424-0564.

Paus, R., Schmelz, M., Biró, T. & Steinhoff, M. (2006). Frontiers in pruritus research: scratching the brain for more effective itch therapy. *J. Clin. Invest., 116*, 1174-1185. ISSN: 1558-8238.

Peter-Bob. (2007). Hypnotic abreaction releases chaotic patterns of electrodermal activity during dissociation. *Intl. Journal of Clinical and Experimental Hypnosis, 55*(435-456). ISSN: 0020-7144.

Picardi, A., Abeni, D., Melchi, C., Puddu, P., & Pasquini, P. (2000). Psychiatric morbidity in dermatological outpatients: an issue to be recognized. *British Journal of Dermatology, 143*(5), 983-991. *ISSN*: 1365-2133.

Picardi, A., Mazzotti, E., Gaetano, P., Cattaruzza, M., Baliva, G., Melchi, C., Biondi, M., & Pasquini, P. (2005). Stress, social support, emotional regulation, and exacerbation of diffuse plaque psoriasis. *Psychosomatics.* (Vol. 46, pp. 556-564). ISSN: 1545-7206.

Picardi, A., Pasquini, P., Cattaruzza, M., Gaetano, P., Melchi, C., Baliva, G., Camaioni, D., Tiago, A, Abeni, D. & Biondi, M. (2003). Stressful Life Events, Social Support, Attachment Security and Alexithymia in Vitiligo A Case-Control Study. *Psychother Psychosom, 72*, 150-158. ISSN: 1423-0348.

Picardi, A., Pasquini, P., Cattaruzza, M. S., Gaetano, P., Baliva, G., Melchi, C. F., Tiago, A., Camaioni, D., Abeni, D., & Biondi, M. (2003). Only limited support for a role of psychosomatic factors in psoriasis: Results from a case-control study. *Journal of Psychosomatic Research, 55*(3), 189-196. ISSN: 0022-3999.

Quiroga Romero, E. & Fuentes Ortega, J. B. (2003). El significado psicológico y metapsicológico de los Modelos Biosocial y Evolucionista de Theodore Millon. *Psicothema, 15*(2), 190-196. ISSN: 1886-144X.

Rabung, S., Ubbelohde, A., Kiefer, E., & Schauenburg, H. (2004). [Attachment security and quality of life in atopic dermatitis]. *Psychother Psychosom Med Psychol, 54*(8), 330-338. ISSN: 0173-7937.

Radmanesh, M., & Shafiei, S. (2001). Underlying Psychopathologies of Psychogenic Pruritic Disorders. *Dermatology and Psychosomatics, 2*, 130-133. *ISSN*: 1424-0564.

Richards, H., & Fortune, D. (2006). Psychological distress and adherence in patients with psoriasis. *Journal of the European Academy of Dermatology and Venereology, 20*(s2), 33-41. *ISSN*: 1468-3083

Richards, H., Fortune, D., Griffiths, C., & Main, C. (2005). Alexithymia in patients with psoriasis Clinical correlates and psychometric properties of the Toronto Alexithymia Scale-20. *Journal of Psychosomatic Research, 58*(1), 89-96. ISSN: 0022-3999.

Richards, H., Ray, D., Kirby, B., Mason, D., Plant, D., Main, C., Fortune, D. G. & Griffiths, C.E.M. (2005). Response of the hypothalamic-pituitary-adrenal axis to psychological stress in patients with psoriasis. *British Journal of Dermatology, 153*(6), 1114-1120. *ISSN*: 1365-2133.

Richards, H. L., Fortune, D. G., Griffiths, C. E. M., & Main, C. J. (2001). The contribution of perceptions of stigmatisation to disability in patients with psoriasis. *Journal of Psychosomatic Research, 50*(1), 11-15. ISSN: 0022-3999.

Robles, T. F. (2007). Stress, Social Support, and Delayed Skin Barrier Recovery. *Psychosomatic Medicine, 69*(8), 807-815.

Russo, P. A. J., Ilchef, R., & Cooper, A. J. (2004). Psychiatric morbidity in psoriasis: a review. *Australasian journal of dermatology, 45*(3), 155-161. ISSN: 1440-0960.

Schmid-Ott, G., Künsebeck, H. W., Jäger, B., Sittig, U., Hofste, N., Ott, R., Malewski, P. & Lamprecht, F. (2005). Significance of the stigmatization experience of psoriasis patients: a 1-year follow-up of the illness and its psychosocial consequences in men and women. *Acta Dermato-Venereologica, 85*(1), 27-32. ISSN: 0001-5555

Schneider, G., Driesch, G., Heuft, G., Evers, S., Luger, T. A., & Stander, S. (2006). Psychosomatic cofactors and psychiatric comorbidity in patients with chronic itch. *Clinical dermatology, 31*(6), 762-767. ISSN: 15075516.

Shafii, M., & Shafii, S. (1979). Exploratory psychotherapy in the treatment of psoriasis. Twelve hundred years ago. *Archives of general psychiatry, 36*(11), 1242. ISSN: 0003990X.

Solomon, G. F. (2001). Psiconeuroinmunología: Sinopsis de su Historia, Evidencia y Consecuencias. Interpsiquis. (In press).

Torello Lotti, Bianchi, B. & Ilaria Ghersetich. (2002). Can the brain inhibit inflammation generated in the skin? The lesson of alfa-malonocyte-stimulating hormone. *Journal of Dermatology, 41*, 311-318. *ISSN*: 1346-8138.

Ulnik, J. C. (2007). *Skin in Psychoanalysis*: Karnac Books. ISBN 10: 1855755165.

Ulnik, J. C. (2004). *Distancias Afectivas en Pacientes con Psoriasis*. Granada: Universidad de Granada.

Valverde, J., Mestanza, M., & Asenjo, C. (2005). Psoriasis relacionada a vulnerabilidad psiquiátrica. *Folia Dermatol, 16*(3), 119-122. *ISSN* 1609-7254.

Van Voorhees, A., & Fried, R. (2009). Depression and quality of life in psoriasis. *Postgraduate medicine, 121*(4), 154. ISSN: 0032-5481.

Verhoeven, E. W. M., De Klerk, S., Kraaimaat, F. W., Van De Kerkhof, P., De Jong, E., & Evers, A. W. M. (2008). Biopsychosocial Mechanisms of Chronic Itch in Patients with Skin Diseases: a Review. *Acta Dermato-Venereologica, 88*(3), 211-218. ISSN: 0001-5555.

Verhoeven, E. W. M., Kraaimaat, F. W., de Jong, E. M. G. J., Schalkwijk, J., van de Kerkhof, P. C. M., & Evers, A. W. M. (2009). Effect of daily stressors on psoriasis: a prospective study. *Journal of Investigative Dermatology, 129*(8), 2075-2077. ISSN: 0022-202X.

Vileikyte, L. (2007). Stress and wound healing. *Clinics in Dermatology, 25*(1), 49-55. ISSN: 0738-081X.

Willemsen, R., Roseeuw, D., & Vanderlinden, J. (2008). Alexithymia and dermatology: the state of the art. *Int J Dermatol, 47*(9), 903-910.

Wittkower, E. D., & Russell, B. (1953). *Emotional factors in skin disease*: PB Hocher. ASIN: B001VGNE7I.

Woodruff, P., Higgins, E., Du Vivier, A., & Wessely, S. (1997). Psychiatric illness in patients referred to a dermatology-psychiatry clinic. *General hospital psychiatry, 19*(1), 29-35. *ISSN*: 0163-8343.

Wright, R. J., Cohen, R. T., & Cohen, S. (2005). The impact of stress on the development and expression of atopy. *Current Opinion in Allergy and Clinical Immunology, 5*(1), 23. *ISSN*:1528-4050.

Yazici A. C., Basterzi, A., Acar, S. T., Ustunsoy, D., Ikizoglu, G., Demirseren, D. & Kanik, A. (2006). Alopecia areata and alexithymia. *Turk Psikiyatri Derg, 17*(2), 101-106. *ISSN*:1300-2163.

Yosipovitch, G., & Samuel, L. (2008). Neuropathic and psychogenic itch. *Dermatologic Therapy, 21*(1), 32-41. ISSN: 1529-8019.

Part 3

Treatment

12

The Role of Immune Response and the Impact of Biological Drugs in Psoriasis Patients

Amedeo Amedei and Mario Milco D'Elios
University of Florence
Italy

1. Introduction

Psoriasis is a chronic immune-mediated skin disease with a intricate pathogenesis and a strong genetic background (Nickoloff et al., 2007a), that affects approximately 1-3% of the worldwide population, with an equal sex distribution (Stern et al., 2004). The main type of psoriasis is chronic plaque psoriasis (Cpp) accounting for approximately 85-90% of all cases. The Cpp is characterized by erythematous scaly plaques, usually on elbows, knees, scalp and buttocks. Plaque size can diverge from minimal to the involvement of the entire skin surface (erythrodermic psoriasis) (C. E. Griffiths et al., 2007; Nestle et al., 2009). Other forms of psoriasis comprise guttate psoriasis, inverse, palmoplantar and generalized pustular psoriasis (C. E. Griffiths & Barker, 2007; Nestle et al., 2009).

The concept of psoriasis as "the disease of healthy people" has long been surpassed, nowadays we know that during the time course of this disease, as a consequence of dysregulated immunity and ensuing inflammation, certain conditions may appear at somewhat unpredictable time points in a progressive fashion; these so-called co-morbidities, although targeting different organs, share common pathogenetic factors. They often become manifest years after the onset of skin manifestations and are often observed in severe forms of psoriasis.

Psoriatic Arthritis (PsA) is traditionally included among common co-morbidities, even if it should be rather considered a component of the clinical spectrum of psoriatic disease. PsA involves peripheral joints, the axial skeleton, sacroiliac joints, nails and enthuses, and is frequently associated with psoriatic skin lesions. The prevalence of PsA ranges from 5 to 40% among psoriatic patients lesions (D. D. Gladman, 2009; Nograles et al., 2009).

Recently, co-morbidities like cardiovascular disease, obesity and metabolic syndrome have been found to be associated with psoriasis, raising the idea that psoriasis might not be only a skin disorder (Gerdes & Mrowietz, 2009; Kimball et al., 2008a; Menter et al., 2008).

Psoriasis patients suffer also from considerable psychological and financial burdens resulting in a significantly impaired quality of life (Rapp, et al., 1999); likewise traditional systemic psoriasis therapies (methotrexate [MTX], cyclosporin A, retinoids or PUVA therapy) have a potential for long-term toxicity and cannot always provide plenty disease improvement (Pathirana et al., 2009; Smith et al., 2009). Thus, the development of agents efficiently targeting key steps in the pathogenesis of psoriasis and co-morbidities is clearly an important goal.

2. Pathogenesis

Psoriasis is thought to be a complex condition resultant by a combination of genetic and environmental factors. The acute forms of psoriasis, guttate and generalized pustular psoriasis (von Zumbusch psoriasis), are both associated with infections (typically b-haemolytic streptococcal or a viral infection). Other triggering factors which may elicit psoriasis in predisposed individuals include trauma (Koebner phenomen) (Eyre & G. G. Krueger, 1984), HIV infection (Reveille et al., 1990), psychogenic stress (Gupta et al., 1989) and definite drugs (e.g. lithium, beta-blockers, interferons and high dose corticosteroids) (Abel et al., 1986).

Histological examination of psoriatic plaques reveals hyperproliferation of keratinocytes (Kcs) with parakeratosis, increased angiogenesis and dermal infiltration of immune cells, predominantly T cells, neutrophils, macrophages and dendritic cells (DCs) (**Figure 1**) (Nestle et al., 2009; Nickoloff et al. 2007b).

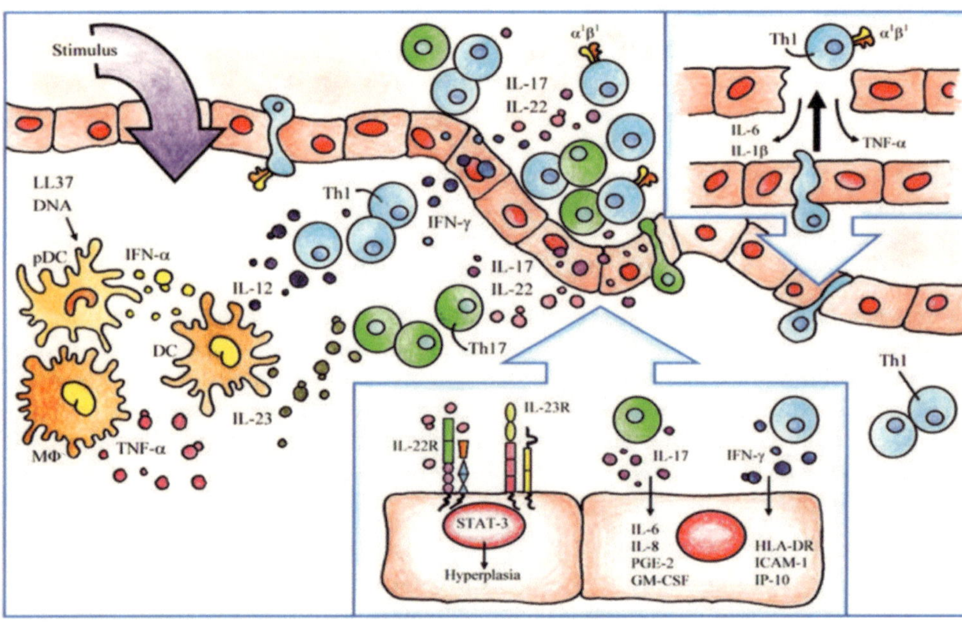

Fig. 1. Psoriatic skin lesions evolution. Different stimuli (e.g. infections, etc.) can trigger an initial episode of psoriasis in genetically predisposed individuals. After starting, the earliest events driving the inflammatory eruption are the secretion of INF-α from pDCs (plasmacytoid dendritic cells) and the production of TNF-α by immune cells of both innate and adaptive response. Large amounts of IFN-α induce activation of the local immune effector cells that secrete pro-inflammatory cytokines. TNF-α is a very active cytokine of the inflammatory infiltrate and is principally secreted by activated macrophages (MΦ), dermal DCs, keratinocytes and T cells. The elevated levels of TNF-α lead to the maturation of DCs into forceful APCs (antigen presenting cells) and, with other cytokines, up-regulates the expression of endothelial E-selectin and ICAM-1 attracting further CLA+ T cells in the skin. Also, the panel of cytokines released by T cells contributes to the stimulation of epidermal keratinocytes and is at least, in some measure, responsible for typical psoriasis skin changes. They induce the expression of ICAM-1, CD40 and MHC-II and trigger keratinocyte hyper-proliferation.

The increased dermis vascularity is driven by angiogenic factors, such as VEGF (vascular endothelial growth factor), highly present in psoriasis plaques (Detmar et al., 1994). Also, the interaction between VEGF and the angiopoietin/Tie signaling pathway is modulated by TNF-a (Tumour necrosis factor-a), that together with interleukin 12 (IL-12) and IL-23 are well known to be crucial immunological mediators in psoriasis. (Holash et al., 1999; Kuroda et al., 2001). Whereas IL-12 induces Th1 (T helper 1) differentiation and thus increases the production of TNF-a, IL-23 stimulates primarily Th17 cells, which secrete most importantly pro-inflammatory cytokines such as IL-17 and IL-22 (Nestle et al., 2009; Toichi et al., 2006; Torti & Feldman, 2007).

Increased concentrations of TNF-a and IL-12/IL-23 have been found as in psoriatic skin (Nestle et al., 2009) as in the synovial fluid and tissue of patients with PsA (FitzGerald & Winchester , 2009; Ritchlin et al, 1998). Their role in psoriasis genesis is highlighted by the successful treatment of psoriasis by agents blocking these cytokines (Boker et al., 2007; Mössner et al., 2008; Scalon et al., 2009). In addition, polymorphisms of IL-23 receptor gene and gene encoding the shared p40 subunit of IL-12 and IL-23 have been linked to psoriasis development (Elder et al., 2010; Hüffmaier et al., 2009; Nestle et al., 2009).

3. Genetics of psoriasis

Family studies have shown that psoriasis has a strong genetic component although the inheritance pattern is still unclear. 71 % of patients with childhood psoriasis have a positive family history (Morris et al., 2001) and analysis of concordance rates in twin studies show a threefold increased risk of psoriasis in monozygotic twins compared to dizygotic twins (Brandrup et al., 1978; Pisani & Ruocco, 1984).

At least ten chromosomal loci have been identified showing statistically significant evidence for linkage to psoriasis (PSORS 1-10). However, the only region that has consistently been identified in genetic screens of families with psoriasis is the major-histocompatibility complex (MHC) region on chromosome 6 named PSORS1 (Capon et al., 2008; Nair et al., 2006), that is responsible for up to 50 % of genetic susceptibility to psoriasis. Within PSORS1 the human leukocyte antigen-C (HLA-C) gene which is the strongest candidate gene for psoriasis , precisely its allele HLACw6 (HLA-Cw*0602) the predominant risk allele (Nair et al., 2006): individuals with this allele have a 10-20-fold increased risk of developing psoriasis (Mallon et al., 1999).

HLA-Cw6 positive and negative psoriasis patients may exhibit distinctive clinical phenotypes (Henseler & Christophers, 1985): guttate psoriasis is mostly confined to HLA-Cw6$^+$ patients meanwhile psoriatic nail disease, palmoplantar pustulosis and psoriatic arthritis are more common in HLA-Cw6$^-$ patients (Fan et al., 2007; Gudjonsson et al., 2006). Furthermore, partial or total remission during pregnancy is much more frequent in HLA-Cw*0602$^+$ women (Gudjonsson et al., 2006).

Despite this strong association, the functional role of HLA-Cw6 remains unknown; as far as we know HLACw6 may exert its effect through the specific or the innate immune system (Figure 2): HLA-Cw6 may act via the adaptive immune system by its antigen presenting capacity and the fact that guttate psoriasis (sturdily associated with HLA-Cw6) is triggered by streptococcal pharyngitis (J. C. Prinz, 2001), supports this hypothesis. HLA-Cw6 may also exert an innate immune response via its interaction with KIRs (killer immunoglobulin-like receptors) of natural killer (NK) and natural killer T (NKT) cells, which are implicated, in psoriasis pathogenesis (Nickoloff, 1999a). KIRs recognize different types of HLA-C molecules leading to either an overall activating or inhibitory immune response. KIRs have been associated with psoriasis and PsA (Martin et al., 2002). HLA-Cw6 is a natural ligand for KIR2DL1 (an inhibitory receptor) and it is possible that interaction between HLA-Cw6 and PaKIR2DL1 would lead to aberrant function of lymphoid cells in psoriasis pathogenesis.

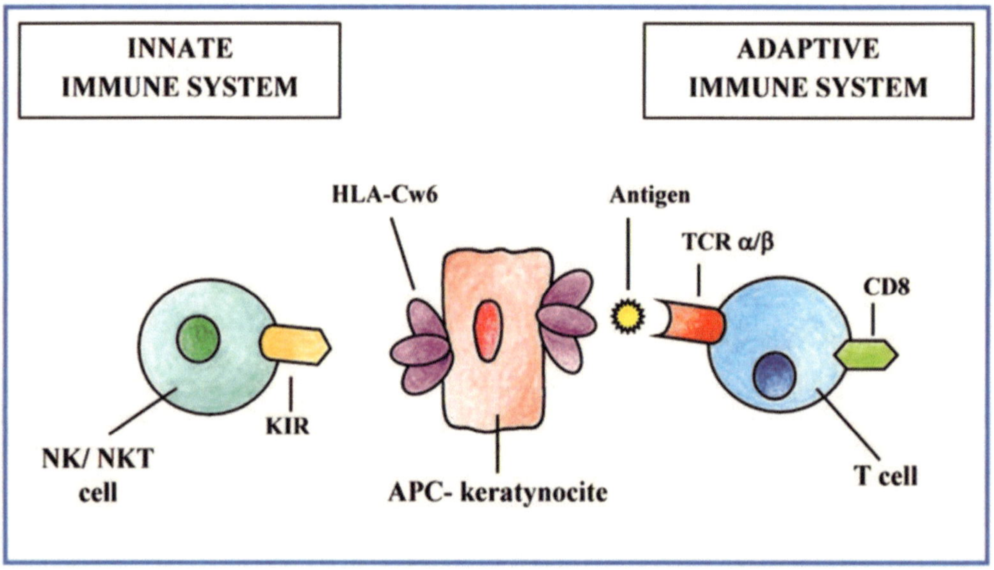

Fig. 2. Hypothetical regulating role of HLA-Cw6 in both specific and innate immune responses.

HLA-Cw6 expressed on APCs can trigger specific immune responses by presentation of processed antigen to the TCR of CD8+ T cells. Also, innate immune response can be elicited by interaction of HLA-Cw6 with its natural Killer immunoglobulin-like receptors expressed on NK and NKT cells.

A new psoriasis susceptibility gene ZNF313/RNF114, which may regulate T cell activation through ubiquitin ligase activity, has been identified (Capon et al., 2008). All these data further supports the concept that multiple gene products share a role in the immune regulation of psoriasis, contributing to disease pathogenesis.

4. Immune response

Although the initial event triggering a psoriatic lesion is still unknown many factors have been shown to play a role in the pathogenesis of psoriasis: physical trauma, infections, stress, drugs, alcohol and smoking can all trigger an initial episode of psoriasis in individuals with genetic predisposition (Bowcock & J. G. Krueger, 2005).

This initial trigger activates dendritic cells, favoring their migration to skin-draining lymph nodes, where antigen-specific T cells (primed by DCs) differentiate into effector T cells, which then traffic to the skin where they induce - in concert with other cells, especially dermal DCs - the creation of a primary psoriatic plaque. During this step some T cells and DCs start to infiltrate the epidermis, where stimulating KCs support the typical epidermal changes (Bowcock & J. G. Krueger, 2005).

Epidermal keratinocytes are able to recruit and activate T cells and most T cells infiltrating psoriatic skin are divided into Th1 ($CD4^+$) and T cytotoxic 1 (Tc1; $CD8^+$) subsets (J. G. Krueger, 2002). Two further T cell subtypes, Th17 cells (McKenzie et al., 2006) and regulatory T cells (Treg) (Sugiyama et al, 2005) have been identified as important contributors to the pathogenesis of autoimmune diseases such as psoriasis (**Figure 3**).

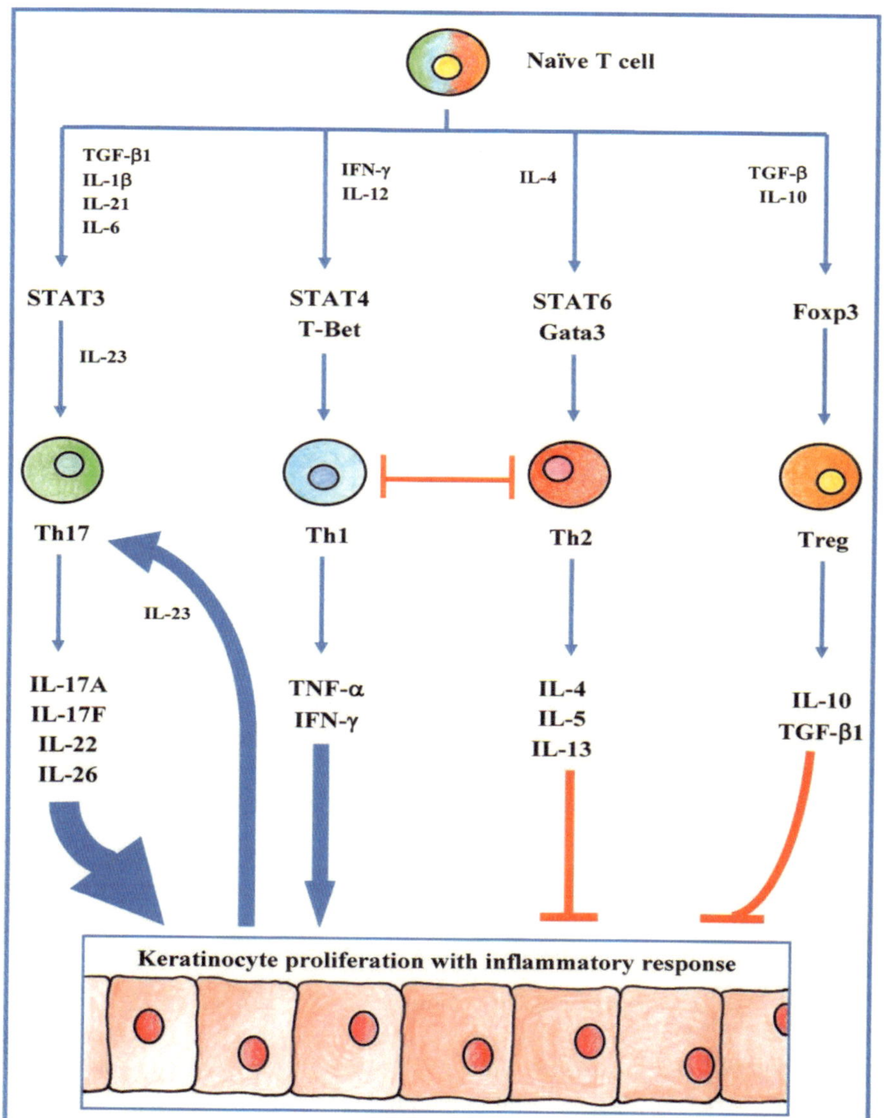

Fig. 3. Role of CD4 T cell subtypes in psoriasis.

Th1 and Th17 pro-inflammatory cytokines mediate keratinocyte hyperproliferation and trigger a 'vicious cycle' of inflammation. IL-23 secreted principally by keratinocytes, dendritic cells and macrophages is critical for maintenance of Th17 function. Low levels of anti-inflammatory cytokines released by Th2 and Tregs potentially counteract but cannot balance the effects of Th1/Th17 cytokines.

From the foregoing it is clear that the contribution of both innate and adaptive immune responses are important in mediating the inflammatory psoriasis cascade (Gaspari, 2006) (**Figure 1**).

4.1 Aberrant activation of the innate fraction of the skin immune system

The present knowledge of the possible role of innate immunity cells (Kcs, Dcs, neutrophils, macrophages, NK and NKT cells) in psoriasis will be discussed.

4.1.1 Keratinocytes in psoriasis

Over the last 20 years it has been regularly discussed if psoriatic skin lesions arise from a primary alteration in epidermal keratinocytes or in T cells (**Figure 1**); the current view is that infiltrating T cells initiate and maintain psoriasis. In this vision, cytokines (e.g., IL-1, IL-6 and IFN-γ) secreted by T cells and other inflammatory cells (DCs, macrophages and neutrophils) would trigger KCs hyperproliferation, inducing epidermal hyperplasia (J. G. Krueger, 2002). In particular, IL-23, whose expression is increased in psoriatic lesion (Piskin et al., 2006), has been implied in the development of epidermal acanthosis, most likely through the induction of IL-22 (Zheng et al., 2007); injection of IL-23 into mouse dermis induces as dermal inflammation as epidermal hyperplasia similarly to features seen in psoriasis (J. R. Chan et al., 2006).

Previous studies (J. G. Krueger, 2002) suggested an additional explanation for the chronic epidermal hyperplasia in psoriatic lesions: the migration of T cells in the epidermis would firstly break the basement membrane, which has been shown to have large areas with reduced staining intensity for collagen IV and laminins (Fleischmajer et al., 2000), and secondly disrupt desmosome connection between KCs. These two events could be interpreted by KCs as an injury and therefore induce a wound repair response. As a consequence many mitogenic cytokines would be released by KCs triggering a regenerative epidermal growth. Hence, T cells in psoriatic epidermis would be responsible for the chronic hyperplasia as by releasing pro-inflammatory cytokines as by disrupting epidermal integrity.

Another evidence against the fundamental role of T cells in psoriasis arise from the observation that HIV^+ patients (which usually have reduced number of $CD4^+$ T cells) develop psoriasis with similar frequency as the rest of the population (Namazi, 2004).

Finally, in 2005 Zenz et al. reported an interesting animal model with psoriasis-like features (Zenz et al., 2005); They knocked out JunB and c-Jun, two components of the AP-1 transcription factor, which control cell proliferation and differentiation , cytokine production, and stress responses in the skin. The importance of this animal model lies in the fact that JunB is located in the PSORS6 locus, which has been shown to be a psoriasis susceptibility region (Hensen et al., 2003). Interestingly, these mice developed not only inflammatory skin lesions but also a form of destructive arthritis. This evidence suggested that alteration in the epidermal Jun-pathway may be sufficient to induce inflammatory reactions in the skin as well as in the joints. At the skin level these mice showed typical hallmarks of psoriasis: hyperkeratosis, enlarged blood vessels, infiltration of T cells and neutrophils, and up-regulation of pro-inflammatory cytokines.

The most intriguing aspect was the examination of the T cells role in development of psoriasis in a genetic model: upon deletion of JunB and c-Jun proteins in Rag2-deficient mice (mice deficient of T/B cells), skin changes like in psoriasis were still induced, though they were milder. These data suggest a minor role for T cells in the etiology of psoriasis-form skin inflammation, and that primary alterations in KCs were sufficient to drive psoriasis-form changes in the mice skin. But before stating that KCs instigate psoriasis in humans, the relevance of this model must be discussed further. A recent study (Haider et al., 2006) showed that the JunBwas expression increased in psoriatic plaques instead of decreased/deleted as in the Zenz mouse model, suggesting a role for JunB as a transcriptional activator of disease-related genes in psoriatic KCs.

The ongoing discussion about the primary instigator of psoriasis reflects the complexity of this disease and the still elusive interplay between KCs and immune cells in driving psoriasis.

This problem was further addressed in a another mouse model, in which STAT-3 was constitutively activated in basal KCs under the control of the keratin 5 promoter (K5.Stat3C) (Sano et al., 2005). As in human psoriatic plaques, induced lesions of K5.Stat3C mice shown a considerable number of $CD4^+$ T and $CD8^+$ T cells in the epidermis. For psoriasis development, this model required both activated STAT-3 in KCs and activated T cells in the dermis and epidermis of the transgenic rodents, suggesting the theory that KCs and T cells could act together in psoriasis pathogenesis.

4.1.2 Neutrophilic granulocytes

Early studies in psoriasis (Jablonska, 1986), in which the initial (pre-pinpoint) lesions were studied histologically,indicated that the primary abnormality in a developing lesion of psoriasis is the perivascular accumulation of neutrophils as well as their epidermis invasion (Kogoj phenomenon). Next, these neutrophils accumulations lead to microscopically detectable microabscesses (Munro abscesses). In many patients with psoriasis, these micropustules may enlarge and become clinically visible as sterile 2–3-mm pustules. In some patients, pustules are the primary visible abnormality, often on an erythematous base.

The presence of neutrophils must be important for the formation of psoriatic skin lesions, in fact agranulocytosis has been reported to result in the remission of psoriasis (Toichi et al., 2000). Next, neutrophils can contribute to the hyperproliferation of keratinocytes by the effects of human leucocyte-derived elastase (Rogalski et al., 2002).

4.1.3 Natural killer T cells

The potential role of cells expressing NK receptors in psoriatic skin was firstly proposed by Nickoloff (Nickoloff et al., 1999b); in further experiments, he showed that a CD94+/CD161+ NKT cell line (isolated from a psoriatic patient) injected in prepsoriatic skin of a SCID mouse, gave rise to creation of psoriatic plaque characterized by diffuse keratinocyte expression of CD1d, CD161+ T cells infiltration and marked presence of mRNA for IFN-c and IL-15 (Nickoloff et al., 2000).

In line with these data, it seems that constitutive CD1d expression on prepsoriatic skin keratinocytes represents a primary prerequisite that ensures their contact with the CD161 molecule on NKT cells. This interaction might also represent one of the critical events in the triggering of psoriasis as CD1d-bearing keratinocytes can present endogenous (self) or exogenous (bacterial, viral) glycolipids to NKT-cells. Consequently to the recognition of glycolipid antigens, NKT cells produce large amounts of IFN-c which induces stronger keratinocyte expression of CD1d; in this way the pathogenic mechanism of psoriatic plaques is not only initiated but also maintained.

Numerous studies have addressed the issue of NKT cells in the lesional skin of psoriasis patients and a constant result evidenced by independent groups of investigators is that CD161+ T cells appear in greater numbers in lesional skin of patients with psoriasis than in normal healthy skin and/or prepsoriatic skin (Bonish et al., 2000; Cameron et al., 2002; Curry et al., 2003; Vissers et al., 2004a).

However, Curry group shown a greater frequency of CD161+ T cells yet in the prepsoriatic skin in comparison with the normal skin, suggesting that certain immune response dysregulations exists in the uninvolved skin and creates a milieu, promoting the psoriatic lesions onset (Curry et al., 2003).

A flow cytometric analysis of psoriatic tissue-infiltrating T cell demonstrated the presence of CD3+ cells expressing also CD16, CD56, CD158b, CD94 or NKG2A and CD4-CD8-, the majority of these is a subset of NKT cells (Liao et al., 2006). In addiction a recent study (Zhao et al., 2008) confirmed that NKT cells as well as CD1d molecules were increased within psoriatic skin.

The supposed pathogenic role of NKT cells in psoriasis is also supported by the effects of different pharmacological treatments, that decreases NKT cell numbers in psoriatic plaques, in particular the clinical efficacy of betamethasone dipropionate (Bovenschen et al., 2007; Vissers et al., 2004b, 2008;) and similarly of alefacept that induce an improvement in plaque severity accompanied by significant reductions of dermal CD94+ and CD161+ (Bovenschen et al., 2007).

In general, these data strongly indicate that lesional CD94+ and CD161+ NKT cells actively participate in the development and/or maintenance of psoriatic lesions, but the relative relevance of each of these subsets remains elusive. However, it might be hypothesized that epidermal NKT cells play a major pathogenic role due to their direct interaction with CD1d+ keratinocytes and the resulting hyperproliferation while the dermal component of NKT cells participates in the immune response through the interaction with CD1d-bearing dermal dendritic cells and monocytes.

Likewise other Th1-mediated autoimmune diseases, psoriasis is associated with decreased numbers of circulating NKT cells (Cameron et al., 2003; Koreck et al., 2002; van der Vliet et al., 2001;); Koreck reported that decreased percentage of NKT cells population in blood of psoriasis patients tended to be even lower in those with frequently relapsing (Koreck et al., 2002). Moreover, different systemic therapy regimens resulted in the recovery of these cells, but their percentage remained significantly lower in comparison with healthy control subjects. In contrast, Langewouters group showed that the number of circulating CD94+ an CD161+ cells was significantly higher in patients with moderate-to-severe as compared to patients with mild psoriasis (Langewouters et al., 2008). It has been also reported that circulating CD161+ NKT cells in people with severe psoriasis belong to Th1 cells (W. L. Chan et al., 2003) and that treatment with alefacept or efalizumab causes significant reduction in their number (Larsen et al., 2007; van Lingen et al., 2008). These observations imply that distinct subsets of NKT cells differentially regulate immune responses and that their relative imbalance might be of importance in the psoriasis pathogenesis, but the precise impact of these findings remains unclear.

4.1.4 Accessory cells (Dendritic cells and macrophages)

DCs are involved in the development of tolerance (Steinman et al., 2003) and are the unique professional antigen-presenting able to take up antigen in the tissue they reside in and to migrate to the draining lymph nodes; here activate naive T cells, generating specific T-cell responses (Teunissen, 2005).

In the peripheral tissues DCs receive all kinds of microenvironment signals, that influence the their maturation process, determining the phenotype and function of mature DCs and their type 1 /type 2 polarizing potential. In case of risk (e.g. infection, cancer), DCs will transform into strong stimulatory antigen presenting cells, whereas under non pathological steady-state conditions DCs do not reach full maturation and they will present self-peptides /MHC complexes in the presence of insufficient costimulatory molecules, inducing T-cell anergy or expansion of regulatory T cells (peripheral tolerance). If this delicate balance of immune reactivity vs. tolerance is broken, chronic inflammatory diseases, like psoriasis, may develop.

In the absence of pathogenic substances, stress signals from neighbouring cells (e.g. necrotic cells) can activate DCs enabling them to stimulate naive T cells (Gallucci et al., 1999). In relation to this, Krueger has expressed an remarkable view concerning traumatic injuries (breaches in the basement membrane and disruption of desmosome connections between adjacent keratinocytes) caused by migrating T cells and DCs in the epidermis, that are possibly involved in the development of psoriasis lesions (J. G. Krueger, 2002). Keratinocytes will respond to these defects by overproduction of cytokines, among others TNF-a, a key cytokine to induce DC migration/maturation.

Another exciting point to mention is the observation that DC development is also affected by mutual interaction with NKT cells (Taniguchi et al., 2003): weak responses by NKT cells to glycolipid /CD1d complexes can be enhanced by DC-derived IL-12, resulting in up-expression of IFN-c by NK T cells. This interaction may be relevant in psoriasis.

DCs are numerous in the dermal part of psoriasis skin and many of them exhibit an activated phenotype (CD80+, CD83+, CD86+ and DC-LAMP+) (Abrams et al., 2000; Teunissen, 2005) and may be an important source of TNF-a (Nickoloff et al., 1991; Zhou et al., 2003).

Recent evidences from different genetic mouse models show that also the macrophages can contribute to T-cell-mediated and epidermis-mediated psoriasis-form skin inflammation and in particular the data from the CD18hypo PL/J psoriasis mouse model demonstrate (Wang et al., 2009) that the psoriasis-form inflammatory skin disorder critically depends on an appropriate activation of macrophages, with ample release of TNF-a.

In human psoriasis, the number of epithelium-lining macrophages was reported to increase in lesional skin. These macrophages can play a role in the regulation of epidermal proliferation and differentiation (van den Oord & de Wolf-Peeters, 1994); also vigorous interactions between macrophages and keratinocytes (Djemadji-Oudjiel et al., 1996) may be involved in the psoriasis pathogenesis (van den Oord & de Wolf-Peeters, 1994).

Macrophages, under different conditions, secrete various pro-inflammatory cytokines: TNF-α, IL-1b, IFN-α/β, IL-6, IL-10, IL-12, and IL-18, (Willment et al., 2003) and notably, in a recent study $CD68^+$ macrophages were identified as important TNF-α source in human psoriasis and upon treatment with anti-TNF-α antibody macrophage levels decreased in the plaque psoriasis, with clinical psoriasis resolution (Marble et al., 2007). In according to this finding, it is also showed that $CD68^+$ macrophages as important TNF-α source in human psoriatic skin, which had distinctly decreased number and TNF-α concentration following bath-PUVA therapy (Wang et al., 2009). This was also found in a T-cell-independent mouse model, with an increase of TNF-α in macrophages (Stratis et al., 2006).

Based on literature data, an emerging model of psoriasis pathogenesis in humans suggests that dermal macrophages, activated by T-cell cytokines, produce large amounts of TNF-α, leading to skin changes (Clark & Kupper, 2006).

4.2 Dysfunction of the adaptive immune response cells

Until the 1990s, psoriasis was thought to be a disease of disordered keratinoctye proliferation and differentiation (G. G. Krueger et al., 1984) and epidermal hyperplasia was the most prominent clinical and histological feature. For this reason, the old psoriasis treatments using antimetabolites including methotrexate which limit epidermal hyperproliferation. However, successive evidence from clinical studies and, experimental models support the theory that psoriasis is a T cell-mediated inflammatory skin disease (Lew et al., 2004) affecting genetically predisposed individuals and the epidermal hyperplasia is an effect of cellular immune infiltration.

4.2.1 Role of T cells

The first evidence resulting in psoriasis being widely considered as a T cell mediated autoimmune disease came from the success in the psoriasis treatment of T cell-targeted therapies such as cyclosporine (Baker et al., 1987), tacrolimus (Jegasothy et al., 1992) or CD4-specific monoclonal antibodies (Moabs) (J. Prinz et al., 1991).

A pivotal study involved the testing of IL-2-diphtheria-toxin fusion protein in psoriasis patients (S. L. Gottlieb et al., 1995). This agent selectively depleting activated T cells that express IL-2 receptors from psoriasis skin lesions and resulted in clinical remission of psoriasis vulgaris.

Subsequently, administration of another fusion protein, cytotoxic T-lymphocyte antigen 4 (CTLA4)-antibody, was shown to reverse the clinical and cellular features of psoriasis

(Abrams et al., 1999). This agent blocks T cell co-stimulation mediated by DCs without directly deplete T cells. Its effectiveness indicated that continuing T cell co-stimulation is required to sustain psoriasis disease activity, including the excessive infiltration of T cells and DCs into the skin (Abrams et al., 2000). All these clinical results confirmed that lesion-associated T cells are central to sustaining disease activity in psoriasis.

Additional evidence highlighting the implication of T cells in psoriasis pathogenesis have been reviewed (Nestle et al., 2009) including the appearance of clonal T cells in psoriatic lesions (Menssen et al., 1995); the development of psoriasis-form phenotype within symptomless psoriatic skin after transplantion onto the xenotransplantation AGR 129 mouse model again underlines the importance of epidermal T cells in psoriasis genesis (Conrad et al., 2007).

Also, based on the findings that expansion of skin resident T cells is important in psoriasis progress in the xenotransplantation AGR mouse model, the function of tissue-specific factors in activation and expansion of resident T cells has been further explored (Conrad et al., 2007). T cells need to pass through the dermo-epidermal junction in order to go into the epidermis and collagen fibrils are an essential part of the dermo-epidermal junction. The most important basement membrane collagen is collagen IV and long-term activation of T cells results in the expression of a receptor for collagen IV, the heterodimeric integrin $\alpha1\beta1$. It has been shown that epidermal accumulation of $\alpha1\beta1^+$ Th1 and Tc1 cells correlate with psoriasis development. Blocking $\alpha1\beta1$ with a neutralizing Moab prevents epidermal T cell accumulation and subsequent psoriasis development in the xenotransplantation AGR mouse model. $\alpha1\beta1$ expression can act as a checkpoint for entry of T cells into epidermis with $\alpha1\beta1^+$ epidermal T cells potentially playing an important role in psoriatic lesion formation.

In conclusion, targeting of these integrins may offer new and effective therapeutic approaches in psoriasis.

4.2.2 The IL-23/Th17 pathway

The IL-23/Th17 pathway is an exciting area in psoriatic pathology (**Figure1**) because it has led to the development of promising innovative treatments which specifically target this pathway (D'Elios et al., 2010). The development, characterization and function of Th17 cells and the role of IL-23 in Th17-cell dependent chronic inflammation in psoriasis have been recently reviewed (Di Cesare et al., 2009). Briefly, IL-23 is a heterodimeric cytokine (Oppmann et al., 2000) composed of the subunits IL-23p19 and IL-12p40 (an IL-12 subunit). Intradermal injection of IL-23 in mice resulted in the development of a psoriasis-form phenotype with histopathological features (Chan et al., 2006). IL-23 can mediate epidermal hyperplasia, acanthosis, hyperparakeratosis and orthohyperkeratosis by way of TNF-α, IL-20R2 and IL-22 (Chan et al., 2006; Zheng et al., 2007). These data are supported by findings in humans including an mRNA over-expression of IL-23p19 and IL-12p40 seen in psoriatic skin lesions, compared to uninvolved skin. Further other results indicate that IL -23 production occurs at inflammatory skin sites and is mediated by tissue-resident and/or recruited immune cells, such DCs and KCs (Piskin et al., 2006).

The pathogenic role of IL-23 in psoriasis is strongly supported by the clinical findings that anti-TNF-α agents can reduce IL-23p19 and IL-12p40 mRNA levels also the reduction of IL-

23 level caused by cyclosporin A, UV therapy and biological agents correlates to clinical improvements in psoriasis patients (A. L. Gottlieb et al., 2005; Haider et al., 2008; Piskin et al., 2004).

Transforming growth factor (TGF)-β1, IL-6 and IL-21 are all required to transform naïve T cells into cells expressing the unique lineage-specific transcription factor, RORC variant 2 and IL-23 receptors with subsequent binding of IL-23 resulting in differentiation into Th17 cells.

Th17 cells in turn produce the pro-inflammatory cytokines IL-17A, IL-17F, IL-22 and IL-26 (Langrish et al., 2005) that activate KCs leading to hyperproliferation and production of proinflammatory cytokines / chemokines, which recruit and activate other immune cells in the inflamed skin, enlarging the inflammatory response and consequently the clinical disease features. Another support for a role of the IL-23/Th17 pathway in psoriasis comes from whole genome studies showing that genetic variants of the IL-23 receptor are associated with psoriasis (Capon et al., 2007).

Regarding the clinical relevance of the IL-23/Th17 pathway, targeting the common subunit p40 of IL-12 and IL-23 demonstrated clinical improvement in psoriasis. Two anti-IL-12p40 Moabs, ustekinumab and ABT-874, have been recently developed as psoriasis cures. As we'll see in more detail later, ustekinumab and ABT-874 are humanized IgG1 Moabs that binding to the p40 subunit of human IL-12 and IL-23, prevents interaction with IL-12Rb1. Phase I (Kauffman et al., 2004) and phase II (Kimball et al., 2008b; G. G. Krueger et al., 2007) studies supported the use of both antibodies as effective treatments for psoriasis.

The safety profile of ustekinumab in psoriasis has been evaluated in 2 phase III studies. Of these, PHOENIX I assessed the efficacy and safety of ustekinumab 45 and 90 mg administered subcutaneously at weeks 0, 4, and then every 12 weeks over 76 weeks of treatment (Leonardi et al., 2008). 67.1 % and 66.4 % of patients who received ustekinumab 45mg and 90 mg respectively, achieved PASI-75 at week 12 compared to placebo control (3.1 %). The observed adverse events were mild, non-life threatening and not significantly different from the placebo group. The most commonly reported adverse events were upper respiratory tract infections, nasopharyngitis, headache, and arthralgia. The PHOENIX II trial (Papp et al., 2008) was conducted to further assess if dosing intensification would increase the response to treatment in partial responder patients (between PASI-50 and PASI-75). It was found that dosing intensification resulted in increased clinical efficacy only in patients receiving 90mg, but not 45mg, of ustekinumab every 8 weeks (PASI-75 in 68.8 % of patients receiving 90mg every 8 weeks versus 33.3 % of patients receiving 90 mg every 12 weeks). The incidence and type of adverse events observed did not differ between PHOENIX I and II studies. Ustekinumab is also effective in the treatment of psoriatic arthritis and this study again confirmed that ustekinumab is well tolerated (A. Gottlieb et al., 2009).

4.2.3 Regulatory T cells

Regulatory T cells (Tregs) are characterized by their ability to suppress the activation and proliferation of effector T cells ($CD4^+/CD8^+$) by direct contact with antigen presenting cells (Gondek et al., 2005) or by releasing IL-10 (Annacker et al., 2003) and/or TGF-β1 (Nakamura et al., 2004) (**Figure 3**).

Tregs express CD4, height CD25 and Foxp3 and are about the 1-5 % of the total population of peripheral $CD4^+$ cells.

Dysfunction of Tregs has been implicated in the pathogenesis of various autoimmune diseases such as multiple sclerosis and rheumatoid arthritis (RA) and in psoriasis; where Treg function and proliferation are both defective (Sugiyama et al., 2005). This combination may result in a failure to limit the activation and proliferation of pathogenic T cells, contributing to the ongoing inflammation seen in psoriasis; for this reason strategies that correct Treg function or increase the Treg/pathogenic T cell ratio may be potential treatments for psoriasis (Sugiyama et al., 2005). Phototherapy, for example, might induce Treg type suppressor cells as well as eliminate pathogenic T cells (Baadsgaard et al., 1990), supporting a possible role of Treg cells in protection against psoriasis.

5. Principal co-morbidities

Today we know that during the time course of psoriasis, certain conditions may appear at somewhat unpredictable time points in a progressive fashion. These so-called co-morbidities, often become manifest years after the onset of skin manifestations and are frequently observed in severe forms of psoriasis.

5.1 Psoriatic arthritis

PsA is traditionally included among common co-morbidities of psoriasis, even if it should be rather considered a component of the clinical spectrum of psoriatic disease. Skin manifestations occur before the onset of arthritis in the large majority of patients (A. B. Gottlieb et al., 2006), and in general, the prevalence of arthritis in psoriasis patients is estimated to be approximately 30% (Gisondi et al., 2005; Zachariae et al., 2002).

In PsA pathogenesis the TNF-α plays a key role, promoting osteoclastogenesis and bone resorption by stimulating the receptor-activator of NFkB, expressed in bone marrow osteoclast precursors (Abu-Amer et al., 2000; Keffer et al., 1991). Moreover, TNF-α has been noted to increase DKK-1 (dickkopf-1), a glycoprotein able to inhibit the bone apposition process by obstructing osteoblast growth (Baron & Rawadi, 2007; Diarra et al., 2007).

Numerous clinical observations support these experimental data, particularly a number of clinical trials showed a significant inhibition of joint damage in patients who underwent anti-TNF therapy, confirming the role of TNF in altered bone remodeling.

Approximately 20% of PsA patients are estimated to suffer from a severe and destructive form of arthritis, that leads to overall increased disability (D. D. Gladman et al., 1990; Queiro-Silva et al., 2003). Interestingly, different results indicate that the DMARDs (disease-modifying antirheumatic drugs) might not be able to inhibit disease progression and osteoarticular damage, even though they are generally useful in providing relief of clinical symptoms (Kana et al., 2003).

There is also convincing evidence of increased mortality in PsA patients, which seems to be related to disease activity, characterized by high erythrosedimentation rate, high medication level, and significant radiological damage at early patient visits (D. D. Gladman et al., 1998). Fortunately, as we shall see later, the mortality in PsA patients has gradually improved by using the biological drugs (Ali et al., 2007).

5.2 Inflammatory bowel disease (IBD)

IBD commonly refers to ulcerative colitis (UC) and Crohn's disease (CD), which are chronic inflammatory diseases of the gastrointestinal tract with unknown etiology. UC and CD have significant clinical differences, however, both diseases share similar pathogenic mechanisms and many extra-intestinal manifestations, and frequently respond to the same treatments.

Many data indicate a stringent correlation between CD and psoriasis (Najarian & A. B. Gottlieb, 2003). Firstly, CD patients have been found to have a seven-fold higher risk of developing psoriasis than control subjects (Mrowietz et al., 2006). This association may be related to the following observations: a) it has been shown that TNF-α has a key role in both conditions, valuing the hypothesis of common inflammatory pathways. This point has been further supported by the therapeutic efficacy of anti-TNF-α antibodies; b) genetic evidences, such as polymorphisms in the TNF-α promoter region and the close position of the susceptibility loci, link psoriasis to CD (Najarian & A. B. Gottlieb, 2003). In particular, a recent study demonstrated a significant association between CD and the IL-23 receptor gene (Duerr et al., 2006) and, as reported previously, IL-23 /IL-17 pathway is involved in psoriasis pathogenesis (Blauvelt, 2008; Rizzo et al., 2011).

On the other hand, the association between psoriasis and UC has been described in only in recent studies, even if the first studies regarding this connection trace back to the 60s and early 70s (Brewerton et al., 1974; McEwen et al., 1971). Most recently, Cohen et coll. (Cohen et al., 2009), in a case-control study with 12,502 psoriasis patients, demonstrated that even though not as high as CD (odds ratio 2.49), UC association is statistically significant and far from being negligible (odds ratio 1.64). This often undervalued correlation is biologically conceivable because chronic systemic inflammation and TNF-α constitute core features of UC, as well as psoriasis (Torres & Rios 2008).

5.3 Metabolic Syndrome (MS) and Cardiovascular Diseases (CVD)

Different overlapping guidelines have been proposed to define the MS: the cardiometabolic risk factors of obesity, impaired glucose tolerance (or type 2 diabetes), insulin resistance, dyslipidemia, and hypertension (Alberti et al., 2006; Grundy et al., 2005; Johnson & Weinstock, 2006). Just like psoriasis, MS is characterized by a pro-inflammatory state, characterized by a complex cytokines network.

In response to various metabolic signals the adipose tissue release the adipokines that modulate flogosis, lipid metabolism, and insulin sensitivity. A cluster of these adipokines is represented by pro-inflammatory cytokines (TNF-α, IL-8 and IL-6) whose overproduction drives the psoriasis pathogenesis, as well as of certain basic features of MS like insulin resistance and diabetes (Arican et al., 2005; Nickoloff & Nestle, 2004; Rondinone, 2006). Consistent with this common pathophysiology, different studies have demonstrated that psoriasis patients show an increased risk of developing the metabolic syndrome (Henseler & Christophers, 1995; Neimann et al., 2006).

The multiple conditions that constitute the MS could very well be the main reasons for CVD in psoriasis patients.

However, in various studies involving patients with psoriasis, the latter was identified as an independent risk factor for myocardial infarction regardless of the presence of the complete MS and an independent risk factor for coronary artery calcification (Gelfand et al., 2006).

Indeed, as of today there is forceful evidence that psoriasis, much like other systemic pro-inflammatory conditions (e.g. RA, SLE), may predispose to an increased CVD risk, following a nontraditional pathway to atherogenesis and premature vascular damage (Kimball et al., 2008c; Saphiro et al., 2007).

In conclusion, basic inflammatory activity in psoriasis could act independently of traditional risk factors, MetS included, and can increase the risk of CVD through its own underlying biological mechanisms (inflammation-driven atherogenesis).

Cell Types	Biological Effects	Clinical Consequences
Leukocytes	Activation/maturation ↑ inflammatory cytokine/expression ROS release	↑ Inflammation Endothelial injury Epidermal Proliferation
Endothelial cells	Suppression of precursor cells/apoptosis ↑ expression of adhesion molecules ↑ release of VEGF Impaired NO Bioavailability Induction of TF expression	↑ Angiogenesis ↑ leukocytes recruitment Endothelian dysfunction Hemostasis impairment
Osteoclast precursors	↑ RANKL expression (↑osteoclast maturation/activation) ↑ DKK-1 level (↓ osteoclast development)	Bone resorption promotion Bone apposition inhibition
Condrocytes/Synoviocytes	Apoptosis ↑ Metalloproteinase synthesis	Articular erosion
Adipocytes	Dysregulation of lipid and glucose metabolism ↑ circulating levels of FFA and LDL	Disadvantageous metabolic response to injury and infection ↑ in traditional CV risk factors
Hepatocytes	Induction of IL-6	Raised CRP serum levels CRP-induced vascular dysfunction
Neural cells	Modulation of cell proliferation NGF-induced	Neurogenic inflammation

↑ = Increase; ↓ = decrease; CRP = C-reactive protein; CV = Cardiovascular; DKK-1 = Dickkopf-1; LDL = Low-density lipoproteins; NGF = Nerve growth factor; NO = Nitric oxide; RANKL = Receptor-Activator of NFkappaB ligand; ROS = Reactive oxygen species; TF = Tissue Factor; VEGF = Vascular endothelial growth factor.

Table 1. Biological effects and clinical consequences of TNF-α stimulation in different cells

Recently, some studies have also shown that in psoriasis patients, the increased risk for myocardial infarction varies by age (higher in younger individuals) and disease severity (higher in severe forms) (Gelfand et al., 2006; Kremers et al., 2007; Mallbris et al., 2004). As such, a young patient with severe psoriasis is burdened by a CVD risk comparable with what is seen in the presence of traditional risk factors such as diabetes and hypertension.

Moreover, a variety of data indicates that psoriasis and CVD (mostly atherosclerosis) share common pathogenic features: both Th1 mediated, with an up-regulation of Th1 cytokines (TNF-α, IFN-γ) and a systemic expression of adhesion molecules, neoangiogenesis factors, and superantigens, these latter potentially able to activate the T cells (Biedermann et al., 2004; Ettehadi et al., 2004; Gudjonsson et al., 2004). The table 1 summarizes the consequences of the TNF-α over-expression in promoting inflammatory conditions such as psoriasis and atherogenesis.

Overlapping of genetic susceptibility loci between psoriasis and atherosclerosis is also worth mentioning, even though its role has yet to be fully understood (Becker et al., 1998).

Lastly, the two conditions also show similar histological aspects, mainly involving T cells, macrophages, mast cells and connective tissue matrix. (Nickoloff et al., 2007a; Nickoloff et al., 2007b).

Alongside the similar pathogenesis, other indirect factors might be responsible for psoriasis-CVD association; in fact some authors have found that a number of conventional systemic psoriasis treatments (e.g. methotrexate, acitretin, cyclosporine) might increase the effects of specific CVD risk factors (Katz et al., 1994; Strober & Menon, 2005; Taler et al., 1999).

6. Disease evaluation

To assess the severity of psoriasis and PsA (baseline/in response to treatment), a number of tools are now available, of which the Psoriasis Activity and Severity Index (PASI) is the most frequently used (Fredriksson & Pettersson, 1978). The PASI combines assessments of the extent of body surface involvement in four anatomical regions (head, trunk, arms and legs) and the severity of desquamation, erythema and plaque induration (thickness) in each region, yielding an overall score of 0 (no psoriasis) to 72 (severe psoriasis) (Fredriksson & Pettersson, 1978). PASI 75 is defined as a 75% reduction in PASI compared with baseline, instead a PASI score of >10 is defined as moderate to severe disease, necessitating systemic therapy (PUVA, UVB 311, MTX, cyclosporin A or biological drugs) (Pathirana et al., 2009)

An additional tool to assess the psoriasis severity is the physician's global assessment (PGA). The PGA takes into account the involvement of the body surface area, induration, scaling and erythema and grades the patient's psoriasis overall, relative to baseline, as 1 (clear), 2 (excellent), 3 (good), 4 (fair), 5 (poor) or 6 (worse) (Pathirana et al., 2009).

In trials investigating patients with PsA, the American College of Rheumatology Criteria (ACR) are most commonly used. The ACR clinical response criteria are defined as percentage reduction [20% (ACR 20), 50% (ACR50) and 70% (ACR 70)] in tender and swollen joint counts and in 3 of the, remaining, 5 ACR core items (patient and physician global assessments, pain, disability and an acute phase reactant) (Montecucco, 2006; Radtke et al., 2009).

A supplementary tool to evaluate clinical remission in psoriatic patients is the Disease Activity Score (DAS) comprising the number of swollen and tender joints, the erythrocyte sedimentation rate and the general health of the patient (measured on a visual analogue scale) (Montecucco, 2006). The DAS measures 44 swollen joints, whereas the modified DAS 28 measures only 28 swollen and tender joints (Prevoo et al., 1995). The effect of psoriasis on the patient's quality of life is measured by the 10-item Dermatology Life Quality Index (DLQI) questionnaire. DLQI scores range from 0 (not at all) to 30 (very much) (Pathirana et al., 2009).

7. Biological drugs

Biological therapies for the treatment of psoriasis are defined by their mode of action and are classified into 3 groups, the inhibitors of TNF-α (adalimumab, certolizumab, etanercept, golimumab, and infliximab), the T-cell modulating agents (such as alefacept) and the inhibitors of IL-12 and IL-23 (ustekinumab and briakinumab).

7.1 TNF-α inhibitors

The TNF-α inhibitors adalimumab, etanercept and infliximab have been approved by the FDA and EMEA for psoriasis and PsA treatment; they have been reviewed quite extensively in the past and the table 2 summarizes the clinical outcome for primary endpoints (e.g. PASI and ACR) in randomized controlled studies.

In this chapter, instead will focus on the new TNF-α blockers such as golimumab and certolizumab (Mössner et al., 2008; Pathirana et al., 2009).

Drug	Disease	Trial Type	Treatment (n° of patients)	Major Results	References
Adalimumab	Psoriasis	12-week RDBPC OLE until week 60	A 40 mg weekly (50) A 40 mg eow (46) Placebo (52)	PASI 75 at week 12: 80 PASI 75 at week 12: 53 PASI 75 at week 12: 4	Gordon *et al.*,2006 *J Am Acad Dermatol* 55: 598–606.
Adalimumab (REVEAL)	Psoriasis	16-week RDBPC OLE until week 52	A 40 mg eow (814) Placebo (398)	PASI 75 at week 16: 71 PASI 75 at week 16: 7	Menter *et al.*, 2008 *J Am Acad Dermatol* 58: 106–115.
Adalimumab (CHAMPION)	Psoriasis	16-week RDBPC	A 40 mg eow (108) MTX (110) Placebo (53)	PASI 75 at week 16: 80 PASI 75 at week 16: 36 PASI 75 at week 16: 19	Saurat *et al.*, 2008 *Br J Dermatol* 158: 558-566.
Adalimumab (ADEPT)	Psoriasis arthritis	24-week RDBPC OLE	A 40 mg eow (151) Placebo (162)	ACR 20 at week 12: 58 ACR 20 at	Mease *et al.*, 2005 *Arthritis Rheum*

		OLE week 48 OLE week 104	OLE A (281)	week 12: 14 ACR 20 at week 48: 58.7 ACR 20 at week 104: 57.3	52: 3279–3289. Gladman *et al.*, 2007 *Arthris Rheum* 56: 476–488. Mease *et al.*, 2009 *Ann Rheum Dis* 68: 702–709.
Adalimumab	Psoriasis arthritis	12-week RDBPC OLE until week 24	A 40 mg eow (51) Placebo (49)	ACR 20 at week 12: 39 ACR 20 at week 12: 16	Genovese *et al.*, 2007 *J Rheumatol* 34: 1040–1050.
Etanercept	Psoriasis	12-week RDBPC	E 25 mg twice weekly (57) Placebo (55)	PASI 75 at week 12: 30 PASI 75 at week 12: 2	Gottlieb *et al.*, 2003 *Arch Dermatol* 139: 1563–1570.
Etanercept CONSORT	Psoriasis	RDBPC	E 25 mg twice weekly (196) E 50 mg twice weekly (194) Placebo (193)	PASI 75 at week 12: 34 PASI 75 at week 12: 49 PASI 75 at week 12: 3	Papp *et al.*, 2005 *Br J Dermatol* 152: 1304–1312.
Etanercept	Psoriasis	RDBPC	E 25 mg weekly (160) E 25 mg twice weekly (162) E 50 mg twice weekly (164) Placebo (166)	PASI 75 at week 12: 14 PASI 75 at week 12: 34 PASI 75 at week 12: 49 PASI 75 at week 12: 4	Leonardi *et al.*, 2003 *N Engl J Med* 349: 2014–2022.
Etanercept	Psoriasis	12-week RDBPC	E 50 mg twice weekly (311) Placebo (307)	PASI 75 at week 12: 47 PASI 75 at week 12: 5	Tyring *et al.*, 2006 *Lancet* 367: 29–35.
Etanercept	Psoriasis arthritis	12-week RDBPC	E 25 mg twice weekly (30) Placebo (30)	ACR 20 at week 12: 73 ACR 20 at week 12: 13	Mease *et al.*, 2000 *Lancet* 356: 385–390.
Etanercept	Psoriasis arthritis	24-week RDBPC OLE until week 48	E 25 mg twice weekly (101) Placebo (104)	ACR 20 at week 12: 59 ACR 20 at week 12: 15	Mease *et al.*, 2004 *Arthritis Rheum* 50: 2264–2272.

Infliximab SPIRIT	Psoriasis	RDBPC	I 3 mg ·kg-1 (99) I 5 mg ·kg-1 (99) Placebo (51)	PASI 75 at week 10: 72 PASI 75 at week 10: 88 PASI 75 at week 10: 6	Gottlieb *et al.*, 2004 *J Am Acad Dermatol* 51: 534–542.
Infliximab EXPRESS I	Psoriasis	RDBPC	I 5 mg ·kg-1 (301) Placebo (77)	PASI 75 at week 10: 80 PASI 75 at week 10: 3	Reich *et al.*, 2005 *Lancet* 366: 1367–1374.
Infliximab	Psoriasis	RDBPC	I 5 mg ·kg-1 (11) I 10 mg ·kg-1 (11) Placebo (11)	PASI 75 at week 10: 82 PASI 75 at week 10: 73 PASI 75 at week 10: 18	Chaudhari *et al.*, 2001 *Lancet* 357: 1842–1847.
Infliximab EXPRESS II	Psoriasis	RDBPC	I 3 mg ·kg-1 (311) I 5 mg ·kg-1 (314) Placebo (208)	PASI 75 at week 10: 70 PASI 75 at week 10: 76 PASI 75 at week 10: 2	Menter *et al.*, 2007 *J Am Acad Dermatol* 56: 31.e1–31.e5.
Infliximab IMPACT	Psoriasis arthritis	16-week RDBPC OLE week 50	I 5 mg ·kg-1 (52) Placebo (52)	ACR 20 at week 16: 65 ACR 20 at week 16: 10	Antoni *et al.*, 2005 *Arthritis Rheum* 52: 1227–1236.
Infliximab IMPACT II	Psoriasis arthritis	24-week RDBPC OLE 52 weeks	I 5 mg ·kg-1 (100) Placebo (100)	ACR 20 at week 24: 54 ACR 20 at week 24: 16	Kavanaugh *et al.*, 2007 *Ann Rheum Dis* 66: 498–505.
Golimumab GO-REVEAL	Psoriasis	24-week RDBPC	G 50 mg q4 wks (146) G 100 mg q4 wks (146) Placebo (113)	PASI 75 at week 14: 40 PASI 75 at week 14: 58 PASI 75 at week 14: 3	Kavanaugh *et al.*, 2009° *Arthritis Rheum* 60: 976–986.
Golimumab GO-REVEAL	Psoriasis arthritis	24-week RDBPC	G 50 mg q4wks (146) G 100 mg q4wks (146) Placebo (113)	ACR 20 at week 14: 51 ACR 20 at week 14: 45 ACR 20 at week 14: 9	Kavanaugh *et al.*, 2009° *Arthritis Rheum* 60: 976–986.

A= Adalimumab; E = Etanercept; I = Infliximab; G = Golimumab; OLE = Open Level Extension; q4 wks = every 4 weeks; RDBPC = Randomized Double-Blind Placebo Controlled Trial

Table 2. Efficacy of anti-TNF-α in the treatment of psoriasis and psoriasis arthritis

Up to now, treatment with MoaB anti-TNF-α has proven to be effective and relatively safe in patients with psoriasis and PsA (Lima et al., 2009).

Since TNF-α has showed an osteoclast stimulating effect, alongside being synergic with DKK-1 in reducing osteoblasts maturation, anti-TNF-α drugs should improve PsA-related bone altering processes, as confirmed by significant inhibition of radiographic progression during treatment with etanercept or infliximab (Antoni et al., 2008; Mease et al., 2006b; van der Heijde et al., 2007).

Equally importantly, anti-TNF-α therapy might have a preventive effect on PsA overlapping in psoriasis patients. In fact, in a case-control study, Gisondi group (Gisondi et al., 2008) has demonstrated that lower limb enthesopathy can be documented in asymptomatic psoriasis patients without any clinical sign of arthropathy. Similar findings were reported in the past concerning entheseal abnormalities (De Filippis et al., 2005) and increased Achilles tendon thickness (Ozcakar et al., 2005); all of which were detected in asymptomatic patients.

Different evidences have proved that anti-TNF-α treatments infliximab and adalimumab are effective in controlling gut inflammation, whereas etanercept is not (Bosani et al., 2009).

There are reports of CD development in patients with ankylosing spondylitis or PsA (Song et al., 2008) and treated with etanercept. However, it is well-known that such patients are burdened with a high risk of chronic IBD development. It is therefore hard to assess whether these cases of CD were really a consequence of anti-TNF-α therapy or rather a coincidental event in predisposed patients.

The reason for the discordant effect of anti-TNF-α treatments on IBD probably lies in different pharmacodynamic features of these drugs, and a number of hypotheses have been expressed in this regard.

Firstly, it has been noted that etanercept, unlike anti-TNF-α Moabs, doesn't induce apoptosis of activated lymphocytes in CD patients (Van den Brande et al., 2003). Given the existing results, it is reasonable to conclude that etanercept has no potential to control or to prevent gut inflammation and hence IBD appearance. A preventive role of anti-TNF-α Moabs against the IBD development in susceptible psoriasis patients cannot be rule out considering the effectiveness of these drugs in both conditions.

About the effects of anti-TNF-a Moabs in MS and CVD, studies regarding the consequence on blood lipids have shown unclear results. A study of RA patients reported a significant decreased atherogenic index of low-density lipoprotein (LDL)/high-densitiy lipoprotein (HDL) ratio after 6 months of therapy with anti-TNF-a (Spanakis et al., 2006); another showed increased HDL levels and reduced C-reactive protein (CRP) and IL-6 levels after 2 weeks (Popa et al., 2005). In contrast, in some cases anti-TNF-a therapy has resulted in a pro-atherogenic effect in RA and PsA patients, with increase of LDL/ HDL ratio and triglycerides levels (Dahlqvist et al., 2004). Another study demonstrated a sudden reduction in HDL levels the day after infliximab infusion, but without any significant variation in the HDL profile (Irace et al., 2004).

No conclusions can be drawn from these inconsistent findings regarding long-term clinical outcomes. As a consequence, many authors seem to agree on the fact that despite the prominent role of TNF-α on lipid regulation, the emerging efficacy of anti-TNF-α therapy

Anti-TNF-a therapy	Frequent side effects	Rare severe side effects	Reference
Adalimumab	• Upper respiratory tract infections • Injection site reactions • Headache	• Severe/ Opportunistic infections • Reactivation/progression of TBC • Onset/exacerbation of CNS demyelinating disorders (e.g. Multiple Sclerosis) • Increased risk of cancer (e.g. Lymphoma) • Drug-induced lupus • Exacerbation of congestive • heart failure • Vasculitis	Pathirana *et al.*, 2009 *J Eur Acad Dermatol Venerol* 23 (Suppl. 2): S5–70. Smith *et al.*, 2009 *Br J Dermatol* 161: 987–1019.
Etanercept	• Upper respiratory tract infections • Injection site reactions • Pruritus	• Severe/ Opportunistic infections • Reactivation/progression of TBC • Onset/exacerbation of CNS demyelinating disorders (e.g. Multiple Sclerosis) • Increased risk of cancer (e.g. Lymphoma) • Drug-induced lupus • Exacerbation of congestive heart failure • Vasculitis • Aplastic anaemia	Pathirana *et al.*, 2009 *J Eur Acad Dermatol Venerol* 23 (Suppl. 2): S5–70. Smith *et al.*, 2009 *Br J Dermatol* 161: 987–1019.
Infliximab	• Upper respiratory tract infections • Acute infusion reaction: • fever, chills, nausea • Headache • Pruritus • Urticaria • Elevated transaminases	• Severe/ Opportunistic infections • Reactivation/progression of TBC • Onset/exacerbation of CNS demyelinating disorders (e.g. Multiple Sclerosis) • Increased risk of cancer (e.g. Lymphoma) • Drug-induced lupus • Exacerbation of congestive heart failure • Vasculitis • Pancytopenia	Pathirana *et al.*, 2009 *J Eur Acad Dermatol Venerol* 23 (Suppl. 2): S5–70. Smith *et al.*, 2009 *Br J Dermatol* 161: 987–1019.

Table 3. Overview of side effects of most prescribed anti-TNF-a treatments in patients with psoriasis

on CV morbidity and mortality is likely independent of the induced blood lipid variations (Soubrier et al., 2008).

Results derived from studies about the effects of anti-TNF-α drugs on insulin resistance in psoriasis patients, appear to show an improvement in insulin sensitivity (Marra et al., 2007). This outcome seems to confirm the beneficial effects of anti-TNF-α Moabs already documented in many RA studies (Huvers et al., 2007; Yazdani-Biuki et al., 2004). In particular, infliximab has proved capable of enhancing insulin sensitivity after the infusion to up to one year (Huvers et al., 2007). Lastly, there have been few isolated cases of psoriasis patients with diabetes developing unpredictable hypo- or hyperglycemia after commencing treatment with TNF inhibitors (Boulton & Bourne, 2007; Wu & Tsai 2008).

In the table 3 are reported the side effects of adalimumab, etanercept and infliximab treatment in psoriasis patients.

7.1.1 Golimumab (CNTO148)

Golimumab is a human immunoglobulin G1K Moab binding both soluble and transmembrane forms of TNF-α, thereby neutralizing their bioactivity by blocking the interaction with receptor (Kavanaugh et al., 2009; Xu et al., 2009).

In a study with 337 patients, the pharmacokinetics of subcutaneously administered golimumab (50 or 100 mg every 4 weeks) were analyzed (Xu et al., 2009) and the following golimumab pharmacokinetic parameters were found: apparent clearance = 1.38 ± 0.04 L per day, apparent volume of distribution = 24.9 ± 1.04 L and absorption rate constant = 0.908 ± 0.121 per day. Significant covariants on apparent clearance were identified as body weight, baseline C-reactive protein level and smoking habits. However, only body weight was found to be a significant covariant on apparent volume of distribution. In addition, golimumab concentrations in patients (50 mg golimumab every 4 weeks) not receiving MTX were 30% lower as compared with patients receiving MTX (Xu et al., 2009). So far, no possible explanation for the different effects of MTX on the serum golimumab concentrations has been provided (Xu et al., 2009).

A randomized, double-blind, placebo-controlled phase III multicenter study was conducted to evaluate the safety and efficacy of golimumab from week 0 to 20 in 405 patients with active PsA (Kavanaugh et al., 2009).

Active PsA was defined as at least three swollen joints and three tender joints as well as active plaque psoriasis with a qualifying lesion of at least 2 cm in diameter. Concomitant MTX, non-steroidal anti-inflammatory drugs (NSAIDs) and corticosteroids were permitted at stable doses.

A significant reduction in PASI 75 among patients receiving golimumab 50 or 100 mg at week 14 (40 and 58%) was observed when compared with patients receiving placebo (3%). PASI 75 scores in patients with golimumab (50 and 100 mg) further improved at week 24 in both golimumab groups (56 and 66%), whereas only 1% of patients in the placebo group reached a PASI 75 (Kavanaugh et al., 2009).

Golimumab significantly ($P < 0.001$) improved signs and symptoms of PsA compared with patients treated with placebo (Kavanaugh et al., 2009). An ACR 20 response at week 14 could be achieved in 51% of patients treated with golimumab 50 mg and in 45% of patients receiving golimumab 100 mg versus only 9% in the placebo group. At week 24, an ACR 20 response was observed in 52% in the golimumab 50-mg group and in 61% in the golimumab 100-mg group versus 12% in the placebo group ($P < 0.001$). ACR 50 and 70 responses were also significantly higher in both golimumab groups than in the placebo group. At week 104, 91.4% of patients in the 50-mg group and 73.1% in the 100-mg group achieved an ACR 20 (Kavanaugh et al., 2009). A good or moderate DAS 28 response was significantly ($P < 0.001$) more often achieved in the golimumab 50 and 100-mg recipients than in the placebo group at week 14 (66 and 67% vs. 24%) and at week 24 (64 and 78% vs. 24%) (Kavanaugh et al., 2009). Assessment of physical function and health-related quality of life were measured by the Health Assessment Questionnaire (HAQ) and Short Form 36 Health Survey (SF-36) and significantly improved in both golimumab groups compared with the placebo group ($P < 0.001$ for HAQ and SF-36 at all comparisons at week 24).Thus, in this study golimumab improved significantly the clinical signs and symptoms of PsA as well as the physical function and quality of life (Kavanaugh et al., 2009).

About the of safety of this treatment, Kavanaugh and coll. (Kavanaugh et al., 2009) reported that 8.6% of patients treated with golimumab shown a serious adverse event up to week 104: serious infectious adverse events comprised sepsis/cholecystitis and abscess formation. about the cancers registered: one basal cell carcinoma, one colon cancer and one small lung cell carcinoma in the golimumab 50-mg group. In the golimumab 100-mg group, three basal cell carcinomas, one prostate cancer and one small lung cancer occurred.

As for adverse events, infections of the upper respiratory tract and nasopharyngitis were most frequently reported.

7.1.2 Certolizumab pegol (CDP870)

Certolizumab pegol, a pegylated Fab-9 fragment of a humanized anti-TNF-a Moab, has been approved for the treatment of patients with CD (Bourne et al., 2008) and it has also been investigated in RA patients (Barnes & Moots, 2007).

It binding to TNF-α, blocks the interaction with specific receptors. Whereas adalimumab, etanercept and infliximab contain an IgG1 Fc region, which can induce antibody-dependent cell-mediated cytotoxicity (ADCC) and complement-dependent cytotoxicity (CDC), certolizumab lacking this Fc region, isn't able of inducing ADCC and CDC (European Medicines Agency [EMEA], 2008).

Pharmacokinetic analysis in the CDP870 trial showed a bioavailability of 85% (EMEA, 2008). Peak plasma concentrations were attained between 54 and 171 h after subcutaneous injection. The mean serum concentration (Cmax) after the subcutaneous administration of 400-mg certolizumab ranged from 46.3 ± 13.1 to 49.5 ± 8.2 mg · mL^{-1}. An increase of Cmax and area under the curve (AUC) was observed with higher doses in a dose-proportional manner. The half-life of certolizumab was found to be approximately 14 days (EMEA, 2008)

Certolizumab pegol has been investigated in patients with moderate to severe psoriasis. In a phase II trial, patients were randomized to receive certolizumab pegol 200 mg, 400 mg or placebo subcutaneously every 2 weeks up to week 12. At week 12, significantly more patients receiving certolizumab pegol 200 or 400 mg achieved PASI 75 than in the placebo group (74.6 and 82.8% vs. 6.8%) (Ortonne et al., 2007). The most frequently reported adverse events comprised headache, nasopharyngitis and pruritus. The frequency of adverse events was similar across all three groups. However, serious adverse events were more common in the 400-mg group (7.0%) than in the 200-mg group (3.3%) and in the placebo-group (1.7%) (Ortonne et al., 2007). According to the data from the phase II study, PASI 75 results and side effects were comparable with those observed in patients treated with the approved TNF-α blockers adalimumab and infliximab. So far, no phase III studies or studies in patients with PsA have been conducted.

7.2 T-cell modulators

In 2003, alefacept and efalizumab were the first biological agents to be approved by the Food and Drug Administration (FDA) for the treatment of psoriasis (Pathirana et al., 2009). In the European Union, only efalizumab was approved for the psoriasis therapy (Pathirana et al., 2009). In 2009, efalizumab was withdrawn from the market in Europe and the United States (EMEA, 2009; Food and Drug Administration [FDA], 2009).

7.2.1 Alefacept

Alefacept, a recombinant dimeric fusion protein, is made up of the terminal portion of leukocyte function antigen-3 (LFA-3). It binds to extracellular human CD2 and the Fc portion of human immunoglobulin IgG1 (Sugiyama et al., 2008). Alefacept blocks signalling between LFA-3 on antigen presenting cells and the CD2 molecule on T cells (primarily $CD45RO^+$).

Subsequently, the activation and proliferation of $CD45RO^+$ T cells, which account for approximately 75% of T lymphocytes in psoriatic lesions, are inhibited. Furthermore, alefacept decreases the number of pathogenic T cells by binding CD2 on $CD45RO^+$ T cells to the FcgIII receptor on natural killer cells, resulting in granzyme-mediated apoptosis of T cells (Gordon et al., 2003; Sobell et al., 2009; Sugiyama et al., 2008). Using a dosage of 15 mg alefacept administered intramuscularly QW, PASI 75 scores at week 12 were found to range between 21 and 35% (Gordon et al., 2003; Pathirana et al., 2009; Sugiyama et al., 2008). Recently, patients receiving alefacept in combination with MTX were shown to improve significantly in ACR 20 at week 24 compared with patients treated with MTX and placebo alone (54% vs. 23%; $P < 0.001$) (Mease et al., 2006a).

7.3 IL-12/IL-23 antagonists

Briakinumab and ustekinumab are both IL-12/IL-23 antagonists. Whereas briakinumab is currently under investigation for the psoriasis treatment in several phase III studies, ustekinumab was recently approved by the EMEA for the therapy of chronic plaque psoriasis.

7.3.1 Briakinumab (ABT874)

Briakinumab is a recombinant fully human, IgG1 Moab targeting the shared p40 subunit of IL-12 and IL-23 (Kimball et al., 2008b). It binds to soluble forms of IL-12 and IL-23, leading to a decreased secretion of pro-inflammatory cytokines: IL-12, IL-6, IFN-γ and TNF-α, as shown in CD patients (Ding et al., 2008).

In a phase I trial with 64 healthy controls, the pharmacokinetics of briakinumab (0.1–5.0 mg $\cdot kg^{-1}$ subcutaneously or intravenously) were evaluated. A linear relationship between the Cmax and AUC (concentration-time) was found with increasing doses. The terminal phase half-life time was about 9 days. No dose dependency was found for the volume distribution at steady state and the clearance of the drug. Subcutaneous and intramuscular application achieved an absolute bioavailability of 42 and 63% respectively (Ding et al., 2008).

A phase II study with briakinumab was conducted (Kimball et al., 2008b) in patients with psoriasis. Patients were randomized in groups of 30 to receive either only one dose of briakinumab 200 mg at week 0, 100 mg briakinumab every other week for 12 weeks, 200 mg weekly for 4 weeks, 200 mg every other week for 12 weeks and 200 mg every week for 12 weeks, or placebo respectively(Kimball et al., 2008b).

PASI 75 was significantly ($P < 0.001$) more often reached in patients in all five briakinumab treatment groups (63, 93, 90, 93, and 90% respectively) compared with the placebo group (3%). Statistically significant improvement to briakinumab therapy was rapid and could be registered in the briakinumab groups as early as at week 1. During the 12-week period, improvement could be sustained in briakinumab-treated patients even for patients in the briakinumab 200 mg x 1 and 200 mg x 4 dosage groups.

Besides injection site reactions, other common side effects the trial study comprised nasopharyngitis and upper respiratory infections. In addition, non-infectious serious adverse events reported in this study included costal chondritis in one patient. Significantly more patients in the briakinumab groups (36%) experienced adverse events compared with the placebo group (10%) (Kimball et al., 2008b).

7.3.2 Ustekinumab (CNTO1275)

Ustekinumab is a human monoclonal antibody binding with high affinity to the p40 subunit of IL 12 and IL 23 and therefore inhibiting the binding to specific receptor (IL-12Rb1) expressed on various cells.

In a phase I study, patients with constant 70% PASI improvement at weeks 8, 12 and 16 shown significant decreases in mRNA expression of different cytokines (IL-8, IL-18 and IFN-γ) as early as week 1 ($P < 0.05$), whereas, in patients without PASI improvement, no significant reduction of cytokine mRNA expression was observed(Wittig, 2007).

The pharmacokinetics of ustekinumab were assessed in different studies (A. B. Gottlieb et al., 2007; Kaufmann et al., 2004; Wittig, 2007): after a single subcutaneous injection, ustekinumab was slowly absorbed into the systemic circulation (mean Tmax about 12 days) and was afterwards slowly eliminated from the circulation (mean t1/2 around 20 days) (A. B. Gottlieb et al., 2007; Wittig, 2007).

The terminal half-life (t1/2) was dose dependent and was found to range from 14.9 ± 4.6 days (0.27 mg $\cdot kg^{-1}$ dose group) to 28.6 ± 9.3 days (2.7 mg $\cdot kg^{-1}$ dose group) (A. B. Gottlieb et al., 2007). Similar results were also observed for t1/2 by Kaufman (Kaufmann et al., 2004), ranging from 18.5 ± 3.6 in the 0.3-mg group to 25.9 ± 3.7 in the 1.0-mg group. An increase of Cmax and AUC was observed with superior dosages (A. B. Gottlieb et al., 2007; Kaufmann et al., 2004).

In the clinical trial conducted by Kaufman (Kaufmann et al., 2004), 18 psoriasis patients were enrolled in four dose groups: 0.1, 0.3, 1.0 and 5.0 mg per kg to assess the clinical response and the safety of a single intravenous administration of ustekinumab. At week 12, PASI 75 was reached in 25, 50, 60 and 100% of patients respectively. In patients responding to ustekinumab treatment, the expression of pro-inflammatory cytokines and chemokines IFN-γ, CXCL-8, CCR2, TNF-α, IL-12p40 and IL-23p19 subunits was decreased, compared with baseline levels (Reddy et al., 2007; Toichi et al., 2006).

In a second double-blind, placebo-controlled study, patients were randomized to receive either a single subcutaneous injection of 0.27, 0.675, 1.35 or 2.7 $mg \cdot kg^{-1}$ ustekinumab or placebo (A. B. Gottlieb et al., 2007). For a second time, patients treated with ustekinumab showed a dose-dependent improvement of their psoriasis. PASI 75 was achieved in 60% of the 0.27 $mg \cdot kg^{-1}$ group, 100% in the 0.675 $mg \cdot kg^{-1}$ group, 50% in the 1.35 $mg \cdot kg^{-1}$ group and 100% in the 2.7 $mg \cdot kg^{-1}$ group, but in none of the patients receiving placebo during the whole study period.

Krueger (G. G. Krueger et al., 2007) evaluated in a double-blind, placebo controlled trial, four subcutaneous dosing regimens of ustekinumab in patients with psoriasis; 320 patients were randomized to receive one of the following treatment regimens: one 45-mg dose, one 90-mg dose, four weekly 45-mg doses and four weekly 90-mg doses of ustekinumab or placebo. The primary endpoint of the study was a 75% improvement in the PASI at week 12. PASI 75 was achieved in 52% of patients receiving ustekinumab 45 mg, in 59% receiving ustekinumab 90 mg, in 67% receiving four weekly 45-mg doses and in 81% of patients receiving four weekly 90-mg doses, whereas only 2% of patients in the placebo group achieved a PASI 75.

Another placebo-controlled double blind randomized crossover study was conducted to evaluate the efficacy of ustekinumab in 146 patients suffering from PsA (A. Gottlieb et al., 2009). Patients were either randomized to receive ustekinumab 90 or 63 mg every week for 4 weeks (weeks 0–3) followed by placebo at weeks 12 and 16 (76 patients, group 1) or placebo (weeks 0–3) and ustekinumab (63 mg) at weeks 12 and 16 (70 patients, group 2). ACR 20 at week 12 (taken as the primary endpoint of the study) was achieved by 42% of patients in group 1 and by 14% in group 2 ($P = 0.0002$). Significantly more patients in group 1 achieved PASI 75 compared with group 2 in week 12 (52% vs. 5%, $P < 0.0001$). However, one should note that the dosages of ustekinumab used in the study were higher (90 and 63 mg, respectively) than those recommended for patients of normal weight (45 mg) with psoriasis (Leonardi et al., 2008).

In conclusion, we report the results of the two double-blind, placebo-controlled phase III studies (Phoenix 1 and Phoenix 2) in patients with psoriasis were performed parallel in USA and Europe. Primary outcome in both studies was PASI 75 at week 12 (Leonardi et al., 2008; 211,). 766 patients of Phoenix 1 trial were randomly assigned to receive either ustekinumab 45 mg or 90 mg at weeks 0 and 4 and afterwards every 12 weeks or placebo at weeks 0 and 4 and to cross over at week 12 to ustekinumab (Leonardi et al., 2008; Papp et al., 2008).

Furthermore, patients initially receiving ustekinumab and reaching a PASI 75 at weeks 28 and 40 were re-randomized at week 40 to either continue therapy with ustekinumab or to withdrawal of the study drug until loss of response. Significantly more patients in both ustekinumab groups (45 and 90 mg) received a PASI 75 at week 12 compared with the placebo group. Patients receiving maintenance therapy up to week 76 significantly better sustained PASI 75 than patients randomized to the drug withdrawal group ($P < 0.0001$).

The design of the Phoenix 2 study closely resembles that of the Phoenix 1 trial (Papp et al., 2008). Of the 1230 patients, 409 patients were randomized to receive ustekinumab 45 mg, 411 to receive ustekinumab 90 mg and 410 to receive placebo at weeks 0 and 4. The efficacy analysis at week 12 revealed the following results for the three groups. The primary endpoint was achieved in 66.7% of the ustekinumab 45-mg group, 75.7% of the ustekinumab 90 mg and 3.7% of the placebo group ($P < 0.0001$ for both ustekinumab 45 and 90 mg vs. placebo).

Quality of life was significantly improved in the patients treated with ustekinumab compared with the placebo groups ($P < 0.0001$) in both Phoenix trials. Patients randomized to maintenance therapy in the Phoenix 1 study were able to sustain improved DLQI scores until the end of the study, whereas in patients withdrawn from the study drug, the DLQI deteriorated again (Leonardi et al., 2008; Papp et al., 2008).

In a randomized active-controlled, parallel three-arm trial (ACCEPT trial), ustekinumab (45 and 90 mg, respectively) was compared versus the anti-TNF-α etanercept (50 mg twice weekly) (C. E. M. Griffiths et al., 2008). The primary endpoint of the study was PASI 75 at week 12. 903 patients were randomized in 3 treatment-arms as follows: 347 patients received etanercept 50 mg subcutaneously twice weekly, 209 patients received ustekinumab 45 mg subcutaneously at weeks 0 and 4, and 347 patients received ustekinumab 90 mg subcutaneously at weeks 0 and 4. PASI 75 at week 12 was achieved by 56.8% of patients in the etanercept group, by 67.5% in the ustekinumab 45-mg group and 73.8% in the ustekinumab 90-mg group. A greater proportion of patients receiving ustekinumab (45 or 90 mg) achieved PASI 75 when compared with the etanercept group ($P = 0.012$ for ustekinumab 45 mg, $P < 0.001$ for ustekinumab 90 mg). Interestingly, PASI 75 values at week 12 in patients receiving etanercept were better than those published in previous studies (Leonardi et al., 2008; Papp et al., 2008).

The table 4 resume the major results obtained using the briakinumab and ustekinumab in psoriasis treatments.

About the major side effects of treatments with ustekinumab; in the phase I studies, no serious adverse events were reported (A. B. Gottlieb et al., 2007; Kaufmann et al., 2004). Adverse events included headaches, abdominal pain and common cold symptoms. Adverse events were comparable in the phase II studies between ustekinumab and placebo groups (79% vs. 72%) (G. G. Krueger et al., 2007). Serious adverse events in patients treated with ustekinumab were infections (2 patients), myocardial infarctions (2 patients), a cerebrovascular accident (1 patient), non-melanoma skin cancer (2 patients) and prostate cancer (1 patient).

In the placebo group, one patient had a basal cell carcinoma and one patient experienced aggravation of his psoriasis requiring hospitalization. In the PsA trial conducted by Gottlieb, the following serious adverse events were reported in the ustekinumab groups: syncope (1 patient), respiratory tract infection (1 patient), haemorrhage (1 patient), stroke (1 patient), congestive heart failure/myocardial infarction/hypertension (1 patient), chest pain (1 patient), gastric ulcer haemorrhage/abdominal pain/back pain (1 patient) and basal cell carcinoma (1 patient) respectively (A. Gottlieb et al., 2009). Two serious infections occurred during the placebo-controlled phase of the two large phase III trials: one case of cellulitis and one case of herpes zoster (both in the ustekinumab 90-mg group) (Ding et al., 2008; Ortonne et al., 2007).

During the placebo-controlled phase of the Phoenix 2 study, a squamous cell carcinoma in a patient in the placebo group and a basal cell carcinoma in a patient in the ustekinumab 90-mg group were observed (Ding et al., 2008). Comparing patients on maintenance therapy with patients randomized to the withdrawal group in Phoenix 1 study did not reveal an increased infection rate between the two groups (Ortonne et al., 2007).

Therapy	**Disease**	**Trial Type**	**Treatment (n° of patients)**	**Major Results**	**Reference**
Briakinumab	Psoriasis	12-week RDBPC	B 200 mg x 1 (30) B 100 mg eow (3) B 200 mg x 4 (30) B 200 mg eow (30) B 200 mg weekly (30) Placebo (30)	PASI 75 at week 12: 63 PASI 75 at week 12: 93 PASI 75 at week 12: 90 PASI 75 at week 12: 93 PASI 75 at week 12: 90 PASI 75 at week 12: 1	Kimball *et al.*, 2008 *Arch Dermatol* 144: 200–207.
Ustekinumab PHOENIX 1	Psoriasis	RDBPC	U 45 mg (255) U 90 mg (256) Placebo (255	PASI 75 at week 12: 67.1 PASI 75 at week 12: 66.4 PASI 75 at week 12: 3.1	Leonardi *et al.*, 2008 *Lancet* 371: 1665 -1674.
Ustekinumab PHOENIX 2	Psoriasis	RDBPC	U 45 mg (409) U 90 mg (411) Placebo (410)	PASI 75 at week 12: 66.7 PASI 75 at week 12: 75.7 PASI 75 at week 12: 3.7	Papp *et al.*, 2008 *Lancet* 371: 1675–1684.
Ustekinumab ACCEPT	Psoriasis	RDBPC	U 45 mg (209) U 90 mg (347) E 2 X 50 mg (347)	PASI 75 at week 12: 67.5 PASI 75 at week 12: 73.8 PASI 75 at week 12: 56.8	Griffiths *et al.*, 2010 *N Engl J Med.* 362: 118-128

B = Briakinumab; E = Etanercept; U = Ustekinumab; RDBPC = Randomized Double-Blind Placebo Controlled Trial

Table 4. Efficacy of anti- IL-12/IL-23 in the psoriasis cure

However, as Th1 and Th17 blockade by ustekinumab might impair cell-mediated immunity, normal KCs host immunity and defence against malignancies, close monitoring in patients on long-term treatment with ustekinumab seems to be appropriate (O'Neill & Kalb, 2009). In the ACCEPT trial, serious adverse events have been observed in 1.2% of patients in the etanercept group, 1.9% in the ustekinumab 45-mg group and 1.2% of patients in the ustekinumab 90 mg group respectively. These included 4 patients in each treatment group: etanercept group: abdominal pain, bacterial meningitis, nephrolithiasis, rotator cuff syndrome; 45-mg ustekinumab group: alcoholic pancreatitis, chest pain/hypertension, psychotic disorder, breast cancer; ustekinumab 90-mg group: urosepsis/renal failure, uveitis, appendicitis and gastroenteritis from food poisoning (C. E. M. Griffiths et al., 2008).

8. Conclusion

Based on a large series of studies, that we discuss in the different paragraphs, current evidence indicates the importance of T cells during psoriasis pathogenesis and demonstre that T cell expansion precedes the development of typical psoriatic changes; the more reasonable conclusion is that psoriasis is the outcome of an inappropriate T cell-based activation event, together with a defect in KCs, whose combination results in the full psoriatic phenotype.

Once recognized the primary role of T cells in psoriasis pathogenesis, several biological therapies have been developed and proposed to counteract immune T response. These treatments consist in blocking the actions of several T cell cytokines that play a key role in sustain the pathogenesis of early and late events of psoriasis, e.g. anti-IL23 and anti-TNF-α.

So far, considering published data from the clinical trials, the new biological agents have been shown to be efficient treatment options for patients suffering from psoriasis and the major comorbidities disease-associated, primarily PsA.

These new biological agents seem to have proven a good risk/benefit ratio. As psoriasis is considered a life-long disease and no causal therapy for the disease is yet available, long-term studies on safe and efficacious treatments are needed and are of major importance.

Taking into account the possibility that uncommon adverse events or events occurring during long-term exposure to these drugs might emerge in the future (e.g. the development of progressive multifocal leukoencephalopathy in long-term patients treated with efalizumab), vigilant and careful post-marketing surveillance in patients treated with biological agents is strongly recommended.

9. Acknowledgment

We thank Dr. Elena Niccolai for editorial support and Dr. Chiara Della Bella for the artworks. We wish to thank Istituto Superiore di Sanità, and Italian Ministry of University and Research for their support of our studies.

10. References

Abel, E. A., DiCicco, L. M., Orenberg, E. K., Fraki, J. E., & Farber, E. M. (1986). Drugs in exacerbation of psoriasis. *J Am Acad Dermatol,* 15, 5 Pt 1, (Nov 1986), 1007–22.

Abrams, J. R., Kelley, S. L., Hayes, E., Kikuchi, T., Brown, M. J., Kang, S., Lebwohl, M. G., Guzzo, C. A., Jegasothy, B. V., Linsley, P. S., & Krueger, J. G. (2000). Blockade of T lymphocyte costimulation with cytotoxic T lymphocyte-associated antigen 4-immunoglobulin (CTLA4Ig) reverses the cellular pathology of psoriatic plaques, including the activation of keratinocytes, dendritic cells, and endothelial cells. *J Exp Med*, 192, 5, (Sep 2000), 681–93, 0022-1007

Abrams, J. R., Lebwohl, M. G., Guzzo, C. A., Jegasothy, B. V., Goldfarb, M. T., Goffe, B. S., Menter, A., Lowe, N. J., Krueger, G., Brown, M. J., Weiner, R. S., Birkhofer, M. J., Warner, G. L., Berry, K. K., Linsley, P. S., Krueger, J. G., Ochs, H. D., Kelley, S. L., & Kang, S. (1999), CTLA4 Igmediated blockade of T-cell costimulation in patients with psoriasis vulgaris. *J Clin Invest*, 103, 9, (May 1999), 1243–52, 0021-9738

Abu-Amer, Y., Erdmann, J., Alexopoulou, L., Kollias, G., Ross, F. P., & Teitelbaum, S. L. (2000). Tumor necrosis factor receptors types 1 and 2 differentially regulate osteoclastogenesis. *J Biol Chem*, 275, 35, (Sep 2000), 27307–27310, 0021-9258

Alberti, K. G., Zimmet, P., & Shaw, J. (2006). Metabolic syndrome - a new world wide definition. A Consensus Statement from the International Diabetes Federation. *Diabet Med*, 23, 5, (May 2006), 469–480, 1262-3636

Ali, Y., Tom, B. D. M., Schentag, C. T., Farewell, V. T., & Gladman, D. D. (2007). Improved survival in psoriatic arthritis (PsA) with calendar time. *Arthritis Rheum*, 56, 8, (Aug 2007), 2708–2714, 0004-3591

Annacker, O., Asseman, C., Read, S., & Powrie, F. (2003). Interleukin-10 in the regulation of T cell-induced colitis. *J Autoimmun*, 20, 4, (Jun 2003), 277–9

Antoni, C. E., Kavanaugh, A., van der Heijde, D., Beutler, A., Keenan, G., Zhou, B., Kirkham, B., Tutuncu, Z., Burmester, G. R., Schneider, U., Furst, D. E., Molitor, J., Keystone, E., Gladman, D. D., Manger, B., Wassenberg, S., Weier, R., Wallace, D. J., Weisman, M. H., Kalden, J. R., & Smolen, J. S. (2008). Two-year efficacy and safety of infliximab treatment in patientswith active psoriatic arthritis: findings of the Infliximab MultinationalPsoriatic Arthritis Controlled Trial (IMPACT). *J Rheumatol*, 35, 5, (May 2008), 569–876, 0315-162X

Arican, O., Aral, M., Sasmaz, S., & Ciragil, P. (2005). Serumlevels of TNFalpha, IFN-gamma, IL-6, IL-8, IL-12, IL-17, and IL-18 in patients with active psoriasis and correlation with disease severity. *Mediators Inflamm* , 2005, 5, (Oct 2005), 273–279,

Baadsgaard, O., Salvo, B., Mannie, A., Dass, B., Fox, D. A., & Cooper, K. D. (1990). In vivo ultraviolet-exposed human epidermal cells activate T suppressor cell pathways that involve CD4+CD45RA+ suppressor-inducer T cells. *J Immunol*, 145, 9, (Nov 1990), 2854–61, 0022-1767

Baker, B. S., Griffiths, C. E., Lambert, S., Powles, A. V., Leonard, J. N., Valdimarsson, H.,& Fry, L. (1987), The effects of cyclosporin A on T lymphocyte and dendritic cell sub-populations in psoriasis. *Br J Dermatol*, 116, 4, (Apr 1987), 503–10, 0007-0963

Barnes, T., & Moots, R. (2007). Targeting nanomedicines in the treatment of rheumatoid arthritis: focus on certolizumab pegol. *Inter J Nanomed*, 2, 1, (2007), 3–7, 1176-9114

Baron, R., & Rawadi, G. (2007). Targeting the Wnt/BCatenin pathway to regulate bone formation in the adult skeleton. *Endocrinology*, 148, 6, (Jun 2007), 2635–2643, 0013-7227

Becker, K. G., Simon, R. M., Bailey-Wilson, J. E., Freidlin, B., Biddison, W. E., McFarland, H. F., & Trent, J. M. (1998). Clustering of non-major histocompatibility complex susceptibility candidate loci in human autoimmune diseases. *Proc Natl Acad Sci USA*, 95, 17, (Aug 1998), 9979–9984, 0027-8424

Biedermann, T., Röcken, M., & Carballido, J. M. (2004). TH1 and TH2 lymphocyte development and regulation of TH cell mediated immune responses of the skin. *J Invest Dermatol*, 9, 1, (Jan 2004), 5–14, 0022-202X

Blauvelt, A. (2008). T-helper 17 cells in psoriatic plaques and additional genetic links between IL-23 and psoriasis. *J Invest Dermatol*, 128, 5, (May 2008), 1064-7, 0022-202X

Boker, A., Kimball, A. B., & Rolz-Cruz, G. (2007). Biologicals in the treatment of psoriasis. *Curr Opin Invest Drugs*, 8, 11, (Nov 2007), 939–946, 1472-4472

Bonish, B., Jullien, D., Dutronc, Y., Huang, B. B., Modlin, R., Spada, F. M., Porcelli, S. A., & Nickoloff, B. J. (2000). Overexpression of CD1d by keratinocytes in psoriasis and CD1d-dependent IFN-gamma production by NK-T cells. *J Immunol*, 165, 7, (Oct 2000), 4076–4085, 0022-1767

Bosani, M., Ardizzone, S., & Porro, G. B. (2009). Biologic targeting in the treatment of inflammatory bowel diseases. *Biologics*, 3, (Jul 2009), 77–97, 1177-5475

Boulton, J. G., & Bourne, J. T. (2007). Unstable diabetes in a patient receiving anti-TNF-alpha for rheumatoid arthritis. *Rheumatology*, 46, 1, (Jan 2007), 178–179, 1462-0324

Bourne, T., Fossati, G., & Nesbitt, A. (2008). A PEGylated Fab' fragment against tumor necrosis factor for the treatment of Crohn's disease: exploring a new mechanism of action. *BioDrugs* 22, 5, (2008), 331–337, 1173-8804

Bovenschen, H. J., Gerritsen, W. J., van Rens, D. W., Seyger, M. M., de Jong, E. M., & van de Kerkhof, P. C. (2007). Explorative immunohistochemical study to evaluate the addition of a topical corticosteroid in the early phase of alefacept treatment for psoriasis. *Arch Dermatol Res*, 298, 9, (Feb 2007), 457–463

Bowcock, A. M., & Krueger, J. G. (2005). Getting under the skin: the immunogenetics of psoriasis. *Nat Rev Immunol*, 5, 9, (Sept 2005), 699–711, 1474-1733

Brandrup, F., Hauge, M., Henningsen, K., & Eriksen, B. (1978). Psoriasis in an unselected series of twins. *Arch Dermatol*, 114, 6, (Jun 1978), 874–878, 0003-987X

Brewerton, D. A., Caffrey, M., Nicholls, A., Walters, D., & James, D. C. (1974). HL-A 27 and arthropaties associated with ulcerative colitis and psoriasis. *Lancet*, 1, 7864, (May 1974), 956–958, 0140-6736

Cameron, A. L., Kirby, B., & Griffiths, C. E. (2003). Circulating natural killer cells in psoriasis. *Br J Dermatol*, 149, 1, (Jun 2003), 160–164, 0007-0963

Cameron, A. L., Kirby, B., Fei, W., & Griffiths, C. E. (2002). Natural killer and natural killer-T cells in psoriasis. *Arch Dermatol Res*, 294, 8, (Nov 2002), 363–369

Capon, F., Bijlmakers, M. J., Wolf, N., Quaranta, M., Huffmeier, U., Allen, M., Timms, K., Abkevich, V., Gutin, A., Smith, R., Warren, R. B., Young, H. S., Worthington, J., Burden, A. D., Griffiths, C. E., Hayday, A., Nestle, F. O., Reis, A., Lanchbury, J., Barker, J. N., & Trembath, R. C. (2008). Identification of ZNF313/ RNF114 as a novel psoriasis susceptibility gene. *Hum Mol Genet*, 17, 13, (Jul 2008), 1938–45

Capon, F., Di Meglio, P., Szaub, J., Prescott, N. J., Dunster, C., Baumber, L., Timms, K., Gutin, A., Abkevic, V., Burden, A. D., Lanchbury, J., Barker, J. N., Trembath, R. C., & Nestle, F. O. (2007). Sequence variants in the genes for the interleukin-23 receptor (IL23R) and its ligand (IL12B) confer protection against psoriasis. *Hum Genet*, 122, 2, (Sep 2007), 201–6

Chan, J. R., Blumenschein, W., Murphy, E., Diveu, C., Wiekowski, M., Abbondanzo, S., Lucian, L., Geissler, R., Brodie, S., Kimball, A. B., Gorman, D. M., Smith, K., de

Waal Malefyt, R., Kastelein, R. A., McClanahan, T. K., & Bowman, E. P. (2006). IL-23 stimulates epidermal hyperplasia via TNF and IL-20R2-dependent mechanisms with implications for psoriasis pathogenesis. *J Exp Med*, 203, 12, (Nov 2006), 2577–87, 0022-1007

Chan, W. L., Pejnovic, N., Liew, T. V., Lee, C. A., Groves, R., & Hamilton, H. (2003). NKT cell subsets in infection and inflammation. *Immunol Lett*, 85, 2, (Jan 2003), 159–163, 0165-2478

Clark, R. A., & Kupper, T. S. (2006). Misbehaving macrophages in the pathogenesis of psoriasis. *J Clin Invest* 116, 8, (Aug 2006), 2084–7, 0021-9738

Cohen, A. D., Dreiher, J., & Birkenfeld, S. (2009). Psoriasis associated with ulcerative colitis and Crohn's disease. *J Eur Acad Dermatol Venereol*, 23, 5, (May 2009), 561–565

Conrad, C., Boyman, O., Tonel, G., Tun-Kyi, A., Laggner, U., de Fougerolles, A., Kotelianski, V., Gardner, H., & Nestle, F. O. (2007). Alpha1beta1 integrin is crucial for accumulation of epidermal T cells and the development of psoriasis. *Nat Med*, 13, 7, (Jun 2007), 836–42, 1078-8956

Curry, J. L., Qin, J. Z., Robinson, J., & Nickoloff, B. J. (2003). Reactivity of resident immunocytes in normal and prepsoriatic skin using an ex vivo skin-explant model system. *Arch Pathol Lab Med*, 127, 3, (Mar 2003), 289–296, 0003-9985

Dahlqvist, S. R., Engstrand, S., Berglin, E., & Johnson, O. (2004). Conversion towards an atherogenic lipid profile in rheumatoid arthritis patients during long-term infliximab therapy. *Scand J Rheumatol*, 35, 2, (Mar-Apr 2004), 107–111

De Filippis, L. G., Caliri, A., Lo Gullo, R., Bartolone, S. , Miceli, G., Cannavò, S. P., Borgia, F., Basile, G., Aloisi, G., Zimbaro, G., Scribano, E., & Bagnato, G. F. (2005). Ultrasonography in the early diagnosis of psoriasis-associated enthesopathy. *Int J Tissue React*, 27, 4 (2005), 159–162, 0250-0868

D'Elios, M. M., Del Prete, G., & Amedei, A. (2010). Targeting IL-23 in human diseases. *Expert Opin Ther Targets*, 14, 7, (Jul 2010), 759-74, 1472-8222

Detmar, M., Brown, L. F., Claffey, K. P., Yeo, K. T., Kocher, O., Jackman, R. W.,. Berse, B., & Dvorak, H. F. (1994). Overexpression of vascular permeability factor/vascular endothelial growth factor and its receptors in psoriasis. *J Exp Med* 180, 3, (Sep 1994), 1141–6, 0022-1007

Di Cesare, A., Di Meglio, P., & Nestle, F. O. (2009). The IL-23/Th17 Axis in the Immunopathogenesis of Psoriasis. *J Invest Dermatol*, 129, 6, (Jun 2009), 1339–50, 0022-202X

Diarra, D., Stolina, M., Polzer, K., Zwerina, J., Ominsky, M. S., Dwyer, D., Korb, A., Smolen, J., Hoffmann, M., Scheinecker, C., van der Heide, D., Landewe, R., Lacey, D., Richards, W. G., & Schett, G. (2007). Dickkopf-1 is a master regulator of joint remodeling. *Nat Med*, 13, 2, (Feb 2007), 156–163. 20, 1078-8956

Ding, C., Xu, J., & Li, J. (2008). ABT-874, a fully human monoclonal anti IL-12/IL-23 antibody for the potential treatment of autoimmune diseases. *Curr Opin Investig Drugs* 9, 5, (May 2008), 515–522, 1472-4472

Djemadji-Oudjiel, N., Goerdt, S., Kodelja, V., Schmuth, M., & Orfanos, C. E. (1996). Immunohistochemical identification of type II alternatively activated dendritic macrophages (RM 3/1+3, MS-1+/_, 25F9-) in psoriatic dermis. *Arch Dermatol Res*, 288, 12, (Nov 1996), 757–64

Duerr, R. H., Taylor, K. D., Brant, S. R., Rioux, J. D., Silverberg, M. S., Daly, M. J., Steinhart, A. H., Abraham, C., Regueiro, M., Griffiths, A., Dassopoulos, T., Bitton, A., Yang,

H., Targan, S., Datta, L. W., Kistner, E. O., Schumm, L. P., Lee, A. T., Gregersen, P. K., Barmada, M. M., Rotter, J. I., Nicolae, D. L., & Cho, J. H. (2006). A genome-wide association study identifies IL23R as an inflammatory bowel disease gene. *Science*, 314, 5804, (Dec 2006), 1461–1463, 0036-8075

Elder, J. T., Bruce, A. T., Gudjonsson, J. E., Johnston, A., Stuart, P. E., Tejasvi, T., Voorhees, J. J., Abecasis, G. R., & Nair, R. P. (2010). Molecular dissection of psoriasis: integrating genetics and biology. *J Invest Dermatol*, 130, 5, (May 2010), 1213-26, 0022-202X

EMEA. (2008). Refusal assessment report for CIMZIA. Procedure No. EMEA/H/C/740. 19 March 2008, available from: <http://www.emea.europa.eu/humandocs/PDFs/EPAR/cimzia/H-740-RAR-en.pdf>

EMEA. (2009). European Medicines Agency recommends suspension of the marketing authorisation of Raptiva (efalizumab). 19 February 2009, available from: <http://www.emea.europa.eu/humandocs/PDFs/EPAR/raptiva/20855709en.pdf >

Ettehadi, P., Greaves, M. W., Wallach, D., Aderka, D., & Camp, R. D. (1994). Elevated tumor necrosis factor-alpha (TNF alpha) biological activity in psoriatic skin lesions. *Clin Exp Immunol*, 96, 1, (Apr 1994), 146–151, 0009-9104

Eyre, R. W., & Krueger, G. G. (1984). The Koebner response in psoriasis, In: *Psoriasis*, Roenigk, H. H., Maibach, H. I., 105-116, Marcel Dekker, 0824772954, New York

Fan, X., Yang, S., Sun, L. D., Liang, Y. H., Gao, M., Zhang, K. Y., Huang, W., & Zhang, X. (2007). Comparison of clinical features of HLA-Cw*0602-positive and-negative psoriasis patients in a Han Chinese population. *Acta Derm Venereol*, 87, 4, 335–40, 0001-5555

FDA. (2009). (2009). FDA statement on the voluntary withdrawal of raptiva from the US market. 8 April 2009, available from: <http://www.fda.gov/bbs/topics/NEWS/2009/NEW01992.html>

FitzGerald, O., & Winchester, R. (2009). Psoriatic arthritis: from pathogenesis to therapy. *Arthritis Res Ther*, 11, 1, (Feb 2009), 214, 1478-6362

Fleischmajer, R., Kuroda, K., Hazan, R., Gordon, R. E., Lebwohl, M. G., Sapadin, A. N., Unda, F., Iehara, N., & Yamada, Y. (2000). Basement membrane alterations in psoriasis are accompanied by epidermal overexpression of MMP-2 and its inhibitor TIMP-2. *J Invest Dermatol*, 115, 5, (Nov 2000), 771–7, 0022-202X

Fredriksson, T., & Pettersson, U. (1978). Severe psoriasis – oral therapy with a new retinoid. *Dermatologica*,157, 4, (1978), 238–244, 0011-9059

Gallucci, S., Lolkema, M., & Matzinger, P. (1999). Natural adjuvants: endogenous activators of dendritic cells. *Nat Med*, 5,11, (Nov 1999), 1249–55, 1078-8956

Gaspari, A. A. (2006). Innate and adaptive immunity and the pathophysiology of psoriasis. *J Am Acad Dermatol*, 54, 3, (Mar 2006), 67–80

Gelfand, J. M., Neimann, A. L., Shin, D. B., Wang, X., Margolis, D. J., & Troxel, A. B. (2006). Risk of myocardial infarction in patients with psoriasis. *JAMA*, 296, 14, (Oct 2006), 1735–1741, 0098-7484

Gerdes, S., & Mrowietz, U. (2009). Impact of comorbidities on the management of psoriasis. *Curr Probl Dermatol*, 38, (Jul 2009), 21–36

Gisondi, P., Girolomoni, G., Sampogna, F., Tabolli, S., & Albeni, D. (2005). Prevalence of psoriatic arthritis and joints complaints in a large population of Italian patients hospitalized for psoriasis. *Eur J Dermatol*, 15, 4, (Jul-Aug 2005), 279–283, 1167-1122

Gisondi, P., Tinazzi, I., El-Dalati, G., Gallo, M., Biasi, D., Barbara, L. M., & Girolomoni, G. (2008). Lower limb enthesopathy in patients with psoriasis without clinical signs of arthropaty: a hospital-based case-control study. *Ann Rheum Dis*, 67, 1, (Jan 2008), 26–30, 0003-4967

Gladman, D. D. (2009). Psoriatic arthritis. *Dermatol Ther*, 22, 1, (Jan-Feb 2009), 40–55, 1396-0296

Gladman, D. D., Farewell, V. T., Husted, J., & Wong, K. (1998). Mortality studies in psoriatic arthritis. Results from a single centre. II. Prognostic indicators for mortality. *Arthritis Rheum*, 41, 6, (Jun 1998), 1103–1110, 0004-3591

Gladman, D. D., Stafford-Brady, F., Chang, C. H., Lewandowski, K., & Russell, M. L. (1990). Longitudinal study of clinical and radiological progression in psoriatic arthritis. *J Rheumatol*, 17, 6, (Jun 1990), 809–812, 0315-162X

Gondek, D. C., Lu, L. F., Quezada, S. A., Sakaguchi, S., & Noelle, R. J. (2005). Cutting edge: contact-mediated suppression by CD4+CD25+ regulatory cells involves a granzyme B-dependent, perforin-independent mechanism. *J Immunol*, 174, 4, (Feb 2005), 1783–6, 0022-1767

Gordon, K. B., Vaishnaw, A. K., O'Gorman, J., Haney, J., Menter, A., & Alefacept Clinical Study Group. (2003). Treatment of psoriasis with alefacept: correlation of clinical improvement with reductions of memory T cell counts. *Arch Dermatol* 139, 12, (Dec 2003), 1563–1570, 0003-987X

Gottlieb, A. B., Chamian, F., Masud, S., Cardinale, I., Abello, M. V., Lowes, M. A., Chen, F., Magliocco, M., & Krueger, J. G. (2005). TNF inhibition rapidly down-regulates multiple proinflammatory pathways in psoriasis plaques. *J Immunol*, 175, 4, (Aug 2005), 2721–9, 0022-1767

Gottlieb, A. B., Cooper, K. D., McCormick, T. S., Toichi, E., Everitt, D. E., Frederick, B., Zhu, Y., Pendley, C. E., Graham, M. A., & Mascelli, M. A. (2007). A phase 1, double-blind, placebo-controlled study evaluating single subcutaneous administration of human interleukin-12/23 monoclonal antibody in subjects with plaque psoriasis. *Curr Med Res Opin*, 23, 5, (May 2007), 1081–1092

Gottlieb, A. B., Mease, P. J., Mark Jackson, J., Eisen, D., Amy Xia, H., Asare, C., & Stevens, S. R. (2006). Clinical characteristics of psoriatic arthritis and psoriasis in dermatologists' office. *J Dermatolog Treat*, 17, 5, (2006), 279–287

Gottlieb, A., Menter, A., Mendelsohn, A., Shen, Y. K., Li, S., Guzzo, C., Fretzin, S., Kunynetz, R., Kavanaugh, A. (2009). Ustekinumab, a human interleukin 12/23 monoclonal antibody, for psoriatic arthritis: randomised, double-blind, placebocontrolled, crossover trial. *Lancet*, 373, 9664, (Feb 2009), 633–40, 0140-6736

Gottlieb, S. L., Gilleaudeau, P., Johnson, R., Estes, L., Woodworth, T. G., Gottlieb, A. B., & Krueger, J. G. (1995). Response of psoriasis to a lymphocyte-selective toxin (DAB389IL-2) suggests a primary immune, but not keratinocyte, pathogenic basis. *Nat Med*, 1, 5, (May 1995), 442–7, 1078-8956

Griffiths, C. E. M., Strober, B., van de Kerkhof, P. C. M., Ho, V., Guzzo, C., Yeilding, N. (2008). A phase 3 multicenter, randomized study comparing ustekinumab and etanercept for the treatment of moderate to severe plaque psoriasis. Proceedings of European Academy of Dermatology and Venerology Annual Congress Paris, July 2008.

Griffiths, C. E., & Barker, J. N. (2007). Pathogenesis and clinical features of psoriasis. *Lancet*, 370, 9583, (Jul 2007), 263–271, 0140-6736

Griffiths, C. E., Christophers, E., Barker, J. N., Chalmers, R. J., Chimenti, S., Krueger, G. G., Leonardi, C., Menter, A., Ortonne, J. P., & Fry, L. (2007). A classification of psoriasis vulgaris according to phenotype. *Br J Dermatol*, G, 2, (Feb 2007), 258-262, 0007-0963

Grundy, S. M., Cleeman, J. I., Daniels, S. R., Donato, K. A., Eckel, R. H., Franklin, B. A., Gordon, D. J., Krauss, R. M., Savage, P. J., Smith. S. C. Jr., Spertus, J. A., Costa, F., American Heart Association, & National Heart, Lung, and Blood Institute. (2005). Diagnosis and management of the metabolic syndrome: an American Heart Association/National Heart, Lung, and Blood Institute Scientific Statement. *Circulation*, 112, 17, (Oct 2005), 2735-2752, 0009-7322

Gudjonsson, J. E., Johnston, A., Sigmundsdottir, H., & Valdimarsson, H. (2004). Immunopathogenic mechanisms in psoriasis. *Clin Exp Immunol*, 135, 1, (Jan 2004), 1-8, 0009-9104

Gudjonsson, J. E., Karason, A., Runarsdottir, E. H., Antonsdottir, A. A., Hauksson, V. B., Jonsson, H. H., Gulcher, J., Stefansson, K., & Valdimarsson, H. (2006). Distinct clinical differences between HLA-Cw*0602 positive and negative psoriasis patients-an analysis of 1019 HLA-C- and HLA-B-typed patients. *J Invest Dermatol*, 126, 4, (Apr 2006), 740-5, 0022-202X

Gupta, M. A., Gupta, A. K., Kirkby, S., Schork, N. J., Gorr, S. K., Ellis, C. N., & Voorhees, J. J. (1989). A psychocutaneous profile of psoriasis patients who are stress reactors. A study of 127 patients. *Gen Hosp Psychiatry*, 11, 3, (May 1989), 166-73

Haider, A. S., Duculan, J., Whynot, J. A., & Krueger, J. G. (2006). Increased JunB mRNA and protein expression in psoriasis vulgaris lesions. *J Invest Dermatol*, 126, 4, (Apr 2006), 912-4, 0022-202X

Haider, A. S., Lowes, M. A., Suárez-Farinas, M., Zaba, L. C., Cardinale, I., Khatcherian, A., Novitskaya, I., Wittkowski, K. M., & Krueger, J. G. (2008). Identification of cellular pathways of "type 1," Th17 T cells, and TNF- and inducible nitric oxide synthaseproducing dendritic cells in autoimmune inflammation through pharmacogenomic study of cyclosporine A in psoriasis. *J Immunol*, 180, 3, (Feb 2008), 1913-20, 0022-1767

Henseler, T., & Christophers, E. (1985). Psoriasis of early and late onset: characterization of two types of psoriasis vulgaris. *J Am Acad Dermatol*, 13, 3, (Sept 1985), 450-6

Henseler, T., & Christophers, E. (1995). Disease concomitance in psoriasis. *J Am Acad Dermatol*, 32, 6, (Jun 1995), 982-986

Hensen, P., Windemuth, C., Hüffmeier, U., Rüschendorf, F., Stadelmann, A., Hoppe, V., Fenneker, D., Ständer, M., Schmitt-Egenolf, M., Wienker, T. F., Traupe, H., & Reis, A. (2003). Association scan of the novel psoriasis susceptibility region on chromosome 19: evidence for both susceptible and protective loci. *Exp Dermatol*, 12,4, (Aug 2003), 490-6

Holash, J., Maisonpierre, P. C., Compton, D., Boland, P., Alexander, C. R., Zagzag, D., Yancopoulos, G. D., & Wiegand, S. J. (1999). Vessel cooption, regression, and growth in tumors mediated by angiopoietins and VEGF. *Science*, 284, 5422, (Jun 1999), 1994-8, 0036-8075

Hüffmaier, U., Lascorz, J., Böhm, B., Lohmann, J., Wendler, J., Mössner, R., Reich, K., Traupe, H., Kurrat, W., Burkhardt, H., & Reis, A. (2009). Genetic variants of the IL-23R pathway: association with psoriatic arthritis and psoriasis vulgaris, but no specific risk factor for arthritis. *J Invest Dermatol*, 129, 2, (Feb 2009), 355-358, 0022-202X

Huvers, F. C., Popa, C., Netea, M. G., van den Hoogen, F. H., & Tack, C. J. (2007). Improved insulin sensitivity by anti-TNFalpha antibody treatment in patients with rheumatic diseases. *Ann Rheum Dis*, 66, 4, (Apr 2007), 558–559, 0003-4967

Irace, C. ,Mancuso, G., Fiaschi, E., Madia, A., Sesti, G., & Gnasso, A. (2004). Effect of anti TNFalpha therapy on arterial diameter and wall shear stress and HDL cholesterol. *Atherosclerosis*, 177, 1, (Nov 2004), 113–118, 0021-9150

Jablonska, S. (1986). Immunological mechanisms in psoriasis: role of polymorphonuclear leukocytes, In: *Psoriasis,* Farber, E. M., Nall, L., Morhenn, V., & Jacobs, P. H., 131-7, Elsevier, 0444012125, New York

Jegasothy, B. V., Ackerman, C. D., Todo, S., Fung, J. J., Abu-Elmagd, K., & Starzl, T. E. (1992). Tacrolimus (FK 506)–a new therapeutic agent for severe recalcitrant psoriasis. *Arch Dermatol*, 128, 6, (Jun 1992), 781–5, 0003-987X

Johnson, L. W., & Weinstock, R. S. (2006). The metabolic syndrome: concepts and controversy. *Mayo Clin Proc*, 81, 12, (Dec 2006), 1615–1620, 0025-6196

Kana, D., Stafford, L., Bresniham, B., & Fitzgerald, O. (2003). A prospective, clinical and radiological study of early psoriatic arthritis: an early synovitis clinic experience. *Rheumatology*, 42, 12, (Dec 2003), 1460–1468, 1462-0324

Katz, H. I., Waalen, J., & Leach, E. E. (1994). Acitretin in psoriasis: an overview of adverse effects. *J Am Acad Dermatol*, 41, 3 Pt 2, (Sep 1994), S7–S12

Kauffman, C. L., Aria, N., Toichi, E., McCormick, T. S., Cooper, K. D., Gottlieb, A. B., Everitt, D. E., Frederick, B., Zhu, Y., Graham, M. A., Pendley, C. E., & Mascelli, M. A. (2004). A phase I study evaluating the safety, pharmacokinetics, and clinical response of a human IL-12 p40 antibody in subjects with plaque psoriasis. *J Invest Dermatol*, 123, 6, (Dec 2004), 1037–44, 0022-202X

Kavanaugh, A., McInnes, I., Mease, P., Krueger, G. G., Gladman, D., Gomez- Reino, J. Papp, K., Zrubek, J., Mudivarthy, S., Mack, M., Visvanathan, S., & Beutler, A. (2009). Golimumab, a new human tumor necrosis factor a, administered every four weeks as a subcutaneous injection in psoriatic arthritis: twenty-four-week efficacy and safety results of a randomized, placebo-controlled study. *Arthritis Rheum,* 60, 4, (Apr 2009), 976– 986, 0003-4967

Keffer, J., Probert, L., Cazlaris, H., Georgopoulos, S., Kaslaris, E., Kioussis, D., & Kollias, G. (1991). Transgenic mice expression human tumor necrosis factor: a predictive genetic model of arthritis. *EMBO J*, 10, 13 (Dec 1991), 4025–4031

Kimball, A. B., Gladman, D., Gelfand, J.M., Gordon, K., Horn, E. J., Korman, N. J., Korver, G., Krueger, G. G., Strober, B. E., Lebwohl, M. G., & National Psoriasis Foundation. (2008a). National Psoriasis Foundation clinical consensus on psoriasis comorbidities and recommendations for screening. *J Am Acad Dermatol,* 58, 6, (Jun 2008), 1031–1042

Kimball, A. B., Gordon, K. B., Langley, R. G., Menter, A., Chartash, E. K., & Valdes, J. (2008b). Safety and efficacy of ABT-874, a fully human interleukin 12/23 monoclonal antibody, in the treatment of moderate to severe chronic plaque psoriasis: results of a randomized, placebo-controlled, phase 2 trial. *Arch Dermatol,* 144, 2, (Feb 2008), 200–7, 0003-987X

Kimball, A. B., Robinson, D. Jr., Wu, Y., Yeilding, N., Paramore, C., Fraeman, K., & Bala, M. (2008c). Cardiovascular disease and risk factors among psoriasis patients in two US healthcare databases, 2001–2002. *Dermatology*, 217, 1, (Mar 2008), 27–37, 1018-8665

Koreck, A., Sura´nyi, A., Szo¨ny, B. J., Farkas, A., Bata-Csörgö, Z., Kemény, L., & Dobozy, A. (2002). CD3+CD56+ NK T cells are significantly decreased in the peripheral blood of patients with psoriasis. *Clin Exp Immunol*, 127, 1, (Jan 2002), 176–182, 0009-9104

Kremers, H. M., McEvoy, M. T., Dann, F. J., & Gabriel, S. E. (2007). Heart disease in psoriasis. *J Am Acad Dermatol*, 57, 2, (Aug 2007), 347-354

Krueger, G. G., Bergstresser, P. R., Lowe, N. J., Voorhees, J. J., & Weinstein, G. D. Psoriasis. (1984). *J Am Acad Dermatol*, 11, 5, (Nov 1984), 937–47

Krueger, G. G., Langley, R. G., Leonardi, C., Yeilding, N., Guzzo, C., Wang, Y., Dooley, L. T., Lebwohl, M., & CNTO 1275 Psoriasis Study Group. (2007). A human interleukin-12/23 monoclonal antibody for the treatment of psoriasis. *N Engl J Med*, 356, 6, (Feb 2007), 580–92, 0028-4793

Krueger, J. G. (2002). The immunologic basis for the treatment of psoriasis with new biologic agents. *J Am Acad Dermatol*, 46, 1, (Jan 2002), 1–23

Kuroda, K., Sapadin, A., Shoji, T., Fleischmajer, R., & Lebwohl, M. (2001). Altered expression of angiopoietins and Tie2 endothelium receptor in psoriasis. *J Invest Dermatol*, 116, 15, (May 2001), 713–20, 0022-202X

Langewouters, A. M., van Erp, P. E., de Jong, E. M., & van de Kerkhof, P. C. (2008). Lymphocyte subsets in peripheral blood of patients with moderate-tosevere versus mild plaque psoriasis. *Arch Dermatol Res* 2008; 300, 3, (Mar 2008), 107–113

Langrish, C. L., Chen, Y., Blumenschein, W. M., Mattson, J., Basham, B., Sedgwick, J. D., McClanahan, T., Kastelein, R. A., & Cua, D. J. (2005). IL-23 drives a pathogenic T cell population that induces autoimmune inflammation. *J Exp Med*, 201, 2, (Jan 2005), 233–40, 0022-1007

Larsen, R., Ryder, L. P., Svejgaard, A., & Gniadecki, R. (2007). Changes in circulating lymphocyte subpopulations following administration of the leucocyte function-associated antigen-3 (LFA-3)/IgG1 fusion protein alefacept. *Clin Exp Immunol*, 149, 1, (Jun 2007), 23–30

Leonardi, C. L., Kimball, A. B., Papp, K. A., Yeilding, N., Guzzo, C., Wang, Y., Li, S., Dooley, L. T., Gordon, K. B., & PHOENIX 1 study investigators. (2008). Efficacy and safety of ustekinumab, a human interleukin-12/23 monoclonal antibody, in patients with psoriasis: 76-week results from a randomised, double-blind, placebo-controlled trial (PHOENIX 1). *Lancet*, 371, 9625, (May 2008), 1665–74, 0140-6736

Lew, W., Bowcock, A. M., & Krueger, J. G. (2004). Psoriasis vulgaris: cutaneous lymphoid tissue supports T-cell activation and "Type 1" inflammatory gene expression. *Trends Immunol*, 25, 6, (Jun 2004), 295–305, 1471-4906

Liao, Y. H., Jee, S. H., Sheu, B. C., Huang, Y. L., Tseng, M. P., Hsu, S. M., & Tsai, T. F. (2006). Increased expression of the natural killer cell inhibitory receptor CD94/NKG2A and CD158b on circulating and lesional T cells in patients with chronic plaque psoriasis. *Br J Dermatol*, 155, 2, (Aug 2006), 318–324, 0007-0963

Lima, X. T., Seidler, E. M., Lima, H. C., & Kimball, A. B. (2009). Long-term safety of biologics in dermatology. *Dermatol Ther*, 22, 1, (Jan-Feb 2009), 2–21, 1396-0296

Mallbris, L., Akre, O., Granath, F., Yin, L., Lindelöf, B., Ekbom, A., & Ståhle-Bäckdahl, M. (2004). Increased risk for cardiovascular mortality in psoriasis inpatients but not in outpatients. *Eur J Epidemiol*, 19, 3, (2004), 225–230

Mallon, E., Newson, R., & Bunker, C. B. (1999). HLA-Cw6 and the genetic predisposition to psoriasis: a metaanalysis of published serologic studies. *J Invest Dermatol*, 113, 4, (Oct 1999), 693–5, 0022-202X

Marble, D. J., Gordon, K. B., Nickoloff, B. J. (2007). Targeting TNFalpha rapidly reduces density of dendritic cells and macrophages in psoriatic plaques with restoration of epidermal keratinocyte differentiation. *J Dermatol Sci*, 48, 2, (Nov 20079, 87–101, 0923-1811

Marra, M., Campanati, A., Testa, R., Sirolla, C., Bonfigli, A. R., Franceschi, C., Marchegiani, F., & Offidani, A. (2007). Effect of etanercept on insulin sensitivity in nine patients with psoriasis. *Int J Immunopathol Pharmacol*, 20, 4, (Oct-Dec 2007), 731–736

Martin, M. P., Nelson, G., Lee, J. H., Pellett, F., Gao, X., Wade, J., Wilson, M. J., Trowsdale, J., Gladman, D., & Carrington, M. (2002). Cutting edge: susceptibility to psoriatic arthritis: influence of activating killer Ig-like receptor genes in the absence of specific HLA-C alleles. *J Immunol*, 169, 6, (Sept 2002), 2818–22, 0022-1767

McEwen, C., DiTata, D., Lingg, C., Porini, A., Good, A., & Rankin, T. (1971). Ankylosing spondylitis and spondylitis accompanying ulcerative colitis, regional enteritis, psoriasis and Reiter's disease. A comparative study. *Arthritis Rheum*, 14, 3, (May-Jun 1971), 291–318, 0004-3591

McKenzie, B. S., Kastelein, R. A., & Cua, D. J. (2006). Understanding the IL-23-IL-17 immune pathway. *Trends Immunol*, 27, 1, (Jan 2006), 17–23, 1471-4906

Mease, P. J., Gladman, D. D., & Keystone, E. C. (2006a). Alefacept with methotrexate for the treatment of psoriatic arthritis: results from a double blind, placebo-controlled study. *Arthritis Rheum* 54, 5, (May 2006), 1638– 1645, 0004-3591

Mease, P. J., Kivitz, A. J., Burch, F. X., Siegel, E. L., Cohen, S. B., Ory, P., Salonen, D., Rubenstein, J., Sharp, J. T., Dunn, M., & Tsuji, W. (2006b). Continued inhibition of radiographic progression in patients with psoriatic arthritis following 2 years of treatment with etanercept. *J Rheumatol*, 33, 4, (Apr 2006), 712–721, 0315-162X

Menssen, A., Trommler, P., Vollmer, S., Schendel, D., Albert, E., Gurtler, L., Riethmüller, G., & Prinz, J. C. (1995). Evidence for an antigenspecific cellular immune response in skin lesions of patients with psoriasis vulgaris. *J Immunol*, 155, 8, (Oct 1995), 4078–83, 0022-1767

Menter, A., Gottlieb, A., Feldman, S. R., Van Voorhees, A. S., Leonardi, C. L., Gordon, K. B., Lebwohl, M. G., Koo, J. Y., Elmets, C. A., Korman, N. J., Beutner, K. R., & Bhushan, R. (2008). Guidelines of care for the management of psoriasis and psoriatic arthritis: section I. Overview of psoriasis and guidelines of care for the treatment of psoriasis with biologics. *J Am Acad Dermatol*, 58, 5, (May 2008), 826–850

Montecucco, C. (2006). Remission, a therapeutic goal in inflammatory arthropathies? Clinical data from adalimumab studies. *Drugs*, 66, 14, (2006), 1783–1795, 0012-6667

Morris, A., Rogers, M., Fischer, G., & Williams, K. (2001). Childhood psoriasis: a clinical review of 1262 cases. *Pediatr Dermatol*, 18, 3, (May-Jun 2001), 188–98

Mössner, R., Schön, M. P., & Reich, K. (2008). Tumor necrosis factor antagonists in the therapy of psoriasis. *Clin Dermatol* 26, 5, (Sep-Oct 2008), 486–502, 0738-081X

Mrowietz, U., Elder, J. T., & Barker, J. (2006). The importance of disease associations and concomitant therapy for the long-term management of psoriasis patients. *Arch Dermatol Res*, 298, 7, (Dec 2006), 309–319

Nair, R. P., Stuart, P. E., Nistor, I., Hiremagalore, R., Chia, N. V., Jenisch, S., Weichenthal, M., Abecasis, G. R., Lim, H. W., Christophers, E., Voorhees, J. J., & Elder, J. T. (2006). Sequence and haplotype analysis supports HLA-C as the psoriasis susceptibility 1 gene. *Am J Hum Genet*, 78, 5, (May 2006), 827–51, 0002-9297

Najarian, D. J., & Gottlieb, A. B. (2003). Connections between psoriasis and Crohn's disease. *J Am Acad Dermatol*, 48, 6, (Jun 2003), 805–821

Nakamura, K., Kitani, A., Fuss, I., Pedersen, A., Harada, N., Nawata, H., & Strober, W. (2004). TGF-beta 1 plays an important role in the mechanism of CD4+CD25+ regulatory T cell activity in both humans and mice. *J Immunol*, 172, 2, (Jan 2004), 834–42, 0022-1767

Namazi, M. R. (2004). Paradoxical exacerbation of psoriasis in AIDS: proposed explanations including the potential roles of substance P and gram-negative bacteria. *Autoimmunity*, 37, 1, (Feb 2004), 67–71

Neimann, A. L., Shin, D. B., Wang, X., Margolis, D. J., Troxel, A. B., & Gelfand, J. M. (2006). Prevalence of cardiovascular risk factors in patients with psoriasis. *J Am Acad Dermatol* 55, 5, (Nov 2006), 829–835

Nestle, F. O., Kaplan, D. H., & Barker, J. (2009). Psoriasis. *N Engl J Med*, 361, 5, (Jul 2009), 496–509, 0028-4793

Nickoloff, B. J. (1999a). Skin innate immune system in psoriasis: friend or foe?. *J Clin Invest*, 104, 9, (Nov 1999), 1161–4, 0021-9738

Nickoloff, B. J., & Nestle, F. O. (2004). Recent insights into the immunopathogenesis of psoriasis provide new therapeutic opportunities. *J Clin Invest*, 113, 12, (Jun 2004), 1664-1675, 0021-9738

Nickoloff, B. J., Bonish, B., Huang, B. B., & Porcelli, S. A. (2000). Characterization of a T cell line bearing natural killer receptors and capable of creating psoriasis in a SCID mouse model system. *J Dermatol Sci*, 24, 3, (Dec 2000), 212–225, 0923-1811

Nickoloff, B. J., Karabin, G. D., Barker, J. N., Griffiths, C. E., Sarma, V., Mitra, R. S., Elder, J. T., Kunkel, S. L., & Dixit, V. M. (1991). Cellular localization of interleukin-8 and its inducer, tumor necrosis factor-alpha in psoriasis. *Am J Pathol*, 138, 1, (Jan 1991), 129–40, 0002-9440

Nickoloff, B. J., Qin, J. Z., & Nestle, F. O. (2007a). Immunopathogenesis of psoriasis. *Clinic Rev Allerg Immunol*, 33, 1-2, (Oct 2007), 45–56, 1080-0549

Nickoloff, B. J., Wrone-Smith, T., Bonish, B., & Porcelli, S. A. (1999b). Response of murine and normal human skin to injection of allogeneic blood-derived psoriatic immunocytes. Detection of T cells expressing receptors typically present on natural killer cells, including CD94, CD158, and CD161. *Arch Dermatol*, 135, 5, (May 1999), 546–552, 0003-987X

Nickoloff, B. J., Xin, H., Nestle, F. O., & Qin, J. Z. (2007b). The cytokine and chemokine network in psoriasis. *Clin Dermatol* 25, 6, (Nov-Dec 2007), 568–573, 0738-081X

Nograles, K. E., Brasington, R.D., & Bowcock, A. M. (2009). New insights into the pathogenesis and genetics of psoriatic arthritis. *Nat Clin Pract Rheumatol*, 5, 2, (Feb 2009), 83–91, 1745-8382

O'Neill, J. L., & Kalb, R. E. (2009). Ustekinumab in the therapy of chronic plaque psoriasis. *Biologics* 3, (Jul 2009), 159–168, 1177-5475

Oppmann, B., Lesley, R., Blom, B., Timans, J. C., Xu, Y., Hunte, B., Vega, F., Yu, N., Wang, J., Singh, K., Zonin, F., Vaisberg, E., Churakova, T., Liu, M., Gorman, D., Wagner, J., Zurawski, S., Liu, Y., Abrams, J. S., Moore, K. W., Rennick, D., de Waal-Malefyt, R., Hannum, C., Bazan, J. F., & Kastelein, R. A. (2000). Novel p19 protein engages IL-12p40 to form a cytokine, IL-23, with biological activities similar as well as distinct from IL-12. *Immunity*, 13, 5, (Nov 2000), 715–25, 1074-7613

Ortonne, J. P., Tassel, C., & Reich, K. (2007). Efficacy of certolizumab pegol, a PEGylated Fab' fragment of an anti-TNF-a monoclonal antibody, in patients previously exposed to biologicals. Preliminary results of a randomised, placebo-controlled phase II clinical trial in psoriasis, *Proceedings of the 16th Congress of the European Academy of dermatology and Venerology*, Vienna, Austria, May 2007.

Ozcakar, L., Cetin, A., Inanici, F., Kaymal, B., Gurer, C. K., & Kolemen, F. (2005). Ultrasonographical evaluation of the Achilles' tendon in psoriasis patients. *Int J Dermatol*, 44, 11, (Nov 2005), 930–932, 0011-9059

Papp, K. A., Langley, R. G., Lebwohl, M., Krueger, G. G., Szapary, P., Yeilding, N., Guzzo, C., Hsu, M. C., Wang, Y., Li, S., Dooley, L. T., Reich, K., PHOENIX 2 study investigators. (2008). Efficacy and safety of ustekinumab, a human interleukin-12/23 monoclonal antibody, in patients with psoriasis: 52-week results from a randomised, double-blind, placebo-controlled trial (PHOENIX 2). *Lancet*, 371, 9625, (May 2008), 1675–84, 0140-6736

Pathirana, A., Ormerod, A. D., Saiag, P., Smith, C., Spuls, P. I., Nast, A., Barker, J., Bos, J. D., Burmester, G. R., Chimenti, S., Dubertret, L., Eberlein, B., Erdmann, R., Ferguson, J., Girolomoni, G., Gisondi, P., Giunta, A., Griffiths, C., Hönigsmann, H., Hussain, M., Jobling, R., Karvonen, S. L., Kemeny, L., Kopp, I., Leonardi, C., Maccarone, M., Menter, A., Mrowietz, U., Naldi, L., Nijsten, T., Ortonne, J. P., Orzechowski, H. D., Rantanen, T., Reich, K., Reytan, N., Richards, H., Thio, H. B., van de Kerkhof, P., & Rzany, B. (2009). European S3-Guidelines on the systemic treatment of psoriasis vulgaris. *J Eur Acad Dermatol Venerol*, 23, 2, (Oct 2009), 1–70

Pisani, M., & Ruocco, V. (1984). 'Twin' psoriasis in monozygotic twins. *Arch Dermatol*, 120, 11, (Nov 1984),1418–9, 0003-987X

Piskin, G., Sylva-Steenland, R. M., Bos, J. D., & Teunissen, M. B. (2006). In vitro and in situ expression of IL-23 by keratinocytes in healthy skin and psoriasis lesions: enhanced expression in psoriatic skin. *J Immunol*; 176, 3, (Feb 2006), 1908–15, 0022-1767

Piskin, G., Tursen, U., Sylva-Steenland, R. M., Bos, J. D., & Teunissen, M. B. (2004). Clinical improvement in chronic plaque-type psoriasis lesions after narrow-band UVB therapy is accompanied by a decrease in the expression of IFN-gamma inducers – IL-12, IL-18 and IL-23. *Exp Dermatol*, 13, 12, (Dec 2004), 764–72

Popa, C., Netea, M. G., Radstake, T., Van der Meer, J. W., Stalenhoef, A. F., van Riel, P. L., & Barerra, P. (2005). Influence of antitumour necrosis factor therapy on cardiovascular risk factors in patients with active rheumatoid arthritis. *Ann Rheum Dis*, 64, 2, (Feb 2005), 303–305, 0003-4967

Prevoo, M. L., van't Hof, M. A., Kuper, H. H., van Leeuwen, M. A., van de Putte, L. B., & van Riel, P. L. (1995). Modified disease activity scores the include twenty-eight joint counts: development and validation in a prospective longitudinal study of patients with rheumatoid arthritis. *Arthritis Rheum*, 38, 1, (Jan 1995), 44–48, 0004-3591

Prinz, J. C. (2001). Psoriasis vulgaris–a sterile antibacterial skin reaction mediated by cross-reactive T cells? An immunological view of the pathophysiology of psoriasis. *Clin Exp Dermatol*, 26, 4, (Jun 2001), 326–32

Prinz, J., Braun-Falco, O., Meurer, M., Daddona, P., Reiter, C., Rieber, P., & Riethmüller, G. (1991). Chimaeric CD4 monoclonal antibody in treatment of generalised pustular psoriasis. *Lancet*, 338, 8762, (Aug 1991), 320–1, 0140-6736

Product Monograph. (2008). Stelara (ustekinumab). Janssen-Ortho Inc, Toronto, Ontario.

Queiro-Silva, R., Torre-Alonso, J. C., Tinture-Eguren, T., & Lopez-Lagunas, I. (2003). A polyarticular onset predicts erosive and deforming disease in psoriatic arthritis. *Ann Rheum Dis,* 62, 1, (Jan 2003), 68–70, 0003-4967

Radtke, B., Reich, K., Blome, C., Rustenbach, S., & Augustin, M. (2009). Prevalence and clinical features of psoriatic arthritis in 2009 patients with psoriasis: results of a German national survey. *J Eur Acad Dermatol Venerol* 23, 6, (Jun 2009), 683–691

Rapp, S. R., Feldman, S.R., Exum, L., Fleischer, A. B., & Reboussin, D. M. (1999). Psoriasis causes as much disability as other major medical diseases. *J Am Acad Dermatol,* 41, 3 Pt 1, (Sep 1999), 401–407

Reddy, M., Davis, C., Wong, J., Marsters, P., Pendley, C., & Prabhakar, U. (2007). Modulation of CLA, IL-12R, CD40L, and IL-2Ralpha expression and inhibition of IL-12 and IL-23 induced cytokine secretion by CNTO 1275. *Cell Immunol,* 247, 1, (May 2007), 1-11, 0008-8749

Reveille, J.D., Conant, M. A., & Duvic, M. (1990). Human immunodeficiency virus-associated psoriasis, psoriatic arthritis, and Reiter's syndrome: a disease continuum?. *Arthritis Rheum,* 33, 10, (Oct 1990), 1574–8, 0004-3591

Ritchlin, C., Haas-Smith, S. A., Hicks, D., Cappuccio, J., Osterland, C. K., & Looney, R. J. (1998). Patterns of cytokine production in psoriatic synovium. *J Rheumatol,* 25, 8, (Aug 1998), 1544–1552, 0315-162X

Rizzo, H. L., Kagami, S., Phillips, K. G., Kurtz, S. E., Jacques, S. L., & Blauvelt, A. (2011). IL-23-mediated psoriasis-like epidermal hyperplasia is dependent on IL-17A. *J Immunol,* 186, 3, (Feb 2011), 1495-502, 0022-1767

Rogalski, C., Meyer-Hoffert, U., Proksch, E., & Wiedow, O. (2002). Human leukocyte elastase induces keratinocyte proliferation in vitro and in vivo. *J Invest Dermatol,* 118, 1, (Jan 2002), 49–54, 0022-202X

Rondinone, C. M. (2006). Adipocyte-derived hormones, cytokines, and mediators. *Endocrine,* 29, 1, (Feb 2006), 81–90, 0969-711X

Sano, S., Chan, K. S., Carbajal, S., Clifford, J., Peavey, M., Kiguchi, K., Itami, S., Nickoloff, B. J., & DiGiovanni, J. (2005). Stat3 links activated keratinocytes and immunocytes required for development of psoriasis in a novel transgenic mouse model. *Nat Med,* 11, 1, (Jan 2005), 43–9, 1078-8956

Saphiro, J., Cohen, A. D., David, M., Hodak, E., Chodik, G., Viner, A., Kremer, E., & Heymann, A. (2007). The association between psoriasis, diabetes mellitus, and atherosclerosis in Israel: a case-control study. *J Am Acad Dermatol,* 56, 4, (Apr 2007), 629–634

Scalon, J. V., Exter, B. P., Steinberg, M., & Jarvis, C. I. (2009). Ustekinumab: treatment of adult moderate to severe chronic plaque psoriasis. *Ann Pharmacother* 43, 9, (Sep 2009), 1456–1465, 1060-0280

Smith, R. L., Warren, R. B., Griffiths, C. E. M., & Worthington, J. (2009). Genetic susceptibility to psoriasis: an emerging picture. *Genome Med* 22, 1, (Jul 2009), 72

Sobell, J. M., Kalb, R. E., & Weinberg, J. M. (2009). Management of moderate to severe plaque psoriasis (part I): clinical update on T-cell modulators and investigational agents. *J Drugs Dermatol,* 8, 3, (Mar 2009), 230–238

Song, I. H., Appel, H., Haibel, H., Loddenkemper, C., Braun, J., Sieper, J., & Rudwaleit, M. (2008). New onset of Crohn's disease during treatment of active ankylosing spondylitis with etanercept. *J Rheumatol,* 35, 3, (Mar 2008), 532–536, 0315-162X

Soubrier, M., Jouanel, P., Mathieu, S., Poujol, D., Claus, D., Dubost, J. J., & Ristori, J. M. (2008). Effects of antitumor necrosis factor therapy on lipid profile in patients with rheumatoid arthritis. *Joint Bone Spine,* 75, 1, (Jan 2008), 22–24, 1297-319X

Spanakis, E., Sidiropoulos, P., Papadakis, J., Ganotakis, E., Katsikas, G., Karvounaris, S., Bizaki, A., Kritikos, H., & Boumpas, D. T. (2006). Modest but sustained increase of serum high density lipoprotein cholesterol levels in patients with inflammatory arthritides treated with infliximab. *J Rheumatol* 33, 12, (Dec 2006), 2440–2446, 0315-162X

Steinman, R. M., Hawiger, D., & Nussenzweig, M. C. (2003). Tolerogenic dendritic cells. *Annu Rev Immunol,* 21, (Dec 2003), 685–711

Stern, R. S., Nijsten, T., Feldman, S. R., Margolis, D. J., & Rolstad, T. (2004). Psoriasis is common, carries a substantial burden even when not extensive, and is associated with widespread treatment dissatisfaction. *J. Invest Dermatol Symp Proc,* G 2, (Mar 2007), 136–139, 1087-0024

Stratis, A., Pasparakis, M., Rupec, R. A., Markur, D., Hartmann, K., Scharffetter-Kochanek, K., Peters, T., van Rooijen, N., Krieg, T., & Haase, I. (2006). Pathogenic role for skin macrophages in a mouse model of keratinocyte-induced psoriasis-like skin inflammation. *J Clin Invest,* 116, 8, (Aug 2006), 2094–104, 0021-9738

Strober, B. E., & Menon, K. (2005). Folate supplementation during methotrexate therapy for patients with psoriasis. *J Am Acad Dermatol,* 53, 4, (Oct 2005), 652–659

Sugiyama, H., Gyulai, R., Toichi, E., Garaczi, E., Shimada, S., Stevens, S. R., McCormick, T. S., & Cooper, K. D. (2005). Dysfunctional blood and target tissue CD4+ CD25 high regulatory T cells in psoriasis: mechanism underlying unrestrained pathogenic effector T cell proliferation. J Immunol, 174, 1, (Jan 2005), 164–73, 0022-1767

Sugiyama, H., McCormick, T. S., Cooper, K. D., & Korman, N. J. (2008). Alefacept in the treatment of psoriasis. *Clin Dermatol,* 26, 5, (Sep-Oct 2008), 50–58, 0738-081X

Taler, S. J., Textor, S. C., Canzanello, V. J., & Schwartz, L. (1999). Cyclosporin-induced hypertension: incidence, pathogenesis and management. *Drug Saf,* 20, 5, (May 1999), 437–449

Taniguchi, M., Seino, K., & Nakayama, T. (2003). The NKT cell system: bridging innate and acquired immunity. *Nat Immunol,* 4, 12, (Dec 2003), 1164–5, 1529-2908

Teunissen, M. B. M. (2005). Langerhans cells and other skin dendritic cells, In: *Skin Immune System: Cutaneous Immunology and Clinical Immunodermatology,* Bos, J. D., 123–82, Boca Raton CRC Press, 0849319595, FL

Toichi, E., Tachibana, T., & Furukawa, F. (2000). Rapid improvement of psoriasis vulgaris during drug-induced agranulocytosis. *J Am Acad Dermatol,* 43, 2, (Aug 2000), 391–5

Toichi, E., Torres, G., McCormick, T. S., Chang, T., Mascelli, M. A., Kauffmann, C. L., Aria, N., Gottlieb, A. B., Everitt, D. E., Frederick, B., Pendley, C. E., & Cooper, K. D. (2006). An anti-IL-12p40 antibody down-regulates type 1cytokines, chemokines, and IL-12/IL-23 in psoriasis. *J Immunol,* 177, 7, (Oct 2006), 4917–4926, 0022-1767

Torres, M. I., & Rios, A. (2008). Current view of the immunopathogenesis in inflammatory bowel disease and its implications for therapy. *World J Gastroenterol,* 14, 13, (Apr 2008), 1972–1980, 1007-9327

Torti, D. C., & Feldman, S. R. (2007). Interleukin-12, interleukin-23, and psoriasis: current prospects. *J Am Acad Dermatol,* 57, 6, (Dec 2007), 1059–1068

van den Brande, J., Braat, H., van den Brink, G. R., Versteeg, H. H., Bauer, C. A., Hoedemaeker, I., van Montfrans, C., Hommes, D. W., Peppelenbosch, M. P., & van

Deventer, S. J. (2003). Infliximab but not etanercept induces apoptosis in lamina propria T-lymphocytes from patients with Crohn's disease. *Gastroenterology*, 124, 7, (Jun 2003), 1774–1785, 0016-5085

van den Oord, J. J., & de Wolf-Peeters, C. (1994). Epithelium-lining macrophages in psoriasis. *Br J Dermatol*, 130, 5, (May 1994), 589–94, 0007-0963

van der Heijde, D., Kavanaugh, A., Gladmann, D. D., Antoni, C., Krueger, G. G., Guzzo, C., Zhou, B., Dooley, L. T., de Vlam, K., Geusens, P., Birbara, C., Halter, D., & Beutler, A. (2007). Infliximab inhibits progression of radiographic damage in patients with active psoriatic arthritis through one year of treatment: results from the induction and maintenance psoriatic arthritis clinical trial 2. *Arthritis Rheum*, 56, 8, (Aug 2007), 2698–2707, 0004-3591

van der Vliet, H. J., von Blomberg, B. M., Nishi, N., Reijm, M., Voskuyl, A. E., van Bodegraven, A. A., Polman, C. H., Rustemeyer, T., Lips, P., van den Eertwegh, A. J., Giaccone, G., Scheper, R. J., & Pinedo, H. M. (2001). Circulating V(alpha24+) Vbeta11+ NKTcell numbers are decreased in a wide variety of diseases that are characterized by autoreactive tissue damage. *Clin Immunol*, 100, 2, (Aug 2001), 144–148, 1521-6616

van Lingen, R. G., Ko¨rver, J. E., van de Kerkhof, P. C., Berends, M. A., van Rens, D. W., Langewouters, A. M., Boezeman, J. B., Seyger, M. M., & de Jong, E. M. (2008). Relevance of compartmentalization of T-cell subsets for clinical improvement in psoriasis: effect of immune-targeted antipsoriatic therapies. *Br J Dermatol*, 159, 1, (Jul 2008), 91–96, 0007-0963

Vissers, W. H., Arndtz, C. H., Muys, L., Van Erp, P. E., de Jong, E. M., & van de Kerkhof, P. C. (2004a). Memory effector (CD45RO+) and cytotoxic (CD8+) T cells appear early in the margin zone of spreading psoriatic lesions in contrast to cells expressing natural killer receptors, which appear late. *Br J Dermatol*, 150, 5, (May 2004), 852–859, 0007-0963

Vissers, W. H., Berends, M., Muys, L., van Erp, P. E., de Jong, E. M., & van de Kerkhof, P. C. (2004b). The effect of the combination of calcipotriol and betamethasone dipropionate versus both monotherapies on epidermal proliferation, keratinization and T-cell subsets in chronic plaque psoriasis. *Exp Dermatol*, 13, 2, (Feb 2004), 106–112

Vissers, W. H., van Vlijmen, I., van Erp, P. E., de Jong, E. M., & van de Kerkhof, P. C. (2008). Topical treatment of mild to moderate plaque psoriasis with 0.3% tacrolimus gel and 0.5% tacrolimus cream: the effect on SUM score, epidermal proliferation, keratinization, T-cell subsets and HLA-DR expression. *Br J Dermatol*, 158, 4, (Apr 2008), 705–712, 0007-0963

Wang, H., Peters, T., Sindrilaru, A., & Scharffetter-Kochanek, K. (2009). Key role of macrophages in the pathogenesis of CD18 hypomorphic murine model of psoriasis. *J Invest Dermatol*, 129, 5, (May 2009), 1100-14, 0022-202X

Willment, J.A., Lin, H. H., Reid, D. M., Taylor, P. R., Williams, D. L., Wong, S. Y., Gordon, S., & Brown, G. D. (2003). Dectin-1 expression and function are enhanced on alternatively activated and GM-CSF-treated macrophages and are negatively regulated by IL-10, dexamethasone, and lipopolysaccharide. *J Immunol*, 171, 9, (Nov 2003), 4569–73, 0022-1767

Wittig, B. M. (2007). Drug evaluation: CNTO 1275, a mAb against IL-12/ IL-23p40 for the potential treatment of inflammatory diseases. *Curr Opin Investig Drugs,* 8, 11, (Nov 2007), 947–954, 1472-4472

Wu, J. J., & Tsai, T. F. (2008). Recurrent hyperglycemia during adalimumab treatment in a patient with psoriasis. *Arch Dermatol,* 144, 10, (Oct 2008), 1403–1404, 0003-987X

Xu, Z., Vu, P., Lee, H., Hu, C., Ling, J., Yan, H., Baker, D., Beutler, A., Pendley, C., Wagner, C., Davis, H. M., & Zhou, H. (2009). Population pharmacokinetics of golimumab an anti-tumor necrosis factor-a human monoclonal antibody, in patients with psoriatic arthritis. *J Clin Pharmacol* 49, 9, (Sep 2009), 1056–1070, 0091-2700

Yazdani-Biuki, B., Stelzl, H., Brezinschek, H. P., Hermann, J., Mueller, T., Krippl, P., Graninger, W., & Wascher, T. C. (2004). Improvement of insulin sensitivity in insulin resistant subjects during prolonged treatment with the anti-TNF-alpha antibody infliximab. *Eur J Clin Invest,* 34, 9, (Sep 2004), 641–642, 0014-2972

Zachariae, H., Zachariae, R., Blomqvist, K., Davidsson, S., Molin, L., Mørk, C., & Sigurgeirsson, B. (2002). Quality of life and prevalence of arthritis reported by 5,795 members of the Nordic Psoriasis Associations. Data from the Nordic Quality of Life Study. *Acta Derm Venereol,* 82, 2, (2002), 108–113, 0001-5555

Zenz, R., Eferl, R., Kenner, L., Florin, L., Hummerich, L., Mehic, D., Scheuch, H., Angel, P., Tschachler, E., & Wagner, E. F. (2005). Psoriasis-like skin disease and arthritis caused by inducible epidermal deletion of Jun proteins. *Nature,* 437, 7057, (Sept 2005), 369–75, 0028-0836

Zhao, Y., Fishelevich, R., Petrali, J. P., Zheng, L., Anatolievna, M. A., Deng, A., Eckert, R. L., & Gaspari, A. A. (2008). Activation of keratinocyte protein kinase C zeta in psoriasis plaques. *J Invest Dermatol,* 128, 9 (Sept 2008), 2190–2197, 0022-202X

Zheng, Y., Danilenko, D. M., Valdez, P., Kasman, I., Eastham-Anderson, J., Wu, J., & Ouyang, W. (2007). Interleukin-22, a T(H)17 cytokine,mediates IL-23-induced dermal inflammation and acanthosis. *Nature,* 445, 7128, (Feb 2008), 648–51, 0028-0836

Zhou, X., Krueger, J. G., Kao, M. C., Lee, E., Du, F., Menter, A., Wong, W. H., & Bowcock, A. M. (2003). Novel mechanism of T-cell and dendritic cell activation revealed by profiling of psoriasis on the 63,100-element oligonucleotide array. *Physiol Genomics,* 13, 1, (Mar 2003), 69–78, 1094-8341

13

Infliximab Therapy for Plaque Psoriasis: The UCL Experience

Pierre-Dominique Ghislain
Dermatology Department, UCL (Université Catholique de Louvain), Brussels Belgium

1. Introduction

Psoriasis is a disease with frequently severe impairment of quality of life. Traditional therapies (topical treatments, UV, cyclosporine, acitretin, methotrexate...) are widely used but are not always sufficient, and may be poorly tolerated or contra-indicated. Among biologicals, firsts on the European dermatological market were etanercept and infliximab. Alefacept use was restricted to the United States of America. Byafter, adalimumab and ustekinumab were launched.

Among all these biotherapies, infliximab is considered a little bit different : known to be one of the most efficient, infliximab treatment requires a mode of administration quite repulsive for some practitioners. It is an intravenous drug, needing a medicalized center of care with good experience and equipment. Infliximab is also known to induce some adverse event, particularly infusion hypersensitivity.

To verify these sentences, we intended to examine our patient cohort treated by infliximab in our Dermatology Unit, with a retrospective study of the first 50 patients beginning infliximab therapy in our Department (excluding patients in phase II or III clinical trials).

Aims :

- to evaluate the proportion of noticeable adverse events, and particularly the therapy discontinuation for adverse events.
- to evaluate in 'real life' the dose and frequency of treatments
- to evaluate the clinical relapses (loss of drug efficacy) and the medical attitude towards this
- to evaluate the reasons for therapy drop-out and/or drug switches
- to evaluate the patient point of view and wishes : drug holidays ? Continuous treatment : good or bad concept for patient psychology ?
- to evaluate the number of temporarily-discontinued treatments and the consequence for re-introduction : adverse event ? Systematic prevention ?

Limitations :

- a retrospective study with 50 patients allows only some observations with no medical evidence

- no comparison is possible
- real life context induces more drop-outs, drug switches and lost to follow-up than controlled clinical studies

2. Retrospective study

2.1 Patients and methods

This is a retrospective study. We revised the list of patients affected with moderate and severe psoriasis and treated with infliximab in our Department since April 2006. Only the first 50 patients were kept, in order to ensure a sufficient trial and analysis period (one year minimum). Four patients were excluded, who were initially treated in the Department but subsequently received follow-up in another hospital. 46 patient files were analyzable in total. Of these, the PASI follow-up data were complete for 41 patients. Analysis of the files was carried out respecting privacy laws, according to the procedures in force for retrospective analyses.

2.2 Results

- Patients were 13 women and 33 men.
- Age range was 19 to 72 years.
- As prior treatment for psoriasis, all patients but 2 (44/46) previously received PUVA therapy and cyclosporine and methotrexate, according to Belgian regulations for the prescription of biological therapy. Two patients did not receive cyclosporine: one due to an absolute renal contra-indication and another who had begun biological therapy in a country where prior treatment with cyclosporine was not required.
- Concerning biological therapy, 15 patients began infliximab as first-line treatment (biotherapy naive patients). 31 took infliximab as second- or third-line treatment.
- The average length of infliximab therapy on day of analysis was 604 days (14 – 1666)
- Best results obtained were PASI 100 (19 patients), PASI 90 (6), PASI 75 (6), PASI 50 (4), PASI <50 (6). Among the 19 patients who achieved PASI 100, 4 had a complete relapse, and 6 a partial relapse. 9 maintained a complete response. Of the patients scoring between 50 and 99%, 8 completely relapsed, and 3 partially.
- As significant adverse events, we noticed 2 cases of arthritis and atypical lupus, 2 typical lupus syndromes, 2 true anaphylactic reactions. We did not see any significant infection. The lupus syndromes required hospitalization and took six months to disappear.
- In clinical follow-up, we did not notice any global tendency to weight loss or gain and no change in blood pressure.
- In the serie, we have one death, by suicide, deemed to be unrelated to the treatment
- Infliximab was used in monotherapy in 41 cases; 5 in combination with methotrexate
- Dosage was secondarily adapted in 8 cases (3 increases in frequency due to insufficient response, 5 dose reductions due to complete and sustained clinical response)
- Temporary interruption and subsequent reintroduction were observed in 10 cases: for non-compliance (2), personal choice (1), intercurrent illness (1), waiting to settle social security (1), extended trip (1), clinical trial (1), temporary treatment switch (3). The reintroduction was accompanied by manifestations of hypersensitivity in one case only.

3. Discussion

3.1 Population

Our patients' demographic data is unremarkable: average weight, alcohol and tobacco habits, comorbidity, and concurrent medication appear to be similar to the general population of psoriasis patients. Only the sex ratio would seem to be non-standard: there are significantly less women than men in our series (13 vs 33). Even if it is not consistent with the general psoriasis sex ratio, it is in accordance with other infliximab case series.

For legal, and social security reimbursement reasons, we do not prescribe infliximab to children and adolescents; our youngest patient is aged 19 years. Subject to a safeguarded general condition, we did not set an upper limit; the oldest patient was aged 72.

3.2 Prior systemic treatment

Prior treatments received for psoriasis are stereotypical: before authorizing biological therapy, Belgian regulations require patients to have tried three therapeutic channels: PUVA therapy, cyclosporine, and methotrexate. It is noted that this refers to PUVA therapy proper, and not just UVB treatment. For cyclosporine, a 'minimum of 2 months of therapy' is stipulated, 'at a minimum of 2.5 mg/kg.day'. For methotrexate, a minimum of 3 months is required, at 15 mg minimum per week. Infringements to either requirement can be made only in the case of documented intolerance or absolute contra-indication.

Among the 46 patients, one was Argentinian and had been able to begin biological therapy in his country without going through the three prior steps; the Belgian authorities therefore authorized him to take infliximab immediately. Another patient had mild renal insufficiency and unstable blood pressure despite the treatment, which was deemed sufficient to certify contra-indication to cyclosporine. The remaining 44 patients all received the three standard treatments, in some cases also UVB, acitretin, or spa treatments. None received fumaric acid (not used in Belgium). Reasons for discontinuing prior treatments included the absence of sufficient clinical results, or an intolerance to the treatment, as well as the prevention of side affects after reaching an excessive cumulative dose. Note: one of the patients had renal insufficiency induced by prolonged cyclosporine therapy.

3.3 Choice of biological therapy

No regulations lay down the use of a specific first-line biological therapy. It would no doubt be logical to begin with a TNF inhibitor, before considering an anti-interleukin, such as ustekinumab, however no objective data exists to support this affirmation. This rationale lies merely in a lack of experience and appraisal with ustekinumab, as opposed to the years of experience with TNF inhibitors, infliximab in particular. There is no way to choose one product over another among TNF inhibitors. Suggestions to begin with etanercept are based on certain data emerging from records, but these are not sufficiently back-up. In the end, the choice of first-line biological therapy currently depends on the habits of the prescriber and discussions with the patient.

In our case series, 15 patients have received infliximab as first-line treatment. The choice was laid out by presenting the patient with the different options, along with their known advantages and disadvantages. Many patients appreciate the simplicity of infliximab's dosage schedule: half a day in hospital every eight weeks seems much easier than more regular injections at home. Patients often say: "at least, with the drip, I can forget about psoriasis and its treatment completely for two whole months". Patients do not have to go to the pharmacy on a regular basis, keep boxes in the family refrigerator, or have a nurse repeatedly visit their house (figure 1).

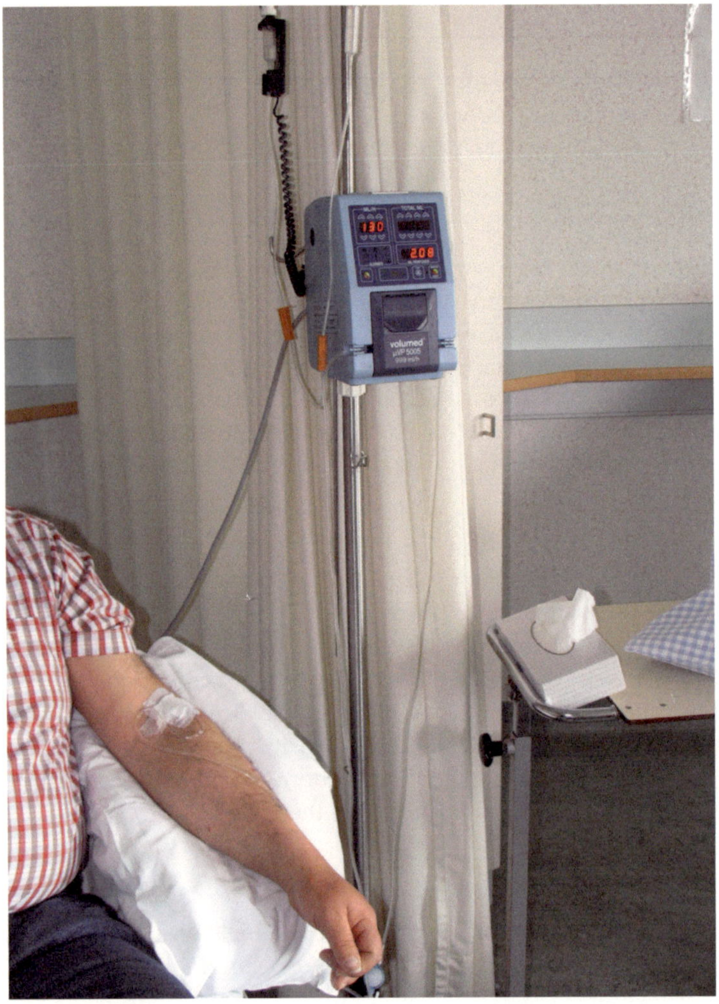

Fig. 1. Infusion in specialized unit

On the other hand, some patients fear the hospital environment and prefer treatments they can manage independently. This explains the figure of 31 patients who began infliximab as second- or third-line treatment. Of these patients, the majority had begun with etanercept, with a clinical response deemed insufficient. Some had begun with adalimumab, with a subsequent secondary clinical relapse. Some patients used these two products before beginning infliximab. One patient had received ustekinumab, with a good clinical result, but the development of a paradoxical eczematous reaction.

When we compared the response to infliximab in biotherapy naive and non-naive patients, we found no significant difference, contrary to our expectations. The two groups have the same numbers of complete responses and there is no difference in the subsequent relapse rate.

3.4 Duration of treatment

The average duration of treatment (stopped on the day of database analysis) is 604 days, with extremes of 14 and 1666 days. This duration is long enough to draw conclusions, at least partial ones. The 14-day duration corresponds to a treatment stopped due to side effects.

3.5 Efficacy of infliximab

Clinical response is often excellent. Primary response must be distinguished from more long-term response. Primary response is immediate efficacy, generally deemed at 10 weeks for infliximab. The more long-term response is the persistence of efficacy, without relapse; there is no defined timeframe for measuring this. We will therefore talk about a 1-year or 2-year response, etc. For this study, we analyzed the long-term response according to the clinical practice at the time of file analysis, so 1 to 4 years after the beginning of treatment.

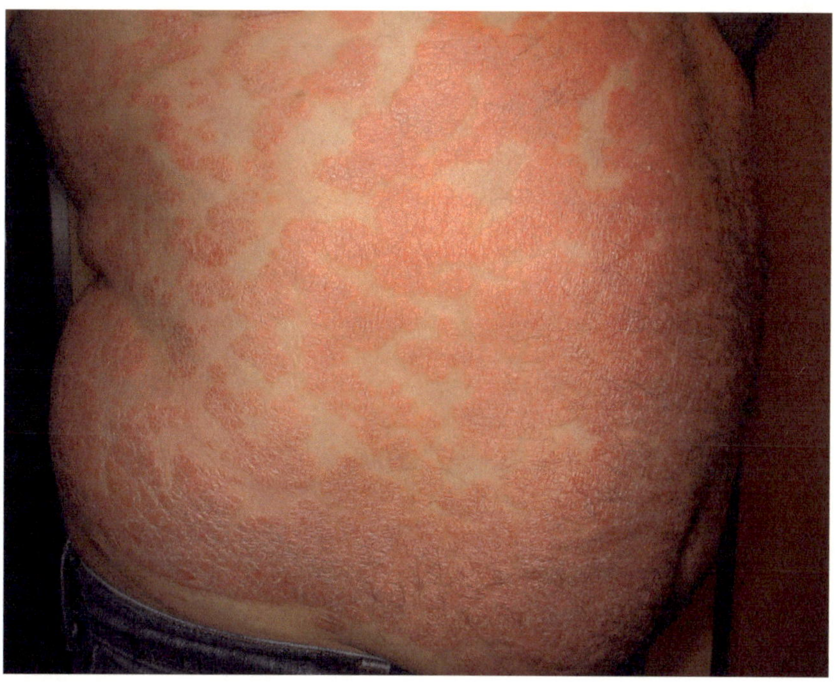

Fig. 2. W0, baseline

A review of the literature indicates excellent clinical response rates to infliximab after 10 weeks: around 80% at PASI 75 (Chaudhari et al., 2001). In other words: four patients out of five achieve a three-quarter response at minimum (reduce their initial PASI by 75% minimum). In our series, this was true for 31 out of 41 assessable patients, so 76%. 19 patients (46%) had a complete response (total clearance of lesions) (table 1). 6 patients achieved a PASI reduction of between 90 and 99%. 6 others reduced their PASI by a percentage between 75 and 89%. Just 4 remained with an improvement of 'only' between 50 and 74%. 6 patients are considered to have a primary resistance to treatment as they have never obtained a 50% reduction in their initial severity. These six patients cannot be distinguished from the others on the basis of age, sex, comorbidity, or prior treatments received. No characteristics predictive of response emerged from our series.

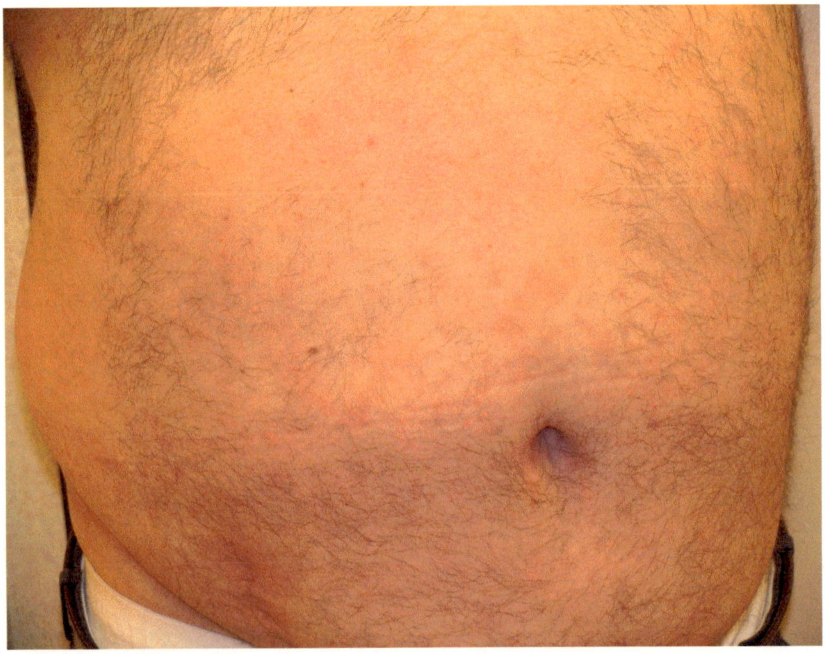

Fig. 3. W10, complete response

	Initial clinical response				
PASI improvement	**100%**	**90-99%**	**75-89%**	**50-74%**	**< 50%**
Number of patients	19	6	6	4	6
%, of patients	(46%)	(15%)	(15%)	(10%)	(15%)

Table 1. Clinical response at 10-12 weeks

Although the initial clinical response is therefore very good, there are concerns about its persistence in the medium and long term. Indeed, in our series there were numerous relapses: of the 35 responders, 12 (34%) experimented complete relapse, and 9 partial losses of efficacy (26%) (table 2). By relapse, we mean relatively rapid or gradual return to initial clinical severity. Each case must be confirmed in time in order to exclude spontaneous fluctuations of the illness. True relapses rarely pose diagnostic problems, and justify treatment abandonment. In contrast, for partial loss of efficacy, the absence of external factors must first be verified. In our series, several patients experienced periods of aggravation, which should be seen in relation to increased alcohol consumption; hygienic, dietary, and psychosomatic care improved several cases. The use of contributory drugs should also be systematically researched.

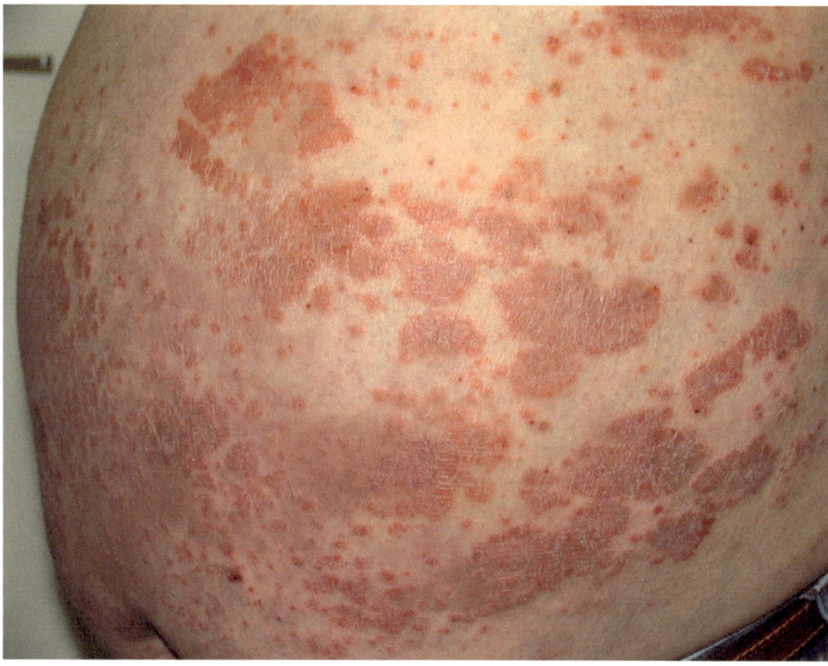

Fig. 4. W46, partial relapse

	Clinical response upon completion (after 1 to 4 years)		
Response evolution	Stable	Partial loss	Complete relapse
Initial responders 100% (19)	9 (47%)	6 (32%)	4 (21%)
Initial responders 50-99% (16)	5 (31%)	3 (19%)	8 (50%)
Total (35 pat.)	*14 (40%)*	*9 (26%)*	*12 (34%)*

Table 2. Clinical response at long-term

Our series shows more relapses than the literature initially reported, but the latter was often based on short observation time periods, or a more frequent combination with methotrexate. However, the most recent publications are in line with our observations. Thus, a Brazilian series demonstrates numbers similar to ours: 32% maintain efficacy, 44% partially recur, 17% completely relapse, and another 6% of patients had a relapse corrected by infusion every six weeks (Duarte et al., 2011). In a series of 120 patients, 93% of patients had an initial response achieving at least PASI 90, however 87% required a higher frequency of treatment than the normal regimen of 5 mg/kg every 8 weeks (Kamili et al., 2011).

In our series, complete relapses occurred most commonly after between 8 and 12 months of treatment; partial relapses could appear up to three years after the start. The responders are highly satisfied and intend to continue treatment, with an improvement in quality of life consistently nearing 100%. We should note that 9 out of 35 patients (26%) maintain a complete clinical response throughout!

An interesting observation is the difference for the long-term result between complete and partial initial responders. Among complete initial responders, half patients maintain the response, and 21% have a complete relapse. In comparison, among partial initial responders, 31% have a stable efficacy, and 50% have a complete relapse.

3.6 Infliximab and methotrexate

We commonly propose infliximab in monotherapy. It is the most common method for treating plaque psoriasis, in contrast to other indications, where combination with methotrexate is systematic. The aim is therefore both to increase treatment efficacy, and to prevent the formation of neutralizing anti-drug antibodies (Poulhalon etal., 2007). The question of more frequently combining infliximab and methotrexate in dermatology has already been raised but never resolved. In our series, 4 patients take methotrexate in parallel with infliximab; they began it after around four months on infliximab, to compensate for insufficient efficacy. 1 other patient began infliximab immediately in parallel with methotrexate.

3.7 Practical attitude in case of relapse

In case of partial relapse, after removing the aggravating factors mentioned above, we usually suggest continuing treatment, this time in combination with methotrexate. The dosage of the latter is in line with usual regulations, adapted to the patient's weight (between 55 and 135 kg, for the present four patients). The medical practice is initially to diminish the dosage relative to methotrexate taken alone, but the clinical facts then dictate the procedure to follow. Tolerance posed no particular problems for three patients. The fourth patient experiences biological perturbations in the liver, which require frequent dose reductions; gastroenterology results are reassuring and allow treatment to be continued, which is furthermore essential due to the severity of the psoriasis and its impact on the patient's life.

We did not try to combine infliximab with other treatments for psoriasis.

Another option would have been to adapt the dosage of infliximab; an increase in frequency has demonstrated success (an infusion every 6 weeks instead of every 8) (Duarte et al., 2011). In Belgium, this is impossible in common practice due to Social Security reimbursement regulations.

If relapse is complete, a combination with methotrexate is not sufficient and the continuation of infliximab is not justified. It could even be deleterious, by analogy with other observations (Korswagen et al., 2011). Among patients with relapse (complete or partial, severe and resistant), 16 were treated with ustekinumab: after a minimum of 10 months, 5 responses at 100%, 7 satisfactory responses (50-99%), and 4 failures were observed. Please note: a naive patient of biological therapy for whom infliximab has never produced a significant improvement (primary non-responder), has then responded optimally to adalimumab.

4. Adaptation of dosage

The official dosage is 5 mg/kg, every eight weeks, after the induction phase. We adapted it in 8 cases. For 3 patients, we increased the frequency of infusions to 1x/6 weeks to try and respond to the loss of efficacy observed. For two of them, response improved temporarily, however the dosage frequency would have had to be increased more, which was not possible. In contrast, for 5 patients, the dose had to be reduced; the clinical response had been complete and stable for 18 months, and these patients questioned the usefulness of continuing the treatment, at least at the initial dosage. Four patients out of the five thus continued their treatment at a reduced dose, without loss of efficacy. In practice, a reduction to 4, and then 3 mg/kg was suggested to them.

4.1 Medical follow-up

The medical follow-up we propose follows English guidelines (Smith et al., 2009): essentially clinical and anamnestic, it is also based on a blood sampling every six months and particular monitoring for tuberculosis risk. For our patients, we have not observed a tendency for weight gain or loss, nor change in blood pressure.

4.2 Adverse events

Few adverse events were observed, but these were occasionally severe.

One death by suicide, of a 30 year old man. The patient had been depressed for a long time, with a first suicide attempt long before the infliximab treatment. The psychological follow-up was good, but the patient was unable to cope with a failed love affair. The doctor considered this suicide as unrelated to the infliximab treatment. Similarly, a 67 year old patient reported an aggravated impotence problem since the first infliximab infusions. He decide to stop the treatment, which left the effect on erectile function unclear. He had reported the same problem during methotrexate treatment, with recovery after discontinuation. Urological examination results were normal.

Overall, we did not observe any significant infection. Specifically, we did not note any opportunistic infection or any tuberculosis. There were no severe infections to justify a deferral of the infliximab infusion, and anti-infective treatment did not need to be increased in any case.

One patient suspended their treatment during cardiac surgery on the mitral valve (condition pre-existing the infliximab treatment).

For six patients, the obligation to discontinue treatment was more acute (see table 3).

The two cases of induced lupus were severe and required hospitalization. Remission was slow. The first patient had already been treated with infliximab, with an excellent initial clinical response but a relapse after one year. The treatment was stopped for 9 months, but the administration of adalimumab was not conclusive, and the patient wished to try infliximab again. Ten days after the first re-introduced infusion, the patient experienced joint pain and swelling, with rapidly-progressive functional disability leading to an incapacity to move, and hospitalization. The second patient, on methotrexate from the start, developed signs of articular lupus from the 9th month of infliximab treatment, with seroconversion. After the 11-month infusion, the seizure was acute, incapacitating, requiring hospitalization and the use of corticosteroids, and then even thalidomide. It was possible to discontinue the latter after six months.

	Age	Sex	Prior biotherapies	Time to onset	Description	Severity	Treatment	Evolution
1	43	F	Infliximab, Adalimumab	1st infusion after a 9-month stop	Lupus syndrome	Severe	Disconti-nuation of infliximab	Complete resolution
2	36	F	Etanercept	9 months	Lupus	Severe	Disconti-nuation of infliximab	Complete resolution
3	40	M	Adalimumab	1st infusion	Arthralgia, ailments	Severe	Disconti-nuation of infliximab	Complete resolution
4	39	M	Etanercept	15 months	Inflammatory joint pain	Moderate	Disconti-nuation of infliximab	Complete resolution
5	41	F	Infliximab, Etanercept	2nd infusion after 2-year stop	Anaphylactic shock	Severe	Prevention for following infusions and progressive desensiti-zation	Good tolerance; reduced efficacy
6	63	M	Etanercept, Adalimumab	4th infusion	Anaphylactic reaction	Moderate	Prevention for following infusions	Good tolerance but clinical relapse

Table 3. Observed adverse events

For patient 3 (see table), resistant to adalimumab from the start, adverse effects arose from the first infliximab infusion: chest pain with normal tracing on the ECG, unremarkable blood pressure and pulse. The second infusion had to be stopped (faintness) and resumed the following week, with premedication. On the following three days, the patient had to visit the emergency department for incapacitating inflammatory joint pain. The patient was off work for 24 hours. The clinical result was good (PASI reduced to 80%). The third infusion gave rise to the same joint pains, increased, diffused, with headaches. The treatment was discontinued and replaced with ustekinumab, with no tolerance problem.

Patient 4, who was resistant to etanercept, initially showed an excellent response to infliximab (98% PASI improvement). After around 10 months, the recurrence preceding each infusion came earlier and earlier. The treatment was discontinued after 17 months, after it had lost all effect and inflammatory, atypical joint pain had developed for several days and then weeks following the last two infusions, despite the use of methotrexate (begun very late).

For patients 5 and 6, the anaphylactic reactions were true. For the first patient, the shock arose on the 2nd infusion after treatment reintroduction. The patient had participated in the Centocor EXPRESS clinical trial (C0168T38) in 2003 and 2004. The treatment had been stopped for 2 years, with use of etanercept. The infliximab treatment could be restarted after the anaphylactic shock, with systematic preventive measures, progressively reduced, but without the possibility of complete cessation. Clinical efficacy was reduced: less complete response, and period of 8 weeks between two infusions became too long. This justified the discontinuation of infliximab 4½ years later. The reaction was less severe for the second patient. The treatment was also continued, with prevention, but a clinical relapse appeared, which became complete six months later (no improvement after infusion). This patient currently has a partial response to ustekinumab.

4.3 Drug holidays

10 patients experienced temporary interruptions to treatment. The reasons varied widely.

Two patients were not compliant: they forgot appointments on several occasions and canceled due to 'lack of time'. Several times, this led to delays of up to three months. This did not affect tolerance for either patient, but one of the two had an insufficient clinical response. The doctor therefore suggested a treatment more in line with their lifestyle.

One patient personally chose to have a drug holiday; he was able to restart treatment successfully and without adverse events, after recurrence of psoriasis.

One patient (already mentioned above) had to interrupt infliximab for nearly six months due to repeated heart surgery.

One patient interrupted treatment for several months, as his Social Security status was unsettled, and he was no longer allowed to claim his treatment fees.

One patient had to go on a extended trip abroad.

One patient interrupted treatment for a clinical drug trial.

Several patients who had received infliximab therapy for several years recently expressed interest in switching to a biological therapy administered subcutaneously, which they had heard about and considered easier to manage. However, the beginning of treatment is often difficult (partial recurrence following the discontinuation of infliximab), and efficacy of the new treatment is not always immediate. Three patients experienced the change badly and tolerated the beginning of the recurrence poorly. Despite medical explanations and the concern for avoiding drug 'shopping', they returned to their prior infliximab treatment. The reintroduction was accompanied by manifestations of hypersensitivity in one case only.

4.4 Adherence to treatment

Infliximab treatment usually involves strong adherence by the patient. When efficacy is maintained in the long-term, the patient is especially grateful for this invariability. All patients consider not having to undergo treatment at home as being very positive. The inconvenience of hospitalized infusion is deemed negligible by most patients. For many, this aspect of full care is even deemed to be positive. One possible problem, in psychological terms, is that the infusions take place in hospitals which treat other ambulatory patients, in particular patients undergoing cancer chemotherapy. This co-existence can be difficult to experience for some patients affected with psoriasis. It is easier to manage in large hospitals, which can organize their wards accordingly.

4.5 Quality of life

We did not have systematically evaluate a score of quality of life. Thus, no analyzis is possible. Only one patient has stopped the treatment because considered too heavy to manage. Four patients complain about the need of hospital infusion. All others were satisfecied by the treatment.

As for other psoriasis treatments, erythematous scars occuring after initial improvement may be of transitory bad perception by the patient (figure 5).

The major problem is to psychologically and medically manage losses of clinical response. But for patients with a sustained complete response, the dermatological quality of life is perfect.

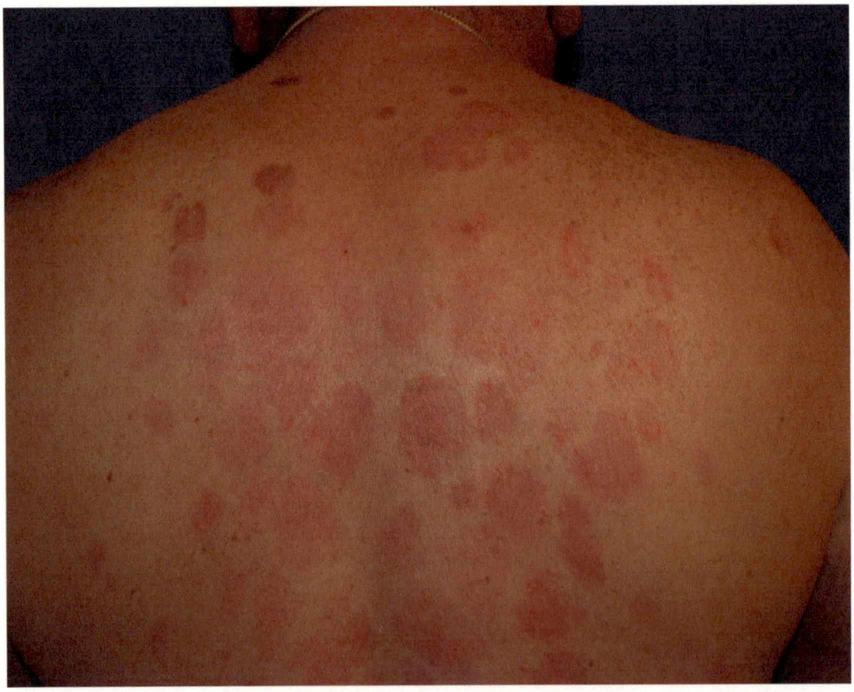

Fig. 5. W6, PASI75 response with erythematous sequelae

5. Conclusion

From this series of 50 patients treated by infliximab, we can confirm the efficacy of the product: PASI 100 (46%), PASI 90-99 (15%), PASI 75-89 (15%), PASI 50-74 (10%). In around half the cases, this efficacy is reduced over time (26%), or completely lost (34%); it is maintained in 40% of cases. In this study, we have a tendency for a more sustained response among complete initial responders in comparison with partial initial responders (47 vs 31%).

We always present infliximab to new patients as the most effective therapy in principle, warning them however about this risk of efficacy loss. The concurrent use of methotrexate could be considered, having proved its worth in indications other than plaque psoriasis (Kamili et al., 2011). Patient satisfaction is increased, despite the need for infusions in specialized and equipped centers. The occurrence of hypersensitivity reactions during infusion must be monitored and the risk of arthritic and lupus reactions must be known.

6. Conflict of interest

The author has participated in clinical trials, given lectures, and participated in expert panels funded by Schering-Plough/Merck. He has also served as consultant for Schering-Plough/Merck.

7. References

Chaudhari U, Romano P, Mulcahy LD, Dooley LT, Baker DG, Gottlieb AB.
Efficacy and safety of infliximab monotherapy for plaque-type psoriasis: a randomised trial. Lancet. 2001 May 9; 357 (9271): 1842-7.

Dalaker M, Bonesrønning JH. Long-term maintenance treatment of moderate-to-severe plaque psoriasis with infliximab in combination with methotrexate or azathioprine in a retrospective cohort. JEADV 2009,23,277–282 .

Duarte AA, Chehin FB. Moderate to severe psoriasis treated with infliximab - 53 patients: patients profile, efficacy and adverse effects. An Bras Dermatol. 2011 Apr; 86 (2): 257-263.

Kamili QU, Miner A, Hapa A, Menter A. Infliximab treatment for psoriasis in 120 patients on therapy for a minimum of one year: a review. J Drugs Dermatol. 2011 May 1; 10 (5): 539-44.

Korswagen LA, Bartelds GM, Krieckaert CL et al. Venous and arterial thromboembolic events in adalimumab-treated patients with antiadalimumab antibodies: a case series and cohort study. Arthritis Rheum. 2011 Apr; 63 (4): 877-83.

Poulalhon N, Begon E, Lebbé C et al. A follow-up study in 28 patients treated with infliximab for severe recalcitrant psoriasis: evidence for efficacy and high incidence of biological autoimmunity. Br J Dermatol. 2007; 156: 329-36.

Puig L. Efficacy of treatment with infliximab in patients with moderate-severe psoriasis and high needs of therapy. A retrospective study of 43 Patients. Actas Dermosifiliogr. 2008;99 Supl 4:30-5.

Smith CH, Anstey AV, Barker JN et al.British Association of Dermatologists' guidelines for biologic interventions for psoriasis 2009. Br J Dermatol. 2009 Nov; 161 (5): 987-1019.

Warren RB,Brown BC, Carmichael AJ, Griffiths CEM. Long-term control of recalcitrant psoriasis with combination infliximab and methotrexate. Clinical and Experimental Dermatology, 34, 415-6.

14

Systemic Cyclosporin in the Treatment of Psoriasis

Delia Colombo* and Antonino Di Pietro
[1]*Ospedale Luigi Marchesi, Via Marchesi, Milano*
Italy

1. Introduction

Cyclosporin was isolated in 1970, by Jean François Borel at Sandoz Laboratories (Basel, Switzerland), from the soil fungus *Tolypocladium inflatum* (Borel et al., 1995; Amor et al., 2010). The compound was initially identified as a possible antifungal agent, but it was subsequently shown to have limited antifungal activity. However, in 1976, the drug demonstrated potent immunosuppressive properties, and two years later, it was successfully shown to prevent renal allograft rejection in renal transplant recipients. A year later, a pilot study showed that cyclosporin improved psoriasis in patients treated for rheumatoid and psoriatic arthritis. Ultimately, in the early 1990s, cyclosporin was approved in Europe for the treatment of psoriasis and atopic dermatitis. In 1997, the United States Food and Drug Administration approved a microemulsion formulation of cyclosporin (Neoral®; Novartis Pharmaceuticals Corporation, East Hanover, NJ, USA) for the treatment of severe psoriasis in adults. Worldwide, cyclosporin has been used extensively in various dermatological disorders: e.g. pyoderma gangrenosum, and refractory chronic idiopathic urticaria (Amor et al., 2010; Vena et al., 2006).

Despite such a distinguished clinical history, some dermatologists have been rather hesitant to use cyclosporin because of concerns about possible adverse effects (Amor et al., 2010; Ryan et al., 2010); however a 'framework' of detailed clinical data now widely supports the effective and safe use of cyclosporin within dermatologists' prescribing guidelines, especially when the drug is used as a 'rescue', or intermittent short-term treatment for severe psoriasis, psoriatic arthritis, or atopic dermatitis (Amor et al., 2010).

Another particularly pertinent consideration is that 'conventional' and generic (including generic microemulsion) formulations of cyclosporin are associated with marked intra- and interindividual variability in absorption, thus creating the potential for subtherapeutic dosing at one extreme and toxicity at the other (Colombo & Egan, 2010; Ryan et al., 2010). For this reason, generic formulations have not yet been approved in several countries. Conversely, the microemulsion Neoral® preparation is associated with low intra- and interpatient variability in cyclosporin absorption and with a consistent dose-exposure relationship. This highlights the importance of prescribing the most clinically appropriate

* Corresponding Author

cyclosporin preparation, and of avoiding any confusion between the various cyclosporin formulations available (Colombo & Egan, 2010). Indeed, a Canadian survey reported that up to 20% of new cyclosporin recipients may be given a cyclosporin formulation different from that actually prescribed (Davies & Gupta 2000).

This chapter will review the following with respect to psoriasis treatment:

- The mechanism of cyclosporin action
- The pharmacokinetic properties of cyclosporin
- The efficacy of cyclosporin in well-designed, randomised controlled trials, with important economic information from certain key clinical trials
- The role of cyclosporin in current combination therapy
- Side effects of the compound.

2. Mechanism of action

Cyclosporin, an 11-amino acid, cyclic polypeptide produced from the fungal species *Beauveria nivea*, is a calcineurin inhibitor that acts selectively on T cells (Amor et al., 2010). Cyclosporin binds to the intracellular immunophilin cyclophilin to form a complex, which then binds to and inhibits the enzymatic activity of calcineurin phosphatase, a serine-

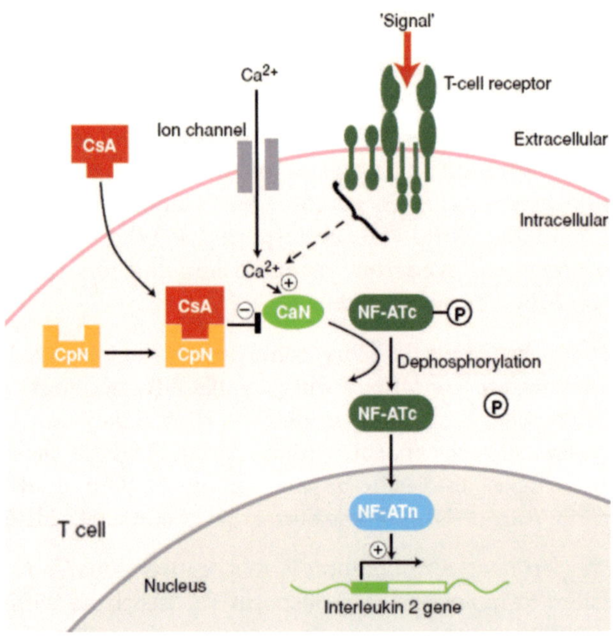

Fig. 1. Mechanism of cyclosporine action. Cyclosporine (CsA) binds to cyclophylin (CpN), forming a complex that binds and blocks the function of the enzyme calcineurin (CaN). As a result, CaN fails to dephosphorylate the cytoplasmic component of the nuclear factor of activated T cells (NF-ATc), and the transport of NF-ATc to the nucleus and the binding of NF-ATc to the nuclear component of the nuclear factor of activated T cells (NF-ATn). The NF-ATc–NF-ATn complex binds to the promoter of the interleukin 2 (IL-2) gene and initiates IL-2 production. Consequently, T cells do not produce IL-2, which is necessary for full T-cell activation.(Modified from Stepkowski, S.M. 2000)

threonine phosphatase that depends on calcium and calmodulin for activity (Amor et al., 2010; Giese et al., 2004; Stepkowski 2000). Consequently, calcineurin cannot dephosphorylate an important transcription factor: the cytoplasmic component of nuclear factor of activated T cells (NF-ATc) [Fig.1]. Transport of NF-ATc to the cell nucleus, and binding of NF-ATc to the promoter region of the IL-2 gene nuclear component of NF-AT (NF-ATn), is therefore blocked and T cells can no longer produce IL-2, a cytokine required for complete activation of the T-cell pathway, granulocyte-macrophage colony-stimulating factor, and interferon-γ production (Amor et al., 2010; Giese et al., 2004). The consequences of cyclosporin action include (Amor et al., 2010):

- Depletion of lymphocytes and macrophages in the epidermis and dermis
- Downregulation of cellular adhesion molecule expression in the dermal capillary endothelium
- Restricted activation of antigen-presenting cells, natural killer cells, and T cells
- Inhibition of keratinocyte hyperproliferation
- Restricted release of histamine from mast cells.

3. Pharmacokinetic properties

Cyclosporin is a lipophilic molecule that is poorly absorbed from 'conventional' orally administered formulations, with major variations in intra- and inter-patient bioavailability (Ryan et al., 2010). A microemulsion preparation (Neoral®; Novartis, East Hanover, New Jersey, USA) was therefore developed with greater hydrophilicity, and higher bioavailability (Colombo & Egan, 2010). There is marked variability among conventional formulations, and for the microemulsion vs conventional formulations : oral forms of cyclosporin are generally not bioequivalent,(Colombo & Egan, 2010) except for Neoral® soft gelatin capsules and Neoral® oral solution, which are bioequivalent (Novartis Pharmaceuticals UK Ltd 2011). Conventional and generic (including generic microemulsion) formulations of cyclosporin are characterised by considerable intra- and inter-individual variability in absorption (Colombo & Egan, 2010; Ryan et al., 2010). By contrast, there is low variability in cyclosporin absorption from the microemulsion Neoral® preparation, which provides a consistent dose-exposure relationship (Colombo & Egan, 2010).

Peak plasma cyclosporin concentrations are attained 1–6 hours after administration of a conventional soft gelatin capsule formulation (Sandimmune®; Novartis Pharmaceuticals Corporation, East Hanover, New Jersey, USA), but 1.5–2.0 hours after oral administration of the microemulsion formulation (Neoral®) (Novartis Pharmaceuticals Corporation 2009; Novartis Pharmaceuticals UK Ltd 2011). Mean peak plasma cyclosporin concentration (C_{max}) after administration of the microemulsion versus conventional preparation is 40–106% greater, and mean area under the plasma concentration versus time curve (AUC) is 20–50% greater (Novartis Pharmaceuticals Corporation 2009; Novartis Pharmaceuticals UK Ltd 2011). After 4 weeks' administration of Neoral® at a mean dosage of 2.48 mg/kg/day in 18 patients with psoriasis, mean C_{max} was 655 ng/mL and mean AUC was 2324 ng•h/mL.(Novartis Pharmaceuticals Corporation 2009)

Cyclosporin is extensively distributed throughout the body, in plasma (33–47% of an administered dose), lymphocytes (4–9%), granulocytes (5–12%), and erythrocytes (41–58%) (Novartis Pharmaceuticals Corporation 2009). In plasma, cyclosporin is extensively bound to proteins (~90%), primarily lipoproteins,(Novartis Pharmaceuticals Corporation 2009) and transfer of the drug may occur between various lipoprotein subfractions, and between albumin and lipoproteins (Ryan et al., 2010). Cyclosporin is excreted in breast milk, such that mothers treated with the compound should not breastfeed (Novartis Pharmaceuticals Corporation 2009).

Cyclosporin is metabolised by the cytochrome P450 (CYP) system, primarily by isozymes CYP3A4 and CYP3A5 in the liver and small intestine; the p-glycoprotein pump also has a major influence on cyclosporin bioavailability and clearance (Novartis Pharmaceuticals Corporation 2009; Ryan et al., 2010). Cyclosporin is eliminated primarily via the bile. The terminal half-life of cyclosporin in plasma has varied from 6–24 hours in various populations,(Novartis Pharmaceuticals UK Ltd 2011; Ryan et al., 2010) but in patients with psoriasis, the value is probably closer to the lower end of this range (Berth-Jones 2005).

4. Clinical efficacy

Cyclosporin is one of the most effective antipsoriatic agents available because of its rapid onset of effect and potent immunosuppressive activity against disease flares (Amor et al., 2010; Ryan et al., 2010). Thus, in patients with severe psoriasis refractory to other agents, cyclosporin can produce rapid remission and serve as a useful 'bridge' to other treatments (Menter et al., 2009).

The efficacy of cyclosporin is dose-dependent, and times to psoriasis remission are shorter at higher doses (Faerber et al., 2001; Timonen et al., 1990). Results from key dose-finding studies and meta-analyses for cyclosporin in psoriatic patients are shown in Table 1. In patients treated with cyclosporin 1.25–5 mg/kg/day for 10–36 weeks, the PASI70 or PASI75 response rate (i.e. the proportion of patients with a decrease in Psoriasis Area and Severity Index [PASI] score of ≥70% or ≥75% from baseline, or with a decrease to a PASI score of ≤8)

Reference	Study design	No. of patients	Cyclosporin dosage (mg/kg/day)	Study duration	Clinical response	
					PASI75[a]	Global disease severity score[b]
Christophers et al., 1992	r, df	217	1.25–5	12–36 wks	18–56	-
Ellis et al., 1991	r, db	85	3–7.5	16 wks	-	59–77
Faerber et al., 2001	ma	597	1.25–5	10–12 wks	16–50[c]	-
Timonen et al., 1990	ma	457	1.25–5	3 mos	24–88	-

[a] Proportion of patients with a decrease in Psoriasis Area and Severity Index (PASI) score of ≥75% from baseline, or with a PASI score ≤8.
[b] Percentage decrease in score from baseline.
[c] PASI70 response.
db = double-blind; df = dose-finding; ma = meta-analysis; mos = months; r = randomised; wks = weeks.

Table 1. Key dose-finding studies and meta-analyses for cyclosporin in psoriatic patients.

was 16–88% (Christophers et al., 1992; Faerber et al., 2001; Timonen et al., 1990). Moreover, in a 16-week study in 85 patients with severe psoriasis, cyclosporin 3–7.5 mg/kg/day reduced global disease severity score by 59–77% (Ellis et al., 1991); however, although major, additional efficacy benefits can be obtained at cyclosporin doses >5 mg/kg/day, these benefits are offset by increased toxicity (Amor et al., 2010).

Psychological distress is common in psoriatic patients (Colombo et al., 2010c; Finzi et al., 2007). A large, observational, follow-up study of more than 1500 psoriatic patients (the PSYCHAE study) revealed that methotrexate and topical corticosteroids were associated with a significantly increased risk of minor psychological distress, whereas cyclosporin significantly reduced such distress, perhaps because of patients' overall perceptions of efficacy and tolerability (Colombo et al., 2010c). This finding has potentially major clinical significance, since it outlines the possibility for markedly improved quality of life during cyclosporin therapy, but the possibility for detrimental effects on quality of life for certain other psoriasis treatments. Additional, comparative investigations are now warranted to clearly define the relative effects of cyclosporin and other antipsoriatic agents on quality of life (see section 8).

4.1 Intermittent short-term therapy

Intermittent short-term therapy for 12–16 weeks is the most widely recommended dosing schedule for psoriasis: that is, short courses of cyclosporin are administered until marked improvement is evident, whereupon treatment is stopped; if relapse manifests, cyclosporin is re-started at the dosage that was earlier effective (Menter et al., 2009).

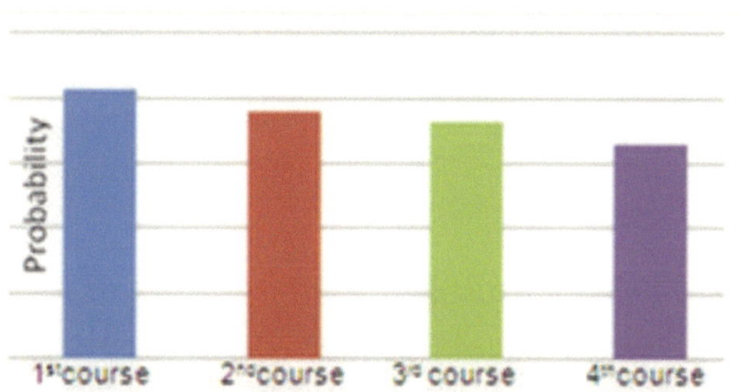

Fig. 2. Maintained efficacy of intermittent short-term cyclosporin therapy during a large, 1-year, multicentre, randomised trial in patients with plaque psoriasis (Ho et al., 1999). Values shown are the probability of a PASI75 response after 12 weeks' treatment with cyclosporin 2.5–5 mg/kg/day.

In a large, multicentre, randomised trial (the Psoriasis Intermittent Short Courses of Efficacy of Sandimmun Neoral® [PISCES] study), 400 patients with plaque psoriasis were initially treated with cyclosporin 2.5–5 mg/kg/day until clearance of psoriasis, or for a maximum of 12 weeks; patients were then randomised to abruptly or gradually discontinue (dosage reduction of 1 mg/kg/day each week) cyclosporin therapy. If relapse occurred, patients received another course of cyclosporin therapy. After 1 year of follow-up, 117 patients had received 3 cyclosporin courses, and 26 had received 4. After the first treatment course, abrupt versus gradual cessation of cyclosporin therapy was associated with a slightly, but significantly, shorter time to disease relapse (median 109 vs 113 days; p=0.038). Overall, the Kaplan-Meier probability of achieving a ≥75% decrease in disease area after 12 weeks' treatment was 83% after the first cyclosporin course, 76% after the second, 73% after the third, and 66% after the fourth [Fig. 2] (Ho et al., 1999).

In an extension of the PISCES trial, 76 patients were followed-up for a total of 2 years. The time in remission during the follow-up period was not significantly different between patients stopping cyclosporin therapy abruptly versus gradually (time in remission: 56.2% vs 61.8%); overall, the mean proportion of follow-up for which patients received cyclosporin was 42.8%. After the first treatment course, the median time to relapse was 115.5 days, but this became progressively shorter with an increasing number of cyclosporin courses (Ho et al., 2001).

4.1.1 Prevention of relapse

The well-designed PREWENT study assessed the efficacy of microemulsion cyclosporin 5 mg/kg/day, administered each weekend for 24 weeks in a total of 243 adults with chronic plaque psoriasis. The primary study endpoint in this multicenter, randomised, double-blind, placebo-controlled trial was relapse rate at 24 weeks: thus, 66.9% of cyclosporin-treated patients versus 53.2% of placebo recipients (p=0.072) had no worsening of psoriasis (i.e. no increase in PASI score to ≥75% of the value recorded before 8–16 weeks' induction therapy with cyclosporin). Although this difference only approached statistical significance, the time to first relapse was significantly longer in the cyclosporin than placebo group (p=0.0233), and in a *post hoc* analysis of patients with mild-to-moderate psoriasis, significantly more cyclosporin-treated patients than placebo recipients had no worsening of psoriasis (69.9% vs 46.3%; p=0.011) [Fig. 3] (Colombo et al., 2010a).

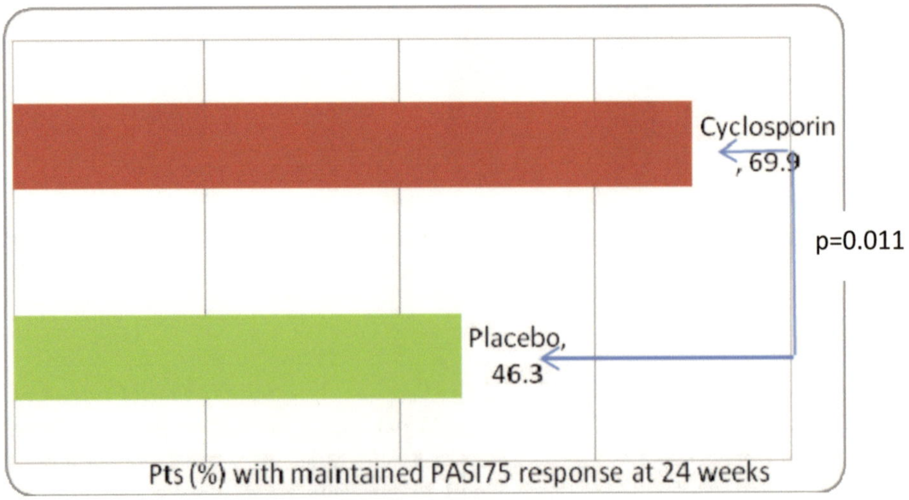

Fig. 3. Weekend cyclosporin therapy (5 mg/kg/day) prevents relapse in patients with mild-to-moderate psoriasis: results from the PREWENT trial (Colombo et al., 2010a).

4.2 Rescue therapy

Short-term cyclosporin therapy has a rapid onset of effect, and can therefore be administered as a rescue or bridging treatment for severe disease flares: that is, until a different maintenance therapy is started. As a bridging therapy, cyclosporin can be 'dovetailed' with the new maintenance regimen (e.g. biological therapy, methotrexate) to avoid clinical deterioration while the new schedule is taking effect. Cyclosporin can then be stopped without a risk of flares, and with a limited risk of adverse effects for only the short time that the cyclosporin bridging schedule and the new maintenance regimen are dovetailed (Amor et al., 2010).

Rescue cyclosporin therapy is especially effective in patients with erythrodermic, generalised, or suberythrodermic pustular psoriasis; a reducing-dosage strategy is employed after starting treatment at 5 mg/kg/day (Menter et al., 2009; Pathirana et al., 2009). In a study of 33 patients with erythrodermic psoriasis, the initial intervention was cyclosporin 4.2 mg/kg/day; after remission, the dosage was reduced by 0.5 mg/kg/day every 2 months. At 2–4 months, two-thirds of patients had attained complete remission, and marginally more than one-quarter had attained significant clinical improvement (Rosenbach et al., 2010).

4.3 Long-term therapy

European guidelines recommend that the maximum period of continuous cyclosporin therapy in patients with psoriasis should be no more than 2 years (Griffiths et al. 2004; Menter et al. 2009; Pathirana et al. 2009). This is primarily because the incidence of renal dysfunction and nonmelanoma skin cancer may increase markedly with high doses of cyclosporin administered for longer periods (Paul et al. 2003; Ryan et al. 2010). In addition, any cyclosporin-related hypertension or renal dysfunction is generally reversible if the dose is maintained at ≤5 mg/kg/day and treatment duration at ≤2 years (Ryan et al. 2010).

Long-term cyclosporin therapy (for up to 2 years or more) maintains its efficacy in most psoriatic patients; however, the principal goal of maintenance therapy is not routine attainment of clinical remission, but rather attainment of marked clinical improvement with the minimum cyclosporin dosage – generally 3-3.5 mg/kg/day (Griffiths et al., 2000). Rather surprisingly, given the long-term nature of psoriasis, and in contrast to European guidelines, US guidelines stipulate that the duration of cyclosporin therapy should be restricted to ≤1 year in psoriatic patients (Amor et al. 2010; Menter et al. 2010). This restriction appears rather strange when it is considered that, only with longer-term treatment (3–5 years or more) may a substantial proportion of patients experience glomerulosclerosis (Menter et al. 2010).

In a large-scale study involving 285 patients with psoriasis, cyclosporin 1.25–5 mg/kg/day administered continuously for 6–30 months reduced mean PASI scores by approximately 75–94% from baseline, but after cyclosporin cessation, approximately 50% of patients experienced a relapse requiring antipsoriatic therapy (Mroweitz et al., 1995). Similarly, in another large-scale study (n=181), 86% of patients treated with cyclosporin at a dosage of ~5 mg/kg/day for 16 weeks had a PASI70 response, and subsequent maintenance therapy with cyclosporin 3 mg/kg/day was associated with a significantly longer median time to relapse than placebo ($p<0.001$); at the end of the 24-week maintenance phase, 42% of patients treated with cyclosporin 3 mg/kg/day compared with 84% of placebo recipients had relapsed (Shupack et al., 1997).

A recent, retrospective evaluation of 193 patients with moderate-to-severe psoriasis revealed that cyclosporin 1.5–3.1 mg/kg/day (mean dosage) administered for 12–36 (mean 14) months reduced mean PASI score from 23.3 to 5.6; the PASI75 response rate was 73.9%. In this trial, 83/193 patients (43%) received cyclosporin monotherapy, whereas the remainder received polytherapy. Among monotherapy recipients, the physician's judgement of therapeutic success (total clearance of lesions) was 71% of patients, whereas that of clinical remission (clearance of lesions with some remaining pigmentation) was 19% of patients. Costs to the Italian healthcare system, based on a mean 1.5 cyclosporin courses administered over 14 months, were estimated at €2,984 per patient overall; the direct costs of cyclosporin acquisition were €2,058 per patient, which are approximately 4½–7 times less than annual treatment courses of etanercept and infliximab (Colombo et al., 2010b). To support and extend these cost findings, the design and execution of comparative economic evaluations of cyclosporin versus biological therapies in patients with moderate-to-severe psoriasis would now be particularly pertinent (see section 8).

In smaller studies, continuous versus intermittent cyclosporin therapy was significantly more effective over a 1-year period in 51 patients with chronic plaque psoriasis (PASI75 response rate: 92% vs 62%, p=0.008), although the mean cumulative annual dose of cyclosporin was 1.4-fold greater for continuous therapy (Chaidemenos et al., 2007). Furthermore, 60 patients with clearance or near clearance of psoriasis during cyclosporin induction therapy (3–7.5 mg/kg/day for 4 months) subsequently received cyclosporin maintenance therapy 1.5 or 3 mg/kg/day, or placebo, for up to 4 months (Ellis et al., 1995). Mean time to relapse was significantly longer in the higher-dose versus lower-dose cyclosporin group (12 vs 9 weeks; p=0.04), and in the higher-dose group versus placebo recipients (12 vs 7 weeks; p=0.002). At study completion, markedly fewer patients in the higher-dose versus lower-dose versus placebo group had relapsed: 43% vs 79% vs 95% (Ellis et al., 1995).

4.4 Rotational therapy

Rotational therapy with various systemic agents (e.g. acitretin, fumaric acid esters, methotrexate, mycophenolate mofetil) has occasionally been advocated as a means of reducing the duration, and any potential toxicity, of cyclosporin therapy (Amor et al., 2010). While most patients require additional antipsoriatic therapy after cyclosporin cessation (Amor et al., 2010), some patients may have an extended period of remission after cyclosporin therapy (Ho et al., 1999, 2001).

5. Indications/dosage

In Europe, cyclosporin is indicated for the treatment of severe psoriasis in patients for whom conventional therapy is ineffective or inappropriate. After starting treatment with oral cyclosporin, psoriatic patients should not be switched to another oral cyclosporin formulation without relevant monitoring of plasma cyclosporin levels, creatinine levels, and blood pressure; indeed, except for Neoral® soft gelatin capsules and Neoral® oral solution, which are bioequivalent, the various oral forms of cyclosporin are not bioequivalent. To avoid any possible confusion among healthcare professionals, and to avoid any potential for major fluctuations in cyclosporin bioavailability, cyclosporin should be prescribed by brand (Neoral® SPC, 2011).

To induce remission of psoriasis, the recommended starting dosage of oral cyclosporin is 2.5 mg/kg actual bodyweight each day, administered in two divided doses; however, when a rapid initial response is required, a starting dosage of 5 mg/kg/day can be used (Neoral® SPC, 2011). If no improvement is evident after 1 month of 2.5 mg/kg/day, the dosage can be gradually increased in 0.5–1 mg/kg increments, at intervals of 2–4 weeks, up to a maximum of 5 mg/kg/day (Menter et al., 2009; Neoral® SPC, 2011). Cyclosporin should be stopped if the response is inadequate after 6 weeks' administration of 5 mg/kg/day. However, after an initially good response, the cyclosporin dosage can be reduced for maintenance therapy in steps of 0.5–1 mg/kg, at intervals of 2 weeks, until the lowest effective dosage level is attained (Amor et al., 2010; Neoral® SPC, 2011). Intermittent cyclosporin therapy may be appropriate for some psoriatic patients: that is, when an initial satisfactory response has been attained, cyclosporin therapy can be stopped and any subsequent relapses treated with reintroduction of cyclosporin at the previously effective dosage (Neoral® SPC, 2011).

Before starting cyclosporin therapy, baseline renal function and blood pressure should be measured. Plasma creatinine should be measured every month. If an increase in plasma creatinine occurs to ≥30% above baseline, cyclosporin dosage should be reduced by 25–50%, even if levels are within the reference range (see section 7.2.2). If such dosage reduction does not successfully reduce plasma creatinine within 1 month, cyclosporin should be stopped. Similarly, if elevated blood pressure occurs and cannot be controlled by cyclosporin dosage reduction, or by intervention with antihypertensive therapy, cyclosporin cessation is advocated (Neoral® SPC, 2011).

6. Combination therapy

6.1 Topical treatments

To improve clinical efficacy, cyclosporin has been administered with various topical therapies (e.g. corticosteroids, dithranol, vitamin D_3 analogues [e.g. calcipotriol]) (Amor et al., 2010). However, data supporting such strategies stem mainly from small-scale, uncontrolled studies (Gottlieb et al., 1995; Griffiths et al., 1989). For example, in 12 psoriatic patients treated with cyclosporin 5 mg/kg/day for up to 18 weeks, and who applied topical dithranol to plaques on half of their bodies, improved clinical efficacy (e.g. significantly reduced severity index) was noted for combination therapy in 58% of patients (Gottlieb et al., 1995). In 13 patients with severe persistent psoriasis, cyclosporin 1–4 mg/kg/day was administered for 12–25 months, and an 81% decrease was noted in mean PASI score; 85% of the patients had received topical corticosteroid therapy after the first 3 months of cyclosporin (Griffiths et al., 1989). A larger randomised, double-blind, placebo-controlled trial in 69 cyclosporin-treated (2 mg/kg/day) patients with severe chronic plaque psoriasis revealed clinical improvement in a significantly greater proportion of patients who used concomitant calcipotriol 50 μg/g ointment versus vehicle: 50% vs 12% of patients ($p=0.0019$) had complete clearing of psoriasis or a ≥90% improvement in PASI score (Grossman et al., 1994).

6.2 Systemic treatments

Combination schedules of cyclosporin plus other systemic antipsoriatic agents (e.g. fumaric acid esters, methotrexate, mycophenolate mofetil) have been used in patients with severe psoriasis to facilitate cyclosporin dosage reduction and to reduce the risk of potential adverse effects (Amor et al., 2010). For instance, in small-scale, uncontrolled trials:

- Cyclosporin plus methotrexate was administered for a mean of up to about 3½ years in 19 patients with severe recalcitrant psoriasis, and the combination schedule produced good control of psoriasis using lower doses of each agent than would have been used for monotherapy; however, 6 patients developed renal impairment, which normalised (n=3), or which improved but did not normalise (n=3), after cyclosporin dosage reduction (Clark et al., 1999).
- Cyclosporin 2.5 mg/kg/day plus mycophenolate mofetil 3 g/day led to moderate or good clinical improvement over 3–11 months' follow-up in 78% of patients with severe recalcitrant psoriasis (Ameen et al., 2001).

Interestingly, in a retrospective assessment of 193 cyclosporin-treated patients with moderate-to-severe plaque psoriasis, 110 patients (57%) had received concurrent therapy with systemic methotrexate or retinoids, or topical and/or phototherapy. In the physician's judgement, a clinical response (therapeutic success or clinical remission) occurred in 80% of combination therapy recipients (Colombo et al., 2010b). Cyclosporin was also investigated in combination with phototherapy. In a study comparing sequential cyclosporin and narrow-band (NB) UVB phototherapy versus NB UVB phototherapy alone in patients with severe psoriasis, both treatments were effective and well tolerated, but the sequential therapy showed a greater efficacy on lesions of UV-shielded body areas and on itching (Calzavara-Pinton et al., 2005). The increased efficacy of the sequential therapy allowed for the reduction of NB UVB dosage and exposure. Nonetheless, it should be remembered that psoriatic patients previously treated with psoralen and ultraviolet A (PUVA), and to a lesser extent UVB, have increased risks of skin malignancies during cyclosporin therapy. Psoriatic patients receiving cyclosporin should not receive concomitant PUVA or UVB therapy (Neoral® Prescribing Information, 2009).

7. Side effects

Side effects, such as hypertension and renal impairment, may be associated with continuous cyclosporin therapy and appear related to treatment duration and dose (Colombo et al., 2010a). Generally, such side effects are reversible after cyclosporin discontinuation, although rarely chronic renal impairment and structural abnormalities in the kidneys may persist and be irreversible (Ryan et al., 2010). To minimise the risk of nephrotoxicity, the most widely recommended cyclosporin regimen in psoriasis is a short-term schedule of 2.5–5.0 mg/kg/day for 12–16 weeks (see section 5); this short course is repeated if subsequent disease flares occur (Amor et al., 2010; Griffiths et al., 2004). Adhering to present guidelines about appropriate dosage and monitoring protocols for cyclosporin use in psoriatic patients will substantially reduce the risk of side effects (Griffiths et al., 2004; Menter et al., 2009; Pathirana et al., 2009).

Although the mechanisms for many cyclosporin-related adverse effects have not been clearly defined, immunophilin inhibition (especially inhibition of immunophilins involved in the regulation of mitochondrial ion channels) and mitochondrial dysfunction may have significant pathogenetic roles (Ryan et al., 2010). Adverse effects reported in large-scale randomised controlled trials and meta-analyses of short-term or longer-term cyclosporin therapy in psoriatic patients are documented in Table 2. As can be seen, in short-term

Study features/AEs[a]	Short-term cyclosporin therapy		Longer-term cyclosporin therapy			
	Ellis et al., 1991	Faerber et al., 2001	Christophers et al., 1992	Krupp & Monka, 1990	Mrowietz et al., 1995	Shupack et al., 1997
No. of patients	85	579	285	631	88	181
Dosage (mg/kg/day)	3–7.5	1.25–5	1.25–5	1.25–5	1.25–5	1.5–6
Duration	16 wks	10–12 wks	12–36 wks	12 wks–16 mos	6–30 mos	40 wks
AEs requiring discontinuation	4.7	4.1	1.6–3.2	5.9	5.7	7.0–11.0
Renal dysfunction	18[e]	≤8	1–13	na	5	17–43
Hypertension	na	5–14	11–26	na	8	9[f]
GI side effects	28–55	3–8	4–5	12	22	12[f]
Headache	20–53	2–4	≤5	6	3	30[f]
Tremor	4–25	na	≤2	1	2	na
Paraesthesias	16–40	na	≤1	11	na	18[f]
Hypertrichosis	24–27	≤5	1–2	7	2	17[f]
Hypercholesterolaemia	na	na	12–25	na	na	na
Hypertriglyceridaemia	na	na	20–53	na	13	na
CV symptoms[b]	5–8	na	na	na	na	na
CNS symptoms[c]	7–25	1–6	na	na	na	na
Fatigue	12–20	≤4	1–2	3	na	11[f]
Influenza-like symptoms	5–20	na	na	na	9	na
Infection[d]	20–27	na	2	na	na	na
Gum hypertrophy	8–15	na	1–2	4	2	na

[a] Percentage of patients, unless otherwise stated.
[b] Chest pain, premature ventricular contraction, tachycardia.
[c] Anxiety, depression, dizziness, insomnia, nervousness, syncope, visual changes, transient ischaemic attack.
[d] Non-influenza-like viral, bacterial, and fungal infections.
[e] ≥15% decrease in glomerular filtration rate.
[f] During 16-wk induction phase (5 mg/kg/day).
AE = adverse effect; CNS = central nervous system; CV = cardiovascular; GI = gastrointestinal; mos = months; na = not available; wks = weeks.

Table 2. Principal side effects reported in large-scale, well-designed clinical trials and meta-analyses of cyclosporin therapy in patients with psoriasis.

studies of up to 16 weeks' duration, about 4–5% of cyclosporin-treated patients had adverse effects requiring treatment discontinuation (Ellis et al., 1991; Faerber et al., 2001). In a meta-analysis of 3 major German studies in approximately 600 patients with severe plaque psoriasis, and across the dosage range 1.25–5.0 mg/kg/day, the principal side effects were hypertension (5–14% of patients), renal dysfunction (≤8%), and gastrointestinal problems (3–8%); increased plasma creatinine levels required intervention in only 3.4% of the total 756 cyclosporin treatment cycles (Faerber et al., 2001).

In longer-term studies of up to 30 months' duration, but across the same dosage range 1.25–6 mg/kg/day, up to 11% of patients discontinued cyclosporin because of adverse effects; hypertension occurred in 8–26% of patients, gastrointestinal problems in 1–22%, and renal dysfunction in 1–43%. Lipid disorders also manifested: hypercholesterolaemia in 12–25% of patients, and hypertriglyceridaemia in 13–53% of patients (Christophers et al., 1992; Krupp & Monika, 1990; Mrowietz et al., 1995; Shupack et al., 1997).

Interestingly, in a recent, well-designed evaluation of relapse rates in patients with chronic plaque psoriasis who had achieved clinical remission after continuous cyclosporin therapy, 243 patients were randomised to 24 weeks of weekend cyclosporin microemulsion therapy 5 mg/kg/day or placebo (the Psoriasis Relapse Evaluation with Week-End Neoral Treatment [PREWENT] study) (Colombo et al., 2010a). In this investigation in a 'real-life' clinical setting, rather than in a group of carefully selected psoriatic patients, cyclosporin was well tolerated: no significant difference was evident in the incidence of adverse events between cyclosporin and placebo recipients (38.4% vs 21.5%). Only one patient (a cyclosporin recipient) had a serious adverse event (breast mass), but this was considered unrelated to study treatment. Furthermore, at no time during the study were mean plasma creatinine levels, or systolic and diastolic blood pressure values, different between the two groups; the incidence of plasma creatinine levels >30% above baseline was similar in the two groups (5.0% vs 3.8% of patients) (Colombo et al., 2010a)

In a retrospective assessment of 193 patients with moderate-to-severe psoriasis who had received a mean cyclosporin dosage of 1.5–3.1 mg/kg/day for 14 months, 83 patients (43%) received cyclosporin as monotherapy (Colombo et al., 2010b). Altogether, marginally more than one-third of patients experienced at least one adverse event. The most frequent events were hypertension (17.6% of patients), hypercholesterolaemia (14.0%), raised plasma creatinine level to >30% above baseline (6.7%), and gastrointestinal symptoms (6.2%). The clinician's assessment of cyclosporin tolerability was 'very good' or 'good' in 90% of cases (Colombo et al., 2010b).

Overall, the possibilities of cyclosporin-induced hypertension and renal dysfunction are perhaps the major tolerability concern among prescribers, and might explain a certain degree of cyclosporin 'under-utilisation' by dermatologists (Ryan et al., 2010). These two side effects are discussed in more detail below, whereas other potential tolerability issues are addressed relatively briefly.

7.1 Hypertension

The incidence of new-onset hypertension during cyclosporin administration to psoriatic patients has varied somewhat in short-term studies (5-14% of patients) and longer-term trials (8–26%; Table 2). Such hypertension is generally reversible after the cyclosporin dosage is reduced, or after antihypertensive medications are added (Ho et al., 1999; Ryan et al., 2010). Importantly, besides specific drug therapy, psoriasis per se may contribute to an increased risk of hypertension, since psoriatic patients have increased incidences of obesity and metabolic syndrome (Gelfand et al., 2006).

Pooled data from 10 studies involving 563 patients with severe psoriasis revealed an overall incidence of new-onset hypertension of 10.6% during cyclosporin therapy (Feutren et al., 1990). However, the occurrence of hypertension was not dose-related (10.0% of patients at 2.5 mg/kg/day; 11.9% at 5.0 mg/kg/day) (Feutren et al., 1990), and this finding agrees with that of several randomised trials (Ryan et al., 2010). The implication, therefore, is that a subset of psoriatic patients exists with heightened sensitivity to cyclosporin, and enhanced susceptibility to hypertension, even at low cyclosporin doses (Ryan et al., 2010). Thus, cyclosporin-induced hypertension may best be managed with antihypertensive therapy rather than with a reduced cyclosporin dosage (Feutren et al., 1990; Ryan et al., 2010).

7.1.1 Management of hypertension

Psoriatic patients have an increased risk of cardiovascular morbidity and mortality (Gelfand et al., 2006). Regular blood pressure monitoring (e.g. weekly self-monitoring) is therefore important in cyclosporin-treated patients with psoriasis. If hypertension occurs, current guidelines advocate a cyclosporin dosage reduction of 25–50%, or commencement of antihypertensive therapy (Griffiths et al., 2004; Pathirana et al., 2009). Dihydropyridine calcium-channel blockers (e.g. amlodipine, isradipine) are generally the interventions of choice, since they confer some degree of nephroprotection (Ryan et al., 2010).

7.2 Renal dysfunction

Though renal dysfuntion is recognized as a cyclosporin-related side effect, the real impact of cyclosporin on kidney function may need to be reassessed. The experience in transplant patients, particularly in kidney transplant recipients where cyclosporin is used at higher doses in life-long regimens shows, that these regimens are well tolerated (Cho & Terasaki, 1988; Opelz, 1994). An Italian study conducted in 573 kidney transplant recipients showed that creatinine plasma levels remain constant and around 1.5 mg/dl over 15 years after the intervention, a clear indication of stable kidney function (Sandrini, data presented at SIN 2003 Bologna).

When renal dysfunction persists during cyclosporin therapy, it is usually related to higher doses (>5 mg/kg/day) or extended treatment (>2 years), and both of these factors may lead to structural renal damage. Renal dysfunction may also comprise functional impairment (i.e. vascular or tubular dysfunction), which may be evident soon after starting treatment. The consequences of vascular dysfunction are reduced glomerular filtration rate and renal blood flow, and reduced creatinine clearance, whereas the consequences of tubular dysfunction may include hypomagnesaemia, reduced plasma bicarbonate levels, hyperuricaemia, and hyperkalaemia. Acute functional impairment is generally reversible when cyclosporin treatment is discontinued; thus, the risk of renal toxicity is minimised when intermittent cyclosporin therapy is prescribed in psoriasis, since such therapy is associated with normalisation of renal function between treatment courses (Ryan et al., 2010).

Besides raised plasma creatinine levels, other predictors of cyclosporin-related nephropathy include advanced age, obesity, new-onset or pre-existing hypertension or renal disorders, and other nephrotoxic treatments. Altogether, as relatively low cyclosporin dosages are now used in psoriasis, tubulopathic changes are rare and reversible (Ryan et al., 2010).

7.2.1 Management of renal dysfunction

If plasma creatinine levels are ≥30% above baseline on two consecutive occasions, 2 weeks apart, the cyclosporin dosage should be reduced by 25–50% for at least 4 weeks; this applies even if creatinine values are within the normal reference range (Griffiths et al., 2004; Menter et al., 2009; Pathirana et al., 2009). After 4 weeks of reduced-dosage treatment, if plasma creatinine levels remain elevated, cyclosporin should be discontinued (Neoral® SPC, 2011).

As a preventive measure against renal dysfunction, it is recommended that psoriatic patients receiving long-term cyclosporin therapy should have glomerular filtration rate measured at least once each year (Griffiths et al., 2004; Pathirana et al., 2009). Guidelines from the European Association of Dermatology and Venereology and from the British Association of Dermatology stipulate that the maximum period of continuous cyclosporin therapy in psoriatic patients should not exceed 2 years (Griffiths et al., 2004; Menter et al., 2009; Pathirana et al., 2009). As a comparison, it should be reminded that in graft recipients, life-long regimens with higher cyclosporin doses are routinely used in clinical practice and have proved well tolerated after many years of use.

Generally, if the cyclosporin dosage is ≤5 mg/kg/day, and if patients are closely monitored so that plasma creatinine levels remain ≤30% above baseline, any renal side effects will be wholly reversible after cyclosporin treatment is stopped (Ryan et al., 2010).

7.3 Central nervous system effects

Headache may occur in up to 53% of cyclosporin-treated patients with psoriasis, paraesthesias in up to 40%, and tremor in up to 25% (Table 2). The latter two effects generally occur during the first few weeks of cyclosporin administration and dissipate after a decrease in cyclosporin dosage; hypomagnesaemia has been postulated as a cause of these effects (Ryan et al., 2010).

Seizures have been reported rarely during cyclosporin therapy, but cyclosporin does have the potential to reduce seizure threshold in epileptic patients; the seizure risk is increased in patients taking concurrent, high-dose corticosteroid therapy. Furthermore, patients taking antiepileptic drugs may have reduced circulating cyclosporin levels because of increased metabolism by the cytochrome P450 system (Ryan et al., 2010).

7.4 Gastrointestinal effects

The rates of cyclosporin-induced gastrointestinal side effects (e.g. abdominal pain, diarrhoea, dyspepsia, nausea, and vomiting) vary markedly: however, a meta-analysis involving 631 psoriatic patients reveals rates of 2.3%, 2.0%, 2.0%, 3.8%, and 1.1%, respectively (Krupp & Monka, 1990).

7.5 Gingival hyperplasia

Gingival hyperplasia may occur in up to 30% of patients taking cyclosporin and is often linked with poor oral hygiene (Ryan et al., 2010). Thanks to increased oral health awareness, improved oral hygiene, and better public health service this condition occurs rarely in developed countries. If it occurs, this side effect usually manifests within the first 3-6 months of treatment.

7.6 Hyperlipidaemia

Hypertriglyceridaemia (>750 mg/dL) occurs in approximately 15% of cyclosporin-treated patients, and hypercholesterolaemia in <3% (Neoral® Prescribing Information, 2011). Importantly, hyperlipidaemia normalizes when cyclosporin therapy is stopped (Shupack et al., 1997).

Severe psoriasis is associated with increased cardiovascular morbidity and mortality (see section 7.1.1); thus, hyperlipidaemia should be actively managed in cyclosporin-treated patients with psoriasis. If cyclosporin therapy is continued, the initial intervention is a lipid-lowering diet. If this is unsuccessful, the cyclosporin dosage should be reduced, or treatment with a lipid-lowering agent started. Fluvastatin was shown to be well tolerated in association with cyclosporin (Holdaas et al., 1995; Launay-Vacher 2005). In general, however, statins should be used with caution because of the risk, albeit very low, of rhabdomyolysis, as reported in a few cases of transplanted patients treated with cyclosporin and lovastatin or simvastatin (Ryan et al., 2010; Corpier et al., 1988).

7.7 Hypertrichosis

In large-scale clinical trials and meta-analyses in cyclosporin-treated patients with psoriasis, the incidence of hypertrichosis has varied widely from 1–27% (Table 2); the cause of this side effect is unclear, but it is unlikely to be an altered endocrine status (Ryan et al., 2010).

7.8 Infections

Cyclosporin-induced infections occur rarely, and are rarely severe; controlled studies in psoriasis report no difference in the incidence of infections between cyclosporin and placebo recipients. Moreover, an overview of 20 years' safety data for cyclosporin in dermatology patients revealed no increases in the risks of opportunistic infections or tuberculosis reactivation (Ryan et al., 2010).

7.9 Malignancies

7.9.1 Lymphomas

B- and T-cell lymphomas have rarely been reported in cyclosporin-treated patients with psoriasis (Ryan et al., 2010). For instance, 2/842 patients (0.2%) developed these lymphomas in a large-scale trial (Krupp & Monka, 1990), whereas no increase in the incidence of lymphomas was noted in another large-scale trial (Paul et al., 2003). Significantly, psoriasis itself leads to chronic immunological overactivation, and to greater risks of lymphoma and other malignancies than in the general population (Ryan et al., 2010).

7.9.2 Nonmelanoma skin cancers

In 1252 patients with severe psoriasis, low-dosage cyclosporin (2.7–3.1 mg/kg/day) was associated with a 6-fold increase in cutaneous squamous cell carcinomas after up to 5 years' follow-up. The greatest risks of these nonmelanoma skin cancers were in patients treated with cyclosporin for >2 years, in patients previously exposed to PUVA, and in patients exposed to other immunosuppressants or methotrexate (Paul et al., 2003). In another large-scale study, 6/842 psoriatic patients (0.7%) developed premalignant or malignant skin lesions during cyclosporin therapy, but nearly all of these patients had received previous treatment with PUVA, ultraviolet B, or methotrexate (Krupp & Monka, 1990).

The current recommendation is that if phototherapy is considered in psoriatic patients, narrowband ultraviolet B should be the first choice; cyclosporin can then be reserved for future therapy, if necessary (Griffiths et al., 2004; Pathirana et al., 2009). Cyclosporin should not be used together with phototherapy, or immediately before or after PUVA (see section 5); in patients with a high total dose of PUVA, or with a history of squamous cell carcinoma or melanoma, cyclosporin should be avoided (Griffiths et al., 2004; Pathirana et al., 2009).

7.9.3 Solid organ tumours

Numerous case reports exist of solid organ tumours developing during cyclosporin treatment in dermatology patients (Ryan et al., 2010). However, no increase in the incidence of solid organ tumours was noted in a study of 1252 psoriatic patients treated with cyclosporin (Paul et al., 2003), and although another large-scale study reported solid organ tumours in 5/842 patients (0.6%), the lead investigator considered any relationship between these tumours and cyclosporin to be unlikely (Krupp & Monka, 1990). Large case-control studies suggest that cyclosporin plus other immunosuppressive therapies may actually have immunoprotective effects against, and reduce the risks of, some tumour types (e.g. breast and rectal cancers) (Ryan et al., 2010).

7.10 Other side effects

Fatigue and influenza-like symptoms may occur in up to 20% of cyclosporin-treated patients (Table 2), and joint pain and muscle aches are also frequently reported (10–40% of patients) (Pathirana et al., 2009).

Hyperbilirubinaemia manifests in up to one-third of cyclosporin recipients (Pathirana et al., 2009), but this effect is usually dose-related, and does not require further investigation if other liver function abnormalities are absent (Ryan et al., 2010). Transaminase elevations may also occur in up to one-third of cyclosporin-treated patients. If plasma bilirubin or transaminase levels are >2 x the upper limit of normal, the cyclosporin dosage should be reduced by 25% (Pathirana et al., 2009).

8. Drug interactions

Several drug interactions have been documented for cyclosporin, which is extensively metabolised by the CYP 3A system in the liver and small intestine. Some of the key interactions include the following: (Novartis Pharmaceuticals Corporation 2009; Ryan et al., 2010)

- Erythromycin should be used with caution in cyclosporin-treated patients with infected eczema, since the former compound can increase cyclosporin toxicity.
- Grapefruit juice inhibits cyclosporin metabolism and should be avoided in cyclosporin recipients.
- Heavy alcohol ingestion should be avoided, as it can increase cyclosporin levels.
- Nephrotoxic drugs, including aminoglycosides, ciprofloxacin, clotrimazole, fibrates, and nonsteroidal anti-inflammatory drugs (NSAIDs), should not be administered, if at all possible, to cyclosporin-treated patients. NSAIDs, especially in dehydrated patients, are likely to potentiate the deleterious effect of cyclosporin on renal function, and importantly, intermittent NSAID use is often not disclosed by patients.
- Cyclosporin may restrict the metabolism of many drugs (e.g. diclofenac, digoxin, methotrexate, prednisolone, repaglinide, simvastatin), thus increasing plasma levels and toxicity.
- Cyclosporin should not be used concomitantly with potassium-sparing diuretics because of the risk of hyperkalaemia, and care should also be exercised if cyclosporin is administered concurrently with potassium-sparing drugs such as angiotensin-converting enzyme inhibitors or angiotensin II receptor antagonists.

9. Conclusions

Cyclosporin was first approved for the treatment of severe psoriasis in the 1990s, and indeed, it is one of the most effective antipsoriatic agents available because of its fast onset of action and potent immunosuppressive activity. Besides psoriasis, other dermatological disorders – most notably, pyoderma gangrenosum and refractory chronic idiopathic urticaria – have seen substantial off-label cyclosporin use in recent years. Nonetheless, concerns remain among some dermatologists about the safety of cyclosporin, even though a growing evidence base exists of a favourable benefit : risk profile for the compound, especially in the management of psoriasis, psoriatic arthritis, and atopic dermatitis.

Perhaps the most frequent safety concerns, and those potentially explaining under-utilisation of cyclosporin by some dermatologists, are hypertension and renal impairment. However, it should be remembered that psoriasis itself is associated with increased cardiovascular morbidity, and any new hypertension emerging during cyclosporin therapy can be managed effectively by dosage reduction and/or antihypertensive therapy. Moreover, persistent renal dysfunction during cyclosporin therapy is usually associated with dosages >5 mg/kg/day, or treatment periods of >2 years; usually, if the dosage is kept at ≤5 mg/kg/day, and if renal function is monitored closely so that plasma creatinine levels remain ≤30% above baseline, any renal side effects occurring during cyclosporin therapy will be reversible when treatment is stopped.

Safety concerns may also exist about possible malignancies during cyclosporin administration. Again, however, it should be emphasised that the disease itself leads to long-term immunological overstimulation, such that psoriatic patients have greater risks of lymphoma and other malignancies compared to the general population. Any risk of nonmelanoma skin cancer during cyclosporin administration appears to be minimised if the duration of continuous therapy is kept to ≤2 years, and if PUVA is avoided; and some studies suggest that cyclosporin plus other immunosuppressant therapy may actually reduce the risks of some cancers (e.g. breast, rectal).

Additional well-designed assessments of various cyclosporin schedules are now warranted in the treatment of psoriasis. Such assessments should include:

- Comparative studies – i.e. vs traditional treatments (e.g. methotrexate) and/or newer agents (e.g. etanercept, infliximab).
- Measures of economic and quality-of-life endpoints, such that relative cost-utility and cost-effectiveness, and important considerations such as effects on psychological distress, can be quantified and clarified.
- Careful evaluation of the clinical potential of specific combination therapy schedules (e.g. cyclosporin plus topical calcipotriol; low-dose cyclosporin plus mycophenolate mofetil, with a possible view to the development of a fixed-dose combination 'pill' with enhanced tolerability). This is particularly pertinent given that most studies of combination therapy to date have been small-scale, uncontrolled evaluations.
- Long-term studies of ≥2 years' duration.

In summary, the immunosuppressive properties of cyclosporin in the transplant and non-transplant settings have been widely recognised for approximately 3½ decades. As such, there is much clinical knowledge and experience of cyclosporin use in non-dermatological settings, but in the dermatological arena, clinical experience is 'catching up'. Cyclosporin has now been used in the treatment of psoriasis for almost 15 years, and with the relatively low doses used, dermatologists appear to be moving beyond any potential safety concerns about the compound, and are increasingly embracing the established antipsoriatic efficacy of the drug. As further clinical, economic, and quality-of-life data accrue from well-conducted clinical trials of cyclosporin monotherapy and combination therapy schedules, dermatologists, policy makers, and patients are likely to gain even more confidence in the favourable efficacy and tolerability profiles of cyclosporin in the treatment of psoriasis and other dermatological disorders.

10. References

Ameen, M., Smith, H.R. & Barker, J.N. Combined mycophenolate mofetil and cyclosporin therapy for severe recalcitrant psoriasis. *Clin Exp Dermatol* 2001;26:480–3.

Amor, K.T., Ryan, C. & Menter A. The use of cyclosporine in dermatology: Part I. *J Am Acad Dermatol* 2010;63:925–46.

Berth-Jones, J,. 2005. The use of ciclosporin in psoriasis. J Dermatolog Treat 16(5-6):258-77.

Borel, J.F., Kjs, Z.L., and Beveridge T. The History of the Discovery and Development of Cyclosporine (Sandimmun®) In: The Search for Anti-inflammatory Drugs.Vincent J., Merluzzi and Julian Adams, Editors, O Birkhauser Boston 1995.

Calzavara-Pinton, P., Leone, G., Venturini, M., et al. A comparative non randomized study of narrow-band (NB) (312 +/- 2 nm) UVB phrototherapy versus sequential therapy with oral administration of low-dose Cyclosporin A and NB-UVB phototherapy in patients with severe psoriasis vulgaris. Eur J Dermatol 2005;15 (6):470-3.

Chaidemenos, G.C., Mourellou, O., Avgoustinaki, N., et al. Intermittent vs. continuous 1-year cyclosporin use in chronic plaque psoriasis. *J Eur Acad Dermatol Venereol* 2007;21:1203–8.

Cho Y.W., Terasaki P.I. Long-term survival. In: Terasaki PI, ed. Clinical transplants, 1988. Los Angeles: UCLA Tissue Typing Laboratory, 1988:277-82.

Christophers, E., Mrowietz, U., Henneicke, H.H., et al. Cyclosporine in psoriasis: a multicenter dose-finding study in severe plaque psoriasis. The German Multicenter Study. *J Am Acad Dermatol* 1992;26:86–90.

Clark, C.M., Kirby, B., Morris, A.D., et al. Combination treatment with methotrexate and cyclosporin for severe recalcitrant psoriasis. *Br J Dermatol* 1999;141:279–82.

Colombo, D. & Egan C.G. Bioavailability of Sandimmun® versus Sandimmun Neoral®: a meta-analysis of published studies. *Int J Immunopathol Pharmacol* 2010;23:1177–83.

Colombo, D., Caputo, A., Finzi, A., et al. Evolution of and risk factors for psychological distress in patients with psoriasis: the PSYCHAE study. *Int J Immunopathol Pharmacol* 2010c;23:297–306.

Colombo, D., Cassano, N., Altomare, G., et al. Psoriasis relapse evaluation with week-end cyclosporine A treatment: results of a randomized, double-blind, multicenter study. *Int J Immunopathol Pharmacol* 2010a;23:1143–52.

Colombo, D., Flori, L., Altomare, G., et al. Clinical outcome evaluation following cyclosporine A treatment in moderate to severe psoriasis: a retrospective study. *Int J Immunopathol Pharmacol* 2010b;23:363–7.

Corpier, CL, Jones PH, Suki WN, et al. Rhabdomyolysis and renal injury with lovastatin use. Report of two cases in cardiac transplant recipients. JAMA 1988;260:239-41.

Davies, E.A. & Gupta, S. A survey on cyclosporine prescribing and dispensing practices. *Nephrol News Issues* 2000;14:S7–10.

Ellis, C.N., Fradin, M.S., Hamilton, T.A. & Voorhees, J.J. Duration of remission during maintenance cyclosporine therapy for psoriasis. Relationship to maintenance dose and degree of improvement during initial therapy. *Arch Dermatol* 1995;131:791-5.

Ellis, C.N., Fradin, M.S., Messana, J.M., et al. Cyclosporine for plaque-type psoriasis. Results of a multidose, double-blind trial. *N Engl J Med* 1991;324:277–84.

Faerber, L., Braeutigam, M., Weidinger, G., et al. Cyclosporine in severe psoriasis. Results of a meta-analysis in 579 patients. *Am J Clin Dermatol* 2001;2:41–7.

Feutren, G., Abeywickrama, K., Friend, D. & von Graffenried, B. Renal function and blood pressure in psoriatic patients treated with cyclosporin A. *Br J Dermatol* 1990;122 Suppl. 36:57–69.

Finzi, A., Colombo, D., Caputo, A., et al. Psychological distress and coping strategies in patients with psoriasis: the PSYCHAE study. *J Eur Acad Dermatol Venereol* 2007;21:1161–9.

Gelfand, J.M., Neimann, A.L., Shin, D.B., et al. Risk of myocardial infarction in patients with psoriasis. *JAMA* 2006;296:1735-41.

Giese, T., Zeier, M., Schemmer, P., et al. Monitoring of NFAT-regulated gene expression in the peripheral blood of allograft recipients: a novel perspective toward individually optimized drug doses of cyclosporine A. *Transplantation* 2004;77:339–44.

Gottlieb, S.L., Heftler, N.S., Gilleaudeau, P., et al. Short-contact anthralin treatment augments therapeutic efficacy of cyclosporine in psoriasis: a clinical and pathological study. *J Am Acad Dermatol* 1995;33:637–45.

Griffiths, C.E., Clark, C.M., Chalmers, R.J., et al. A systematic review of treatments for severe psoriasis. *Health Technol Assess* 2000;4:1–125.

Griffiths, C.E., Dubertret, L., Ellis, C.N., et al. Ciclosporin in psoriasis in clinical practice: an international consensus statement. *Br J Dermatol* 2004;150 Suppl. 67:11–23.

Griffiths, C.E., Powles, A.V., McFadden, J., et al. Long-term cyclosporin for psoriasis. *Br J Dermatol* 1989;120:253–60.

Grossman, R.M., Thivolet, J., Claudy, A., et al. A novel therapeutic approach to psoriasis with combination calcipotriol ointment and very low-dose cyclosporine: results of a multicenter placebo-controlled study. *J Am Acad Dermatol* 1994;31:68–74.

Ho, V.C., Griffiths, C.E., Albrecht, G., et al. Intermittent short courses of cyclosporin (Neoral®) for psoriasis unresponsive to topical therapy: a 1-year multicentre, randomized study. The PISCES Study Group. *Br J Dermatol* 1999;141:283–91.

Ho, V.C., Griffiths, C.E., Berth-Jones, J., et al. Intermittent short courses of cyclosporine microemulsion formulation for the long-term management of psoriasis: a 2-year cohort study. *J Am Acad Dermatol* 2001;44:643–51.

Holdaas, H., Hartmann, A., Stenstrom, J., et al. Effect of fluvastatin for safely lowering atherogenic lipids in renal transplant patients receiving cyclosporine. Am J Cardiol 1995;76:102A-106A.

Krupp, P. & Monka, C. Side-effect profile of cyclosporin A in patients treated for psoriasis. *Br J Dermatol* 1990;122 Suppl. 36:47–56.

Launay-Vacher, V., Izzedine, H., Deray ,G. Statins' dosage in patients with renal failure and cyclosporine drug-drug interactions in transplant recipient patients. Int J Cardiol 2005;101:9-17.

Menter, A., Korman, N.J., Elmets, C.A., et al. Guidelines of care for the management of psoriasis and psoriatic arthritis: section 4. Guidelines of care for the management and treatment of psoriasis with traditional systemic agents. *J Am Acad Dermatol* 2009;61:451–85.

Menter, A., Korman, N.J., Elmets, C.A., et al. Guidelines of care for the management of psoriasis and psoriatic arthritis: section 5. Guidelines of care for the treatment of psoriasis with phototherapy and photochemotherapy. *J Am Adad Dermatol* 2010;62:114–35.

Mrowietz, U., Färber, L., Henneicke-von Zepelin, H.H., et al. Long-term maintenance therapy with cyclosporine and posttreatment survey in severe psoriasis: results of a multicenter study. German Multicenter Study. *J Am Acad Dermatol* 1995;33:470–5.

Neimann, A.L., Shin, D.B., Wang, X., et al. Prevalence of cardiovascular risk factors in patients with psoriasis. *J Am Acad Dermatol* 2006;55:829–35.

Neoral® Prescribing Information. Available from: http://www.pharma.us.novartis.com/product/pi/pdf/neoral.pdf [accessed May 5, 2011].

Neoral® Summary of Product Characteristics. Available from: http://www.medicines.org.uk/EMC/medicine/1307/SPC/Neoral+Soft+Gelatin+Capsules%2c+Neoral+Oral+Solution/[Accessed May 9, 2011].

Novartis Pharmaceuticals Corporation. 2009. Neoral® (cyclosporine) soft gelatin capsules oral solution: full US prescribing information [online]. Available from: http://www.pharma.us.novartis.com/product/pi/pdf/neoral.pdf [Accessed 17 May 2011].

Novartis Pharmaceuticals UK Ltd. 2011. Neoral® (ciclosporin) soft gelatin capsules, oral solution: summary of product characteristics [online]. Available from: http://www.medicines.org.uk/EMC/medicine/1307/SPC/Neoral+Soft+Gelatin+Capsules%2c+Neoral+Oral+Solution/ [Accessed 17 May 2011].

Opelz, G. Effect of the maintenance immunosuppressive drug regimen on kidney transplant outcome. Transplantation 1994;58:443-446

Pathirana, D., Ormerod, A.D., Saiag, P., et al. European S3-guidelines on the systemic treatment of psoriasis vulgaris. *J Eur Acad Dermatol Venereol* 2009;23 Suppl. 2:1–70.

Paul, C.F., Ho, V.C., McGeown, C., et al. Risk of malignancies in psoriasis patients treated with cyclosporine: a 5 y cohort study. *J Invest Dermatol* 2003;120:211–6.

Rosenbach, M., Hsu, S., Korman, N.J., et al. Treatment of erythrodermic psoriasis: from the medical board of the National Psoriasis Foundation. *J Am Acad Dermatol* 2010;62:655–62.

Ryan, C., Amor, K.T. & Menter, A. The use of cyclosporine in dermatology: part II. *J Am Acad Dermatol* 2010;63:949–72.

Sandrini, S. Creatinine plasma levels in kidney transplant recipients over 15 years data presented at SIN meeting 2003 Bologna.

Shupack, J., Abel, E., Bauer, E., et al. Cyclosporine as maintenance therapy in patients with severe psoriasis. *J Am Acad Dermatol* 1997;36(3 Pt 1):423–32.

Stepkowski, S.M. Molecular targets for existing and novel immunosuppressive drugs. *Expert Rev Mol Med* 2000;2:1–23.

Timonen, P., Friend, D., Abeywickrama, K., et al. Efficacy of low-dose cyclosporin A in psoriasis: results of dose-finding studies. *Br J Dermatol* 1990;122 Suppl. 36:33–9.

Vena, G.A., Cassano, N., Colombo, D., et al. Cyclosporine in chronic idiopathic urticaria: a double-blind, randomized, placebo-controlled trial. *J Am Acad Dermatol* 2006;55:705–9.

15

Topical Therapies for Psoriasis

Amitava Mitra[1*] and Ercem Atillasoy[2]
[1]*Biopharmaceutics, Product Value Enhancement, Pharmaceutical Sciences and Clinical Supply, West Point, PA, Merck Research Laboratories*
[2] *Global Regulatory Affairs, Upper Gwynedd, PA, Merck Research Laboratories*
USA

1. Introduction

Psoriasis is a chronic and recurring inflammatory condition of the skin that affects approximately 2% of the western population (Nestle et al., 2009). The most common form is plaque type psoriasis, the treatment of which is the focus of this chapter. Patients with psoriasis often present with scaly, painful and disfiguring skin lesions (Nestle et al., 2009). Although, it is seldom life-threatening, psoriasis is associated with a high degree of morbidity - patients are embarrassed about the appearance of their skin. There are significant psychosocial issues affecting these patients, often they experience social isolation, stigmatization, alcoholism and depression. In addition, patients with psoriasis, like those with other major medical disorders, have reduced levels of employment and income as well as a decreased quality of life (Horn et al., 2007). The combined costs of long-term therapy and social costs of the disease have a major impact on healthcare systems and on society in general. There are several co-morbidities that have been linked to psoriasis and it has been hypothesized that psoriasis as a disease has important systemic manifestations (Nestle et al., 2009). The shared conditions include the metabolic syndrome, depression, and cancer. Psoriasis can also occur in association with inflammatory bowel disease (Wolf et al., 2008), diabetes mellitus (Wolf et al., 2008) and HIV infection (Maurer, 2005). Although cases have been reported, it is unclear whether cancer particularly lymphoma and skin cancer, is related to psoriasis or the long term consequences of its treatment (Gelfand et al., 2006a). The relationship between psoriasis and the risk of cardiovascular disease is of emerging significance (Gelfand et al., 2006b). While patients with mild psoriasis appears to be in no excess risk, the moderate and severe form of the disease is associated with an increase in frequency of myocardial infarction and an increase in mortality, in large part because of cardiovascular events (Gelfand et al., 2006b). If confirmed, these findings would have major implications for future preventive and therapeutic strategies. Further, it is estimated that a significant population of juvenile guttate psoriasis cases are preceded by streptococcal infections (Campalani & Barker, 2005).

For treatment purposes, psoriasis can be categorized into localized and generalized forms, based upon body surface area (BSA) involvement. For localized, mild to moderate disease, usually defined as lesions covering <10% of body surface area, topical therapy is often

---

[*] Corresponding Author

sufficient (Nestle et al., 2009). For generalized disease, systemic therapy approaches such as oral therapy, immunotherapy and UVB phototherapy are effective treatment options. In any case, the treatment plan should include obtaining rapid control of the disease and maintaining that control. In this chapter, the authors provide an overview of current guidances for topical management of psoriasis, novel mono- and combination topical therapies as well as combination regimens of topical and phototherapy. Several of the well-established traditional topical medications such as coal tar, salicylic acid and anthralins are only briefly reviewed here. Interested readers are referred to the following references (Su & Fang, 2008; Witman 2001) for information. An overview of the topical antipsoriatic medications is summarized in Table 1. Most of the trade names used throughout this chapter represent those marketed in United States (US).

Drug	Formulation	Disease Type
	Monotherapy	
Corticosteroids		
Clobetasol propionate	Ointment, spray, foam, lotion, shampoo	Plaque and scalp psoriasis
Halobetasol propionate	Ointment	Plaque psoriasis
Betamethasone	Cream, gel, lotion, foam	Plaque and scalp psoriasis
Mometasone	Cream, ointment, gel	Plaque and scalp psoriasis
Vitamin D3 analogues		
Calcipotriol	Ointment, cream, solution	Plaque, scalp and nail psoriasis
Calcitriol	Ointment	Plaque psoriasis
Tacalcitol	Ointment	Plaque psoriasis
Retinoids		
Tazarotene	Gel, cream	Plaque psoriasis
Coal tar	Ointment, gel, solution, shampoo, soap	Plaque and scalp psoriasis
Anthralin	Ointment, cream	Plaque psoriasis
Calcineurin inhibitors *(investigational use)*		
Tacrolimus	Ointment	Face, genitelia and intertriginous psoriasis
Pimecrolimus	Cream	Intertriginous psoriasis
PDE4 inhibitors		
AN-2728	Ointment	Plaque psoriasis
	Combination Product	
Calcipotriol + betamethasone dipropionate	Ointment	Plaque, scalp and nail psoriasis
Betamethasone dipropionate + salicylic acid	Ointment, cream, lotion	Plaque, scalp and nail psoriasis

Table 1. A summary of topical medications for psoriasis.

2. Guidances for effective management of psoriasis

Although there is no cure for psoriasis, several available therapies can help control skin lesions and associated symptoms. Some treatments can also induce remission for months or longer. Despite availability of numerous topical and systemic treatment options, there is a lack of patient satisfaction with the available treatments and high rates of non-compliance. In order to optimize topical treatment of psoriasis, guidelines have been developed for more effective management of psoriasis. Some of the available guidances for topical treatment are discussed in this section:

The American Academy of Dermatology (AAD) has published a six part series of guidelines in 2009, on the management of psoriasis and psoriatic arthritis. The third section of this series discusses the use of topical medications for the treatment of psoriasis (Menter et al., 2009). This guidance discusses the efficacy and safety of as well as offer recommendations for the use of topical corticosteroids such as vitamin D analogues, tazarotene, tacrolimus, pimecrolimus, emollients, salicylic acid, anthralin, coal tar, as well as combination therapy. The authors concluded that patients with localized psoriasis can be treated with topical agents, which generally provide a high efficacy-to-safety ratio. Topical agents may also be used adjunctively in patients with more extensive psoriasis who are undergoing therapy with either ultraviolet light, systemic or biologic medications. However, the use of topical agents as monotherapy in the generalized form of the disease or in the setting of limited, but recalcitrant, disease was not recommended.

The Cochrane Skin Group in UK published a review of topical therapies for chronic plaque psoriasis following examination of 131 studies (Mason et al., 2009). They concluded that vitamin D analogues showed similar efficacy as potent or very potent corticosteroids when used on the body, whereas topical corticosteroids proved the most effective treatment for scalp psoriasis. Combination of topical corticosteroids and vitamin D analogues were more effective than either agent as single formulation. Although the overall safety of topical therapies was high, topical corticosteroids were associated with lower incidence of local adverse events than vitamin D analogues. Warren et. al. (Warren et al., 2010) has published a review summarizing the guidances on the use of topical, systemic and biological therapies for the treatment of psoriasis; co-morbidities associated with psoriasis; and complementary therapies for psoriasis. The UK National Health Service provides an annual evidence update on psoriasis and has included new guidelines and systematic reviews on psoriasis published or indexed from November 2008 to October 2009 in the *2009 Annual Evidence Update on Psoriasis* from NHS Evidence - Skin Disorders.

In Germany, Nast et. al. have developed an evidence based guidelines for topical treatment (Nast et al., 2007). The guidelines focus on induction therapy in cases of mild, moderate, and severe plaque-type psoriasis in adults and contain a series of therapeutic recommendations. A similar guideline is also available for systemic treatment of psoriasis (Pathirana et al., 2009).

A guide has also been developed to optimize and harmonize the amount of topical medications to be applied on children (Long et al., 1998). Study conducted in children aged between 6 months to 9 years, showed that the amount of an ointment applied on children was similar to that predicted in accordance with these guidelines (Long et al., 1998).

3. Topical antipsoriatic medications

3.1 Corticosteroids

Topical corticosteroids, particularly high-potency corticosteroids, have been a mainstay in the topical treatment of psoriasis for decades (Bagel 2009). Their efficacy may be attributed to multiple mechanisms of action, including their anti-inflammatory, immunosuppressive and antiproliferative effects. Topical corticosteroids are often classified into seven classes in United States and four in UK and Germany based on potency. A detailed classification system has been discussed else where (Horn et al., 2010). In the United States, topical corticosteroids are classified as following: class I (superpotent), class II (potent), class III (upper mid strength), class IV (mid strength), class V (lower mid strength), class VI (mild) and class VII (least potent). Typically corticosteroids of lower potency are mainly used on the face and groin, and in infants and children. Mid-potency corticosteroids are typically used as initial therapy on all other areas in adults. Potent and superpotent corticosteroids are often used for stubborn, cutaneous plaques or lesions on the scalp, extremities, including palms, and/or soles as well as for initial therapy to achieve quick resolution of lesions. In this section detailed discussion of a few representative steroids are provided, however there are several other corticosteroids which are effective against psoriasis topically. Some steroids which are widely used in topical psoriasis treatment but have not been discussed in this section include, methylprednisolone aceponate (Ruzicka 2006), which has shown good efficacy against chronic therapy-resistant psoriasis, including both progressive and stationary phases. Although topical corticosteroids are effective in maintenance of the disease, these therapies can cause many potential local adverse effects including cutaneous atrophy, formation of telangiectasia, development of striae, steroid rosacea, perioral dermatitis, and skin infections (Horn et al., 2010). Risks of systemic adverse effects increase with prolonged use, or use of higher potency steroids, particularly with greater percent of BSA to which the topical steroid drug is applied. These risks include metabolic disturbances such as hypothalamic-pituitary-adrenal (HPA) axis suppression, Cushing like syndrome, osteonecrosis of the hip and immunosuppression are other rare but possible serious adverse events. Tachyphylaxis or tolerance often occurs with prolonged use, leading to less durable potency or lower effectiveness of topical steroids. Therefore, several strategies have been proposed to improve safety for long-term use of topical corticosteroids (Horn et al., 2010) such as, 1) using rotational treatment regimens that minimize side effects, 2) combination with other topical medications, 3) following package inserts on the maximum usage per week, and 4) caution when using in vulnerable body areas (such as face) and in children.

3.1.1 Clobetasol

Clobetasol propionate is a super high-potency glucocorticosteroid, initially approved for treatment of steroid-responsive dermatosis. Clobetasol propionate is traditionally formulated in an ointment base for treatment of psoriasis. However, several novel formulation of clobetasol propionate are now available such as spray, foam, lotion, and shampoo formulations, which may provide for improved convenience and acceptance in many patients with similar efficacy, safety, and tolerability as the traditional ointment and cream formulations (Feldman and Yentzer, 2009). While there are very few direct clinical comparison studies between clobetasol propionate in different vehicles, the efficacy rates of obtaining clear or almost clear of psoriasis are high for the novel formulations with most patients achieving success after 2-4 weeks of treatment in well controlled clinical trials, but the response rates are similar for all presentations. Small differences in vasoconstrictor potency or cutaneous absorption have been noted among the formulations, but the clinical significance of these observations is difficult to discern.

The development of a foam formulation of clobetasol propionate 0.05% (e.g. Olux®) provides an effective and cosmetically appealing treatment option for patients with plaque-type psoriasis because it spreads easily and is cosmetically elegant. Olux is based on VersaFoam® platform, a thermolabile and low-residue foam. A randomised, placebo-controlled, double-blinded study of 279 patients aged 18 years or older with mild-to-moderate plaque-type psoriasis demonstrated the efficacy and tolerability of clobetasol propionate foam (Gottlied et al., 2003). After 2 weeks of twice-daily applications of clobetasol propionate foam versus vehicle foam, 68% of patients in the active treatment arm were clear of lesions versus 21% of patients receiving placebo. The treatment was well tolerated with 5% of patients receiving clobetasol propionate foam and 7% of those receiving placebo reported burning at the site of application. Although the efficacy of the clobetasol propionate foam can partially be attributed to patient adherence, the foam also delivers the active drug more efficiently than other formulations that have been compared. This may be due to the easier spread of foam onto the skin. In *in vitro* skin penetration studies, application of foam to donor skin resulted in higher drug accumulation and increased rate of permeation into skin layers (Huang et al., 2005).

A study comparing two novel formulations containing 0.05% clobetasol propionate, Clobex® spray and Olux® foam clearly highlighted the difference in efficacy from two products containing the same active ingredient (Mraz et al., 2008). In a study of 77 randomized patients aged 18 years or older with moderate to severe plaque psoriasis the products were applied as per the product labeling. At the end of the treatment period (2 weeks for foam and 4 weeks for spray), patients treated with clobetasol propionate spray showed a significantly greater median reduction in affected body surface area compared to the clobetasol propionate foam. Improvements in quality of life were statistically significantly greater at all time points for patients treated with clobetasol propionate spray compared to patients treated with the foam formulation. The majority of adverse events for both products were mild in severity (Mraz et al., 2008).

Clobex® shampoo containing 0.05% clobetasol propionate is a once-daily, short-contact, shampoo treatment for moderate-to-severe scalp psoriasis (Feldman & Yentzer, 2009). The efficacy and safety of clobetasol propionate 0.05% shampoo was evaluated in a randomized, double-blind, vehicle-controlled clinical trial of 142 patients aged 12 years and older with moderate-to-severe scalp psoriasis (Jarratt et al., 2004). Patients applied clobetasol propionate shampoo or vehicle shampoo once daily for 15 minutes for four weeks. Treatment success (defined as a global psoriasis rating of "clear" or "minimal") was obtained for 42% of patients who used clobetasol propionate shampoo versus 2% of patients who used vehicle shampoo. Recurrence of the scalp psoriasis, assessed during a two week follow-up period, showed that the clobetasol propionate shampoo was more effective than the vehicle shampoo in preventing recurrence after treatment was discontinued. Similar safety profile was established between the clobetasol propionate shampoo and vehicle shampoo. No skin atrophy, telangiectasia, acne or severe adverse events were noted for either treatment group (Jarratt et al., 2004).

3.1.2 Mometasone

Mometasone furoate (Elocon® cream) is a potent synthetic glucocorticoid, which is commonly used in dermatological conditions (Prakash & Benfield 1998). It is available as cream, ointment and lotion formulations for the treatment of patients with atopic dermatitis, seborrhoeic dermatitis, scalp psoriasis and psoriasis vulgaris. Although mometasone demonstrates greater anti-inflammatory activity and a longer duration of action than betamethasone, it has low potential to cause adverse systemic effects such as suppression of the hypothalamic-pituitary-adrenal (HPA) axis. Moreover, its atrophogenic potential is low and no greater than that of other glucocorticoids in its class, such as betamethasone valerate. Transient, mild to moderate, local adverse effects such as burning, stinging, folliculitis, dryness, acneiform eruptions and signs of skin atrophy have been reported with mometasone. Mometasone has shown a low risk of primary sensitization and cross-reactions in preliminary patch test studies.

In clinical studies with patients aged between 12 and 90 years, with moderate to severe scalp psoriasis (Swinehart et al., 1989; Vanderploeg et al., 1989) or psoriasis vulgaris (Bressinck et al., 1988; Svensson et al., 1992), who had not used topical glucocorticoids for 2 weeks or taken systemic glucocorticoids for 6 weeks prior to enrolment showed that in general, mometasone (0.1% lotion, ointment or cream applied once or twice daily) was significantly superior to topical glucocorticoid preparations of similar and weaker potency. The ointment formulation of mometasone was significantly superior to once-daily hydrocortisone 1.0% ointment (Bressinck et al., 1988; Katz et al., 1989), twice-daily betamethasone valerate 0.1% ointment (Svensson et al., 1992; Medansky et al., 1987), triamcinolone acetonide 0.1% ointment (Medansky et al., 1988), and 3 times daily fluocinolone acetonide 0.025% ointment (Medansky et al., 1988).

The effectiveness of alternate-day treatment with mometasone 0.1% ointment in maintenance therapy of psoriasis vulgaris was evaluated in a randomized, double-blind, 3-week study in 48 adult patients with moderate psoriasis vulgaris. After 1 week (n = 48) of once-daily application of mometasone 0.1% ointment, patients either continued with daily application (n = 25) or applied mometasone 0.1% ointment on alternate days (n =19) for 2 weeks. At the end of the study period both regimens were effective in treating disease signs and symptoms with no detectable difference between the treatment groups (Prakash & Benfield 1998).

In patients with scalp psoriasis, the effects of mometasone lotion were significantly superior to those of twice-daily application of betamethasone valerate 0.1% lotion or triamcinolone acetonide 0.1% lotion (Swinehart et al., 1989; Vanderploeg et al., 1989).

A study in 24 patients with moderate to severe psoriasis evaluated the response to mometasone 0.1% ointment applied once daily on the face and intertriginous areas and other affected body areas (Lebwohl et al., 1993) After 2 weeks, the face and intertriginous areas showed a quicker and significantly superior response to treatment as compared with other body areas (Lebwohl et al., 1993).

3.1.3 Betamethasone

Betamethasone dipropionate (BDP, Diprolene®) is a mid-potency synthetic fluorinated corticosteroid and is commonly used in combination with vitamin D3 analogues (Saraceno et al., 2009). Betamethasone dipropionate is commonly formulated as a gel. Several attempts have been made to increased betamethasone dipropionate skin permeation by encapsulating in liposomes. The liposomal formulations achieved improved corticosteroid dermal delivery (Fresta & Puglisi 1997). However, in a double blind randomized trial comparing a liposomal formulation containing 0.039% betamethasone dipropionate against the gel containing 0.064% betamethasone dipropionate, showed that the gel was more effective in reducing psoriatic plaques than the liposome after application for 14 days (Korting et al., 1990). Hence, liposome encapsulation of betamethasone dipropionate may increase the anti-inflammatory action but not the antiproliferative effect.

Betamethasone valerate (BMV) is also available as a foam formulation (Luxiq®) containing 0.12% betamethasone valerate for use as a treatment for psoriasis affecting the scalp (Feldman et al., 2001) and non-scalp (Stein et al., 2001) regions of the body. Betamethasone valerate foam formulated in a thermolabile hydroethanolic foam vehicle is absorbed more rapidly, and demonstrated 2-fold greater skin penetration in a human cadaver skin model, than the betamethasone valerate lotion (Franz et al., 1999). Safety and efficacy of the betamethasone valerate foam was evaluated in a randomized, multicenter, double-blind, active- and placebo-controlled trial in adult patients with moderate to severe scalp psoriasis (Franz et al., 1999). At the end of 28-days of treatment, patients on betamethasone valerate foam showed significantly better clearing of plaques than those on betamethasone valerate lotion and placebo. Further, there was no evidence of increased toxicity for betamethasone valerate foam (Franz et al., 1999).

3.1.4 Halobetasol

Halobetasol propionate (HP) is a high potency corticosteroid available as 0.05% ointment and cream (Rivera & Hsu 2005). Halobetasol is a synthetic trihalogenated corticosteroid structurally similar to clobetasol propionate but with an additional fluorine atom (Rivera & Hsu 2005).

The efficacy and safety of 0.05% halobetasol ointment (Ultravate®) in the treatment of patients aged 18 years or older with moderate plaque psoriasis was demonstrated in two multicenter, randomized, double-blind, and placebo controlled studies in 204 patients (Bernhard et al., 1991). In both studies the medication and placebo were applied twice daily for 2 weeks. At the end of the treatment period, 0.05% halobetasol ointment was found to be more effective over placebo. No systemic adverse events or findings of skin atrophy were reported in these studies. Reports of "stings" or "burns" were equally divided between halobetasol formulation and its vehicle. These two studies demonstrated that 0.05% halobetasol ointment was clinically beneficial and without evidence of significant adverse events during the treatment period.

Three clinical studies separately compared the 0.05% halobetasol propionate ointment to 0.05% clobetasol propionate ointment (Goldberg et al., 1991), 0.05% betamethasone dipropionate (BDP) ointment (Mensing et al., 1991) and 0.1% betamethasone valerate (BMV) ointment (Blum & Yawalkar 1991) in plaque psoriasis. The efficacy of the halobetasol propionate ointment was significantly superior to those of the other products in these studies. Neither skin atrophy nor systemic adverse effects were observed for halobetasol propionate during 4 weeks. However, because of the risks associated with prolonged use reported in upto

13% of patients, the daily application of halobetasol propionate should be limited to a maximum of 14 days with a maximum dose of 50 g per 2 weeks (Rivera & Hsu 2005).

3.2 Vitamin D3 analogues

The active form of vitamin D3 is known to play an important role in the regulation of intestinal calcium absorption, bone mineralization and the prevention of rickets. In addition to these actions, vitamin D3 has several additional biological effects including the stimulation of cellular differentiation, inhibition of proliferation and immunomodulation (Muller & Bendtzen, 1996). This makes vitamin D3 a potential candidate for treatment of psoriasis. However, parent vitamin D3 might not be suitable for treating psoriasis due to potential for hypercalcemia. Hence, several vitamin D3 analogues have been developed for treatment of psoriasis (Tanghetti 2009). Vitamin D analogues bind to the vitamin D receptor, thus causing biological actions on both corneocytes and on immune-competent cells in the skin. Analogues such as calcipotriol, calcitriol, tacalcitol and maxacalcitol inhibit corneocyte proliferation and stimulate corneocyte differentiation *in vitro*. In addition, these analogues have only minimal effects on calcium levels and calcium excretion (Barker et al., 1999). However, due to concerns with elevating the serum calcium levels with extensive application to large body surface area, these analogues usually have a limit on total amount used per week.

3.2.1 Calcipotriol (Calcipotriene)

Calcipotriol is a synthetic vitamin D3 analogue formulated as a cream and scalp solution (Dovonex®) at a drug loading of 0.005%. The calcipotriol cream is effective in treatment of plaque psoriasis and statistically significantly better than the placebo alone (Staberg et al., 1989). In addition, a solution has been developed for scalp psoriasis (Klaberg et al., 1994), and calcipotriol ointment has also been investigated for nail psoriasis (Tosti et al., 1998).

A comparison of calcipotriol ointment with a combination of betamethasone dipropionate and salicylic acid ointment (Diprosalic®) showed that calcipotriol was as effective as the combination product for treating nail psoriasis (Tosti et al., 1998). Comparisons of 0.005% calcipotriol ointment and 5% coal tar ointment in conjunction with sun exposure in 10 adult patients with stable plaque psoriasis showed that both calcipotriol and coal tar ointment had comparable efficacies in treating stable plaque psoriasis when used simultaneously with sun exposure, although the initial response to calcipotriol was faster (Kaur et al., 2001).

The calcipotriol cream formulation is less greasy than the ointment formulation and hence has better patient acceptability. It was the impression that the effect of calcipotriol is more pronounced on lesional infiltration and scaling, whereas the effect is less pronounced on the vascular component of psoriasis, as determined by redness. Finally, the therapeutic response to calcipotriol ointment can be increased by occlusion with a polyethylene film (Boyrke et al., 1993).

3.2.2 Calcitriol

Calcitriol is a synthetic form of the active metabolite of vitamin D3. It has anti-proliferative, prodifferentiating and immunomodulating effects on human keratinocytes (Lehmann 2009).

A calcitriol ointment (Vectical®) for mild-to-moderate plaque psoriasis was approved by the US Food and Drug Administration (FDA) in 2009 (Kowalzick 2009). Multicenter and randomized clinical trials have shown calcitriol ointment to be efficacious, safe and cosmetically acceptable as compared to placebo and other topical psoriasis therapies (Kircik 2009). Pharmacokinetic studies in patients with psoriasis and healthy control subjects have demonstrated that topical calcitriol ointment produced minimal systemic absorption of calcitriol and does not alter systemic calcium homeostasis significantly even when applied to approximately one third of the body surface area (Kircik 2009). However, the Vectical® prescribing information limits the use to 200 gm per week due to concern of disturbance in calcium metabolism. The efficacy and safety of topical calcitriol ointment were examined in two placebo-controlled, randomized, multicenter, parallel-group double blind clinical trials of identical design in a total of 839 patients aged 18 years or older with mild-to-moderate plaque psoriasis (Lebwohl et al., 2007). Both studies showed that at the end of the treatment period, the patients in the calcitriol group showed significantly better clearing of psoriatic plaques than those in the vehicle group. The incidence of treatment related adverse events such as mild skin discomfort, pruritus, and erythema was similar for the calcitriol and the vehicle groups in both studies (Lebwohl et al., 2007).

3.3 Retinoids

Retinoids provide a distinct class of treatment option within antipsoriatic therapies, which are largely dominated by immunomodulatory effects. The mechanism of action of retinoids in psoriasis may include direct suppression of inflammation as well as inhibition of proliferation and normalization of differentiation in the epidermal layer (van de Kerkhof 2006). In the US topical retinoid for psoriasis is approved as tazarotene gel and cream (Tazorac®) available in 0.05% and 0.1% formulations. It is recommended that treatment commences with the 0.05% formulation, and the concentration increased if necessary and tolerated. Tazarotene is applied once daily in the evening. All formulations and strengths can be used for plaque psoriasis. In general, gels and the more-concentrated strengths tend to have higher incidences of irritation, pruritus, erythema, stinging and desquamation (Yamauchi et al., 2004). The cream formulations are being marketed as less irritating (Linden & Weinstein 1999). A recent improvement in tazarotene therapy was a reduction of skin irritation by short contact applications or concurrent steroid use (Veraldi & Schianchi 2003). These side effects are most apparent on initial application, but are generally alleviated with continued usage. Tazarotene is contraindicated in pregnant women and in women who are not taking adequate birth control in view of its teratogenic potential, category X pregnancy status. In addition, tazarotene use should be avoided in nursing women, and patients who have substantial sun exposure, who do not use adequate sun protection and who use photosensitisers or have photodermatitis (Veraldi & Schianchi 2003).

The efficacy of once-daily topical tazarotene has been studied in four randomized, double or single blinded clinical trials; two trials on the tazarotene gel formulation (Lebwohl et al., 1998; Weinstein et al., 1997) and two trials on tazarotene cream formulation (Weinstein et al., 2003) in patients at least 18 years old and having plaque psoriasis in at least 2% of the total body surface area. The duration of active treatment was 12 weeks and an additional 12 weeks follow-up period without active treatment was incorporated in these studies. These studies showed that as early as at week 1, tazarotene 0.1% formulation showed a statistically significant improvement as compared to the vehicle, with the 0.05% tazarotene formulations showing statistically significant improvement at week 4. Twelve weeks after the discontinuation of therapy (post-treatment phase), both 0.1% and 0.05% tazarotene cream were significantly better as compared to the vehicle (Weinstein et al., 2003). Comparative studies between calcipotriol and tazarotene monotherapy have been carried out, showing superior efficacy of calcipotriol during the first 8 weeks but equal efficacy after 12 weeks' treatment (Tzung et al., 2005). The penetration of tazarotene through human skin is limited. The systemic availability after topical tazarotene 0.05% or 0.1% gel is < 1% after single application, and 2.6% and 5.3%, respectively, after once-daily applications following 2 weeks of treatment. After 12 weeks of treatment, the systemic availability of tazarotene 0.05% was 1.8% and for the 0.1% tazarotene preparation it was 3.9% (Tang-Liu et al., 1999).

3.4 Other topical agents

While tars, anthralins and salicylic acid containing products have been used for decades in the United States for the treatment of plaque psoriasis, recent innovative delivery technologies have provided new versions of these products, offering the prospect of enhanced tolerability, convenience and compliance. Some of these novel topical products are discussed in this section.

3.4.1 Anthralins

A timed-release cream of anthralin (Psoriatec®) has been developed with the potential to reduce skin irritations that are sometimes observed with generic anthralin. Psoriatec can be a relatively convenient formulation to reduce side effects, such as irritation and skin staining, by following instructions for short contact anthralin therapy (SCAT).

3.4.2 Coal tar

An emollient foam formulation of coal tar (Scytera™) has been developed for convenient usage to relief of the symptoms of psoriasis. This formulation is neither intended for use for prolonged periods nor in areas such as rectum, genital area, or eyes. As with other tar containing products, skin exposure to sunlight should be avoided after application and it has the potential to stain clothing, contact lenses, and hair. Some tar products are also available as co-packaged kits, one such example is Clobeta Plus®. This product is co-packaging of clobetasol cream and coal tar solution.

3.4.3 Salicylic acid

Salicylic acid as a topical agent aids in the removal of excessive keratin in hyperkeratotic skin disorders, including psoriasis (including body, scalp, palms and soles) (Beani 2002). Salicylic acid has been shown to produce desquamation of the horny layer of skin while not effecting qualitative or quantitative changes in the structure of the viable epidermis. It has been used as monotherapy or as combination therapy to reduce the size and scale of psoriatic plaques. Recent development of foam formulations of salicylic acid such as Salvax® and Salkera® may lead to broader use of this agent. In children under 12 years of age and those patients with renal or hepatic impairment, the area to be treated should be limited and the patient monitored closely for signs of salicylate toxicity. Contact with eyes and other mucous membranes should be avoided.

4. Novel agents for topical treatment of psoriasis

4.1 Calcineurin Inhibitors

These agents inhibit the activity of calcineurin phosphatase, an enzyme important for the translocation of the pluripotent transcription factor, nuclear factor of activated T cell, from the cytoplasm to the nucleus where it activates a number of proinflammatory cytokines associated with T-cell activation. Hence, these agents have potential for treatment of skin diseases mediated by calcineurin phosphatase (Luger & Paul 2007). Currently these calcineurin inhibitors are approved for use in mild to moderate atopic dermatitis only, any use in psoriasis is off-label, and therefore not within approved US-FDA prescribing information. A black box warning has been added to the labels of these medications stating that the long-term safety of topical calcineurin inhibitors has not been established and that rare cases of cancer have been reported in patients who used the medications, although a causal relationship in human beings has not been established. Apart from topical tacrolimus and pimecrolimus, another new oral calcineurin inhibitor, voclosporin is also in clinical development for treatment of plaque psoriasis (Papp & Carey 2010).

4.1.1 Tacrolimus

Tacrolimus is an immunosuppressive drug whose main use is after allogenic organ transplant to reduce the activity of the patient's immune system and hence reduce the risk of organ rejection. It is also used in a topical ointment preparation (Protopic®) for the treatment of severe atopic dermatitis, vitiligo and psoriasis. Tacrolimus ointment was approved in the United States in 2000, and Europe in 2001 for atopic dermatitis. However, new research has proven the potential use of tacrolimus in psoriasis (Luger & Paul 2007; Beck 2005). The introduction of tacrolimus ointment marked the advent of a new, nonsteroidal drug class, topical immunomodulators, for the management of inflammatory dermatoses.

Tacrolimus ointment seems most effective in treating psoriasis where the skin is thin, that is on the face, genitelia and intertriginous areas (Martín Ezquerra et al. 2006). In one study 21 patients with facial psoriasis lesions applied tacrolimus (0.1%) ointment twice a day for 4 weeks without occlusion. A complete or good response was obtained in majority of the patients (Yamamoto & Nishioka 2003).

The efficacy and tolerability of tacrolimus ointment has also been investigated for the treatment of male genital psoriasis (Bissonnette et al., 2008). In an open-label study in 12 adult male patients with genital psoriasis, patients received topical tacrolimus 0.1% ointment twice daily for 8 weeks followed by a 4-week observational period. Psoriasis severity also improved significantly for the glans, shaft of the penis, and scrotum. The ointment was very well tolerated, with only mild pruritus or burning sensation of limited duration reported (Bissonnette et al., 2008).

The safety and efficacy of tacrolimus (0.1 %) ointment for the treatment of psoriasis on the face, intertriginous areas, or both were evaluated in an open-label, clinical trial of 21 patients with psoriasis (Freeman et al., 2003). A total of 81 percent of patients experienced complete clearance at day 57 (end of treatment). Only 2 patients reported adverse events, which were limited to itching and the feeling of warmth at the application site (Freeman et al., 2003).

4.1.2 Pimecrolimus

Pimecrolimus is a non-steroidal immunosuppressant derived from ascomycin. Pimecrolimus 1% cream (Elidel®) was approved in the United States, the European Union, and Japan as second-line therapy for the short-term and non-continuous chronic treatment of mild to moderate atopic dermatitis in patients, who have failed to respond adequately to other topical prescription treatments, or when those treatments are not advisable (Fabroni & Wollina 2009). Pimecrolimus also has an enormous potential as topical treatment for numerous inflammatory skin diseases like psoriasis and dermatitis (Fabroni & Wollina 2009).

Pimecrolimus is not effective in plaque-type psoriasis when used as the commercially available formulation without occlusion (Wollina et al., 2006). However, pimecrolimus has been shown to be effective in intertriginous psoriasis (Wollina et al., 2006). A double-blind, randomised, vehicle-controlled study was performed in 57 patients aged 18 years or older with moderate-to-severe intertriginous psoriasis. By week 8 of treatment, 82% of patients using pimecrolimus scored their disease as being equally well, or completely controlled, compared with 41% of the vehicle group. The pimecrolimus treatment was also well tolerated (Gribetz et al., 2004).

4.2 Phosphodiesterase 4 (PDE4) Inhibitors

PDE4 is the predominant cyclic AMP degrading enzyme, present in a variety of inflammatory cells including eosinophils, neutrophils, macrophages, T cells and monocytes. In addition, this enzyme is expressed in non-immune cells such as keratinocytes and fibroblasts. Due to the broad anti-inflammatory and immuno-modulatory action of PDE4 inhibitors, it has been proposed that PDE4 inhibitors might also be efficacious for skin disorders such as psoriasis and atopic dermatitis (Bäumer et al., 2007). These PDE4 inhibitors displayed strong anti-inflammatory action in models of allergic contact dermatitis in mice, in the arachidonic acid induced skin inflammation in mice and in ovalbumin sensitized guinea pigs. The determination of cytokines in skin homogenates revealed that both Th1 as well as Th2 cytokines are suppressed by PDE4 inhibitors, indicating an anti-inflammatory activity in both the Th2 dominated acute phase as well as the Th1 dominated chronic phase of atopic dermatitis. Due to the suppression of Th1 cytokines, activity can also be expected in psoriasis (Bäumer et al., 2007). Consequently PDE4 inhibitors are currently in clinical development for treatment of psoriasis both topically (AN-2728 from Anacor Pharmaceuticals) and orally (CC-10004 from Celgene Corporation).

4.2.1 AN-2728

A recent publication gives a comprehensive summary of preclinical, phase I and phase II data for topical AN-2728 (Nazarian & Weinberg 2009). Till date 3 phase IB, 1 Phase IIA and 1 phase IIB trials have been completed for AN-2728, and results suggest that AN-2728 is well tolerated with significantly better efficacy in plaque psoriasis as compared to placebo controls. A phase IIB, randomized, double-blind, placebo-controlled, parallel-assignment, single-center, safety and efficacy clinical trial assessed AN-2728 ointment (5% bid for 12 weeks) in 30 patients with plaque psoriasis (Nazarian & Weinberg 2009). Preliminary data revealed that psoriatic plaques treated with AN-2728 exhibited a reduced overall target plaque severity score compared with plaques treated with vehicle alone at 8 weeks of treatment. In addition, AN-2728 topical therapy has also been reported to be well tolerated. In the phase IIA trial, no treatment-related adverse events or laboratory anomalies were reported; one patient reported mild gingivitis and diarrhea, but these effects were not considered to be related to the trial medication (Nazarian & Weinberg 2009).

4.3 Janus-Associated Kinase (JAK) inhibitors

The JAK family is composed of four tyrosine kinases - JAK1, JAK2, JAK3, and tyrosine kinase 2 (TYK2) (Fridman et al., 2011). Members of the JAK family are essential for signaling by many cytokines and growth factors following their binding to specific receptors on the cell surface. The interaction activates one or more JAKs, JAKs in turn activate the signal transducer and activator of transcription (STAT) proteins that transmit the growth and activation signals to the nucleus. JAK signaling is involved in a number of biologic processes, including the formation and development of blood cells and the regulation of immune function. Hyperactivation of JAKs has been associated with a number of disease states, including chronic myeloproliferative disorders and inflammatory diseases such as rheumatoid arthritis (RA) and psoriasis (Fridman et al., 2001). As a result, JAK inhibitors are currently in clinical development for treatment of psoriasis both topically (INCB18424 from Incyte Corporation) and orally (Tofacitinib from Pfizer).

A 28-day phase Ib/IIa dose escalation trial of topical INCB18424 in patients with mild-to-moderate psoriasis demonstrated rapid onset of action, reduction in total lesion area, and improvement in lesion thickness, erythema, and scaling (Mesa 2010).

5. Combination topical therapies

The commonly used topical medications described in this chapter provide efficacy through varying and divergent pathways. As these agents act through different mechanisms, there is a scientific rationale for their use in combination therapy. The rationale assumes that agents are selected on the basis of their individual mechanisms of action, which may offer the possibility of additive or synergistic efficacy, reduction in the dose of either or both products, and reduction in the occurrence of side effects (Norris 2005). Several studies have proven the advantages of using a combination of topical medications for treatment of psoriasis. Recently, a fixed dose combination ointment containing 50 μg/g calcipotriol and 0.5 mg/g betamethasone dipropionate (approved in US as Taclonex®) was found to be effective against psoriasis vulgaris (Claréus et al., 2009). This ointment formulation combines the keratinocyte differentiation and antiproliferative action of the vitamin D_3 analogues (calcipotriol) with the anti-inflammatory effect of steroids (betamethasone dipropionate), thus enhancing effectiveness while reducing the side-effect profile of the individual agents (Saraceno et al., 2009). It was found that the combination product had a more rapid onset of action (Papp et al., 2003) than calcipotriol or betamethasone alone and was more effective (Douglas et al., 2002) than calcipotriol or betamethasone alone. In a clinical trial with 1605 randomized patients aged 18 years or older showed that the combination product (Taclonex®) was significantly more effective than betamethasone, calcipotriol and placebo. The local adverse reactions were also low compared to the other drugs. It was concluded that two different treatment regimens (i.e. application once or twice daily) employing the two-compound product provided rapid and marked clinical efficacy as compared to calcipotriol or betamethasone alone and also were safe therapies for psoriasis vulgaris (Saraceno et al., 2009). Combination of calcipotriol and betamethasone has also been shown to have significant advantages in treatment of scalp and nail psoriasis (Saraceno et al., 2009). More recently, a combination of 0.005% calcipotriol and 0.064% betamethasone dipropionate (Taclonex Scalp® in US and Xamiol® in Europe) has been approved for the treatment of moderate to severe scalp psoriasis vulgaris in adults. This once-daily therapy has a quick onset of action and greater efficacy than monotherapy with either ingredient. At 8 weeks, the combination product had a safety profile comparable with betamethasone dipropionate and was associated with significantly fewer adverse events than calcipotriol (Guenther 2009).

A combination of betamethasone dipropionate and salicylic acid (Diprosalic®) is available as ointment and lotion formulations. Faster improvement in scaling, itching, and redness has been observed with Diprosalic® as compared to betamethasone dipropionate alone (Guenther 2004). It has also been shown that the combination ointment has similar efficacy to clobetasol and calcipotriene (calcipotriol) ointments.

A multicentre, randomised, double-blind, vehicle-controlled, parallel-group study was carried out to study the effect of the addition of calcipotriol ointment to methotrexate in patients aged 18 years or older with psoriasis vulgaris (De Jong 2003). From this study, it was concluded that the combined use of calcipotriol with methotrexate resulted in a methotrexate-sparing effect, while still maintaining the efficacy. Calcipotriol treatment increased the time to relapse of psoriasis following discontinuation of methotrexate. The combination of calcipotriol and methotrexate was safe and well tolerated. The combination resulted in lower cumulative doses of methotrexate as compared to monotherapy, thus significantly reducing the risk of methotrexate side effects (De Jong 2003).

The combination of calcipotriol ointment (twice daily) and tazarotene gel (once daily) was compared with clobetasol ointment (twice daily) in the treatment of psoriasis (Bowman et al., 2002). The vitamin D3 analogue plus retinoid treatment had comparable efficacy to that of the potent topical steroid. Similarly a comparison of twice-daily calcipotriol ointment against the combination of tazarotene gel and 0.1% mometasone furoate cream was superior during the first 2 weeks of treatment. However, by 8 weeks of treatment, both groups exhibited similar responses (van de Kerkhof 2006).

6. Combination of topical therapy with phototherapy

Phototherapy for psoriasis includes narrowband and broadband UVB phototherapy; psoralens combined with UVA, targeted excimer laser phototherapy, and combination treatments (Nguyen et al., 2009). The combination of phototherapy with topical products has long been used for treatment of plaque psoriasis. In the 1920s, William Goeckerman combined the use of UVB phototherapy with topical application of tars (Su & Fang 2008; Witman 2001). This in-patient psoriasis regimen, known as the Goeckerman regimen, is still occasionally used in major dermatologic centers.

Psoralen photochemotherapy uses a combination of topical application (or ingestion) of 8-methoxypsoralen followed by exposure of the affected skin area to long-wavelength UV (320 - 400 nm) (Nguyen et al., 2009). Other psoralen derivatives such as 5-methoxypsoralen and 4,5,8-trimethylpsoralen are also used in topical PUVA therapy. Bath psoralen UVA combination involves immersion of either localised areas (such as the hands or feet) or the whole body in water containing dissolved 8-methoxypsoralen prior to UVA exposure (Nguyen et al., 2009).

Photodynamic therapy is another non-invasive technique used in the treatment of skin diseases. 5-aminolevulinic acid is a prodrug that is metabolized intracellularly to form the photosensitizing molecule protoporphyrin IX. When protoporphyrin IX is activated by light, cytotoxic reactive oxygen species and free radicals are generated. This phototoxic effect may be used for treatment of malignant and non-malignant hyperproliferative tissue (Gupta & Ryder 2003). Photodynamic therapies using 5-aminolaevulinic acid in plaque psoriasis has also been reported (Gupta & Ryder 2003), however these are not approved regimens. Side effects of the aforementioned regimens include short and long term adverse effects of visible and UV light, such as acute phototoxicity, and longer term effects such as photoaging and photocarcinogenesis. Protective clothing, sunblock and sunglasses should be used to protect unaffected areas of the body.

7. Sequential therapy

Sequential therapy is a strategy to treat psoriasis using a specific combination of therapeutic agents in a particular sequence with the aim of achieving initial efficacy followed by a safe maintenance regimen (Koo 1999). This treatment strategy maximizes efficacy of each medication while minimizing long term side effects. The strategy involves three main steps - 1) clearing phase, 2) transitional phase and 3) maintenance phase (Koo 1999). A combination of topical, systemic and phototherapy agents can be used to achieve the desired outcome, depending on the severity of the disease (Lebwohl et. al., 2004).

The clearing phase involves the use of a rapid acting agent such as a potent or super-potent topical steroid at the maximum dermatologic dose with the main aim of promptly controlling an acute outbreak of psoriasis. This is followed by the transitional phase, in which a well tolerated maintenance agent such as acitrein or vitamin D analogue is introduced and administered along with the clearing agent. The clearing agent is slowly tapered off in this phase of treatment. The transitional phase can be challenging as it requires prevention of breakthrough of the disease, while tapering off the clearing agent and adjusting dose of the maintenance agent to ensure long term control with minimal side effects. Finally, in the third phase of the treatment, the patient is retained on the maintenance therapy, with additional therapy such as phototherapy, as needed (Koo 1999).

Several combinations of therapeutic agents and regimen for sequential therapy have been proposed in literature (Lebwohl et. al., 2004; Bhutani et. al., 2011). However the choice of treatment agents needs careful consideration based on the severity and type of the disease, and the need to balance safety and efficacy. Recently, a sequential treatment regimen of clobetasol and calcitriol has been shown to be efficacious and safe for the management of moderate-to-severe plaque psoriasis (Brodell et. at., 2011). In a multicentre, open-label study in subjects aged 18-80 years with moderate-to-severe plaque psoriasis, the patients applied clobetasol propionate (0.05% spray) twice daily for up to four weeks. At the end of four weeks, if the patient's overall disease severity was assessed as clear, almost clear, mild or moderate, the patients were treated with calcitriol (3 µg/g ointment) twice daily for an additional eight weeks (upto week 12) or unless the patient's disease was assessed as severe or returned to the baseline score, at which time the treatment was discontinued. Patients were evaluated at baseline and at 2, 4, 8 and 12 weeks. In 84% of the patients who completed the 12 week study, this treatment resulted in at least one grade improvement in disease severity and hence was considered successful as per predefined criteria. There was a significant decrease in the percent body surface area affected, from 7.1% at baseline to 3.9% at week 12. The sequential treatment regimen was also well tolerated with no unexpected adverse events. Most reported adverse events and skin irritations were mild in severity (Brodell et. at., 2011).

8. Challenges in developing topical medications for psoriasis

The unique nature of drug delivery across the skin also presents with several unique challenges in development of topical products, such as:

1. Optimization of both drug property and formulation composition to enhance the rate and extent of drug diffusion through the stratum corneum;
2. Reduced drug concentration and increase in data variability due to presystemic metabolism in the skin;
3. Switch of topical formulations during clinical development that can be very challenging, hence only minimal formulation changes can be usually made during development;
4. No control on deep tissue penetration through formulation approaches, which is primarily influenced by protein binding and dermal blood flow;
5. Lack of confidence in dose projection due to difficulty in establishing robust skin pharmacokinetic-pharmacodynamic relationship;
6. High variability in *in vitro* and *in vivo* skin permeability remains a major obstacle in using these tools in formulation development;
7. Guidances from regulatory agencies often call for clinical comparisons of innovative drugs with approved active comparators, thus increasing the challenges for development and licensure of novel products;
8. Regulatory standards call for demonstration of benefit for each component within a fixed dose combination product, the so-called "Combination Rule", another challenge in development of a combination product.

In addition to these general challenges in topical formulation development, there are several challenges specific to psoriasis and the development of antipsoriatic topical products, such as:

1. Psoriatic lesions can have both thickened and markedly thinned epidermis, this heterogeneity in the skin morphology can increase the variability in drug permeation and systemic absorption, thus increasing challenges in formulation development;
2. A significant number of psoriasis patients feel that the current therapies are either not sufficiently efficacious or aggressive. Hence, a primary challenge is to develop new

therapies which can be once daily application and show quick response, such as within the first four weeks of treatment;

3. Effective management of psoriasis frequently necessitates combining therapies in order to achieve optimum response while minimizing any side-effects. Thus any new topical therapy should have appropriate safety and efficacy when used in combination with another topical medication, systemic therapy and/or phototherapy;
4. In order to increase patient adherence to therapy, new topical formulations should have appropriate cosmetic elegance such as ease of use, no or minimal staining potential on clothing and bedding, quick absorption on application and being less greasy;
5. Formulations which can be used on many areas of the body including hair-bearing sites are preferred as patients often have psoriasis plaques in multiple areas;
6. Due to the availability of a wide variety of therapies and presence of generic products in the market, competitive cost of any new medication is paramount in influencing physician's and patient's choice of product.

9. Conclusion

As is summarized in this chapter, there are several treatment options for psoriasis and exciting novel targets (e.g. PDE4 and JAK) are being investigated as potential topical treatment options. Also, combination topical products and combination of topical and phototherapy have been shown to provide more effective treatment options. The epidermal hyperproliferation in psoriatic patients may increase the variability in drug penetration across the skin. Hence novel drug delivery approaches such as liposomes, iontophoresis, and electroporation are being investigated for improved delivery. Recent research has emphasized the importance of treatment adherence in the management of psoriasis. Adherence to treatment is likely to be a far more important determinant of success than are small differences in drug delivery, especially in actual clinical use as opposed to the well controlled environment of clinical trials. Several guidances have been developed to optimize topical treatment of psoriasis and hence enable more effective management of psoriasis. Since patients prefer a less messy vehicle, adherence and outcomes are likely to be better with the more novel formulation options such as foams and sprays compared with the traditionally recommended ointment.

10. Declaration of interest

The authors are employees of Merck Research Laboratories, a division of Merck Sharp and Dohme Corporation, which markets certain topical therapies discussed in the chapter.

11. References

Bagel J. (2009). Topical therapies for the treatment of plaque psoriasis. *Cutis*, 84, Suppl 4, 3-13.

Barker JN, Ashton RE, Marks R, Harris RI, Berth-Jones J. (1999). Topical maxacalcitol for the treatment of psoriasis vulgaris: a placebo controlled, double-blind, dose finding study with active comparator. *Br J Dermatol*, 141, 2, 274-278.

Bäumer W, Hoppmann J, Rundfeldt C, Kietzmann M. (2007). Highly selective phosphodiesterase 4 inhibitors for the treatment of allergic skin diseases and psoriasis. *Inflamm Allergy Drug Targets*, 6, 17-26.

Beani C. (2002). Salicylic acid as a keratolytic agent. *Ann Dermatol Venereol*. 2002, 129, 6, 933-935.

Beck LA. (2005). The efficacy and safety of tacrolimus ointment: a clinical review. *J Am Acad Dermatol*, 53, 2 Suppl 2, S165-S170.

Bernhard J, Whitmore C, Guzzo C, Kantor I, Kalb RE, Ellis C, Urbach F, Schwartzel EH, Gibson JR. (1991). Evaluation of halobetasol propionate ointment in the treatment of plaque psoriasis: report on two double-blind, vehicle-controlled studies. *J Am Acad Dermatol*, 25, 1170-1174.

Bhutani T, Zitelli KB, Koo J. (2011). Yin-yang strategy: proposing a new, effective, repeatable, sequential therapy for psoriasis. *J. Drug Dermatol*, 10, 831-834.

Bissonnette R, Nigen S, Bolduc C. (2008). Efficacy and tolerability of topical tacrolimus ointment for the treatment of male genital psoriasis. *J Cutan Med Surg*, 12, 230-234.

Blum G, Yawalkar S. (1991). A comparative multicenter double blind trial of 0.05% halobetasol propionate ointment and 0.1% betamethasone valerate ointment in the treatment of patients with chronic localized plaque psoriasis. *J Am Acad Dermatol*, 25, 1153-1156.

Bowman PH, Maloney JE, Koo JY. (2002). Combination of calcipotriene (Dovonex) ointment and tazarotene (Tazorac) gel versus clobetasol ointment in the treatment of plaque psoriasis: a pilot study. *J Am Acad Dermatol*, 46, 907-913.

Boyrke JF, Berth-Jones J, Hutchinson PE. (1993). Occlusion enhances the efficacy of topical calcipotriol in treatment of psoriasis vulgaris. *Clin Exp Dermatol*, 18, 504-506.

Bressinck R, Williams J, Peets E. (1988). Comparison of effect of mometasone furoate ointment 0.1%, and hydrocortisone ointment 1%, on adrenocortical function in psoriasis patients. *Today's Ther Trends*, 5, 4, 25-35.

Brodell RT, Bruce S, Hudson CP, Weiss JS, Colon LE, Johnson LA, Gottachalk RW. (2011). A multi-center, open-label study to evaluate the safety and efficacy of a sequential treatment regimen of clobetasol propionate 0.05% spray followed by calcitriol 3 mg/g ointment in the management of plaque psoriasis. *J Drugs Dermatol*, 10, 2, 158-164.

Campalani E, Barker J.N. (2005). The clinical genetics of psoriasis. *Current Genomics*, 6, 51-60.

Claréus BW, Houwing R, Sindrup JH, Wigchert S. (2009). The DESIRE study - psoriasis patients' satisfaction with topical treatment using a fixed combination of calcipotriol and betamethasone dipropionate in daily clinical practice. *Eur J Dermatol*, 19, 581-585.

De Jong EMGJ, Mørk NJ, Seijger MM. (2003). The combination of calcipotriol and methotrexate compared with methotrexate and vehicle in psoriasis: results of a multicentre placebo controlled randomized trial. *Br J Dermatol*, 148, 318-325.

Douglas WS, Poulin Y, Decroix J. (2002). A new calcipotriol/betamethasone formulation with rapid onset of action was superior to monotherapy with betamethasone dipropionate or calcipotriol in psoriasis vulgaris. *Acta Derm Venereol*, 82, 131-135.

Fabroni C, Lotti T. (2009). Pimecrolimus in dermatology. *G Ital Dermatol Venereol*, 144, 321-325.

Feldman SR, Ravis SM, Fleischer AB. (2001). Betamethasone valerate in foam vehicle is effective with both daily and twice a day dosing: a single-blind, open-label study in the treatment of scalp psoriasis. *J Cutan Med Surg*, 5, 386-389.

Feldman SR, Yentzer BA. (2009). Topical clobetasol propionate in the treatment of psoriasis: a review of newer formulations. *Am J Clin Dermatol*, 10, 397-406.

Franz TJ, Parsell DA, Halualani RM, Hannigan JF, Kalbach JP, Harkonen WS. (1999). Betamethasone valerate foam 0.12%: a novel vehicle with enhanced delivery and efficacy. *Int J Dermato*, 38, 628-632.

Freeman AK, Linowski GJ, Brady C. (2003). Tacrolimus ointment for the treatment of psoriasis on the face and intertriginous areas. *J Am Acad Dermatol,* 48, 564-568.

Fresta M, Puglisi G. (1997). Corticosteroid dermal delivery with skin lipid liposomes. *J Control Rel,* 44, 141-151.

Fridman JS, Scherle PA, Collins R, Burn T, Neilan CL, Hertel D, Contel N, Haley P, Thomas B, Shi J, Collier P, Rodgers JD, Shepard S, Metcalf B, Hollis G, Newton RC, Yeleswaram S, Friedman SM, Vaddi K. (2011). Preclinical evaluation of local JAK1 and JAK2 inhibition in cutaneous inflammation. *J Invest Dermatol.* (Epub ahead of print).

Gelfand JM, Shin DB, Neimann AL, Wang X, Margolis DJ, Troxel AB. (2006a). The risk of lymphoma in patients with psoriasis. *J Invest Dermatol,* 126, 10, 2194-2201.

Gelfand JM, Neimann AL, Shin DB, Wang X, Margolis DJ, Troxel AB. (2006b). Risk of myocardial infarction in patients with psoriasis. *JAMA,* 296, 14, 1735-1741.

Goldberg B, Hartdegen R, Presbury D, Smith EH, Yawalkar S. (1991). A double blind multicenter comparison of 0.05% halobetasol propionate ointment and 0.05% clobetasol propionate ointment in patients with chronic localized plaque psoriasis. *J Am Acad Dermatol,* 25, 6, 1145-1148.

Gottlieb AB, Ford RO, Spellman MC. (2003). The efficacy and tolerability of clobetasol propionate foam 0.05% in the treatment of mild to moderate plaque-type psoriasis of nonscalp regions. *J Cutan Med Surg,* 7, 185-192.

Gribetz C, Ling M, Lebwohl M. (2004). Pimecrolimus cream 1% in the treatment of intertriginous psoriasis: a double-blind, randomized study. *J Am Acad Dermatol,* 51, 731-738.

Guenther LC. (2004). Fixed-dose combination therapy for psoriasis. *Am J Clin Dermatol,* 5, 2, 71-77.

Guenther LC. (2009). Treatments for scalp psoriasis with emphasis on calcipotriol plus betamethasone dipropionate gel (Xamiol). *Skin Therapy Lett,* 14, 1-4.

Gupta AK, Ryder JE. (2003). Photodynamic therapy and topical aminolevulinic acid: an overview. *Am J Clin Dermatol,* 4, 699-708.

Horn EJ, Fox KM, Patel V, Chiou CF, Dann F, Lebwohl, M. (2007). Association of patient reported psoriasis severity with income and employment. *J Am Acad Dermatol,* 57, 6, 963-971.

Horn EJ, Domm S, Katz HI. (2010). Topical corticosteroids in psoriasis: strategies for improving safety. *J Eur Acad Dermatol Venereol,* 24, 119-124.

Huang X, Tanojo H, Lenn J, Deng CH, Krochmal L. (2005). A novel foam vehicle for delivery of topical corticosteroids. *J Am Acad Dermatol,* 53, 1 Suppl 1, S26-38.

Jarratt M, Breneman D, Gottlieb AB, Poulin Y, Liu Y, Foley V. (2004). Clobetasol propionate shampoo 0.05%: a new option to treat patients with moderate to severe scalp psoriasis. *J Drugs Dermatol,* 3, 367-373.

Katz HI, Prawer SE, Watson MJ. (1989). Mometasone furoate ointment 0.1% vs. hydrocortisone ointment 1.0% in psoriasis. *Int J Dermatol,* 28, 342-344.

Kaur I, Saraswat A, Kumar B. (2001). Comparison of calcipotriol and coal tar in conjunction with sun exposure in chronic plaque psoriasis: a pilot study. *J Dermatol,* 28, 448-450.

Kircik L. (2009). Efficacy and safety of topical calcitriol 3 microg/g ointment, a new topical therapy for chronic plaque psoriasis. *J Drugs Dermatol,* 8, Suppl 8, s9-s16.

Klaber MR, Hutchinson PE, Pedvis-Leftick A, Kragballe K, Reunala TL, Van de Kerkhof PC, Johnsson MK, Molin L, Corbett MS, Downess N. (1994). Comparative effects of calcipotriol solution (50 micograms/ml) and betamethasone 17-valerate solution (1 mg/ml) in the treatment of scalp psoriasis. *Br. J. Dermatol*, 131, 5, 678-683.

Koo J. (1999). Systemic sequential therapy of psoriasis: A new paradign for improved therapeutic results. *J. Am. Acad. Dermatol*, 41, S25-28.

Korting HC, Zienicke H, Schäfer-Korting M, Braun-Falco O. (1990). Liposome encapsulation improves efficacy of betamethasone dipropionate in atopic eczema but not in psoriasis vulgaris. *Eur J Clin Pharmacol*, 39, 4, 349-351.

Kowalzick L. (2009). Novel topical therapy for mild-to-moderate plaque psoriasis: focus on calcitriol. *Clin Cosmet Investig Dermatol*, 16, 2, 153-159.

Lebwohl M, Peets E, Chen V. (1993). Limited application of mometasone furoate on the face and intertriginous areas: analysis of safety and efficacy. *Int J Dermatol*, 32, 11, 830-831.

Lebwohl M, Ast E, Callen JP, Cullen SI, Hong SR, Kulp-Shorten CL, Lowe NJ, Phillips TJ, Rosen T, Wolf DI, Quell JM, Sefton J, Lue JC, Gibson JR. (1998). Once-daily tazarotene gel versus twice-daily fluocinonide cream in the treatment of plaque psoriasis. *J Am Acad Dermatol*, 38, 5, 705-711.

Lebwohl M, Menter A, Koo J, Feldman SR. (2004). Combination therapy to treat moderate to severe psoriasis. *J. Am. Acad. Dermatol*, 50, 416-430.

Lebwohl M, Menter A, Weiss J, Clark SD, Flores J, Powers J, Balin AK, Kempers S, Glinert RJ, Fleming T, Liu Y, Graeber M, Pariser DM. (2007). Calcitriol 3 microg/g ointment in the management of mild to moderate plaque type psoriasis: results from 2 placebo-controlled, multicenter, randomized double-blind, clinical studies. *J Drugs Dermatol*, 6, 4, 428-435.

Lehmann B. (2009). Role of the vitamin D3 pathway in healthy and diseased skin-facts, contradictions and hypotheses. *Exp Dermatol*, 18, 97-108.

Linden KG, Weinstein GD. (1999). Psoriasis: current perspectives with emphasis on treatment. *Am J Med*, 107, 595-605.

Long CC, Mills CM, Finlay AY. (1998). A practical guide to topical therapy in children. *Br J Dermatol*,138, 293-296.

Luger T, Paul C. (2007). Potential new indications of topical calcineurin inhibitors. *Dermatology*, 215, Suppl 1:45-54.

Martín Ezquerra G, Sánchez Regaña M, Herrera Acosta E. (2006). Topical tacrolimus for the treatment of psoriasis on the face, genitalia, intertriginous areas and corporal plaques. *J Drugs Dermatol*, 5, 334-336.

Mason AR, Mason J, Cork M. (2009). Topical treatments for chronic plaque psoriasis. *Cochrane Database Syst Rev*, 2, CD005028.

Maurer TA. (2005). Dermatologic manifestations of HIV infection. *Top HIV Med*, 13, 5, 149-154.

Medansky RS, Brody NI, Kanof NB. (1987). Clinical investigations of mometasone furoate – a novel nonfluorinated, topical corticosteroid. *Semin Dermatol*. 6, 2, 94-100.

Medansky RS, Bressinck R, Cole GW. (1988). Mometasone furoate ointment and cream 0.1% in treatment of psoriasis: comparison with ointment and cream formulations of flucinolone acetonide 0.025% and triamcinolone acetonide 0.1%. *Cutis*. 42, 480-485.

Mensing H, Korsukewitz G, Yawalkar S. (1991). A double blind multicenter comparison of 0.05% halobetasol propionate ointment and 0.05% betamethasone dipropionate ointment in chronic plaque psoriasis. *J Am Acad Dermatol*, 25, 1166-1169.

Menter A, Korman NJ, Elmets CA, Feldman SR, Gelfand JM, Gordon KB, Gottlieb A, Koo JY, Lebwohl M, Lim HW, Van Voorhees AS, Beutner KR, Bhushan R. (2009). Guidelines of care for the management of psoriasis and psoriatic arthritis. Section 3.

Guidelines of care for the management and treatment of psoriasis with topical therapies. *J Am Acad Dermatol*, 60, 4, 643-659.
Mesa RA. (2010). Ruxolitinib, a selective JAK1 and JAK2 inhibitor for the treatment of myeloproliferative neoplasms and psoriasis. *IDrugs*, 13, 6, 394-403.
Mraz S, Leonardi C, Colón LE. (2008). Different treatment outcomes with different formulations of clobetasol propionate 0.05% for the treatment of plaque psoriasis. *J Dermatolog Treat*, 19, 354-359.
Muller K, Bendtzen K. (1996). 1,25-dihydroxyvitamin D3 as a natural regulator of human immune functions. *J Invest Dermatol Symp Proc*, 1, 1, 68-71.
Nast A, Kopp I, Augustin M. (2007). German evidence-based guidelines for the treatment of psoriasis vulgaris (short version). *Arch Dermatol Res*, 299, 111–138.
Nazarian R, Weinberg JM. (2009). AN-2728, a PDE4 inhibitor for the potential topical treatment of psoriasis and atopic dermatitis. *Curr Opin Investig Drugs*, 10, 1236-1242.
Nestle FO, Kaplan DH, Barker J. (2009). Psoriasis. *New Engl J Med*, 361, 496-509.
Nguyen T, Gattu S, Pugashetti R, Koo J. (2009). Practice of phototherapy in the treatment of moderate-to-severe psoriasis. *Curr Probl Dermatol*, 38, 59-78.
Norris DA. (2005). Mechanisms of action of topical therapies and the rationale for combination therapy. *J Am Acad Dermatol*, 53, 1 Suppl 1, S17-S25.
Papp KA, Guenther L, Boyden B, et al. (2003). Early onset of action and efficacy of a combination of calcipotriene and betamethasone dipropionate in the treatment of psoriasis. *J Am Acad Dermatol*, 48, 48-54.
Papp KA, Carey W. (2010). Psoriasis care: new and emerging pharmacologic trends. *J Cutan Med Surg*, 14, 3, 119-129.
Pathirana D, Ormerod AD, Saiag P, Smith C, Spuls PI, Nast A, Barker J, Bos JD, Burmester GR, Chimenti S, Dubertret L, Eberlein B, Erdmann R, Ferguson J, Girolomoni G, Gisondi P, Giunta A, Griffiths C, Hönigsmann H, Hussain M, Jobling R, Karvonen SL, Kemeny L, Kopp I, Leonardi C, Maccarone M, Menter A, Mrowietz U, Naldi L, Nijsten T, Ortonne JP, Orzechowski HD, Rantanen T, Reich K, Reytan N, Richards H, Thio HB, van de Kerkhof P, Rzany B. (2009). European S3-Guidelines on the systemic treatment of psoriasis vulgaris. *J Eu Acad Dermatol Venereology*, 23, Suppl 2, 5-70.
Prakash A, Benfield P. (1998). Topical Mometasone: A Review of its pharmacological properties and therapeutic use in the treatment of dermatological disorders. *Drugs*, 55, 145-163.
Rivera AM, Hsu S. (2005). Topical halobetasol propionate in the treatment of plaque psoriasis: a review. *Am J Clin Dermatol*, 6, 311-316.
Ruzicka T. (2006). Methylprednisolone aceponate in eczema and other inflammatory skin disorders-a clinical update. *Int J Clin Pract*, 60, 85–92.
Saraceno R, Gramiccia T, Frascione P, Chimenti, S. (2009). Calcipotriene/betamethasone in the treatment of psoriasis: a review article. *Expert Opin Pharmacother*, 10, 14, 2357-2365.
Staberg B, Roed-Petersen J, Menne T. (1989). Efficacy of topical treatment in psoriasis with MC903, a new vitamin D analogue. *Acta Derm Vevereol*, 69, 147-150.
Stein LF, Sherr A, Solodkina G, Gottlieb AB, Chaudhari U. (2001). Betamethasone valerate foam for treatment of nonscalp psoriasis. *J Cutan Med Surg*, 5, 4, 303-307.
Su Y-H, Fang J-Y. (2008). Drug delivery and formulations for topical treatment of psoriasis. *Exp Opin Drug Deliv*, 5, 235-249.

Svensson A, Reidhav, Gisslen, H. (1992). A comparative study of mometasone furoate ointment and betamethasone valerate ointment in patients with psoriasis vulgaris. *Curr Ther Res*, 52, 390-396.

Swinehart JM, Barkoff JR, Dvorkin D, Fisher G, Peets E. (1989). Mometasone furoate lotion once daily versus triamcinolone acetonide lotion twice daily in psoriasis. *Int J Dermatol*, 28, 680-681.

Tang-Liu DD, Matsumoto RM, Usansky JI. (1999). Clinical pharmacokinetics and drug metabolism of tazarotene: a novel topical treatment for acne and psoriasis. *Clin Pharmacokinet*, 37, 273-287.

Tanghetti EA. (2009). The role of topical vitamin D modulators in psoriasis therapy. *J Drugs Dermatol*, 8, Suppl, s4-8.

Tosti A, Piraccini BM, Cameli N, Kokely F, Plozzer C, Cannata GE, Benelli C. (1998). Calcipotriol ointment in nail psoriasis: a controlled double blind comparison with betamethasone dipropionate and salicylic acid. *Br J Dermatol*, 139, 4, 655-659.

Tzung TY, Wu JC, Hsu NJ. (2005). Comparison of tazarotene 0.1% gel plus petrolatum once daily versus calcipotriol 0.005% ointment twice daily in the treatment of plaque psoriasis. *Acta Derm Venereol*, 85, 236-239.

van de Kerkhof PC. (2006). Update on retinoid therapy of psoriasis in an update on the use of retinoids in dermatology. *Dermatol Ther*, 19, 252-263.

Vanderploeg DE, Cornell RC, Binder R. (1989). Clinical trial in scalp psoriasis. Mometasone furoate 0.1% applied once daily vs betamethasone valerate lotion 0.1% applied twice daily. *Acta Ther*, 15, 145-152.

Veraldi S, Schianchi R. (2003). Short contact therapy with tazarotene in psoriasis vulgaris. *Dermatology*, 206, 347-348.

Warren RB, Brown BC, Grindlay DJC, Griffiths CEM. (2010). What's new in psoriasis? Analysis of the clinical significance of new guidelines and systematic reviews on psoriasis published in 2008 and 2009. *Clinical and Experimental Dermatology*, 35, 7, 688-692.

Weinstein GD, Krueger GG, Lowe NJ. (1997). Tazarotene gel, a new retinoid, for topical therapy of psoriasis: vehicle-controlled study of safety, efficacy, and duration of therapeutic effect. *J Am Acad Dermatol*, 37, 85-92.

Weinstein GD, Koo JY, Krueger GG, Lebwohl MG, Lowe NJ, Menter MA, Lew-Kaya DA, Sefton J, Gibson JR, Walker PS; (2003). Tazarotene cream in the treatment of psoriasis: Two multicenter, double-blind, randomized, vehicle-controlled studies of the safety and efficacy of tazarotene creams 0.05% and 0.1% applied once daily for 12 weeks. J Am Acad Dermatol, 48, 5, 760-767.

Witman PM. (2001). Topical therapies for localized psoriasis. *Mayo Clin Proc*, 76, 943-949.

Wolf N, Quaranta M, Prescott NJ, Allen M, Smith R, Burden AD, Worthington J, Griffiths CE, Mathew CG, Barker JN, Capon F, Trembath FC. (2008). Psoriasis is associated with pleiotropic susceptibility loci identified in type II diabetes and Crohn disease. *J Med Genet*, ;45, 2, 114-116.

Wollina U, Hansel G, Koch A, Abdel-Naser MB. (2006). Topical pimecrolimus for skin disease other than atopic dermatitis. *Expert Opin Pharmacother*, 7, 1967-1975.

Yamamoto T, Nishioka K. (2003). Topical tacrolimus: an effective therapy for facial psoriasis. *Eur J Dermatol*, 13, 471-473.

Yamauchi PS, Rizk D, Lowe NJ. (2004). Retinoid therapy for psoriasis. *Dermatol Clin*, 22, 467-476.

16

Biotech on the Rise: The Treatment of Psoriasis with Biological Drugs

Daria Capece et al.*
Department of Experimental Medicine,
University of L'Aquila, L'Aquila
Italy

1. Introduction

Psoriasis is a chronic inflammatory skin disorder affecting 1-3% of the general population worldwide. Up to one-third of psoriatic patients have concomitant psoriatic arthritis (Gerdes et al, 2009). Multiple studies and clinical trials support an important role for dysregulation of the immune system in the development of psoriasis. In recent years, the improved understanding of the molecular basis underlying psoriasis has led to the introduction of biological drugs, providing a new effective treatment option for this disease. Biologics target key steps in the pathogenesis of psoriasis, and can be classified into three main categories: TNFα inhibitors, T cell inhibitors and IL-12/IL-23 inhibitors (Weger, 2010). In this chapter we discuss the state of the art of biological therapies for psoriasis and psoriatic arthritis and give a brief overview of the new biological approaches that are currently undergoing evaluation for the treatment of both diseases.

2. TNFα Inhibitors

TNFα is a proinflammatory cytokine that plays key roles in both innate and adaptive immunity. At high concentrations, it can trigger an excessive inflammatory response ending in organ damage. The development of anti-TNFα biologics originated from a study by Brennan et al., which showed that the expression of pro-inflammatory cytokines by synoviocytes in rheumatoid arthritis patients was inhibited by TNF-neutralizing antibodies (Brennan et al, 1989). To date, the role of TNFα in psoriasis and psoriatic arthritis has been fully investigated (Schottelius et al, 2004). Increased levels of TNFα and a differential expression of TNFα receptors I and II have been found in lesional psoriatic skin compared with normal-appearing skin; in addition, in psoriatic patients, the plasma concentration of TNFα is higher and the mRNA expression of this cytokine is increased in peripheral blood

* Valeria Iansante[1], Mariafausta Fischietti[1], Daniela Verzella[1], Maria Concetta Fargnoli[2], Ketty Peris[2], Roberto Giacomelli[3], Francesca Zazzeroni[1] and Edoardo Alesse[1]
[1]*Department of Experimental Medicine, University of L'Aquila, L'Aquila, Italy*
[2]*Department of Sciences and Biomedical Technology, University of L'Aquila, L'Aquila, Italy*
[3]*Department of Internal Medicine and Public Health, University of L'Aquila, L'Aquila, Italy*

mononuclear cells. Currently, four TNFα antagonists are approved for the treatment of psoriasis and/or psoriatic arthritis, namely etanercept, infliximab, adalimumab and golimumab; a new TNFα inhibitor (certolizumab pegol) is currently undergoing a phase III trial for the treatment of psoriatic arthritis.

2.1 Etanercept

Etanercept is a recombinant human fusion protein consisting of a dimer of the extracellular portion of TNFα receptor II linked to the Fc portion of IgG1 (Amgen, Inc, 2011). Etanercept binds to both the trimeric form of soluble TNFα and to the transmembrane form, antagonizing their biological actions (Bachmann et al, 2010). Several studies reported a reduction of different inflammatory cell types in psoriatic lesions during etanercept treatment, such as T cells, natural killer cells, neutrophils, macrophages and plasmocytoid dendritic cells (de Groot et al, 2010). Etanercept also blocks downstream T-cell mediated events inducing apoptosis of CD11c+ myeloid dendritic cells (Malaviya et al, 2006). In addition, etanercept has been shown to down-regulate Th17 cell markers, as well as Th17 cell products and effector molecules (Antiga et al, 2010; Zaba et al, 2007). Etanercept is FDA- and EMA-approved for the treatment of psoriasis and psoriatic arthritis. It is also approved for the treatment of other autoimmune conditions such as rheumatoid arthritis, juvenile idiopathic arthritis and ankilosing spondilytis (Amgen, Inc., 2011).

2.1.1 Administration

Etanercept is administered subcutaneously at a dose of 50 mg twice a week in patients with plaque psoriasis or at 25 mg twice a week in patients with psoriatic arthritis during the first 12 weeks of treatment. After the initiation phase, the dosage for plaque psoriasis is reduced to 25 mg twice a week or 50 mg weekly during the maintenance phase (Amgen, Inc., 2011). Etanercept can be administered either continuously or intermittently. Gordon et al reported no loss of efficacy with intermittent therapy, with a similar response between retreatment and initial therapy in psoriatic patients (Gordon et al, 2006a). However, a multicenter European open-label study showed that both regimens provide a significant improvement in quality of life, with a greater improvement in the continuous treatment group (Dauden et al, 2009). Non-neutralizing anti-etanercept antibodies have been observed by several authors, but the relevance of them is still debated (Bachmann et al, 2010).

2.1.2 Clinical efficacy

Several high-quality clinical trials (Cassano et al, 2010; Gottlieb et al, 2003; Leonardi et al, 2003, 2010; Papp et al, 2005; Tyring et al, 2007; van de Kerkhof et al, 2008) have evaluated both the short-term and long-term efficacy of etanercept in the treatment of psoriasis. In clinical trials, the severity of psoriasis is assessed by the Psoriasis Area and Severity Index (PASI). PASI 75 is defined as a 75% reduction in PASI score compared with baseline. An initial randomized, double-blind, placebo-controlled, multicenter trial of 112 patients demonstrated a PASI 75 response in 30% of patients receiving 25 mg etanercept twice a week compared with 2% of placebo-treated patients after 12 weeks. After 24 weeks, PASI 75 response increased to 56% in the etanercept-treated arm compared with 5% in the placebo group (Gottlieb et al, 2003). Leonardi et al. demonstrated that the efficacy of etanercept is dose-related, reporting a PASI 75 response in 34% and 49% of patients treated with 25 mg and 50 mg twice weekly after 12 weeks of treatment, respectively. The improvement continued through week 24, with 44% and 59% of patients achieving a PASI 75, respectively (Leonardi et al, 2003). The same high-dose etanercept regimen was used in a recent study by Griffiths et al., who reported a PASI 75 response in 57% of patients after 12 weeks of treatment (Griffiths et al, 2010). In a further multicentre 24-week study, the efficacy of etanercept during the initial treatment phase and after dose reduction were evaluated (Papp et al, 2005). Patients were treated with a dose of 50 mg etanercept, 25 mg etanercept or placebo twice weekly for the first 12 weeks. During the second 12 weeks of treatment, the dosage was reduced to 25 mg twice weekly. Papp et al. reported a PASI 75 in 49% of patients treated with 50 mg twice weekly and in 34% of patients receiving 25 mg twice weekly of etanercept compared with 3% in the placebo group at week 12, and demonstrated that the effect obtained with the higher dose could be preserved in most patients after dose reduction (Papp et al, 2005). A further increase of the dose of etanercept to 100 mg did not demonstrate an improvement in efficacy (Cassano et al, 2006). Recent data by van de Kerkhof et al. demonstrated that etanercept 50 mg once weekly for 24 weeks was effective, with a PASI 75 response of 38% after 12 weeks, which increased to 71% after 24 weeks (van de Kerkhof et al, 2008). Similar results were reported by Sterry et al. (Sterry et al, 2010). Regarding long-term efficacy, etanercept response has been demonstrated to last up to 96 weeks, resulting in a statistically significant improvement (Tyring et al, 2007; Esposito et al, 2010). Etanercept is the only biological drug that has shown efficacy and safety in pediatric patients with moderate to severe plaque psoriasis (Paller et al, 2008). Paller et al. reported a PASI 75 response in 57% of children and adolescents treated with etanercept (0.8 mg/kg body weight) compared with 11% in placebo patients after 12 weeks. The efficacy of the treatment was maintained through 96 weeks (Paller et al, 2010). Treatment with etanercept also provides an improvement in the quality of life of patients, as measured by the Dermatology Life Quality Index (DLQI) (Leonardi et al, 2003; van de Kerkhof et al, 2008).

Two pivotal studies have demonstrated the efficacy of etanercept in the treatment of psoriatic arthritis. In these studies, the American College of Rheumatology (ACR) criteria is the most frequently parameter used to assess the severity of psoriatic arthritis. A double-blind, placebo-controlled study enrolling 60 patients suffering from psoriatic arthritis showed achievement of ACR 20, ACR 50 and ACR 70 response in 73%, 50% and 13% of patients after 12 weeks of treatment with etanercept, compared with 13%, 3% and 0% in the placebo group (Mease et al, 2000). Furthermore, the same authors reported an additional double-blind, placebo-controlled clinical trial in 250 patients with psoriatic arthritis. At 12 weeks, an ACR 20 response was observed in 59% of etanercept-treated patients compared with 15% of the placebo group. This study also reported an improvement in quality of life measured by the Health Assessment Questionaire (HAQ) (Mease et al, 2004). The improvements observed were maintained for up to 2 years (Mease et al, 2010). A recent study by Saougou et al. reported a PASI 90 response in 68% of etanercept-treated patients affected by psoriatic arthritis after 5 years (Saougou et al, 2011).

Although highly effective as monotherapy, few studies have been published on the combination of etanercept with cyclosporine, narrowband UVB, acitretin and methotrexate (reviewed in Foley et al, 2010). Preliminary data from short-term analysis support the use of etanercept in combination therapy which does not seem to be associated with additional toxicities. This provides an attractive option for patients inadequately responding to monotherapy. However, further long-term studies are needed to confirm the safety of combination therapy.

2.2 Infliximab

Infliximab is a chimeric IgG anti-TNFα monoclonal antibody constiting of a human constant (75%) region and murine variable (25%) regions (Centocor Ortho Biotech, Inc., 2011). *In vivo*, infliximab binds to human TNFα and forms stable complexes, resulting in the loss of biological activity of this pro-inflammatory cytokine (Scallon et al, 1995). Infliximab is able to neutralize both soluble and trans-membrane TNFα and induces the elimination of TNFα bearing cells, such as macrophages, dermal dendritic cells, and T cells (Gisondi et al, 2004; Zaba et al, 2007). Recently, it has been suggested that infliximab induces p53-related keratinocytes apoptosis, highlighting another effect of this drug in psoriasis (Raho et al, 2011). Infliximab is FDA- and EMA-approved for the treatment of psoriasis, psoriatic arthritis, rheumatoid arthritis, ankylosing spondylitis, adult and pediatric Crohn's disease and ulcerative colitis (Centocor Ortho Biotech, Inc., 2011).

2.2.1 Administration

Infliximab is administered as a 2-3 hour intravenous infusion at a dose of 5mg/kg. The infusions are given at weeks 0, 2 and 6 (induction period) and then every 8 weeks (maintenance period) (Centocor Ortho Biotech, Inc., 2011). The efficacy of continuous versus intermittent treatment was evaluated in the clinical trial EXPRESS II, reporting that continuous treatment achieved better results than intermittent therapy to maintain PASI response and to reduce the occurrence of anti-infliximab antibodies, the most common cause of decreased drug efficacy (Haraoui et al, 2006; Menter et al, 2007; Vena & Cassano, 2007).

2.2.2 Clinical efficacy

Several pivotal clinical trials demonstrated the clinical efficacy of infliximab in the treatment of plaque psoriasis (Chaudhari et al, 2001; Gottlieb et al, 2004; Reich et al, 2005, 2006). Two phase II studies evaluated the efficacy of infliximab at different doses, 5 and 10 mg/kg and 3 and 5 mg/kg, respectively (Chaudhari et al, 2001; Gottlieb et al, 2004). In the first study of 33 psoriatic patients, a PASI 75 response was observed in 82% and 73% of patients receiving 5 and 10 mg/kg of infliximab, respectively, and in 8% of the patients receiving placebo after 10 weeks. In the second study (SPIRIT) of 249 plaque psoriasis patients, 72% and 88% of patients receiving 3 and 5 mg/kg of infliximab, respectively, achieved PASI 75 at week 10 compared with 6% of the placebo-treated patients. These results demonstrated a high short-term efficacy of infliximab and identified 5 mg/kg as the ideal dosage regimen in the treatment of psoriasis. The rapid response induced by infliximab decreased after 50 weeks (Reich et al, 2005). The phase III multi-center, double-blind, placebo-controlled trial EXPRESS enrolled 378 patients with plaque psoriasis and showed a PASI 75 response in 80% of the patients after 10 weeks compared with 3% in placebo group. The response was maintained through week 24 and decreased to 61% by week 50. Nevertheless, the retrospective analysis of the EXPRESS trial showed that infliximab continuous therapy for 1 year resulted in a sustained improvement in PASI score (Reich et al, 2010). Moreover, infliximab provides a substantial improvement in quality of life, with a meaningful decrease in DLQI both in short-term and long-term treatment (Feldmann et al, 2005; Gottlieb et al, 2004; Menter et al, 2007; Reich et al, 2006, 2010).

The IMPACT trial evaluated the efficacy of infliximab in 104 patients with psoriatic arthritis (Antoni et al, 2005a). At week 16, 65% of patients achieved ACR 20 compared with 10% of the placebo group and 46% and 29% achieved ACR 50 and ACR 70, respectively. The efficacy of infliximab has been evaluated in a larger cohort of patients (n=200) in the IMPACT 2 trial. At week 14, 64% of infliximab-treated patients showed a PASI 75 response and 58% achieved ACR 20; in addition ACR 20 criteria were maintained up to 1 year (Antoni et al, 2005b; Kavanaugh et al, 2007). The long-term efficacy of infliximab was evaluated by a two-year extension of the IMPACT trial (Antoni et al, 2008). At week 98, maintenance of the ACR 20 criteria was observed in 68% of infliximab-treated patients and 64% of them achieved PASI 75.

Regarding combination therapy, the concomitant administration of methotrexate has been reported to prolong the long-term efficacy of infliximab by decreasing the development of human anti-infliximab neutralizing antibodies (Klotz et al, 2007).

2.3 Adalimumab

Adalimumab is the first fully humanized recombinant anti-TNFα monoclonal antibody. Adalimumab is able to bind both soluble and membrane-bound TNFα in a dose-dependent manner (Abbott Laboratories, 2011). It has been shown that adalimumab lyses TNFα-bearing cells in the presence of complement and induces apoptosis *in vitro*; in addition adalimumab affects the biological responses controlled by TNFα, such as the expression of adhesion molecules, serum concentration of cytokines, reactive oxygen species and dendritic cells in psoriatic plaques (Papoutsaki et al, 2007). Moreover, adalimumab is able to modulate Toll-like receptors expression on basal keratinocytes (De Pità et al, 2011). Adalimumab is FDA- and EMA-approved for the treatment of psoriasis, psoriatic arthritis, rheumatoid arthritis, Crohn's disease, juvenile idiopathic arthritis and ankylosing spondylitis (Abbott Laboratories, 2011).

2.3.1 Administration

Adalimumab is administered as a subcutaneous injection and the recommended dose for psoriasis is a loading dose of 80 mg at week one, followed by 40 mg at week two and continuous 40 mg injection every other week (eow) for maintenance. In psoriatic arthritis the ideal dosage regimen is 40 mg every second week (Abbott Laboratories, 2011). The continuous therapy with adalimumab seems to be more effective than intermitted therapy to provide a sustained response (Menter et al, 2008). Recently, encouraging results have been obtained in the retreatment of patients who relapsed after interruption of adalimumab therapy (Papp et al, 2011) and patients who lost efficacy during treatment with another TNFα antagonist (Van et al, 2008). Development of anti-adalimumab antibodies may occur, as demonstrated in patients with rheumatoid arthritis (Bartelds et al, 2010).

2.3.2 Clinical efficacy

The clinical efficacy of adalimumab was analyzed by three main clinical trials (Gordon et al, 2006b; Menter et al, 2008; Saurat et al, 2008). In an earlier phase II study enrolling 147 psoriatic patients, two dose regimens of adalimumab were evaluated. Gordon et al. reported a PASI 75 improvement in 80% of patients treated with 40 mg weekly and in 53% of patients receiving 40 mg eow compared with 4% of patients in the placebo group at week 12. At week 60, PASI 75 response was observed in 64% and 56% of patients treated with 40 mg weekly or 40 mg eow, respectively (Gordon et al, 2006b). The phase III placebo-controlled randomized trial by Menter et al. of 1212 patients with plaque psoriasis evaluated the efficacy of adalimumab 40 mg eow. The authors reported a PASI 75 response rate in 71% of the patients after 16 weeks and in 70% after 24 weeks of 40 mg eow adalimumab therapy; the efficacy decreased during weeks 33 to 52 (Menter et al, 2008). The first head-to-head trial CHAMPION compared adalimumab vs methotrexate and reported a PASI 75 response in 80% of patients in the adalimumab 40 mg eow group, in 36% of patients in the methotrexate group and in 19% of those in the placebo group (Saurat et al, 2008). An improvement in DLQI after treatment with adalimumab has been reported by several studies (Menter et al, 2010; Revicki et al, 2008; Saurat et al, 2008; Shikiar et al, 2007).

The clinical efficacy of adalimumab in psoriatic arthritis has also been described (Genovese et al, 2007; Gladman et al, 2007; Mease et al, 2005, 2009). The ADEPT trial involving 315 psoriatic arthritis patients tested the long-term clinical efficacy of adalimumab through 2 years. Mease et al. reported that 58% of patients treated with adalimumab achieved the ACR 20 after 12 weeks compared with 14% of the patients in the placebo group and that similar percentages were maintained up to week 104 (Mease et al, 2005, 2009). These data were confirmed by Genovese et al. who reported an ACR 20 response in 65% of adalimumab-treated patients after week 24 (Genovese et al, 2007).

Recently, the use of adalimumab in combination with traditional therapies was evaluated in psoriasis. Adalimumab with methotrexate results in a lower discontinuation rate of the TNFα antagonist (Heiberg et al, 2008); the concomitant administration of adalimumab with phototherapy seems to be clinically effective, but further investigations in controlled clinical trials are needed (Bagel, 2011). The use of topical agents in combination with adalimumab results in a higher short-term efficacy that decreases after 4 weeks (Thaçi et al, 2010).

2.4 Golimumab

Golimumab is a new TNFα antagonist and, like adalimumab, is a fully human anti-TNFα IgG monoclonal antibody, which binds to both soluble and transmembrane forms of TNFα. Golimumab has been recently FDA- and EMA-approved for the treatment of psoriatic arthritis as monotherapy or in combination with methotrexate. Golimumab is also approved for controlling symptoms of rheumatoid arthritis and ankylosing spondylitis (Centocor Ortho Biotech, Inc., 2010).

2.4.1 Administration

Golimumab is the first patient-administered once-monthly anti-TNFα drug. The recommended dosage is 50 mg subcutaneously every 4 weeks (Centocor Ortho Biotech, Inc., 2010).

2.4.2 Clinical efficacy

The phase III GO-REVEAL clinical trial evaluated the efficacy of golimumab in 405 patients suffering from active psoriatic arthritis (Kavanaugh et al, 2009a). Patients received 50 mg, 100 mg or placebo once every 4 weeks. Achievement of ACR 20 criteria at week 14 was the primary end-point and was observed in 51% of patients treated with 50 mg, in 45% of patients receiving 100 mg of golimumab and in 9% of patients in the placebo group. At 24 weeks, Kavanaugh et al. reported further improvement, with 52% and 61% of patients treated with 50 mg and 100 mg achieving ACR 20 criteria, respectively, compared with only 12% of patients in the placebo group. At week 14, a PASI 75 was achieved in 40% and in 58% of patients receiving 50 mg and 100 mg golimumab, respectively, compared to 3% of patients receiving placebo (Kavanaugh et al, 2009a). Long-term efficacy of golimumab was evaluated in a 2-year trial (Kavanaugh et al, 2009b). At week 52, the percentage of patients treated with 50 mg of golimumab achieving ACR 20 and PASI 75 responses was 78% and 62%, respectively. At week 104, the proportion of patients with the aforementioned clinical responses increased to 91% and 69%, respectively. With regard to the group of patients who received 100 mg of golimumab, Kavanaugh et al. observed an ACR 20 response in 81% and in 73% of patients at week 52 and 104, respectively. At the same time points, the percentage of patients achieving a PASI 75 was 70% and 76%, respectively (Kavanaugh et al, 2009b). The authors also reported an improvement in physical function and quality of life (Kavanaugh et al, 2009a).

2.5 Certolizumab pegol

Certolizumab Pegol is another TNFα antagonist approved for the treatment of rheumatoid arthritis and Crohn's disease (UCB, Inc., 2010). It is a pegylated Fab fragment of a humanized anti-TNFα antibody. The presence of polyethylene glycol prolongs serum half-life of the drug. Certolizumab pegol is unable to induce antibody-dependent cell-mediated cytotoxicity and complement-dependent cytotoxicity because of the lack of the Fc region (Bourne et al, 2008). Preliminary data from two phase II clinical trials showed that certolizumab pegol is effective in patients with moderate to severe plaque psoriasis (Ortonne et al, 2007, 2008a, 2008b). In these studies the efficacy and safety at two different dose regimens were evaluated. Patients were treated with 200 mg, 400 mg of certolizumab pegol or placebo every two weeks subcutaneously. At week 12, a PASI 75 response was observed in 74.6% of patients receiving 200 mg and in 82.8% of 400 mg treated-patients compared with 6.8% of patients in the placebo group (Ortonne et al, 2007). The same authors showed that at week 12 a higher number of patients achieved PASI 90 and had a greater improvement in health-related quality of life (Ortonne et al, 2008a, 2008b). A phase III trial of certolizumab pegol for psoriatic arthritis is ongoing (UCB, Inc., 2010).

2.6 Safety of TNF inhibitors

The aforementioned clinical trials show that TNFα antagonists are well tolerated and safe. The commonest side effect associated with etanercept, adalimumab and golimumab treatment is a reaction at the site of injection, including redness, itching, bruising, pain, swelling and/or irritation as well as allergic reactions such as latex allergy (Kerbleski & Gottlieb, 2011). Treatment with infliximab is associated with infusion reactions, occurring in around 20% of patients, including pruritus, headache, rash, urticaria, fever or anaphylactic reactions (Leman & Burden, 2008). For all TNFα inhibitors, the primary concern is the increased risk for viral, bacterial and fungal infections, mainly of the upper respiratory tract (Kunz, 2009). Therapy with anti-TNF agents can lead to reactivation of latent tuberculosis, more frequently with infliximab (associated with the highest risk) and adalimumab than etanercept (Dixon et al, 2006). Another safety issue is the development of malignancies. The use of TNFα inhibitors is associated with an increased risk of non-melanoma skin cancer (NMSC); the occurence of NMSC may be due to the previous use of phototeraphy and immunosuppressive agents, even if a potential risk to develop cancer after anti-TNFα therapy cannot be excluded (Kerbleski & Gottlieb, 2011). A paradoxical side effect of anti-TNF therapies is the new onset and worsening of psoriasis, which have been reported in some cases (Ko et al, 2009). Infliximab, adalimumab and golimumab have been shown to cause hepatotoxicity (Kavanaugh et al, 2009a; Reich et al, 2005). On the contrary, etanercept seems to be effective and safe in the treatment of psoriatic patients with chronic hepatitis C virus-infection (Piccolo et al, 2008; Zeinn et al, 2005). Moreover, TNF inhibitors can potentially worsen congestive heart failure (Chung et al, 2009). The TNF blockade can lead to development of antinuclear antibodies and anti-double-stranded DNA antibodies. A lupus-like syndrome may occur with TNF antagonists, but it is a rare event that reverts after discontinuation of therapy (Ramos-Casals et al, 2008). Other rare events associated with TNF antagonists are the development of serious hematological diseases, such as leukopenia, neutropenia, thrombocytopenia, pancytopenia or aplastic anemia and the development or worsening of peripheral and central demyelinating disorders (Montane et al, 2007; Roberts & McColl, 2004). Rare dermatological diseases such as erythema multiforme, Steven's Johnson syndrome and toxic epidermal necrolysis have been reported during etanercept, infliximab and adalimumab treatment (Kerbleski & Gottlieb, 2011).

3. T-cell inhibitors

Psoriasis is defined as a T cell-mediated autoimmune disease based on the advanced understanding of its pathogenesis. Primarily, a deregulated Th1/Th17 response has been reported in psoriatic skin (Lowes et al, 2008). Due to the primary role that T cells play in this disease, a new class of biologics has been designed to interfere with T-cell activation and functions. Currently, alefacept is the only T cell inhibitor drug approved for the treatment of psoriasis. Efalizumab was withdrawn from the market because of the associated risk of progressive multifocal leukoencephalopathy. Two other T-cell modulators are currently being evaluated for their use in psoriasis and psoriatic arthritis.

3.1 Alefacept

Alefacept is a recombinant human fusion protein consisting of the soluble lymphocyte function-associated antigen-3 (LFA-3) and the IgG1 Fc fragment (Biogen Inc., 2003). The LFA-3 portion binds to CD2, highly expressed on CD4+ and CD8+ memory-effector T cells (CD45RO+), while the IgG1 portion binds to Fc receptors on cytotoxic cells (da Silva et al, 2002). Alefacept inhibits T-cell activation and proliferation, by interfering with the downstream activation of cytokines by interfering with the binding between CD2 on T lymphocytes and LFA-3 on antigen-presenting cells (da Silva et al, 2002). Since CD2 is highly expressed on CD45RO+ T cells, alefacept mainly inhibits memory-effector T cells, which represent the majority of T lymphocytes in psoriatic lesions, and preserves naïve cells

(Krueger, 2002). Alefacept also causes the depletion of CD45RO+ memory T cells via cytotoxic cell-mediated apoptosis; this occurs between CD2 on target T lymphocytes and Fc receptors, primarily FcγRIII+, on natural killer cells and macrophages (Cooper et al, 2002). Alefacept was the first FDA-approved biologic agent in 2003 for the treatment of moderate to severe chronic plaque psoriasis in patients who are candidates for systemic treatment or phototherapy (Biogen Inc., 2003) but it is not currently approved for the treatment of psoriasis by EMA. It is also being investigated for the treatment of other conditions caused by T-cell dysregulation, such as psoriatic arthritis (Kraan et al, 2002; Mease & Reich, 2009).

3.1.1 Administration

The recommended administration of alefacept is a once-weekly 15 mg intramuscular injection (IM) for 12 weeks (Biogen Inc., 2003), although intravenous bolus injection (IV) has also been evaluated in several studies. A comparison of the pharmacokinetic and biologic activity of IM and IV administration showed that an adequate dose of IM alefacept leads to similar bioavailability and efficacy compared to IV administration and it is associated with minimal adverse effects (Vaishnaw & TenHoor, 2002). Retreatment with an additional 12-week course may be initiated if CD4+ T-lymphocyte counts are within the normal range, and a minimum of a 12-week interval has passed since the previous course of treatment (Biogen Inc., 2003).

3.1.2 Clinical efficacy

A series of clinical trials showed significant improvement in the PASI score in patients treated with alefacept. The first multicenter, randomized, controlled phase II trial was conducted in 229 patients who received alefacept 0.025, 0.075 and 0.150 mg/kg IV or placebo weekly for 12 weeks, with a 12-week follow-up (Ellis & Krueger, 2001). Patients achieved a reduction in PASI by 38%, 53% and 53%, respectively, compared with 21% reduction by placebo. A significant improvement in quality of life was also reported, and long-term follow-up showed a sustained response for a median of 10 months (Ellis & Krueger, 2001).

Two phase III clinical trials showed similar results (Krueger et al, 2002; Lebwohl et al, 2003). In these trials, patients with chronic plaque psoriasis received a once-weekly administration of alefacept IV or IM for 12 weeks, with a 12-week follow-up. In the first study (Krueger et al, 2002), a total of 553 patients was randomized to receive 7.5 mg of IV alefacept or placebo, while in the second trial (Lebwohl et al, 2003) 507 patients were treated with 10 or 15 mg of IM alefacept or placebo. Both trials showed a significant clinical improvement in psoriatic patients: a PASI 75 was achieved by 28% in IV-treated patients compared to 8% in placebo-treated patients, and by 28% and 33% in 10 or 15 mg IM-treated patients, respectively, compared to 13% in the placebo group. Most responder patients maintained a 50% or greater reduction in PASI in the follow-up period. Other studies have been performed to investigate alefacept efficacy and safety in the long-term treatment of plaque psoriasis. Treatment of up to 5 courses provided incremental efficacy in responders, while maintaining the safety profile (Menter et al, 2006; Roberts et al, 2010). Although these studies are limited by the decreasing number of patients over multiple treatment courses or the lack of appropriate controls, but do they suggest that multiple courses of alefacept are well tolerated and maintain clinical improvement in responder patients.

Several studies evaluated the effect of alefacept in combination with other therapies, including topical agents, methotrexate, cyclosporine, acitretin, systemic retinoids, or phototherapy (Krueger et al, 2008). The results suggest that the combination of alefacept with other psoriasis therapies is efficacious and well tolerated but larger studies are needed to confirm these results and evaluate long-term effects.

3.1.3 Safety

Alefacept is one of the safest biologic drugs for psoriasis. Clinical trials have demonstrated that it is well tolerated (Gottlieb, 2004; Krueger et al, 2002; Lebwohl et al, 2003; Roberts et al, 2010). The main concern is T lymphocyte depletion so that monitoring of CD4+ T cells is required during treatment and administration should be withheld if the CD4+ T-cell count falls below 250 cells/mL (Biogen Inc., 2003). The most common side effects are pharyngitis, headache, rhinitis, bronchitis and flu (Ellis & Krueger, 2001; Gottlieb et al, 2003; Krueger et al, 2002; Lowe et al, 2003). These infections are not severe, and there is no evidence to date to suggest a predisposition to malignancies associated with alefacept.

3.2 Abatacept

Abatacept is a fusion protein composed of an Fc fragment of IgG1 and the extracellular domain of CTLA-4 (cytotoxic lymphocyte antigen-4) that inhibits T-cell costimulation. Abatacept is currently approved for the treatment of rheumatoid arthritis (Bristol-Myers Squibb, 2009). A phase II study has been terminated for psoriatic arthritis and it showed that 10 mg/kg may be an effective treatment (Mease et al, 2011).

3.3 Rituximab

Rituximab is a chimeric monoclonal antibody that selectively binds the CD20 antigen of B cells. Rituximab is currently used in the treatment of non Hodgkin's lymphoma and rheumatoid arthritis (Genentech USA, Inc., 2011). A phase I trial is ongoing to assess the efficacy and safety of rituximab in patients with psoriatic arthritis (Swedish Medical Center, 2009).

4. IL-12/IL-23 inhibitors

A third class of biologics classified as IL-12/IL-23 inhibitors has been developed for treating psoriasis. These two cytokines, mainly produced by activated dendritic cells, lead to differentiation of Th cells into the Th1 and Th17 subsets, respectively (Nestle et al, 2009). Moreover, elevated levels of IL-12 and IL-23 have been observed in psoriatic skin lesions (Yawalcar et al, 2009). Currently, ustekinumab is FDA- and EMA-approved for the treatment of chronic plaque psoriasis, whereas briakinumab, has recently had its approval application withdrawn in the US and Europe to conduct further analysis and clinical trials (Centocor Ortho Biotech, 2009; Kurzeia et al, 2011).

4.1 Ustekinumab

Ustekinumab is a fully human monoclonal antibody that binds to the p40 subunit that is shared by IL-12 and IL-23 (Centocor Ortho Biotech, 2009). IL-12 activates natural killer and T cell responses, including CD4+ T cell differentiation toward the Th1 phenotype, while IL-23 leads to Th17 differentiation, regulates T memory cells, and activates macrophages to maintain chronic autoimmune inflammation (Aggarwal et al, 2003; Trinchieri, 2003). Ustekinumab prevents the interaction of these cytokines with the IL-12Rβ1 receptor, neutralizing their immune-mediated responses. A single administration of anti-IL-12p40 demonstrated significant changes in psoriatic skin lesions after 2 weeks, including the reduction of a type 1 cytokine (IFN-γ) and chemokines (IL-8, IFN-γ-inducible protein-10, and MCP-1), and a decrease of TNFα and infiltrating T cells (Toichi et al, 2006).

Ustekinumab was approved by the FDA in September 2009 for the treatment of adult patients with moderate-to-severe plaque psoriasis who are candidates for phototherapy or systemic therapy (Centocor Ortho Biotech, 2009). Early-stage clinical trials have also demonstrated its therapeutic potential in psoriatic arthritis (Gottlieb et al, 2009).

4.1.1 Administration

Ustekinumab is administered by subcutaneous injections at the recommended dose of 45 mg for patients who weigh ≤100 kg and 90 mg for those who weight ≥100 kg, at week 0 and then at week 4, followed by one injection every 12 weeks as maintenance treatment (Centocor Ortho Biotech, 2009). Clinical response to ustekinumab is associated with serum ustekinumab concentration and patient body weight. Two phase III clinical trials demonstrated that efficacy of the 45 and 90 mg doses of ustekinumab was similar in patients weighing ≤100 kg, while the 90 mg dose was more effective than the 45 mg dose in patients weighing >100 kg (Leonardi et al, 2008; Papp et al, 2008).

4.1.2 Clinical efficacy

The first phase II trial was performed in 320 patients with moderate-to-severe plaque psoriasis who were randomized to receive one of four subcutaneous dosing regimens of ustekinumab (one 45 mg dose, one 90 mg dose, 4-weekly 45 mg doses, or 4-weekly 90 mg doses) or placebo (Krueger et al, 2007). At week 12, a PASI 75 was achieved by 52%, 59%, 67%, and 81%, respectively, of the aforementioned groups, compared to 2% of placebo patients. Other measures of clinical outcome, including DLQI and Physician's Global Assessment (PGA) showed significant improvements in responders compared with placebo patients at both weeks 12 and 24. Two important clinical trials for the assessment of ustekinumab efficacy and safety are PHOENIX-1 and PHOENIX-2. Both are large-scale, randomized, placebo-controlled phase III trials designed to evaluate the efficacy and safety of ustekinumab in patients with moderate-to-severe plaque psoriasis over a period of five years. In the PHOENIX-1 study, 766 patients were randomized to subcutaneous injections of 45 mg or 90 mg of ustekinumab at weeks 0 and 4 and then every 12 weeks, or placebo at weeks 0 and 4, with crossover to ustekinumab at week 12 (Leonardi et al, 2008). At week 12, a PASI 75 was achieved by 67.1%, 66.4%, and 3.1% of patients receiving 45 mg, 90 mg or placebo, respectively. Results at week 28 demonstrated durable effects of ustekinumab with 71.2% and 78.6% of patients treated with 45 mg or 90 mg achieving or maintaining a PASI 75 score. Patients that achieved PASI 75 were re-randomized to maintenance ustekinumab or withdrawal from treatment at week 40. A PASI 75 response was better maintained in patients receiving maintenance ustekinumab than in those who were withdrawn from treatment. The median time to loss of PASI 75 in patients withdrawn from therapy was 15 weeks. The PHOENIX-2 study enrolled 1230 patients (Papp et al, 2008). Its design and results were similar to the PHOENIX-1 study: a PASI 75 was achieved by 66.7% of patients in the 45 mg group, by 75.7% in the 90 mg group, by 3.7% in the placebo group, at week 12. However, a dosing intensification was added for those subjects who did not respond fully to ustekinumab (PASI 50 to <75). At week 28, partial responders were re-randomized to continue dosing regimen every 12 weeks or to increase dosing frequency to every 8 weeks. In the 90 mg group, 22 of 33 partial responders achieved PASI 75 after increasing dosage frequency to every 8 weeks. Conversely, dosing intensification did not improve clinical outcomes in the 45 mg group. The authors concluded that intensification of dosing to once every 8 weeks with ustekinumab 90 mg might be necessary to achieve a full response in partial responders. The ACCEPT study is a randomized phase III clinical trial that directly compares ustekinumab to etanercept in 903 patients with psoriasis (Griffiths et al, 2010). Patients were randomized to receive ustekinumab 45 or 90 mg at week 0 and 4, or etanercept 50 g twice weekly for 12 weeks. At week 12 PASI 75 was achieved by 74% of the patients in the ustekinumab 90 mg group, by 68% of patients in the ustekinumab 45 mg group, and by 57% of those in the etanercept group. Patients who were unresponsive to etanercept were switched to ustekinumab, with almost a 50% response rate within the first 12 weeks. There were no significant safety differences between ustekinumab and etanercept in the ACCEPT trial. Both drugs were generally well tolerated. This head-to-head comparison clearly showed a significant superiority of ustekinumab over etanercept for the treatment of patients with moderate-to-severe psoriasis. However, this trial only evaluated 12 weeks of therapy, a short period to have an adequate comparison of the drugs, especially for their safety profiles.

4.1.3 Safety

In general, ustekinumab is well tolerated with only mild adverse events experienced in clinical trials. The most common adverse events have been equally observed between the treatment and placebo groups and included upper respiratory infections, headache, nasopharyngitis, arthralgia, back pain, and injection site reactions (Leonardi et al, 2008; Papp et al, 2008). Safety concerns exist for risks of infection and suppression of tumor immune surveillance. Individuals congenitally deficient in IL-12p40 or IL-12Rβ1 are known to have an increased susceptibility to intracellular pathogens, including tuberculosis and salmonella (Döffinger et al, 2002). However, in the PHOENIX 1 and 2 studies only two serious infections occurred in the ustekinumab group treated with the 90 mg dose. No mycobacterial or salmonella infections were reported. The risk of malignancy did not appear to be significant. Cutaneous malignancies were reported in two patients in the PHOENIX 2 study, a squamous cell carcinoma in the placebo group and a basal cell carcinoma in the 90 mg treatment group. No malignancies were reported in the PHOENIX 1 trial. The rate of malignancies reported in ustekinumab-treated patients was comparable to the rate in the general population. Patients with psoriasis have an increased risk of cardiovascular events. In the phase II trial of ustekinumab two patients experienced myocardial infarction and one suffered a stroke (Krueger et al, 2007). However, subsequent larger phase III studies revealed no apparent increased risk of cardiovascular side effects. Further studies are needed to assess long-term ustekinumab safety in patients treated for extended periods.

4.2 Briakinumab

Briakinumab is a recombinant fully human IgG1 monoclonal antibody directed against the shared p40 subunit of IL-12 and IL-23 (Kimball et al, 2008). Due to its binding to the aforesaid cytokines, briakinumab causes a decrease in secretion of IL-6, IL-12, INF-γ and TNFα, as demonstrated in patients with Crohn's disease (Ding et al, 2008). In a phase II study, 180 patients suffering from psoriasis were treated with placebo or briakinumab at one of the following doses: one 200 mg dose at week 0, 100 mg eow for 12 weeks, 200 mg weekly for 4 weeks, 200 mg eow for 12 weeks, 200 mg weekly for 12 weeks. At week 12, an improvement in PASI 75 was reported for all briakinumab-treated groups compared with placebo (Kimball et al, 2008). The retreatment efficacy and the long-term safety of briakinumab through 48 weeks have been evaluated by the same authors (Kimball et al, 2009). Kimball et al. reported that the efficacy of briakinumab was higher in the first 12 weeks compared with the re-treatment phase, although more patients showed a PASI 75 response during this period. The most frequent adverse events observed during the treatment with briakinumab were injection site reactions, upper respiratory infections and nasopharyngitis.

5. Perspectives

In the last decade, the detailed comprehension of the molecular mechanisms involved in psoriasis has led to the development of new biological drugs, such as monoclonal antibodies, recombinant proteins and small RNA drugs, which are currently under evaluation for psoriasis and/or psoriatic arthritis.

5.1 Anti-interleukin 17

IL-17 is a pro-inflammatory cytokine produced by Th17 T cells, one of the key players in the pathogenesis of psoriasis. Due to its role in psoriasis, IL-17 is a new emerging target for biological therapy.

AMG 827 is a fully human IgG2 anti IL-17 receptor monoclonal antibody investigated in phase II trials for psoriasis, rheumatoid arthritis and Crohn's disease (Amgen, 2011). Preliminary data from a small study showed that psoriatic patients treated with 700 mg AMG 827 IV had a significant improvement in terms of histopathological features and PASI score (Russell et al, 2010).

AIN457 is a recombinant fully human anti-IL-17 monoclonal antibody that selectively binds and neutralizes IL-17. The efficacy and safety of AIN457 has been evaluated in a phase II trial (Jancin, 2009) which enrolled 36 patients suffering from chronic plaque psoriasis. A PASI 75 response was observed in 44% of patients receiving 3 mg/kg AIN457 IV compared with 9% of placebo group. AIN457 is currently undergoing phase II studies for psoriasis, psoriatic arthritis and rheumatoid arthritis and a phase III study for uveitis (Novartis, 2010).

LY2439821 is a new humanized IgG4 anti-IL-17 monoclonal antibody in a phase II trial for psoriasis and rheumatoid arthritis (Eli Lilly and Company, 2011).

5.2 Anti-interleukin 22

IL-22 is a pro-inflammatory cytokine produced by both Th17 and a new group of T cells known as Th22 cells; Th22 cells are known to induce epidermal hyperplasia and dermal inflammation via several transcription factors such as STAT3 (Nograles et al, 2009). ILV-094 is a fully human anti IL-22 monoclonal antibody. A phase I study to evaluate the efficacy and safety of ILV-094 in psoriasis has been recently completed, while it is currently ongoing a phase II trial for rheumatoid arthritis (Pfizer, 2010).

5.3 Chaperonin 10

Chaperonin 10 belongs to the heat shock proteins family and acts as a molecular chaperon, regulating protein folding. Several studies support its anti-inflammatory activity and its role in down-regulating the excessive immune response (van Eden, 2008). Recombinant Chaperonin 10 (Cpn10) mimics these activities and its efficacy in psoriasis has been evaluated by a single-center, double-blind exploratory study, showing a significant improvement in Cpn10-treated patients (Williams et al, 2008). Phase II trials have been completed for psoriasis, rheumatoid arthritis and multiple sclerosis (Golant & Gutman-Yassky, 2011).

5.4 Small RNA drugs

The use of RNA interference as a drug is one of the possible therapeutic strategies to target the pro-inflammatory cytokines involved in psoriasis, as shown by several phase I and II ongoing clinical trials (reviewed in Jackson et al, 2006). On the basis of their role in psoriasis, suitable mRNA targets are TNFα, IL-20 and IL-23. A recent study showed that local small RNA therapy against TNFα provided amelioration in psoriasis in a xenograft transplantation model (Jakobsen et al, 2009). These results indicate that RNA interference is a potential therapy in the treatment of inflammatory skin diseases. Nevertheless the main challenge for this kind of therapy remains the delivery of small RNA.

6. Conclusion

The introduction of biological drugs in clinical practice has revolutionized the treatment of psoriasis and psoriatic arthritis in the last decade. Biologics have shown to be effective and to have an acceptable safety profile, but there is still a need to assess long-term toxicity through clinical experience and careful post-marketing surveillance.

7. References

Abbott Laboratories. (March, 2011). HUMIRA package insert Abbott Laboratories. In: *www.humira.com*, 28.05.2011, available from: *http://www.rxabbott.com/pdf/humira.pdf.*

Aggarwal, S., Ghilardi, N., Xie, M.H., de Sauvage, F.J. & Gurney, A.L. (2003). Interleukin-23 promotes a distinct CD4 T cell activation state characterized by the production of interleukin-17. *The Journal of Biological Chemistry,* Vol.278, No.3, pp.1910-1914.

Amgen , Inc. (2011). Pipeline. In: *www.amgen.com*, 28.05.2011, available from: *http://www.amgen.com/science/pipe.html*

Amgen, Inc. (February, 2011). Enbrel package Insert. In: *www.enbrel.com,* 28.05.2011, available from: *http://pi.amgen.com/united_states/enbrel/derm/enbrel_pi.pdf.*

Antiga, E., Volpi, W., Chiarini, C., Cardilicchia, E., Filì, L., Manuelli, C., Parrochi, P., Fabbri, P. & Caproni, M. (2010). The role of etanercept on the expression of markers of T helper 17 cells and their precursors in skin lesions of patients with psoriasis vulgaris. *International Journal of Immunopathology and Pharmacology,* Vol.23, No.3, pp.767-774.

Antoni, C., Kavanaugh, A., Kirkham, B., Tutuncu, Z., Burmester, G.R., Schneider, U., Furst, D.E., Molitor, J., Keystone, E., Gladman, D., Manger, B., Wassenberg, S., Weier, R., Wallace, D.J., Weisman, M.H., Kalden, J.R. & Smolen, J. (2005a). Sustained benefits of infliximab therapy for dermatologic and articular manifestations of psoriatic arthritis: results from the infliximab multinational psoriatic arthritis controlled trial (IMPACT). *Arthritis and Rheumatism,* Vol.52, No.4, pp.1227-1236.

Antoni, C., Krueger, G.G., de Vlam, K., Birbara, C., Beutler, A., Guzzo, C., Zhou, B., Dooley, L.T. & Kavanaugh, A. (2005b). Infliximab improves signs and symptoms of psoriatic arthritis: results of the IMPACT 2 trial. *Annals of the Rheumatic Diseases,* Vol.64, No.8, pp.1150-1157.

Antoni, C.E., Kavanaugh, A., van der Heijde, D., Beutler, A., Keenan, G., Zhou, B., Kirkham, B., Tutuncu, Z., Burmester, G.R., Schneider, U., Furst, D., Molitor, J., Keystone, E., Gladman, D.D., Manger, B., Wassenberg, S., Weier, R., Wallace, D.J., Weisman, M.H., Kalden, J.R. & Smolen, J.S. (2008). Two-year efficacy and safety of infliximab treatment in patients with active psoriatic arthritis: findings of the Infliximab Multinational Psoriatic Arthritis Controlled Trial (IMPACT). *The Journal of Rheumatology,* Vol.35, No.5, pp.869-876.

Bachmann, F., Nast, A., Sterry, W. & Philipp, S. (2010). Safety and efficacy of the tumor necrosis factor antagonists. *Seminars in Cutaneous Medicine and Surgery,* Vol.29, No.1, pp.35-47.

Bagel, J. (2011). Adalimumab plus narrowband ultraviolet B light phototherapy for the treatment of moderate to severe psoriasis. *Journal of Drugs Dermatology,* Vol.10, No.4, pp.366-371.

Bartelds, G.M., Wijbrandts, C.A., Nurmohamed, M.T., Stapel, S., Lems, W.F., Aarden, L., Dijkmans, B.A., Tak, P.P. & Wolbink, G.J. (2010). Anti-infliximab and anti-adalimumab antibodies in relation to response to adalimumab in infliximab switchers and anti-tumour necrosis factor naive patients: a cohort study. *Annals of the Rheumatic Diseases,* Vol.69, No.5, pp.817-821.

Biogen, Inc. (2003). Amevive package insert. In: *www.clinicaltrials.gov,* 28.05.2011, available from: *http://www.fda.gov/downloads/Drugs/DevelopmentApprovalProcess/HowDrugsareDevelopedandApproved/ApprovalApplications/TherapeuticBiologicApplications/ucm086009.pdf.*

Boehncke, W.H. (2007). Efalizumab in the treatment of psoriasis. *Biologics,* Vol.1, No.3, pp. 301-309.

Brennan, F.M., Chantry, D., Jackson, A., Maini, R. & Feldmann M. (1989). Inhibitory effect of TNF alpha antibodies on synovial cell interleukin-1 production in rheumatoid arthritis. *The Lancet,* Vol.2, No.8657, pp.244-247.

Bristol-Myers Squibb. (August, 2009). Orencia package insert. In: *www.orencia.com,* 28.05.2011, available from: *http://packageinserts.bms.com/pi/pi_orencia.pdf.*

Cassano, N., Loconsole, F., Galluccio, A., Miracapillo, A., Pezza, M. & Vena, G.A. (2006). Once-weekly administration of high-dosage Etanercept in patients with plaque psoriasis: results of a pilot experience (power study). *International Journal of Immunopathology and Pharmacology,* Vol.19, No.1, pp.225-229.

Cassano, N., Loconsole, F., Miracapillo, A., Travaglini, M., Di Giuseppe, M.D., Congedo, M., Galluccio, A., Buquicchio, R., Mastrandrea, V., Filieri, M., Raho, G., Pezza, M. & Vena, G.A. (2010). The role of etanercept on the expression of markers of T helper 17 cells and their precursors in skin lesions of patients with psoriasis vulgari Treatment of psoriasis with different dosage regimens of etanercept: preliminary results from the Taranta Plastic Study Groups. *International Journal of Immunopathology and Pharmacology,* Vol.23, No.3, pp.797-802.

Centocor Ortho Biotech, Inc. (2009). Stelara medication label. In: *www.fda.gov,* 28.05.2011, available from: *http://www.accessdata.fda.gov/drugsatfda_docs/label/2009/125261lbl.pdf.*

Centocor Ortho Biotech, Inc. (December, 2010). Simponi package insert. In: *www.simponi.com,* 28.05.2011, available from: *http://www.simponi.com/sites/default/files/pdf/prescribing-information.pdf.*

Centocor Ortho Biotech, Inc. (February, 2011). Remicade package insert. In: *www.remicade.com,* 28.05.2011, available from: *http://www.remicade.com/remicade/assets/hcp_ppi.pdf.*

Chaudhari, U., Romano, P., Mulcahy, L.D., Dooley, L.T., Baker, D.G. & Gottlieb, A.B. (2001). Efficacy and safety of infliximab monotherapy for plaque-type psoriasis: a randomised trial. *The Lancet,* Vol.357, No.9271, pp.1842-1847.

Chung, E.S., Packer, M., Lo, K.H., Fasanmade, A.A. & Willerson, J.T. (2009). Randomized, double-blind, placebo-controlled, pilot trial of infliximab, a chimeric monoclonal antibody to tumor necrosis factor-alpha, in patients with moderate-to-severe heart failure: results of the anti-TNF Therapy Against Congestive Heart Failure (ATTACH) trial. *Circulation,* Vol.107, No.25, pp.3133-3140.

Cooper, J.C., Morgan, G., Harding, S., Subramanyam, M., Majeau, G.R., Moulder, K. & Alexander, D.R. (2003). Alefacept selectively promotes NK cell-mediated deletion of CD45R0+ human T cells. *European Journal of Immunology,* Vol.33, No.3, pp.666-675.

da Silva, A.J., Brickelmaier, M., Majeau, G.R., Li, Z., Su, L., Hsu, Y.M. & Hochman, P.S. (2002). Alefacept, an immunomodulatory recombinant LFA-3/IgG1 fusion protein, induces CD16 signaling and CD2/CD16-dependent apoptosis of CD2(+) cells. *Immunology,* Vol.168, No.9, pp.4462-4471.

Dauden, E., Griffiths, C., Ortonne, J.P., Kragballe, K., Molta, C.T., Robertoson, D., Pedersen, R., Estojak, J. & Boggs, R. (2009). Improvements in patient-reported outcomes in moderate-to-severe psoriasis patients receiving continuous or paused etanercept treatment over 54 weeks: the CRYSTEL study. *Journal of the European Academy of Dermatology and Venereology,* Vol.23, No.12, pp.1374-82.

de Groot, M., Teunissen, M.B.M., Picavet, D.I., de Rie, M.A. & Bos, J.D. (2010). Reduction of different inflammatory cell types of the innate immune system in psoriatic skin during etanercept treatment. *Experimental Dermatology,* Vol.19, pp.754-756.

De Pità, O., Nardis, C., Lupi, F., Luci, C.A., Frezzolini, A. & Pallotta, S. (2011). Modulation of Toll-like receptors in psoriatic patients during therapy with adalimumab. *International Journal of Immunopathology and Pharmacology,* Vol.24, No.1, pp.185-188.

Ding, C., Xu, J. & Li, J. (2008). ABT-874, a fully human monoclonal anti-IL-12/IL-23 antibody for the potential treatment of autoimmune diseases. *Current Opinion in Investigational Drugs,* Vol. 9, No.5, pp.515-522.

Dixon, W.G., Watson, K., Lunt, M., Hyrich, K.L., Silman, A.J. & Symmons, D.P. (2006). Rates of serious infection, including site-specific and bacterial intracellular infection, in rheumatoid arthritis patients receiving anti-tumor necrosis factor therapy: results from the British Society for Rheumatology Biologics Register. *Arthritis and Rheumatism,* Vol.54, No.8, pp.2368-2376.

Döffinger, R., Dupuis, S., Picard, C., Fieschi, C., Feinberg, J., Barcenas-Morales, G. & Casanova, J.L. (2002). Inherited disorders of IL-12- and IFNgamma-mediated immunity: a molecular genetics update. *Molecular Immunology,* Vol.38, No.12-13, pp.903-909.

Eli Lilly and Company. (April, 2011). A Study in Patients With Moderate to Severe Psoriasis. In:*www.clinicaltrials.gov,*28.05.2011, available from: *http://clinicaltrials.gov/ct2/show/NCT01107457?term=LY2439821&rank=3.*

Ellis, C.N. & Krueger, G.G. (2001). Treatment of chronic plaque psoriasis by selective targeting of memory effector T lymphocytes. *New England Journal of Medicine,* Vol.345, No.4, pp.248-255.

Esposito, M., Giunta, A., Mazzotta, A., Babino, G., Talamonti, M., Chimenti, M.S. & Chimenti, S. (2010). Continuous treatment of plaque-type psoriasis with etanercept: an observational long-term experience. *International Journal of Immunopathology and Pharmacology,* Vol.23, No.2, pp.503-509.

Feldman, S.R., Gordon, K.B., Bala, M., Evans, R., Li, S., Dooley, L.T., Guzzo, C., Patel, K., Menter, A. & Gottlieb, A.B. (2005). Infliximab treatment results in significant improvement in the quality of life of patients with severe psoriasis: a double-blind placebo-controlled trial. *The British Journal of Dermatology,* Vol.152, No.5, pp.954-960.

Foley, P.A., Quirk, C., Sullivan, J.R., Dolianitis, C., Hack, S.P., Thirunavukkarasu, K. & Cooper, J. (2010). Combining etanercept with traditional agents in the treatment of psoriasis: a review of the clinical evidence. *Journal of the European Academy of Dermatology and Venereology,* Vol.24, pp.1135-1143.

Genentech USA, Inc. (April, 2011). Rituxan package insert. In:*www.rituxan.com,* 28.05.2011, available from: *http://www.gene.com/gene/products/information/pdf/rituxan-prescribing.pdf.*

Genentech, Inc. (2009). Voluntary U.S. market withdrawal of Raptiva® (efalizumab). In: *www.fda.gov,* 28.05.2011, available from: *http://www.fda.gov/downloads/Safety/MedWatch/SafetyInformation/SafetyAlertsforHuman MedicalProducts/UCM149681.pdf.*

Genovese, M.C., Mease, P.J., Thomson, G.T., Kivitz, A.J., Perdok, R.J., Weinberg, M.A., Medich, J. & Sasso, E.H. (2007). Safety and efficacy of adalimumab in treatment of patients with psoriatic arthritis who had failed disease modifying antirheumatic drug therapy. *The Journal of Rheumatology,* Vol.34, No.5, pp.1040-1050.

Gerdes, S. & Mrowietz, U. (2009). Impact of comorbidities on the management of psoriasis. *Current Problems in Dermatology*, Vol.38, pp.21-36.

Gisondi, P., Gubinelli, E., Cocuroccia, B. & Girolomoni, G. (2004). Targeting tumor necrosis factor-alpha in the therapy of psoriasis. *Current Drug Targets - Inflammation & Allergy*, Vol.3, No.2, pp.175-183.

Gladman, D.D., Mease, P.J., Ritchlin, C.T., Choy, E.H., Sharp, J.T., Ory, P.A., Perdok, R.J. & Sasso, E.H. (2007). Adalimumab for long-term treatment of psoriatic arthritis: forty-eight week data from the adalimumab effectiveness in psoriatic arthritis trial. *Arthritis & Rheumatism*, Vol.56, No.2, pp.476-488.

Golant, A.K. & Guttman-Yassky, B.S.E. (2011). Psoriasis Treatments: A review of the current research pipeline. *Psoriasis Forum*, Vol.17, No.1, pp.11-23.

Gordon, K.B., Gottlieb, A.B., Leonardi, C.L., Elewski, B.E., Wang, A., Jahreis, A. & Zitnik, R. (2006a). Clinical response in psoriasis patients discontinued from and then reinitiated on Etanercept therapy. *Journal of Dermatological Treatment*, Vol.17, No.1, pp. 9-17.

Gordon, K.B., Langley, R.G., Leonardi, C., Toth, D., Menter, M.A., Kang, S., Heffernan, M., Miller, B., Hamlin, R., Lim, L., Zhong, J., Hoffman, R. & Okun, M.M. (2006b). Adalimumab therapy for moderate to severe psoriasis: A randomized, controlled phase III trial. *Journal of American Academy of Dermatology*, Vol.55, No.4, pp.598-606.

Gottlieb, A.B., Krueger, J.G., Wittkowski, K., Dedrick, R., Walicke, P.A. & Garovoy, M. (2002). Psoriasis as a model for T-cell-mediated disease: immunobiologic and clinical effects of treatment with multiple doses of efalizumab, an anti-CD11a antibody. *Archives of Dermatology*, Vol.138, No.5, pp. 591-600.

Gottlieb A.B., Matheson, R.T., Lowe, N., Krueger, G.G., Kang, S., Goffe, B.S., Gaspari, A.A., Ling, M., Weinstein, G.D., Nayak, A., Gordon, K.B. & Zitnik, R. (2003). A randomized trial of etanercept as monotherapy for psoriasis. *Archives of Dermatology*, Vol.139, No.12, pp.1627-1632.

Gottlieb, A.B., Evans, R., Li, S., Dooley, L.T., Guzzo, C.A., Baker, D., Bala, M., Marano, C.W. & Menter, A. (2004). Infliximab induction and maintenance therapy for moderate-to-severe psoriasis: a phase III, multicenter, double-blind trial. *Journal of American Academy of Dermatology*, Vol.51, No.4, pp.534-542.

Gottlieb, A., Menter, A., Mendelsohn, A., Shen, Y.K., Li, S., Guzzo, C., Fretzin, S., Kunynetz, R. & Kavanaugh, A. (2009). Ustekinumab, a human interleukin 12/23 monoclonal antibody, for psoriatic arthritis: randomised, double-blind, placebo-controlled, crossover trial. *The Lancet*, Vol.373, No.9664, pp.633-640.

Griffiths, C.E., Strober, B.E., van de Kerkhof, P., Ho, V., Fidelus-Gort, R., Yeilding, N., Guzzo, C., Xia, Y., Zhou, B., Li, S., Dooley, L.T., Goldstein, N.H. & Menter, A. (2010). Comparison of ustekinumab and etanercept for moderate-to-severe psoriasis. *New England Journal of Medicine*, Vol.362, No.2, pp.118-128.

Haraoui, B., Cameron, L., Ouellet, M. & White, B. (2006). Anti-infliximab antibodies in patients with rheumatoid arthritis who require higher doses of infliximab to achieve or maintain a clinical response. *Journal of Rheumatology*, Vol.33, No.1, pp.31-36.

Heiberg, M.S., Koldingsnes, W., Mikkelsen, K., Rødevand, E., Kaufmann, C., Mowinckel, P. & Kvien, T.K. (2008). The comparative one-year performance of anti-tumor necrosis factor alpha drugs in patients with rheumatoid arthritis, psoriatic arthritis, and ankylosing spondylitis: results from a longitudinal, observational, multicenter study. *Arthritis and Rheumatism,* Vol.59, No.2, pp.234-240.

Jackson, A.L., Burchard, J., Schelter, J., Chau, B.N., Cleary, M., Lim, L. & Linsley, P.S. (2006). Widespread siRNA "off-target" transcript silencing mediated by seed region sequence complementarity. *RNA,* Vol. 12, No.7, pp.1179-1187.

Jakobsen, M., Stenderup, K., Rosada, C., Moldt, B., Kamp, S., Dam, T.N., Jensen, T.G. & Mikkelsen, J.G. (2009). Amelioration of psoriasis by anti-TNF-alpha RNAi in the xenograft transplantation model. *Molecular Therapy,* Vol. 17, No.10, pp.1743-1753.

Jancin, B. (2009). IL-17A Blocker Shows Early Promise for Psoriasis. *Skin and Allergy News,* Vol.40, No.11, pp.5.

Kavanaugh, A., Krueger, G.G., Beutler, A., Guzzo, C., Zhou, B., Dooley, L.T., Mease, P.J., Gladman, D.D., de Vlam, K., Geusens, P.P., Birbara, C., Halter, D.G. & Antoni, C. (2007). Infliximab maintains a high degree of clinical response in patients with active psoriatic arthritis through 1 year of treatment: results from the IMPACT 2 trial. *Annals of the Rheumatic Diseases,* Vol.66, No.4, pp.498-505.

Kavanaugh, A., McInnes, I., Mease, P., Krueger, G.G., Gladman, D., Gomez-Reino, J., Papp, K., Zrubek, J., Mudivarthy, S., Mack, M., Visvanathan, S. & Beutler, A. (2009a). Golimumab, a new human tumor necrosis factor alpha antibody, administered every four weeks as a subcutaneous injection in psoriatic arthritis: Twenty-four-week efficacy and safety results of a randomized, placebo-controlled study. *Arthritis and Rheumatism,* Vol.60, No.4, pp.976-986.

Kavanaugh, A., Mease, P., Krueger, G.G. et al. (2009b). Golimumab, a new human TNF alpha antibody, administered subcutaneously every 4 week in psoriatic arthritis patients: 104-week efficacy and safety results of the randomized, placebo-controlled GO-REVEAL study. Abstract presented at the 2009 European League Against Rheumatism (EULAR) Annual Congress. June 10-13, Copenhagen.

Kerbleski, J.F. & Gottlieb, A.B. (2011). Dermatological complications and safety of anti-TNF treatments. *Gut,* Vol.58, No.8, pp.1033-1039.

Kimball, A.B., Gordon, K.B., Langley, R.G., Menter, A., Chartash, E.K. & Valdes, J. (2008). Safety and efficacy of ABT-874, a fully human interleukin 12/23 monoclonal antibody, in the treatment of moderate to severe chronic plaque psoriasis: results of a randomized, placebo-controlled, phase 2 trial. *Archives of Dermatology,* Vol. 144, No.2, pp.200-207.

Kimball, A.B., J. Zhong, J., Valdes, J.M. & Gordon, K. (2009). Retreatment efficacy and long-term safety of the fully human, interleukin-12/23 monoclonal antibody ABT-874 in the treatment of moderate to severe psoriasis: 48 week results from a phase II trial to severe psoriasis: 48 week results from a phase II trial. *Journal of the American Academy of Dermatology* Vol.60, Ab.168, San Francisco, 67th Annual Meeting of the American Academy of Dermatology (AAD), March 6-10.

Klotz, U., Teml, A. & Schwab, M. (2007). Clinical pharmacokinetics and use of infliximab. *Clinical Pharmacokinetics,* Vol.46, No.8, pp.645-660.

Ko, J.M., Gottlieb, A.B. & Kerbleski, J.F. (2009). Induction and exacerbation of psoriasis with TNF-blockade therapy: a review and analysis of 127 cases. *Journal of Dermatological Treatement,* Vol.20, No.2, pp.100-108.

Kothary, N., Diak, I.L., Brinker, A., Bezabeh, S., Avigan, M. & Pan, G.D. (2011). Progressive multifocal leukoencephalopathy associated with efalizumab use in psoriasis patients. *Journal of American Academy of Dermatology*, 21 April.

Kraan, M.C., van Kuijk, A.W., Dinant, H.J., Goedkoop, A.Y., Smeets, T.J., de Rie, M.A., Dijkmans, B.A., Vaishnaw, A.K., Bos, J.D. & Tak, P.P. (2002). Alefacept treatment in psoriatic arthritis: reduction of the effector T cell population in peripheral blood and synovial tissue is associated with improvement of clinical signs of arthritis. *Arthritis & Rheumatism,* Vol.46, No.10, pp.2776-2784.

Krueger, G.G. (2002). Selective targeting of T cell subsets: focus on alefacept - a remittive therapy for psoriasis. *Expert Opinion on Biological Therapy,* Vol.2, No.4, pp.431-441.

Krueger, G.G., Papp, K.A., Stough, D.B., Loven, K.H., Gulliver, W.P. & Ellis, C.N. (2002). A randomized, double-blind, placebo-controlled phase III study evaluating efficacy and tolerability of 2 courses of alefacept in patients with chronic plaque psoriasis. *Journal of American Academy of Dermatology,* Vol.47, No.6, pp.821-833.

Krueger, G.G., Langley, R.G., Leonardi, C., Yeilding, N., Guzzo, C., Wang, Y., Dooley, L.T. & Lebwohl, M. (2007). A human interleukin-12/23 monoclonal antibody for the treatment of psoriasis. *The New England Journal of Medicine,* Vol.356, No.6, pp.580-592.

Krueger, G.G., Gottlieb, A.B., Sterry, W., Korman, N. & Van De Kerkhof, P. (2008). A multicenter, open-label study of repeat courses of intramuscular alefacept in combination with other psoriasis therapies in patients with chronic plaque psoriasis. *The Journal of Dermatological Treatment,* Vol.19, No.3, pp.146-155.

Kunz M. (2009). Current treatment of psoriasis with biologics. *Current Drug Discovery Technologies,* Vol.6, No.4, pp.231-240.

Kurzeja, M., Rudnicka, L. & Olszewska, M. (2011). New interleukin-23 pathway inhibitors in dermatology: ustekinumab, briakinumab, and secukinumab. *Am J Clin Dermatol.* Vol.12, No.2, pp.113-125.

Lebwohl, M., Christophers, E., Langley, R., Ortonne, J.P., Roberts, J. & Griffiths, C.E. (2003). An international, randomized, double-blind, placebo-controlled phase 3 trial of intramuscular alefacept in patients with chronic plaque psoriasis. *Archives of Dermatology,* Vol.139, No.6, pp.719-727.

Leman, J. & Burden, A. (2008). Treatment of severe psoriasis with infliximab. *Journal of Therapeutics and Clinical Risk Management,* Vol.4, No.6, pp.1165-1175.

Leonardi, C.L., Powers, J.L., Matheson, R.T., Goffe, B.S., Zitnik, R., Wang, A. & Gottlieb, A.B. (2003). Etanercept as monotherapy in patients with psoriasis. *The New England Journal of Medicine,* Vol.349, No.21, pp.2014-2022.

Leonardi, C.L., Kimball, A.B., Papp, K.A., Yeilding, N., Guzzo, C., Wang, Y., Li, S., Dooley, L.T. & Gordon, K.B. (2008). Efficacy and safety of ustekinumab, a human interleukin-12/23 monoclonal antibody, in patients with psoriasis: 76-week results from a randomised, double-blind, placebo-controlled trial (PHOENIX 1). *The Lancet,* Vol.371, No.9625, pp.1665-1674.

Leonardi, C., Strober, B., Gottlieb, A.B., Elewski, B.E., Ortonne, J.P., van de Kerkhof, P., Chiou, C.F., Dunn, M. & Jahreis, A. (2010). Long-term safety and efficacy of etanercept in patients with psoriasis: an open-label study. *Journal of Drugs in Dermatology,* Vol.9, No.8, pp.928-937.

Lowes, M.A., Chamian, F., Abello, M.V., Fuentes-Duculan, J., Lin, S.L., Nussbaum, R., Novitskaya, I., Carbonaro, H., Cardinale, I., Kikuchi, T., Gilleaudeau, P., Sullivan-Whalen, M., Wittkowski, K.M., Papp, K., Garovoy, M., Dummer, W., Steinman, R.M. & Krueger, J.G. (2005). Increase in TNF-alpha and inducible nitric oxide synthase-expressing dendritic cells in psoriasis and reduction with efalizumab (anti-CD11a). *Proceedings of the National Academy of Sciences,* Vol.102, No.52, pp. 19057-19062.

Lowes, M.A., Kikuchi, T., Fuentes-Duculan, J., Cardinale, I., Zaba, L.C., Haider, A.S., Bowman, E.P. & Krueger, J.G. (2008). Psoriasis vulgaris lesions contain discrete populations of Th1 and Th17 T cells. *The Journal of Investigative Dermatology,* Vol.128, No.5, pp.1207-1211.

Malaviya, R., Sun, Y., Tan, J.K., Wang, A., Magliocco, M., Yao, M., Krueger, J.G. & Gottlieb, A.B. (2006). Etanercept induces apoptosis of dermal dendritic cells in psoriatic plaques of responding patients. *Journal of the American Academy of Dermatology,* Vol.55, No.4, pp.590-597.

Mease, P.J., Goffe, B.S., Metz, J., VanderStoep, A., Finck, B. & Burge, D.J. (2000). Etanercept in the treatment of psoriatic arthritis and psoriasis: a randomised trial. *The Lancet,* Vol.356, No.9227, pp.385-390.

Mease, P.J., Kivitz, A.J., Burch, F.X., Siegel, E.L., Cohen, S.B., Ory, P., Salonen, D., Rubenstein, J., Sharp, J.T. & Tsuji, W. (2004). Etanercept treatment of psoriatic arthritis: safety, efficacy, and effect on disease progression. *Arthritis & Rheumatism,* Vol.50, No.7, pp.2264-2272.

Mease, P.J., Gladmanm D.D., Ritchlinm C.T., Rudermanm E.M., Steinfeldm S.D., Choy, E.H., Sharp, J.T., Ory, P.A., Perdok, R.J. & Weinberg, M.A. (2005). Adalimumab for the treatment of patients with moderately to severely active psoriatic arthritis: results of a double-blind, randomized, placebo-controlled trial. *Arthritis & Rheumatism,* Vol.52, No.10, pp.3279-3289.

Mease, P.J., Ory, P., Sharp, J.T., Ritchlin, C.T., Van den Bosch, F., Wellborne, F., Birbara, C., Thomson, G.T., Perdok, R.J., Medich, J., Wong, R.L. & Gladman, D.D. (2009). Adalimumab for long-term treatment of psoriatic arthritis: 2-year data from the Adalimumab Effectiveness in Psoriatic Arthritis Trial (ADEPT). *Annals of the Rheumatic Diseases,* Vol.68, No.5, pp.702-709.

Mease, P.J. & Reich, K. (2009). Alefacept with methotrexate for treatment of psoriatic arthritis: open-label extension of a randomized, double-blind, placebo-controlled study. *Journal of American Academy of Dermatology,* Vol.60, No.3, pp.402-411.

Mease, P.J., Woolley, J.M., Singh, A., Tsuji, W., Dunn, M. & Chiou, C.F. (2010). Patient-reported outcomes in a randomized trial of etanercept in psoriatic arthritis. *The Journal of Rheumatology,* Vol.37, No.6, pp.1221-1227.

Mease, P., Genovese, M.C., Gladstein, G., Kivitz, A.J., Ritchlin, C., Tak, P.P., Wollenhaupt, J., Bahary, O., Becker, J.C., Kelly, S., Sigal, L., Teng, J. & Gladman, D. (2011). Abatacept in the treatment of patients with psoriatic arthritis: results of a six-month, multicenter, randomized, double-blind, placebo-controlled, phase II trial. *Arthritis and Rheumatism,* Vol. 63, No.4, pp.939-948.

Menter, A., Cather, J.C., Baker, D., Farber, H.F., Lebwohl, M. & Darif, M. (2006). The efficacy of multiple courses of alefacept in patients with moderate to severe chronic plaque psoriasis. *Journal of American Academy of Dermatology,* Vol.54, No.1, pp.61-63.

Menter, A., Feldman, S.R., Weinstein, G.D., Papp, K., Evans, R., Guzzo, C., Li, S., Dooley, L.T., Arnold, C. & Gottlieb, A.B. (2007). A randomized comparison of continuous vs. intermittent infliximab maintenance regimens over 1 year in the treatment of moderate-to-severe plaque psoriasis. *Journal of American Academy of Dermatology,* Vol.56, No.1, pp.31.e1-15.

Menter, A., Tyring, S.K., Gordon, K., Kimball, A.B., Leonardi, C.L., Langley, R.G., Strober, B.E., Kaul, M., Gu, Y., Okun, M. & Papp, K. (2008). Adalimumab therapy for moderate to severe psoriasis: A randomized, controlled phase III trial. *Journal of American Academy of Dermatology,* Vol.58, No.1, pp.106-115.

Menter, A., Augustin, M., Signorovitch, J., Yu, A.P., Wu, E.Q., Gupta, S.R., Bao, Y. & Mulani, P. (2010). The effect of adalimumab on reducing depression symptoms in patients with moderate to severe psoriasis: a randomized clinical trial. *Journal of American Academy of Dermatology,* Vol.62, No.5, pp.812-818.

Montané, E., Sallés, M., Barriocanal, A., Riera, E., Costa, J. & Tena, X. (2007). Antitumor necrosis factor-induced neutropenia: a case report with double positive rechallenges. *Clinical Rheumatology,* Vol.26, No.9, pp.1527-1529.

Nestle, F.O., Kaplan, D.H. & Barker, J. (2009). Psoriasis. *New England Journal of Medicine,* Vol.361, No.5, pp.496-509.

Nograles, K.E., Brasington, R.D. & Bowcock, A.M. (2009). New insights into the pathogenesis and genetics of psoriatic arthritis. *Nature Clinical Practice Rheumatology,* Vol.5, No.2, pp.83-91.

Novartis. (July, 2010). Research and development: clinical pipeline. In: *www.novartis.com,* 16.05.2011, available from: *http://www.novartis.com/downloads/investors/presentations-events/pipeline-update/2010/2010-11-17-making-science_happen.pdf.*

Ortonne, J.P., Reich, K., Sterry, W. & Terpstra, I. (2008a). Safety and efficacy (PASI 90 and global evaluation) of subcutaneous certolizumab pegol in patients with moderate to severe chronic plaque psoriasis: results from a doubleblind, placebo-controlled trial. *Journal of the American Academy of Dermatology,* Vol.58, Ab.4, San Antonio, 66th Annual Meeting of the American Academy of Dermatology (AAD), February 1-5.

Ortonne, J.P., Reich, K. & Keininger, D.L. (2008b). Certolizumab pegol improved health-related quality of life in patients with psoriasis: data from a phase II study. *Journal of the American Academy of Dermatology,* Vol.58, Ab.121, San Antonio, 66th Annual Meeting of the American Academy of Dermatology (AAD), February 1-5.

Paller, A.S., Siegfried, E.C., Langley, R.G., Gottlieb, A.B., Pariser, D., Landells, I., Hebert, A.A., Eichenfield, L.F., Patel, V., Creamer, K. & Jahreis, A. (2008). Etanercept treatment for children and adolescents with plaque psoriasis. *New England Journal of Medicine,* Vol.358, No.3, pp.241-251.

Paller, A.S., Siegfried, E.C., Eichenfield, L.F., Pariser, D., Langley, R.G., Creamer, K. & Kricorian, G. (2010). Long-term etanercept in pediatric patients with plaque psoriasis. *Journal of the American Academy of Dermatology,* Vol.63, No.5, pp.762-768.

Papoutsaki, M., Chimenti, M.S., Costanzo, A., Talamonti, M., Zangrilli, A., Giunta, A., Bianchi, L. & Chimenti, S. (2007). Adalimumab for severe psoriasis and psoriatic arthritis: an open-label study in 30 patients previously treated with other biologics. *Journal of the American Academy of Dermatology,* Vol.57, No.2, pp.269-275.

Papp, K., Tyring, S., Lahfa, M., Prinz, J., Griffiths, CE., Nakanishi, A.M., Zitnik, R., van de Kerkhof, P.C. & Melvin, L. (2005). A global phase III randomized controlled trial of etanercept in psoriasis: safety, efficacy, and effect of dose reduction. *The British Journal of Dermatology,* Vol.152, No.6, pp.1304-1312.

Papp, K.A., Caro, I., Leung, H.M., Garovoy, M. & Mease, P.J. (2007). Efalizumab for the treatment of psoriatic arthritis. *Journal of Cutaneous Medicine and Surgery,* Vol.11, No.2, pp.57-66.

Papp, K.A., Langley, R.G., Lebwohl, M., Krueger, G.G., Szapary, P., Yeilding, N., Guzzo, C., Hsu, M.C., Wang, Y., Li, S., Dooley, L.T. & Reich, K. (2008). Efficacy and safety of ustekinumab, a human interleukin-12/23 monoclonal antibody, in patients with psoriasis: 52-week results from a randomised, double-blind, placebo-controlled trial (PHOENIX 2). *The Lancet,* Vol.371, No.9625, pp.1675-1684.

Papp, K., Crowley, J., Ortonne, J.P., Leu, J., Okun, M., Gupta, S.R., Gu, Y. & Langley, R.G. (2011). Adalimumab for moderate to severe chronic plaque psoriasis: efficacy and safety of retreatment and disease recurrence following withdrawal from therapy. *The British Journal of Dermatology,* Vol.164, No.2, pp.434-441.

Pfizer. (January, 2010). Pfizer pipeline. In: *www.pfizer.com,* 16.05.2011, available from: *http://www.pfizer.com/files/research/pipeline/2010_0127/pipeline_2010_0127.pdf.*

Piccolo, D., Di Cesare, A., Fargnoli, M.C., Paolini, M., Vecchiotti, S. & Peris, K. (2008). Effective control of psoriasis by etanercept in a patient with HCV-related diseases. *European Journal of Dermatology,* Vol.18, No.4, pp.459-482.

Raho, G., Vena, G.A., Bizzoca, A., Cassano, N., Garofalo, E., Congedo, M. & Gennarini, G. (2010). Influence of infliximab on keratinocyte apoptosis in psoriasis patients. *Immunopharmacology and Immunotoxicology,* Vol.33, No.1, pp.227-231.

Ramos-Casals, M., Brito-Zerón, P., Soto, M.J., Cuadrado, M.J. & Khamashta, M.A. (2008). Autoimmune diseases induced by TNF-targeted therapies. *Best Practice & Research Clinical Rheumatology,* Vol.22, No.5, pp.847-861.

Reich, K., Nestle, F.O., Papp, K., Ortonne, J.P., Evans, R., Guzzo, C., Li, S., Dooley, L.T. & Griffiths, C.E. (2005). Infliximab induction and maintenance therapy for moderate-to-severe psoriasis: a phase III, multicentre, double-blind trial. *The Lancet,* Vol.366, No.9494, pp.1367-1374.

Reich, K., Nestle, F.O., Papp, K., Ortonne, J.P., Wu, Y., Bala, M., Evans, R., Guzzo, C., Li, S., Dooley, L.T. & Griffiths, C.E. (2006). Improvement in quality of life with infliximab induction and maintenance therapy in patients with moderate-to-severe psoriasis: a randomized controlled trial. *The British Journal of Dermatology,* Vol.154, No.6, pp.1161-1168.

Reich, K., Ortonne, J.P., Kerkmann, U., Wang, Y., Saurat, J.H., Papp, K., Langley, R. & Griffiths, C.E. (2010). Skin and nail responses after 1 year of infliximab therapy in patients with moderate-to-severe psoriasis: a retrospective analysis of the EXPRESS Trial. *Dermatology,* Vol.221, No.2, pp.172-178.

Revicki, D., Willian, M.K., Saurat, J.H., Papp, K.A., Ortonne, J.P., Sexton, C. & Camez, A. (2008). Impact of adalimumab treatment on health-related quality of life and other patient-reported outcomes: results from a 16-week randomized controlled trial in patients with moderate to severe plaque psoriasis. *The British Journal of Dermatology,* Vol.158, No.3, pp.549-557.

Roberts, L. & McColl, G.J. (2004). Tumour necrosis factor inhibitors: risks and benefits in patients with rheumatoid arthritis. *Internal Medicine Journal,* Vol.34, No.12, pp.687-693.

Roberts, J.L., Ortonne, J.P., Tan, J.K., Jaracz, E. & Frankel, E. (2010). The safety profile and sustained remission associated with response to multiple courses of intramuscular alefacept for treatment of chronic plaque psoriasis. *Journal of American Academy of Dermatology,* Vol.62, No.6, pp.968-978.

Russell, C.B., Kerkhof, K., Bigler, J., Timour, M., Welcher, A.A., Novitskaya, I., Khatcherian, A., Krueger, J., Rand, H., Martin, D.A. & Zeichner, J.A. (2010). Blockade of IL-17R with AMG 827 leads to rapid reversal of gene expression. *Journal of Investigative Dermatology,* Vol.130, No.S1, S46.

Saougou, I., Markatseli, T.E., Papagoras, C., Voulgari, P.V., Alamanos, Y. & Drosos, A.A. (2011). Sustained Clinical Response in Psoriatic Arthritis Patients Treated with Anti-TNF Agents: A 5-year Open-Label Observational Cohort Study. *Seminars in Arthritis and Rheumatism,* Vol.40, No.5, pp.398-406.

Saurat, J.H., Stingl, G., Dubertret, L., Papp, K., Langley, R.G., Ortonne, J.P., Unnebrink, K., Kaul, M. & Camez, A. (2008). Efficacy and safety results from the randomized controlled comparative study of adalimumab vs. methotrexate vs. placebo in patients with psoriasis (CHAMPION). *The British Journal of Dermatology,* Vol.158, No.3, pp.558-566.

Scallon, B.J., Moore, M.A., Trinh, H., Knight, D.M. & Ghrayeb, J. (1995). Chimeric anti-TNF-alpha monoclonal antibody cA2 binds recombinant transmembrane TNF-alpha and activates immune effector functions. *Cytokine,* Vol.7, No.3, pp.251-259.

Schottelius, A.J., Moldawer, L.L., Dinarello, C.A., Asadullah, K., Sterry, W. & Edwards, C.K. 3rd. (2004). Biology of tumor necrosis factor-alpha- implications for psoriasis. *Experimental Dermatology,* Vol.13, No.4, pp.193-222.

Shikiar, R., Heffernan, M., Langley, R.G., Willian, M.K., Okun, M.M. & Revicki, D.A. (2007). Adalimumab treatment is associated with improvement in health-related quality of life in psoriasis: patient-reported outcomes from a phase II randomized controlled trial. *Journal of Dermatological Treatment,* Vol.18, No.1, pp.25-31.

Sterry, W., Ortonne, J.P., Kirkham, B., Brocq, O., Robertson, D., Pedersen, R.D., Estojak, J., Molta, C.T. & Freundlich, B. (2010). Comparison of two etanercept regimens for treatment of psoriasis and psoriatic arthritis: PRESTA randomised double blind multicentre trial. *The British Medical Journal,* Feb 2; 340:c147. doi: 10.1136/bmj.c147.

Swedish Medical Center (September, 2009). Rituxan With or Without Methotrexate in Psoriatic Arthritis. In: *www.clinicaltrials.gov,* 16.05.2011, available from: *http://clinicaltrials.gov/ct2/show/NCT00509678.*

Thaçi, D., Ortonne, J.P., Chimenti, S., Ghislain, P.D., Arenberger, P., Kragballe, K., Saurat, J.H., Khemis, A., Sprøgel, P., Esslinger, H.U., Unnebrink, K. & Kupper, H. (2010). A phase IIIb, multicentre, randomized, double-blind, vehicle-controlled study of the efficacy and safety of adalimumab with and without calcipotriol/betamethasone topical treatment in patients with moderate to severe psoriasis: the BELIEVE study. *The British Journal of Dermatology,* Vol.163, No.2, pp.402-411.

Toichi, E., Torres, G., McCormick, T.S., Chang, T., Mascelli, M.A., Kauffman, C.L., Aria, N., Gottlieb, A.B., Everitt, D.E., Frederick, B., Pendley, C.E. & Cooper, K.D. (2006). An anti-IL-12p40 antibody down-regulates type 1 cytokines, chemokines, and IL-12/IL-23 in psoriasis. *The Journal of Immunology,* Vol.177, No.7, pp.4917-4926.

Trinchieri, G. (2003). Interleukin-12 and the regulation of innate resistance and adaptive immunity. *Nature Reviews. Immunology,* Vol.3, No.2, pp.133-146.

Tyring, S., Gordon, K.B., Poulin, Y., Langley, R.G., Gottlieb, A.B., Dunn, M. & Jahreis, A. (2007). Long-term safety and efficacy of 50 mg of etanercept twice weekly in patients with psoriasis. *Archives of Dermatology,* Vol.143, No.6, pp.719-726.

UCB, Inc. (December, 2010). Cimzia package insert. In: *www.cimzia.com,* 28.05.2011, available *from: http://www.cimzia.com/pdf/Prescribing_Information.pdf.*

Vaishnaw, A.K. & TenHoor, C.N. (2002). Pharmacokinetics, biologic activity, and tolerability of alefacept by intravenous and intramuscular administration. *Journal of Pharmacokinetics and Pharmacodynamics,* Vol.29, No.5-6, pp.415-426.

van de Kerkhof, P.C., Segaert, S., Lahfa, M., Luger, T.A., Karolyi, Z., Kaszuba, A., Leigheb, G., Camacho, F.M., Forsea, D., Zang, C., Boussuge, M.P., Paolozzi, L. & Wajdula, J. (2008). Once weekly administration of etanercept 50 mg is efficacious and well tolerated in patients with moderate-to-severe plaque psoriasis: a randomized controlled trial with open-label extension. *The British Journal of Dermatology,* Vol.159, No.5, pp.1177-1185.

van Eden, W. (2008). XToll, a recombinant chaperonin 10 as an anti-inflammatory immunomodulator. *Current Opinion in Investigational Drugs,* Vol. 9, No.5, pp.523-533.

van, L., Modi, S.V., Yang, D.J. & Hsu, S. (2008). Sustained efficacy and safety of adalimumab in psoriasis treatment: a retrospective study of 49 patients with and without a history of TNF-alpha antagonist treatment. *Archives of Dermatology,* Vol.144, No.6, pp.804-806.

Vena, G.A. & Cassano, N. (2007). Anti-tumor necrosis factor therapies for psoriasis. *Expert Review of Dermatology,* Vol.2, pp.335-349.

Weger, W. (2010). Current status and new developments in the treatment of psoriasis and psoriatic arthritis with biological agents. *The British Journal of Pharmacology,* Vol.160, No.4, pp.810-20.

Williams, B., Vanags, D., Hall, S., McCormack, C., Foley, P., Weiss, J., Johnson, B., Latz, E. & Feeney, D. (2008). Efficacy and safety of chaperonin 10 in patients with moderate to severe plaque psoriasis: evidence of utility beyond a single indication. *Archives of Dermatology,* Vol. 144, No.5, pp.683-685.

Yawalkar, N., Tscharner, G.G., Hunger, R.E. & Hassan, A.S. (2009). Increased expression of IL-12p70 and IL-23 by multiple dendritic cell and macrophage subsets in plaque psoriasis. *Journal of Dermatological Science,* Vol.54, No.2, pp.99-105.

Zaba, L.C., Cardinale, I., Gilleaudeau, P., Sullivan-Whalen, M., Suárez-Fariñas, M., Fuentes-Duculan, J., Novitskaya, I., Khatcherian, A., Bluth, M.J., Lowes, M.A. & Krueger, J.G. (2007). Amelioration of epidermal hyperplasia by TNF inhibition is associated with reduced Th17 responses. *The Journal of Experimental Medicine,* Vol.204, No.13, pp.3183-3194.

Zeinn, N.N. & Etanercept Study Group. (2005). Etanercept as an adjuvant to interferon and ribavirin in treatment-naive patients with chronic hepatitis C virus infection: a phase 2 randomized, double-blind, placebo-controlled study. *Journal of Hepatology*, Vol.42, No.3, pp.315-322.

17

Food, Nutrition and Diet Therapy in Psoriasis

Maria Lucia Diniz Araujo, Paulla Suylane Santos Fernandes Costa and Maria Goretti Pessoa de Araujo Burgos
Federal University of the Pernambuco
Brazil

1. Introduction

Diet has been suggested to play a role in the etiology and pathogenesis of psoriasis (Araujo et al., 2009; Wolters, 2005). Periods of fasting, a hypocaloric and vegetarian diet have been associated with an improvement in symptoms due to changes in the metabolism of polyunsaturated fatty acids (PUFAs) and an influence on the profile of eicosanoids, leading to suppression of the inflammatory process (Lithell et al., 1983; Rucevic et al., 2003; Wolters, 2005). The consumption of alcoholic beverages is prevalent among patients with psoriasis and is the greatest cause of the high mortality rate among individuals with moderate to severe forms of the disease and should therefore be avoided (Chistophers, 2001; Poikolainen et al., 1990; Smith & Fenske, 2000; Wolters, 2005). According to several authors, calcitriol (the active form of vitamin D) and its analogs have anti-proliferation, pro-differentiation and immune-regulating properties that may inhibit the growth and maturation of keratinocytes, with oral supplementation often suggested for patients who do not topically use calcitriol (Andorini, 2002; Holick, 2003; Wolters, 2005).

The skin acts as an interface between the body and surrounding environment, thus the skin is constantly exposed to both endogenous and exogenous pro-oxidants, leading to the generation of harmful oxidant species. Oxidative stress and the generation of excessive free radicals have been related to skin inflammation in psoriasis. Patients with this condition have reduced plasma levels of β-carotene and α-tocopherol as well as a decline in serum selenium and high concentrations of malondialdehyde, which is a marker of lipid peroxidation in the plasma and red blood cells (Briganti & Picardo, 2003; Azzini et al., 1995; Serwin et al., 2003).

Data from literature indicates that the topical application or oral administration of antioxidants is suggested as preventive therapy for the natural aging of the skin and cancer caused by ultraviolet rays (Briganti & Picardo, 2003). With regard to lipids, studies have demonstrated the anti-inflammatory effect of fish oil in individuals with psoriasis, as diets rich in omega 3 modify the metabolism of PUFAs, thereby influencing the profile of eicosanoids, which leads to the suppression of the inflammatory process (Smith & Fenske, 2000). A number of authors report an association between latent sensitivity to gluten (pre-celiac disease state) and different skin diseases, including psoriasis, suggesting a gluten-free diet may provide beneficial effects (Duggan, 2004; Humbert et al., 2006; Leffler et al., 2003; Michaelsson et al., 2003; Nelson, 2002; Wolters, 2005).

The aforementioned data underscore the importance of studies on psoriasis, especially with regard to the influence of nutrition on the etiopathogenesis and treatment of this condition.

2. Influence of calorie intake, periods of fasting and vegetarian diet

A number of studies report that symptoms of inflammatory disease, such as rheumatoid arthritis, can improve with a hypocaloric diet or during periods of fasting (Muller et al., 2001; Palmblad et al., 1991). Similarly, the prevalence and severity of psoriasis were shown to improve during periods of fasting and a hypocaloric diet,suggesting diet to be an important consideration for theprevention and treatment of the moderate non-pustular form of the disease (Rucevic et al., 2003; Wolters, 2005)

While various mechanisms have been discussed, the direct cause of these positive effects on the symptoms of psoriasis remains unknown (Wolters, 2005). The most important reason is likely a reduction in arachidonic acid (AA) intake, resulting in a lower production of inflammatory eicosanoids. During the fasting state, a reduction in the activation of TCD4 cells and an increase in the number and/or function of the anti-inflammatory cytokine interleukin 4 have been observed; Calorie restriction leads to a reduction in oxidative stress (Fraser et al., 1999; Wolters, 2005). However, the few studies that have addressed the effect of caloric restriction on psoriasis offer inconsistent data on the benefits of this conduct over a long period of time (Lithell et al., 1983; Rucevic et al., 2003). The results of evaluations carried out during World War I revealed that individuals with psoriasis experienced significant improvement during calorie restriction, with the recurrence of skin lesions after the reintroduction of a normal diet (Ricketts et al., 2010).

A vegetarian diet may be beneficial to all patients with psoriasis due to the reduction in AA intake and consequent reduction in the formation of inflammatory eicosanoids (Fraser et al., 1999).

3. Polyunsaturated fatty acids

Lipids are macronutrients that perform energy, structural and hormonal functions in organisms. Fatty acids are monocarboxylic acids with a hydrocarbon chain of variable size and double bonds between carbon atoms. These substances are classified as monounsaturated and polyunsaturated, depending on the number of double bonds they contain. Fatty acids are integral compounds of nearly all lipids. Two series of PUFAs are differentiated, depending on the location of the first double carbon bond at the methyl radical. Linoleic acid, which is an essential fatty acid, belongs to the omega 6 family and is found in a large quantity of oleaginous seeds; this acid can be converted into AA, which is prinicipally derived from meat and egg sources (Dutra-de-Oliveira, 2000). Eicosapentaenoic acid (EPA) and docosahexaenoic acid are the most abundant omega 3 fatty acids in food and are found mainly in cold-water fish, such as mackerel, sardine, salmon, herring, etc. (Wolters, 2005).

Besides their function in the phospholipid membrane, PUFAs are needed for the formation of eicosanoids, which are metabolic regulators (Jones & Papamandjaris, 2001). AA is a precursor of prostaglandins, leukotrienes and other compounds that have important functions in inflammation and the regulation of immunity, whereas EPA derivatives exhibit anti-inflammatory properties (Calder, 2001). High concentrations of AA and its pro-inflammatory metabolites have been observed in psoriatic lesions as well as in other auto-immune and inflammatory disorders. Therefore, one treatment option for psoriasis may be the replacement of AA with an alternative fatty acid, especially EPA, which is metabolized through the same enzymatic pathways as AA (Mayser et al., 2002; Wolters, 2005).

Fish oil (omega 3), has been observed to change the serum and lipid composition of epidermal and blood cell membranes, which rationalizes its use in the treatment of psoriasis. High levels of AA are found in psoriatic lesions and it is believed that its metabolite, leukotriene B4, may be the mediator of inflammation in psoriasis (Ricketts et al., 2010). Thus, when omega 3 fatty acids are metabolized by cyclooxygenase or lipoxygenase in place of AA in the cell membranes, these substances may assist in reducing inflammation (Ricketts et al., 2010).

Conflicting results are reported regarding the effect of the oral supplementation of omega 3 on this disease and there are no clear findings regarding the dose to be employed (Mayser et al., 2002; Wilkinson, 1990). In vitro studies report that the addition of fish oil to the diet of individuals with psoriasis leads to an increase in EPA in relation to AA in the plasma and platelets, with a significant reduction in the synthesis of leukotriene B4 (Ricketts et al., 2010)

Initial studies involving different amounts of EPA ranging from 3.6 to 14 grams per day for periods of six weeks to six months report some clinical improvement with minimal side effects; however, lower doses for a shorter period of time are reported to offer no significant improvement (Maurice et al., 1987; Ziboh et al., 1986; Kragballe & Fogh, 1989; Kojima et al., 1989). The majority of studies report positive results; however, less effective results are reported in randomized, controlled trials (Wolters, 2005). Despite the inconsistent results, the consumption of fish rich in omega 3 is recommended. Moreover, parenteral infusions of omega 3 may be beneficial to patients hospitalized with acute psoriasis (Wolters, 2005).

4. Gluten

Celiac disease is an enteropathy associated with different extra-intestinal manifestations, such as anemia, transaminase elevation, osteopenia, neurological conditions, emotional and psychiatric disorders, auto-immune disease and dermatological problems. This disease is characterized by an allergy to gluten (a protein found in wheat, oats, rye and barley), leading to malabsorption and atrophy of the intestinal villi, which improves with a gluten-free diet (Abenavoli et al., 2006).

This gluten-sensitive enteropathy tends to bemildly symptomatic and even asymptomatic, which may explain the association between latent gluten sensitivity and psoriasis (Wolters, 2005). A number of studies report an association between celiac disease and psoriasis (Michaelsson et al., 2000; Woo et al., 2004). According to some authors, however, this association is controversial due to currently limited data (Addolorato et al., 2003; Collin & Reunal, 2003). Since both celiac disease and psoriasis are related to T helper 1 (Th1) cytokines, this association could be caused by the activation of Th1 by the interleukins IL1 and IL8, stemming from the rapid division of keratinocytes (Ojetti et al., 2003).

There is no consensus among current literature regarding the high prevalence of patients with psoriasis and antibodies associated to celiac disease (Ricketts et al., 2010). Thus, there is a need for prospective studies in order to determine the incidence of celiac disease and the real percentage of increased levels of antigliadin, antiendomysial and anti-tissue transglutaminase antibodies in patients with psoriasis (Ricketts et al., 2010).

A gluten-free diet can improve skin lesions even in patients without celiac disease but with the antigliadin antibodies IgA and IgG, which are important to the diagnosis of celiac disease (Michaelsson et al., 2003). Likewise, studies indicate that a gluten-free diet leads to an improvement in rheumatoid arthritis, which is another chronic inflammatory disease (Hafstrom et al., 2001). Data remains scarce in regards to the mechanisms involved in the association between celiac disease, psoriasis and a gluten-free diet in skin lesions. A number of hypotheses have been raised, such as an alteration in intestinal permeability, immune mechanisms and vitamin D deficiency (Abenavoli et al., 2006).

5. Oxidative stress and antioxidants

The skin is constantly exposed to oxidants, which leads to the formation of harmful reactive oxygen species (Briganti & Picardo, 2003). Oxidative stress and the increased formation of free radicals have been related to skin inflammation and are reported to be among the most important factors in the pathogenesis of psoriasis (Kiymat et al., 2003; Rocha et al., 2004; Relhan et al., 2002; Wolters, 2005). Studies demonstrate that individuals with psoriasis have high concentrations of malondialdehyde, OuvirLer foneticamentea marker of lipid peroxidation, and is compromised antioxidant status, with reduced levels of β-carotene, α-tocopherol and selenium (Azzini et al., 1995; Briganti & Picardo, 2003; Serwin et al., 2003).

High alcohol intake (stemming from the psychosocial impact of the disease) and either active or passive smoking are among some of the factors that can increase oxidative stress and reduce levels of natural antioxidants in individuals with a history of the disease for more than three years (Lecomte et al., 1994; Mckenzie, 2000; Monk & Neil, 1986; Naldi et al., 1992). The consumption of fruit and vegetables may be beneficial to such individuals due to the high antioxidant content, such as karotenoids, flavonoids and vitamin C, as an adequate antioxidant status is considered useful to the prevention of imbalance between oxidative stress and antioxidant defense (Naldi et al., 1996; Wolters, 2005). However, few studies have investigated the effects of antioxidant supplementation on the symptoms of psoriasis (Wolters, 2005).

6. Selenium

Selenium is an essential trace element with immune-modulating and anti-proliferative properties, with an influence over the immune response whether through a change in the expression of cytokines and respective receptors or by making immune cells more resistant to oxidative stress (Celerier et al., 1995; Roy et al., 1992; Spallholtz et al., 1990). Moreover, data indicates that patients with inflammatory skin diseases, skin cancer, malignant melanoma and cutaneous T-cell lymphoma have low concentrations of selenium (Clark et al., 1984; Deffuant et al., 1984; Hinks et al., 1987; Michaelsson & Edqvist, 1984).

The low concentration of selenium found in patients with psoriasis may be a risk factor for the development of the disease. However, there are few studies on the role of this element in the pathogenesis (Hinks et al., 1987; Fairris et al., 1989; Michaelsson et al., 1989; Harvima et al., 1993; Pinton et al., 1995; Azzini et al., 1995). Low levels of selenium are related to the severity of psoriasis and may occur due to low food intake or excessive flaking of the skin (Serwin et al., 2003). Serwin et al. (2003) found that selenium levels were significantly lower in patients with a diagnosis of psoriasis for more than three years in comparison to healthy volunteers (38.69 vs 48.41; $p < 0.05$).

Kharaeva et al. (2009) demonstrated for the first time that the combination of conventional therapy and supplementation with vitamin E, co-enzyme Q10 and selenium resulted in an improvement in the clinical condition of patients with severe psoriasis as well as a reduction in oxidative stress. Supplementation using inorganic forms of selenium (sodium selenite and selenate) is also reported to lead to clinical improvement in patients with psoriasis (Fairris et al., 1989; Pinton et al., 1995).

7. Vitamin D

Vitamin D is a pro-hormone that can be produced from 7-dehydrocholesterol through the exposure of skin to ultraviolet B rays of the sun. Besides its importance in the homeostasis of calcium and bone metabolism, calcitriol (the active form of vitamin D) has effects on more than 30 types of tissue, including skin (Wolters, 2005). Vitamin D plays an important role in reducing the risk of a number of chronic diseases, such as auto-immune diseases, infectious diseases, cardiovascular diseases and some forms of cancer (breast, colon-rectal and prostate cancer) (Fu &Vender, 2011).

Vitamin D plays an essential role in cell proliferation, differentiation, apoptosis and angiogenesis.Vitamin D also has beneficial effects on inflammatory diseases medicated by Th1 lymphocytes, such as diabetes, psoriasis, Crohn's disease and multiple sclerosis (Cantorna et al., 2004; Holick, 2007; Ikeda et al., 2010). Vitamin D has proven to be highly effective in the treatment of psoriasis, as patients having received vitamin D for the treatment of osteoporosis exhibited an improvement in psoriasis (Abramovits, 2009; Smith et al., 2009; Van De Kerkhof, 2005). Due to the function of calcitriol and its analogs in psoriasis, oral supplementation with vitamin D should be considered in patients who do not make use of topical treatment with this vitamin, as vitamin D deficiency is frequent in these individuals (Holick, 2003; Wolters, 2005).

8. Vitamin B12

Data from the literature demonstrates the efficacy of using intramuscular and systemic vitamin B12 in patients with psoriasis in addition to the positive effects of topical vitamin B12 (Ricketts et al., 2010).

9. Zinc

Zinc deficiency has been associated with the presence of psoriatic plaque (Smith et al., 2009). However, there is little evidence on the benefits of oral supplementation as of yet (Burrows et al., 1994). Moreover, there are no recommendations regarding the amount or chemical form that offers the best beneficial effects.

10. Alcoholic beverages

The first studies on the association between psoriasis and the consumption of alcoholic beverages emerged in 1963. While some investigations have failed to demonstrate such an association, recent studies have shown a significant correlation (Wolf et al., 1999). Besides contributing to the development of psoriatic plaque, alcohol intake is involved in triggering periods of exacerbation, associated with a reduced response to treatment and the risk of liver toxicity associated to the use of methotrexate (Gupta et al., 1993; Higgins et al., 1994; Liu et al., 2010; Qureshi et al., 2010; Smith & Fenske, 2000).

The exact mechanism by which alcohol causes or aggravates psoriasis is not yet fully clarified. Some authors propose that alcohol induces immunological dysfunction, leading to immunosuppression, and increases the production of inflammatory cytokines and cell cycle activators, such as cyclin D1 and keratinocyte growth factor, which could lead to epidermal over-proliferation (Farkas et al., 2003; Ockenfels et al., 1996; Smith & Fenske, 2000). Moreover, the greater susceptibility to superficial infection observed in alcoholics, such as those caused by Streptococcus and trauma, has also been suggested in the development of psoriasis (Farkas et al., 2003).

Data from literature indicates that alcohol is a risk factor for psoriasis in young and middle-aged men and, while not a risk factor in women, alcohol intake aggravates the condition in this gender (Poikolainen et al., 1994). Patients with psoriasis are recommended to exercise with caution when consuming alcohol, especially during periods of exacerbation. Moreover, due to all possible effects, a number of authors recommend abstention (Behnam et al., 2005; Wolters, 2005). Thus, identifying this risk factor in patients with psoriasis could contribute toward a reduction in episodes of exacerbation, thereby achieving better treatment results (Kazakevich et al., 2011).

11. Obesity

The first associations between psoriasis and obesity were reported in large epidemiological studies carried out in Europe (Duarte et al., 2010). A pioneering American study conducted in the state of Utah reports a 34% prevalence of obesity among individuals with psoriasis, which is much higher than the 18% reported in the general population (Herron et al., 2005)

Obesity is known to cause a state of chronic inflammation, with high levels of TNF-α, IL-6 and C-reactive protein, which are associated to the progressive increase in body mass index (BMI). In this state of chronic inflammation, alterations in resistance/sensitivity to insulin and greater oxidative stress, with the production of free radicals, lead to a greater likelihood of the development of diabetes and metabolic syndrome as well as the influence of these pro-inflammatory cytokines in the course and presentation of psoriasis (Hamminga et al., 2006; Wakkee et al., 2007). The association between obesity and psoriasis has been well established, as obesity can increase the risk of developing psoriasis and preexisting psoriasis can increase the risk of patients becoming obese (Farías et al., 2011).

Non-pharmacological treatment aimed at changes in lifestyle should be offered to all patients, especially those with a BMI ≥ 25 kg/m^2, for whom the goal is controlled, healthy weight loss (Farías et al., 2011). A low-calorie diet is recommended, following the Step I diet (Obesity Society, 2000) (Table 1), with a calorie restriction of 500 to 1000 kilocalories per day, based on the patient's energy expenditure, which can be determined through measurement techniques such as indirect calorimetry or through mathematical formulas such as the Harris-Benedict equation (Table 2) (Frankenfield et al., 1998). For greater compliance to treatment and patient follow up, the participation of a nutritionist is needed to individualize the treatment, considering all socioeconomic and cultural aspects. Farías et al (2011) suggests the recommendations of the Nutrition Committee of the American Heart Association (Table 3 e Table 4).

Nutrient	Recommendation intake
Reducing calories	Approximately 500 to 1,000 kilocalories / day
Total fat	< 30% of total calories
Saturated fat	8 a 10% of total calories
Monounsaturated fat	≤15% of total calories
Polyunsaturated fat	≤10% of total calories
Total cholesterol	<300 mg / day
Proteins	Approximately 15% of total calories
Carbohydrates	At least 55% of total calories
Sodium	100 mmol / day (approximately 2.4 g of sodium)
Calcium	1.000 to 1.500 mg/Day
Fiber	20 a 30 g/Day

Table 1. Diet Step 1 (Obesity Society, 2000).

Women	BMR = 655 + (4.35 x weight in pounds) + (4.7 x height in inches) - (4.7 x age in years)
Men	66 + (6.23 x weight in pounds) + (12.7 x height in inches) - (6.8 x age in years)

Table 2. Basal metabolic rate according to the Harris Benedict formula.

Balance calorie intake and physical activity to achieve or maintain a healthy body weight.
Consume a diet rich in vegetables and fruits.
Choose whole-grain, high-fiber foods
Consume fish, especially oily fish, at least twice a week.
Limit your intake of saturated fat to _7% of energy, *trans* fat to _1% of energy, and cholesterol to _300 mg per day by -Choosing lean meats and vegetable alternatives; – Selecting fat-free (skim), 1%-fat, and low-fat dairy products; and – Minimizing intake of partially hydrogenated fats.
Minimize your intake of beverages and foods with added sugars.
Choose and prepare foods with little or no salt.
If you consume alcohol, do so in moderation.
When you eat food that is prepared outside of the home, follow the AHA Diet and Lifestyle Recommendations.

Table 3. Diet and Lifestyle Recommendations for Cardiovascular Disease Risk Reduction (American Heart Association Commitee Nutrition, (AHA) 2006).

Lifestyle	• Know your caloric needs to achieve and maintain a healthy weight. • Know the calorie content of the foods and beverages you consume. • Track your weight, physical activity, and calorie intake. • Prepare and eat smaller portions. • Track and, when possible, decrease screen time (eg, watching television, surfing the Web, playing computer games). • Incorporate physical movement into habitual activities. • Do not smoke or use tobacco products. • If you consume alcohol, do so in moderation (equivalent of no more than 1 drink in women or 2 drinks in men per day).
Food choices and preparation	• Use the nutrition facts panel and ingredients list when choosing foods to buy. • Eat fresh, frozen, and canned vegetables and fruits without high-calorie sauces and added salt and sugars. • Replace high-calorie foods with fruits and vegetables. • Increase fiber intake by eating beans (legumes), whole-grain products, fruits, and vegetables. • Use liquid vegetable oils in place of solid fats. • Limit beverages and foods high in added sugars. Common forms of added sugars are sucrose, glucose, fructose, maltose, dextrose, corn syrups, concentrated fruit juice, and honey. • Choose foods made with whole grains. Common forms of whole grains are whole wheat, oats/oatmeal, rye, barley, corn, popcorn, brown rice, wild rice, buckwheat, triticale, bulgur (cracked wheat), millet, quinoa, and sorghum. • Cut back on pastries and high-calorie bakery products (eg, muffins, doughnuts). • Select milk and dairy products that are either fat free or low fat. • Reduce salt intake by - comparing the sodium content of similar products (eg, different brands of tomato sauce) and choosing products with less salt; - choosing versions of processed foods, including cereals and baked goods, that are reduced in salt; and - limiting condiments (eg, soy sauce, ketchup). • Use lean cuts of meat and remove skin from poultry before eating. • Limit processed meats that are high in saturated fat and sodium. • Grill, bake, or broil fish, meat, and poultry. • Incorporate vegetable-based meat substitutes into favorite recipes. • Encourage the consumption of whole vegetables and fruits in place of juices.

Table 4. Practical Tips to Implement AHA 2006 Diet and Lifestyle Recommendations.

12. Psoriasis and metabolic syndrome

Metabolic syndrome is a set of metabolic alterations, particularly insulin resistance, which, together, lead to a greater risk of pro-inflammatory and pro-thrombotic alterations. A number of studies have suggested an increase in the prevalence of the components of metabolic syndrome in patients with psoriasis (Cohen et al., 2008; Neimann et al., 2006; Sommer et al., 2006).

Patients with psoriasis have a greater prevalence of metabolic syndrome in comparison to those with other dermatological conditions (30.1% vs 20.6%; OR: 1.65; 95%CI: 1.16 to 2.35) (Gisondi et al., 2007). However, few studies have considered the possibility of associating the treatment for psoriasis with the components of metabolic syndrome (Fu &Vender, 2011). A case report of a patient with psoriasis and metabolic syndrome suggests that the treatment program designed by nutritionists and endocrinologists through the modification of diet and treatment of comorbidities provided an improvement in blood glucose, cholesterol and BMI, along with a clinical improvement in psoriasis (Saraceno et al., 2008).

13. Conclusion

Diet is an important factor in the etiology and pathogenesis of psoriasis. Low-calorie and vegetarian diets may be beneficial to the treatment of this condition. Although the results regarding the oral supplementation of fish oil are inconsistent, patients are recommended to consume fish rich in omega 3 PUFAs and parenteral infusions of PUFAs are recommended for patients hospitalized with acute psoriasis. Further studies are needed to clarify the role of a gluten-free diet, which may improve the severity of the disease in patients with IgA and/or IgG antigliadin antibodies. Moreover, the consumption of fruit and vegetables may be beneficial due to their high antioxidant content. Vitamin D is an important treatment option due to its immuno-regulating and anti-proliferation activity. Patients with psoriasis should not consume alcoholic beverages in order to avoid exacerbation of the disease.

14. References

Abenavoli, L.; Proietti, I.; Leggio, L.; Ferrulli, A.; Vonghia, L.; Capizzi, R.; Rotoli, M.; Amerio, P.L.; Gasbarrini, G. & Addolorato, G. (2006). Cutaneous manifestations in celiac disease. *World Journal of Gastroenterology*, Vol.12, pp.843-52, ISSN 1007-9327.

Abramovits, W. (2009).Calcitriol 3 microg/g ointment: an effective and safe addition to the armamentarium in topical psoriasis therapy. *Journal of Drugs in Dermatology*, Vol. 8, supplement 8, pp. s17–s22, ISSN 1545-9616.

Addolorato, G.; Parente, A.; De Lorenze, G.; D'angelo Di Paola ,M.E.; Abenavoli, L.; Leggio, L.; Capristo, E.; De Simone, C.; Rotoli, M.; Rapaccini, G.L. & Gasbarrini, G. (2003). Rapid Regression of psoriasis in a coeliac patient after gluten-free diet. A case report and review of the literature. *Digestion*, Vol. 68, No.1, pp.9-12, ISSN 0012-2823.

American Heart Association Nutrition Committee. (2006). Diet and lifestyle recommendations revision 2006: a scientific statement from the American Heart Association Nutrition Committee. Vol.;114, pp.82–96, Access in June 27, 2011, Retrieved from < http:// circ.ahajournals.org/cgi/reprint/CIRCULATIONAHA.106.176158>.

Andorini, L. (2002). Immunorregulatory effects of vitamin D receptors ligands in autoimmune diseases. *International Immunopharmacology*, Vol. 2, pp.1017-28, ISSN 1878-1705.

Araujo, M.L.D.; Burgos, M.G.A.P. & Moura,, I.S.C.M.(2009). Nutritional influences in psoriasis. *Anais Brasileiros de Dermatologia*, Vol. 84, No.1, pp.90-2, ISSN 1806-4841.

Azzini M, Girelli D, Olivieri O, Guarini P, Stanzial AM, Frigo A, Milanino, R.; Bambara, L.M. & Corrocher, R. (1995). Fatty acids and antioxidant micronutrients in psoriatic arthritis. *Journal of rheumatology*, Vol.22, pp.103-8, ISSN 0315-162X.

Behnam, S.M.; Behnam, S.E. & Koo, J.Y. (2005). Alcohol as a risk factor for plaque-type psoriasis. *Cutis*, Vol.76, pp.181-5, ISSN 0011-4162.

Briganti, S. & Picardo, M. (2003). Antioxidant activity, lipid peroxidation and skin disease. What´s new. *Journal of the European Academy of Dermatology and Venereology*, Vol.17, pp.663-9, ISSN 1468-3083.

Burrows, N.P.; Turnbull, A.J.; Punchard, N.A.; Thompson, R.P.H. & Jones, R.R.(1994). A trial of oral zinc supplementation in psoriasis. *Cutis*, Vol.54, pp. 117-8, ISSN 0011-4162.

Calder, P.C. (2001). Polyunsaturated fatty acids, inflammation, and immunity. *Lipids*, Vol.36, pp.1007-24, ISSN 0024-4201.

Cantorna, M. T..; Zhu, Y, Froicu, M., & Wittke, A. (2004). "Vitamin D status, 1,25-dihydroxyvitamin D3, and the immune system."*American Journal of Clinical Nutrition*, Vol. 80, supplement, pp. 1717S–1720S, ISSN: 1938-3207.

Celerier, P.; Richard, A.; Litoux, P. & Dreno, B. (1995). Modulatory effects of selenium and atrontium salts on keratinocyte-derived inflammatory cytokines. *Archives of Dermatological Research*, Vol.287, No. 7,pp. 680-682, ISSN 1432-069X.

Chistophers, E. (2001). Psoriasis - epidemiology and clinical espectrum. Clinical and Experimental Dermatology, Vol.26, pp.314-20, ISSN 1365-2230.

Clark, L.C.; Graham, G.F.; Crounse, R.G.; Grimson, R.; Hulka, B. & Shy, C.M. (1984). Plasma selenium and skin neoplasms: a case control study. *Nutrition and Cancer*, Vol.6, No.1, pp.13-21, ISSN 1532-7914.

Cohen, A.D.; Sherf, M.; Vidavsky, L.; Vardy, D.A. & Shapiro, J. (2008). Meyerovitch.Association between psoriasis and the metabolic syndrome. *Dermatology*, Vol.216, pp.152-5, ISSN 1018-8665.

Collin, P. & Reunala, T. (2003). Recognition and management of the cutaneous manifestations of coeliac disease: a guide for dermatologists. *American Journal of Clinical Dermatology*, Vol.4, pp.13-20, ISSN 1175-0561.

Deffuant C, Celerier P, Boiteau L, Litoux P, Dreno B. (1984). Serum selenium in melanoma and epidemotropic cutaneous T-cell lymphoma. *Acta Dermato- Venearologica* , Vol.64, No.1, pp.:9-14, ISSN 0001-5555.

Duarte, G.V.; Follador, I.; Cavalheiro, C.M.A.; Silva, T.S. & Oliveira, M.F.S.P.(2010). Psoriasis and obesity: literature review and recommendations for management. *Anais Brasileiros de Dermatologia*, Vol.85,No.3,pp:355-60, ISSN 1806-4841.

Duggan, J.M. (2004). Coeliac Disease: the great imitator. *The Medical Journal of Australia*, Vol.180, pp.524-6, ISSN 0025-. 729X.

Dutra-de-Oliveira,J.E.(2000).Lipids. IN:*Nutritional Sciences*, 87-95, Sarvier, ISSBN: 9788573781830 ,São Paulo, Brazil.

Fairris, G.M.; Lloyd, B.; Hinks, L.; Pekins, P.J. & Clayton, B.E. (1989). The effect of supplementation with selenium and vitamin E in psoriasis. *Annals of Clinical Biochemistry*, Vol. 26, pp. 83-8, ISSN 1758-1001.

Farías, M.M.; Serrano, V. & De La Cruz, C. (2011). Psoriasis y obesidad:revisión y recomendaciones prácticas. *Actas Dermo-Sifiliográficas*, doi:10.1016/j.ad.2011.03.010, ISSN 0001-7310.

Farkas, A.; Kemeny, L.; Szell, M.; Dobozy, A. & Bata-Csörgo, Z.(2003). Ethanol and acetone stimulate the proliferation of HaCaT keratinocytes: the possible role of alcohol inexacerbating psoriasis. *Archives of Dermatological Research*, Vol.295, No.2, pp.56-62, ISSN 1432-069X.

Frankenfield, D.; Muth, E. & Rowe, W. (1998). The Harris-Benedict studies of human basal metabolism: history and limitations. *Journal of the American Dietetic Association*, Vol.98, pp.439-45, ISSN 0002-8223.

Fraser, D.A.; Thoen, J.; Reselend, J.E.; Forre, O. & Kjeldsen-Kragh, J. (1999). Decreased CD4+ lymphocyte activation and increased interleukin production in peripheral blood of rheumatoid arthritis patients after acute starvation. *Clinical Rheumatology*, Vol.18, pp.394-401, ISSN 1434-9949.

Fu, L.W. & Vender, R. Systemic Role for Vitamin D in the Treatment of Psoriasis andMetabolic Syndrome. *Dermatology Research and Practice*, Vol. 2011, ISSN 1687-6105.

Gisondi, P.; Tessari, G.; Conti, A.; Piaserico, S.; Schianchi ,S.; Peserico, A.; Giannetti, A. & Girolomoni, G. (2007). Prevalence of metabolic syndrome in patients with psoriasis: a hospital-based case-control study. *British Journal of Dermatology*, Vol.157, No.1, pp.68-73, ISSN 1365-2133.

Gupta, M.A.; Schork, N.J.; Gupta, A.K. & Ellis, C.N (1993). Alcohol intake and treatment responsiveness of psoriasis: a prospective study. *Journal of the American Academy of Dermatology*, Vol. 28, pp.730-2, ISSN 0190-9622.

Hafstrom, I.; Ringertz, B.; Spangberg, A.; Von Zweigbergk, L.; Brannemark, S.; Nylander, I.; Rönnelid , J.; Laasonen, L. & Klareskog , L. .(2001). A vegan diet free of gluten improves the signs and symptoms of rheumatoid arthritis: the effects on arthritis correlate with a reduction in antibodies to food antigens. *Rheumatology*,Vol.40, No.10, pp.1175-9, ISSN 1531-6963.

Hamminga, E.A.; Van der Lely, A.J.; Neumann, H.A.M. &Thio, H.B. (2006). Chronic inflammation in psoriasis and obesity: Implications for therapy. *Medical Hypotheses*, Vol. 67, pp.768-73, ISSN 0306-9877.

Harvima, R.J.; Jagerroos, H.; Kajander, E.O.; Harvima, I.T.; Aalto, M.L.; Neittaanmaki H.; Naukkarinen, A.; Kantola, M.; Miettinen, U.K. & Horsmanheimo, M. (1993).

Screening of effects of selenomethionine-enriched yeast supplementation on various immunological and chemical parameters of skin and blood in psoriatic patients. *Acta Dermato- Venearologica,* Vol.73, No.2, pp.88-91, ISSN 0001-5555.

Herron, M.D.; Hinckley, M.; Hoffman, M.S, Papenfuss J, Hansen CB, Callis CP, Krueger GG. (2005). Impact of Obesity and Smoking on Psoriasis Presentation and Management. *Archives of Dermatology,* Vol.141, No.12, pp.1527-34, ISSN 0003-987X.

Higgins, E.A. & Du Vivier, A.W.P. (1994). Alcohol abuse and treatment resistance in skin disease. *Journal of the American Academy of Dermatology,* Vol. 30, No.6, pp.1048, ISSN 0190-9622.

Hinks, L.J.; Young, S. & Clayton, B.E. (1987). Trace element status in eczema and psoriasis. *Clinical and Experimental Dermatology,* Vol.12, No.2, pp.93-7, ISNN 1365-2230.

Holick, M. (2007)."Medical progress: vitamin D deficiency". *The New England Journal of Medicine,* vol. 357, no. 3, pp. 266–281, ISSN 0028-4793.

Holick, M.F. (2003). Vitamin D: a millennium perspective. *Journal of Cellular Biochemistry,* Vol.88, pp.296-307, ISSN 1097-4644.

Humbert, P.; Pelletier, F.; Dreno, B.; Puzenat, E. & Aubin, F. (2006) Gluten intolerance and skin diseases. *European Journal of Dermatology,* Vol.16, pp.4-11, ISSN 1952-4013.

Ikeda, U.; Wakita,T.Ohkuri, D.; Chamoto, K.; Kitamura, H.; Iwakura, Y. & Nishimura, T. (2010). "1α,25-dihydroxyvitamin D3 and all-trans retinoic acid synergistically inhibit the differentiation and expansion of Th17 cells," *Immunology Letters,* Vol.134, No.1, pp 7-16, ISSN 0165- 2478.

Jones, P.J.H. & Papamandjaris, A.A. (2001). Lipids: cellular metabolism. In: Bowman, B.A. & Russel,l R.M. *Present knowledge in nutrition,* 9th Ed, Vol.1, 104-14, ISBN 9781578811991, Washigton, United States.

Kazakevich, N.; Moody, M.N.; Landau, JM. & Goldberg, L.H. (2011). Alcohol and Skin Disorders: With a Focus on Psoriasis. Retrieved from http://www.skintherapyletter.com/2011/16.4/2.html.

Kharaeva, Z.; Gostova, E.; De Luca, C.; Raskovic, D. & Korkina, L. (2009). Clinical and biochemical effects of coenzyme Q10, Vitamin E, and Selenium supplementation to psoriasis patients. *Nutrition* , Vol.25, pp. 295-302, ISSN 0899-9007.

Kiymat Baz, M.; Kokturk, B.C.A.; Yazici, A.C.; Eskandari, G.; Guliz, I.H. & Api Atik, U. (2003). Oxidant /antioxidant status in patients with psoriasis. *Yonsei Medical Journal,* Vol .44;No. 6, pp. 987 – 990, ISSN 0513-5796.

Kojima T, Terano T, Tanabe E, Okamoto S, Tamura Y, Yoshida S.Effect of highly purified eicosapentaenoic acid on psoriasis. (1989).*Journal of the American Academy of Dermatology,* Vol.21, pp.150-1, ISSN 0190-9622.

Kragballe, K. & Fogh, K. Low-fat diet supplemented with dietary fish oil (MAX-EPA) and results in improvement of psoriasis and in formation of leukotriene B5. (1989). *Acta Dermato- Venearologica,* Vol.69, pp.23-8, ISSN 0001-5555.

Lecomte, E; Herbert, B.; Pirollet, P.; Chancerelle, Y.; Arnaud, J.; Musse, N.; Paille, F.; Siest, G. & Artur, Y. (1994). Effect of alcohol consumption on blood antioxidant nutrients and oxidative stress indicators. *The American Journal of Clinical Nutrition* ,Vol.60, No.2, pp.255-61, ISSN: 1938-3207.

Leffler, D.; Saha, S. & Farrel, R.J. (2003). Celiac Disease. *American Journal of Managed Care*, Vol.9, pp.825-31, ISSN 1936-2692.

Lithell, H.; Bruce, A.; Gustafsson, I.B.; Hoglund, N.J.; Karlstrom, B.; Ljunghall, K.; Sjölin, K.; Venge, P.; Werner, I. & Vessby, B. (1983). A fasting and vegetarian diet treatment trial on chronic inflammatory disorders. *Acta Dermato- Venearologica*, Vol.63, No.5, pp.397-403, ISSN 0001-5555.

Liu, S.W.; Lien, M.H. & Fenske, N.A. (2010). The effects of alcohol and drug abuse on the skin. *Clinical Dermatology* , Vol.28, No.4, pp.391-9, ISSN: 15075516.

Maurice, P.D.; Allen, B.R.; Barkley, A.S.; Cockbill, S.R.; Stammers, J.; Bather P.C. (1987). The effects of dietary supplementation with fish oil in patients with psoriasis. *British Journal of Dermatology*, Vol.117, pp.599-606, ISSN 1365-2133.

Mayser, P.; Grinn, H. & Gringer, F. (2002). Omega-3 fatty acids in psoriasis. *British Journal of Dermatology*,V.87, Suppl 1, s.77-82, ISSN 1365-2133.

Mckenzie, R.C. (2000). Selenium, ultraviolet radiation and the skin. *Clinical and Experimental Dermatology*, Vol.25, No.8, pp.631-6, ISSN 1365-2230.

Michaelsson, G. & Edqvist, L.E. (1984). Erytrocyte glutathione peroxidase activity in acne vulgaris and the effect of selenium and vitamin E treatment. *Acta Dermato-Venearologica*, Vol.64, No.1, pp.9-14, ISSN 0001-5555.

Michaelsson, G.; Ahs, S.; Hammarstrom, I.; Lundin, I.P. & Hagforsen, E. (2003). Gluten-free diet in psoriasis patients with antibodies to gliadin results in decreased expression of tissue transglutaminase and fewer Ki67+ cells in the dermis. *Acta Dermato-Venearologica*, Vol.83, pp.425-9, ISSN 0001-5555.

Michaelsson, G.; Berne, B.; Carlmark, B. & Strand, A. (1989).Selenium in whole blood and plasma is decreased in patients with moderate and severe psoriasis. *Acta Dermato-Venearologica*, Vol. 69, No.1; pp.:29-34 ,ISSN 0001-5555.

Michaelsson, G.; Gerden, B.; Hagforsen, E.; Nilsson, B.; Pihl-Lundin, I.; Kraaz, W.; Hjelmquist ,G. & Lööf L. (2000). Psoriasis pacients with antibodies to gliadin can be improved by a gluten-free diet. *British Journal of Dermatology*, Vol.142, pp.44-51, ISSN1365-2133.

Michaelsson, G.; Gerdén, B.; Ottoson, M.; Parra, A.; Sjoberg, O.; Hjelmguist, G. & Lööf, L.(2006). Patients with psoriasis often have increased serum levels of IgA antibodies to gliadin. *British Journal of Dermatology*, Vol.129, pp. 667-73, ISSN 1365-2133.

Monk, B.E. & Neil, S.M. (1986). Alcohol consumption and psoriasis. Dermatologica ,Vol.173, No.2, pp.57-60, ISSN 0011-9075.

Muller, H.; De Toledo, F.W. & Resch, K.L. (2001). Fasting followed by vegetarian diet in patients with rheumatoid arthritis: a systematic review. *Scandinavian Journal of Rheumatology*, Vol.30, pp.1-10, ISSN 1502-7732.

Naldi, L.; Parazzini, F.; Brevi, A.; Peserico,, A.; Veller Fornasa, C.; Grosso,G.; Rossi, E.; Marinaro, P.; Polenghi, M.M.; Finzi, A.; Galbiati, G.; Recchia, G.; Cristofolini, M.; Schena, D. & Cainelli, T. (1992). Family history, smoking habits, alcohol consumption and the risk of psoriasis. *British Journal of Dermatology*, Vol. 127, No.3, pp. 212-217 , ISSN 1365-2133.

Naldi, L.; Parazzini, F.; Peli, L.; Chatenoud, L. & Cainelli, T. (1996) Dietary Factors and the risk of psoriasis. Results of an Italian case-control study.British *Journal of Dermatology*, Vol.134, pp.101-6, ISSN 1365-2133.

Neimann, A.L.; Shin, D.B.; Wang, X.; Margolis, D.; Troxel, A.B. & Gelfand, J.M. (2006). Prevalence of cardiovascular risk factors in patients with psoriasis. *Journal of the American Academy of Dermatology*, Vol.55, pp. 829-35, ISSN 0190-9622.

Nelson, DA. (2002). Gluten-sensitive enteropathy (celiac disease): more common than you think. *American Family Physician*, Vol. 66, pp.2259-66, ISSN 0002-838X.

Obesity Society. (2000). The Practical Guide: Identification, Evaluation, and Treatment of Overweight and Obe- sity in Adults. Access in June 27, 2011, Retrieved from < http://www.nhlbi.nih. gov/guidelines/obesity/prctgd b.pdf>.

Ockenfels, H.M.; Keim-Maas, C.; Funk, R.; Nussbaum, G. & Goos, M. (1996). Ethanol enhances the IFN-gamma, TGF-alpha and IL-6 secretion in psoriatic co-cultures. *British Journal of Dermatology*, Vol.135, No.5, pp.746-51.

Ojetti, V.; Aguilar Sanchez, J.; Guerriero, C.; Fossati, B.; Capizzi, R.; De Simone, C.; Migneco, A.; Amerio, P.; Gasbarrini, G. & Gasbarrini, A. (2003). High prevalence of celiac disease in psoriasis.*The American Journal of Clinical Nutrition*, Vol.98, pp.2574-5, ISSN 1938-3207.

Palmblad, J.; Hafstrom, I. & Ringertz, B. (1991). Antirheumatic effects of fasting. *Rheumatic Disease Clinics of North America*,Vol. 17, pp.351-62, ISSN 0889-857X.

Pinton, J.; Friden, H.; Kettaneh-Wold, N.; Wold, S.; Dreno, B.; Richard, A. & Bieber, T. (1995). Clinical and biological effects of balneotherapy with selenium-rich spa water in patients with psoriasis vulgaris. *British Journal of Dermatology*, Vol.133, No.2, pp.344-7, ISSN 1365-2133.

Poikolainen, K.; Reunala, T. & Karvonen, J. (1994). Smoking alcohol and life events related to psoriasis among women. *British Journal of Dermatology*, Vol.130, pp.437-7, ISSN 1365-2133.

Poikolainen, K.; Reunala, T.; Karvonen, J.; Lauharanta, J. & Karkkainen, P. (1990). Alcohol intake: A risk factor for psoriasis in young and midlle aged men? *British Journal of Dermatology*, Vol.300; pp.780-3, ISSN 1365-2133.

Qureshi, A.A.; Dominguez, P.L.; Choi, H.K.; Han, J. & Curhan, G. Alcohol intake and risk of incident psoriasis in US women: a prospective study. (2010). *Archives of dermatology*, Vol.146, No.12, pp.1364-9 , ISSN 0003-987X.

Relhan, V.; Gupta, S.; Dayal, S.; Pandde, R. & Lal, H. (2002). Blood thiol and Malondialdehyde level in psoriasis. *The Journal of Dermatology*, Vol.29, pp.399 – 403, ISSN 1346-8138.

Ricketts, J.R.; Rothe, M.J. & Grant-Kels, J.M.(2010). Nutrition and psoriasis. *Clinics in Dermatology* , Vol. 28, pp. 615–626, ISSN 15075516.

Rocha, P.P.; Silva, R.A S.; Figuniredo, A.; Quinitanilha, A. & Texeira, F. (2004).The Inflammatory response in mild and in severe psoriasis. *British Journal of Dermatology*, Vol. 150, No.5, pp. 917 - 928, ISSN 1365-2133.

Roy, M.; Kiremidjan-Schumacher, L.; Wishe, H.I.; Cohen, M.W. & Stotsky, G. (1992). Effect of selenium on the expression of high affinity interleukin 2 receptors. *Proceedings of the Society for Experimental Biology and Medicine*, Vol. 200, No.1, pp.36-43, ISSN: 0037-9727.

Rucevic, I.; Perl, A.; Barisic- Drusko, V. & Adam Perl, M. (2003). The role of low energy diet in psoriasis vulgaris treatment. *International Journal Collegium Antropologicum*, Vol.27, Suppl. 1, s.41-8, ISSN 0350-6134.

Saraceno, R.; Ruzzetti, M.; De Martino MU, Di Renzo, L.; Cianci, R.; De Lorenzo, A. & Chimenti, S. (2008). Does metabolic syndrome influence psoriasis? *European Review for Medical and Pharmacological Sciences* , Vol.12, No.5, pp.339-41, ISSN 1128-3602.

Serwin, A.B.; Wasowicz, W.; Gromadzinska, J. & Chodynicka, B. (2003). Selenium status in psoriasis and its relation to the duration and severity of the disease. *Nutrition*, Vol.19, pp.301-4, ISSN 0899-9007.

Smith, K.E. & Fenske, N.A. (2000). Cutaneous manifestations of alcohol abuse. *Journal of the American Academy of Dermatology* ,Vol.43, pp.1-16, ISSN 0190-9622.

Smith, N,; Weymann, A.; Tausk, F.A. & Gelfand, J.M. (2009). Complementary and alternative medicine for psoriasis: A qualitative review of the clinical trial literature. *Journal of The American Academy of Dermatology*, Vol.61, No.5, pp.841-56, ISSN 0190-9622.

Sommer, D.M.; Jenisch, S.; Suchan, M.; Christophers, E. & Weichenthal, M. (2006). Increased prevalence of the metabolic syndrome in patients with moderate to severe psoriasis. *Archives of Dermatological Research*, Vol. 298, pp.321-8, ISSN 1432-069X.

Spallholtz, J.E.; Boylan, L.M. & Larsen, H.S. (1990). Advances in understanding selenium role in the immune system. *Annals of the New York Academy of Sciences* , Vol.587, pp.123-39, ISSN 1749-6632.

Van De Kerkhof, P. C. M. (2005). The topical treatment of psoriasis. *Clinical and Experimental Dermatology*, Vol. 30, No. 2, pp. 205–208, ISSN 1365-2230.

Wakkee, M.; Thio, H.B.; Prens, E.P.; Sijbrands, E.J.G. & Neumann, H.A.M. (2007). Unfavorable cardiovascular risk profiles in untreated an treated psoriasis patients. Atherosclerosis. Vol.190, pp.1-9, ISSN 0021-9150.

Wilkinson, D.I. (1990). Do dietary supplements of fish oils improve psoriasis? *Cutis*. Vol.46, pp.334-6, ISSN 0011-4162.

Wolf, R.; Wolf, D. & Ruocco, V. (1999). Alcohol intake and psoriasis. *Clinical Dermatology*, Vol.17, pp.423-30, ISSN: 15075516.

Wolters, M. (2005). Diet and psoriasis - experimental clinical and evidence. *British Journal of Dermatology*, Vol.153, pp. 706-14, ISSN 1365-2133.

Woo, W.K.; McMillan, S.A.; Watson, R.G.; McCluggage, W.G.; Sloan, J.N. & McMillan, J.C. (2004). Coeliac disease - associated antibodies correlate with psoriasis activity. *British Journal of Dermatology*, Vol.151, pp.891-4, ISSN1365-2133.

Ziboh, V.A.; Cohen, K.A, Ellis, C.N, Miller, C.; Hamilton, T.A.; Kragballe, K.; Hydrick, C.R. & Voorhees, J.J. (1986). Effects of dietary supplementation of fish oil on neutrophil and epidermal fatty acids. Modulation of clinical course of psoriatic subjects. *Archives of Dermatology*, Vol.122, pp.1277-82, ISSN 0003-987X.